CARDIAC COMPUTED TOMOGRAPHY

A Companion to BRAUNWALD'S HEART DISEASE

CARDIAC COMPUTED TOMOGRAPHY

A Companion to BRAUNWALD'S HEART DISEASE

RON BLANKSTEIN, MD, FACC, FASNC, MSCCT, FASPC
Associate Director, Cardiovascular Imaging Program
Director, Cardiac Computed Tomography
Co-Director, Cardiovascular Imaging Training Program
Senior Physician, Preventive Cardiology
Brigham and Women's Hospital
Professor of Medicine and Radiology
Harvard Medical School
Boston, Massachusetts

ELSEVIER

Elsevier
1600 John F. Kennedy Blvd.
Ste 1800
Philadelphia, PA 19103-2899

CARDIAC COMPUTED TOMOGRAPHY: A COMPANION TO BRAUNWALD'S HEART DISEASE

ISBN: 978-0-443-10618-7

For accessibility purposes, images in electronic versions of this book are accompanied by alt-text descriptions provided by Elsevier. For more information, see https://www.elsevier.com/about/accessibility.

Books and Journals published by Elsevier comply with applicable product safety requirements. For any product safety concerns or queries, please contact our authorized representative, Elsevier B.V., at productsafety@elsevier.com.

Publisher's note: Elsevier takes a neutral position with respect to territorial disputes or jurisdictional claims in its published content, including in maps and institutional affiliations.

Notice

Practitioners and researchers must always rely on their own experience and knowledge in evaluating and using any information, methods, compounds, or experiments described herein. Because of rapid advances in the medical sciences, in particular, independent verification of diagnoses and drug dosages should be made. To the fullest extent of the law, no responsibility is assumed by Elsevier, authors, editors, or contributors for any injury and/or damage to persons or property as a matter of product liability, negligence or otherwise, or from any use or operation of any methods, products, instructions, or ideas contained in the material herein.

Senior Content Strategist: Melanie Tucker
Senior Content Development Specialist: Himanshi Chauhan
Publishing Services Manager: Deepthi Unni
Senior Project Manager: Manchu Mohan
Design Direction: Renee Duenow

Printed in India

Last digit is the print number: 9 8 7 6 5 4 3 2 1

This book is dedicated to
my wife, Rachel,
and our daughters, Jordana and Eliana,
for their love, support, and inspiration.

Contributors

Stephan Achenbach, MD, MSCCT
Chairman and Professor of Cardiology
Department of Cardiology
Friedrich-Alexander University of Erlangen–Nuremberg
Erlangen, Germany

Ayaz Aghayev, MD
Cardiovascular Radiologist
Department of Radiology
Brigham and Women's Hospital
Harvard Medical School
Boston, Massachusetts

Nandan S. Anavekar, MBBCh
Professor of Medicine
Department of Cardiovascular Diseases and Radiology
Mayo Clinic
Rochester, Minnesota

Charalambos Antoniades, MD, PhD, FESC, FRCP, FMedSci
Chair of Cardiovascular Medicine
Acute Multidisciplinary Imaging and Interventional Centre
Division of Cardiovascular Medicine
University of Oxford
Oxford, United Kingdom

Alexios S. Antonopoulos, MD, PhD
Assistant Professor of Cardiology
1st Cardiology Department
National and Kapodistrian University of Athens
Greece

Daniel S. Berman, MD
Director
Cardiac Imaging
Department of Cardiology
Cedars Sinai Medical Center
Los Angeles, California

Marcio S. Bittencourt, MD, MPh, PhD
Associate Professor
Department of Medicine
University of Pittsburgh
Pittsburgh, Pennsylvania

Michael J. Blaha, MD, MPH
Professor
Department of Medicine
Division of Cardiology
Johns Hopkins Ciccarone Center
Baltimore, Maryland

Philipp Blanke, MD
Associate Professor
Department of Radiology
University of British Columbia and St. Paul's Hospital
Vancouver, Canada

Ron Blankstein, MD, FACC, FASNC, MSCCT, FASPC
Associate Director, Cardiovascular Imaging Program
Director, Cardiac Computed Tomography
Co-Director, Cardiovascular Imaging Training Program
Senior Physician, Preventive Cardiology
Brigham and Women's Hospital
Professor of Medicine and Radiology
Harvard Medical School
Boston, Massachusetts

Roger S. Blumenthal, MD
Kenneth Jay Pollin Professor of Cardiology
Department of Medicine/Cardiology
Johns Hopkins Medical Institutions
Director
Johns Hopkins Ciccarone Preventive Cardiology Center
Baltimore, Maryland

Michael A. Bolen, MD
Staff Radiologist
Department of Cardiothoracic Radiology
Cleveland Clinic
Cleveland, Ohio

Matthew J. Budoff, MD
Professor of Medicine
Department of Internal Medicine
UCLA School of Medicine
Torrance, California

Filippo Cademartiri, MD, PhD
Director
Advanced Cardiovascular Imaging
IRCCS SYNLAB SDN
Naples, Italy
Centro Diagnostico Italiano
Milan, Italy
Department of Radiology
Erasmus Medical Center University
Rotterdam, Netherlands

Rhanderson Cardoso, MD, FACC
Assistant Professor of Medicine
Division of Cardiology
Brigham and Women's Hospital, Harvard Medical School
Boston, Massachusetts

João L. Cavalcante, MD, FACC, FASE, FSCCT, FSCMR
Section Head
Department of Cardiac Imaging
Allina Health Minneapolis Heart Institute
Director
Cardiovascular Imaging Research Center and Core Lab
Minneapolis Heart Institute Foundation
Minneapolis, Minnesota

Kavitha M. Chinnaiyan, MD
Cardiologist
Department of Cardiovascular Medicine
Corewell Health
Royal Oak, Michigan

Andrew D. Choi, MD, FACC, MSCCT
Professor of Medicine and Radiology
Director
Noninvasive Cardiology; Co-Director, Multimodality Cardiac Imaging
Department of Radiology
Division of Cardiology
The George Washington University School of Medicine
Washington, District of Columbia

Paul C. Cremer, MD
Associate Professor of Medicine and Radiology
Bluhm Cardiovascular Institute
Northwestern University Feinberg School of Medicine
Chicago, Illinois

Ricardo C. Cury, MD, MBA
Professor and Chairman
Department of Radiology
Florida International University Herbert Wertheim College of Medicine
Chairman
Department of Radiology
Baptist Health of South Florida
Coral Gables, Florida

Timothy Andrew Fairbairn, MBChB, PhD
Consultant Cardiologist
Department of Cardiology
Liverpool Heart and Chest Hospital
Associate Professor
Department of Life Sciences
University of Liverpool
Liverpool, United Kingdom

Maros Ferencik, MD, PhD, MCR
Professor of Medicine and Radiology
Knight Cardiovascular Institute
Oregon Health and Science University
Portland, Oregon

Aloke V. Finn, MD
Medical Director
Department of Pathology
CVPath Institute Inc.
Gaithersburg, Maryland

Brian Burns Ghoshhajra, MD, MBA
Associate Chair, Operations Analytics
Academic Director, Cardiovascular Imaging
Department of Radiology
Massachusetts General Hospital
Associate Professor
Department of Radiology
Harvard Medical School
Boston, Massachusetts

Jelani K. Grant, MD, MHS
Department of Medicine
Division of Cardiology
Johns Hopkins Ciccarone Center
Baltimore, Maryland

Sumit Gupta, MBBS, PhD
Staff Radiologist
Department of Radiology
Divisions of Cardiovascular/Thoracic Imaging
Brigham and Women's Hospital
Boston, Massachusetts

Abdul Rahman Ihdayhid, MBBS (Hons), PhD, FRACP
Associate Professor
Curtin Medical School
Curtin University
Associate Professor
Department of Cardiology
Fiona Stanley Hospital
Perth, Australia
Associate Professor
Harry Perkins Institute of Medical Research
Perth, Australia

Kenji Kawai, MD, PhD
Research Fellow
Department of Cardiovascular Pathology
CVPath Institute
Gaithersburg, Maryland

Omar K. Khalique, MD, FACC, FSCCT, FSCAI, FSCMR, FASE
Director, Division of Cardiovascular Imaging
Division of Cardiovascular Imaging
St Francis Hospital and Heart Center
Roslyn, New York

Jonathon A. Leipsic, MD, FRCPC
Professor and Chair
Department of Radiology
UBC
Vancouver, British Columbia, Canada
Professor
Department of Medicine (Cardiology)
UBC
Vancouver, British Columbia, Canada

Andrew Lin, MBBS, BMedSc, PhD
Cardiologist
Monash Victorian Heart Institute and Monash Health Heart
Victorian Heart Hospital
Melbourne, Victoria, Australia

Fay Y. Lin, MD
Clinical Associate Professor
Department of Population Health
Icahn School of Medicine at Mount Sinai
New York, New York

Juan Lopez-Mattei, MD
Medical Director
Department of Cardiac Imaging
Lee Health Heart Institute
Fort Myers, Florida

Davide Margonato, MD
Department of Cardiovascular Imaging
IRCCS San Raffaele
Milano, Italy
Research Scholar
Cardiovascular Imaging Research Center
Minneapolis Heart Institute and Foundation
Minneapolis, Minnesota

Christopher D. Maroules, MD, FSCCT
Director of Cardiac Imaging
SimonMed Imaging
Scottsdale, Arizona
Chief Operating Officer
Innovation Health Services
Norfolk, Virginia

Mohamed Marwan, MD, FSCCT
Professor of Cardiology
Department of Cardiology
Friedrich-Alexander University of Erlangen–Nuremberg
Erlangen, Germany

Pál Maurovich-Horvat, MD, PhD, MPH, DSc
Professor
Department of Radiology
Semmelweis University
Budapest, Hungary

Aloha Meave González, MD
Cardiac Radiologist
Chair, Cardiac Magnetic Resonance Unit
Instituto Nacional Cardiología, Ignacio Chávez
México City, México

Nehal N. Mehta, BA, MD, MSCE
Professor of Medicine
Department of Cardiology
The George Washington University School of Medicine and Health Sciences
Washington, District of Columbia
Adjunct Associate Professor of Medicine
Department of Cardiovascular Medicine
University of Pennsylvania Perelman School of Medicine
Philadelphia, Pennsylvania

Lindsey R. Mitrani, MD
Cardiologist
Department of Cardiology
Mount Sinai Hospital and Northern Westchester Hospital at Northwell Health
New York, New York

Khurram Nasir, MD, MPH, MSc
Chief of Division of Cardiovascular Prevention and Wellness
Department of Cardiology
Houston Methodist DeBakey Heart & Vascular Center
Houston Methodist-Rice Digital Health Institute
Houston, Texas

David E. Newby, BA BSc (Hons), PhD, BM, DM, FRCP, FESC, FRSE, FMedSci
British Heart Foundation Duke of Edinburgh Professor of Cardiology
British Heart Foundation Centre for Cardiovascular Diseases
University of Edinburgh
Edinburgh, United Kingdom

Koen Nieman, MD, PhD
Professor
Departments of Medicine and Radiology
Stanford University
Stanford, California

Roosha Parikh, MD, FACC, FASE, FSCCT, FSCMR, FASNC, RPVI
Associate Director
Cardiac CT
Associate Program Director
Advanced Cardiovascular Imaging Fellowship
St. Francis Hospital and Heart Center
Roslyn, New York

Amit R. Patel, MD
Professor
Department of Medicine
University of Virginia
Charlottesville, Virginia

Nidhi H. Patel
Department of Medicine
Division of Cardiology
Emory University School of Medicine
Atlanta, Georgia

Ronen Rubinshtein, MD, FACC, FESC, MSCCT
Director
Heart Institute
Edith Wolfson Medical Center
Holon, Israel
Associate Professor
Tel Aviv University
Tel Aviv, Israel

Robert D. Safian, MD, FACC, MSCAI, FSCCT, FSVM
The Lucia Zurkowski Endowed Chair
The Center for Innovation and Research in Cardiovascular Diseases
William Beaumont University Hospital-Corewell Health East
Professor of Medicine
Department of Cardiovascular Medicine
Oakland University William Beaumont School of Medicine
Royal Oak, Michigan

Leslee J. Shaw, PhD
Professor
Department of Medicine
Icahn School of Medicine at Mount Sinai
New York, New York

Arthur Shiyovich, MD
Associate Physician
Brigham and Women's Hospital
Assistant Professor of Medicine
Harvard Medical School
Boston, Massachusetts

Michael L. Steigner, MD
Cardiovascular Radiologist
Medical Director 3D Lab
Department of Radiology
Brigham and Women's Hospital
Associate Professor
Department of Radiology
Harvard Medical School
Boston, Massachusetts

Todd C. Villines, MD
Professor
Department of Medicine
Division of Cardiovascular Medicine
Vice-Chair
Clinical Services
Cardiovascular Division
University of Virginia
Charlottesville, Virginia

Renu Virmani, MD
President Emeritus and Founder
Department of Pathology
CVPath Institute, Inc.
Gaithersburg, Maryland

Eric E. Williamson, MD
Chair, Department of Radiology
Chief Medical Information Officer
Mayo Clinic
Rochester, Minnesota

Foreword

Cardiac computed tomography (CT) has undergone a remarkable transformation since the development of the first CT scanner in the early 1970s by Sir Godfrey Hounsfield, whose work earned the Nobel Prize in 1979. Although early CT systems were too slow for imaging moving structures like the heart, the advent of electron-beam CT (EBCT) in the 1980s enabled rapid acquisition and laid the foundation for performing coronary artery calcium (CAC) scoring. The introduction of multidetector CT (MDCT) in the early 2000s—initially with 4-slice and later 64-slice scanners—marked a turning point by enabling high-resolution coronary CT angiography (CCTA), which allowed direct visualization of coronary artery stenosis and plaque morphology. Subsequent technical innovation, including the use of dual-source detectors, led to improved spatial and temporal resolution and a reduction in patient radiation dose, which further improved the diagnostic accuracy of CCTA and enabled the visualization of coronary stents. The advent of photon counting CT (PCCT) promises to revolutionize coronary CT by increasing resolution, potentially lowering radiation doses, reducing blooming artifact, and—very importantly—providing spectral information not furnished by conventional CT.

In parallel with these technological advances, there have also been multiple clinical trials that confirmed the diagnostic accuracy and clinical impact of using cardiac CT for evaluating patients with acute or stable chest pain, or those who are being evaluated for various structural heart disease interventions. As a result, numerous clinical guidelines around the world now strongly endorse the use of CCTA as a first-line testing option for evaluating patients with known or suspected coronary heart disease. Certainly, every cardiologist needs to know how to use cardiac CT appropriately and how to use the results in clinical practice most effectively. Accordingly, this book—with chapters that have been authored by many of the leaders in the field—is geared toward general cardiologists, cardiology fellows, and cardiovascular imagers who seek to understand all the latest developments in the field of cardiac CT.

This Companion to *Heart Disease* is edited by Dr. Ron Blankstein, who is one of the pioneers in the field of cardiac CT. With over 20 years of experience in the field, his research has informed strategies for radiation dose reduction, established the prognostic value of CCTA, introduced the technique of CT perfusion, and helped validate new approaches to quantitative plaque analysis in clinical trials. His work has contributed significantly to the integration of coronary artery calcium scoring and CCTA into clinical decision-making algorithms for both symptomatic and asymptomatic individuals. Through leadership roles as President of the Society of Cardiovascular Computed Tomography and Chair of the Cardiovascular Imaging Section Leadership Council of the American College of Cardiology, and as Director of the Cardiac CT Program at Brigham and Women's Hospital, he has taught several hundred trainees in cardiac CT and has helped define standards for image acquisition, interpretation, and clinical reporting. He has also led multiple training guidelines that have defined the knowledge and skills necessary for advanced training in cardiac CT. His research on image-guided risk stratification and use of cardiac CT in clinical trials has been foundational in bridging imaging science with preventive cardiovascular care. In recognition of his contributions to the fields of preventive cardiology and cardiac CT, he was awarded the 2025 Arthur S. Agatston Award by the Society of Cardiovascular Computed Tomography.

Eugene Braunwald
Boston, Massachusetts

Robert O. Bonow
Chicago, Illinois

Douglas L. Mann
St. Louis, Missouri

Gordon F. Tomaselli
Baltimore, Maryland

Deepak L. Bhatt
New York, New York

Scott D. Solomon
Boston Massachusetts

Peter Libby
Boston, Massachusetts

Contents

Braunwald's Heart Disease Family of Books

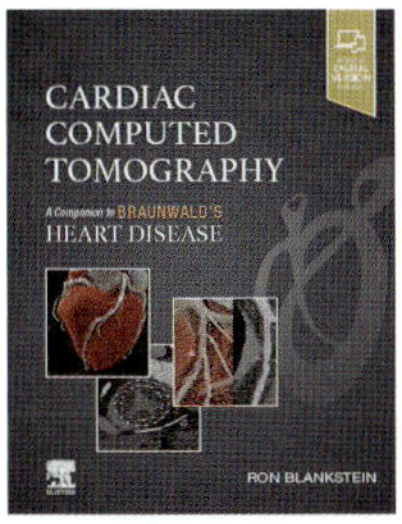

BLANKSTEIN
Cardiac Computed Tomography

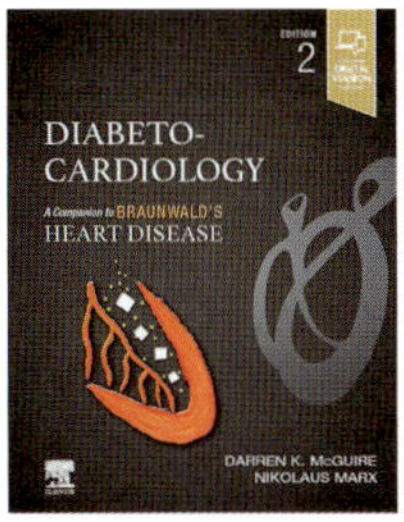

MCGUIRE AND MARX
Diabeto-Cardiology

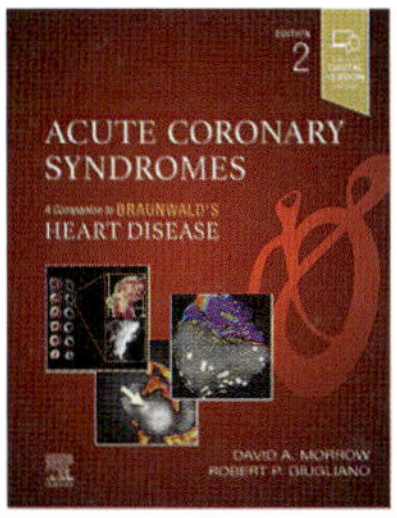

MORROW
Acute Coronary Syndromes

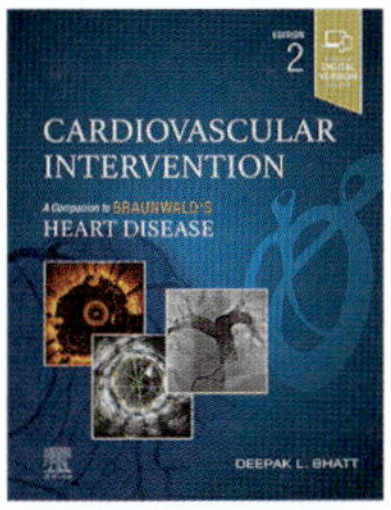

BHATT
Cardiovascular Intervention

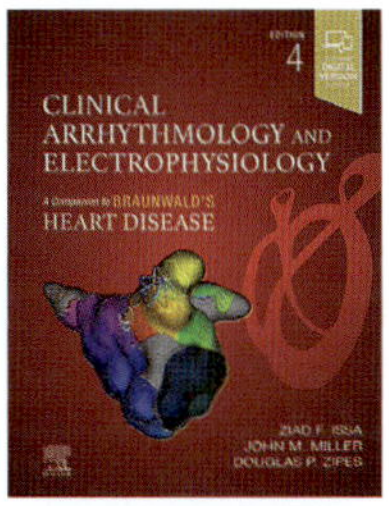

ISSA, MILLER, ZIPES
Clinical Arrhythmology and Electrophysiology

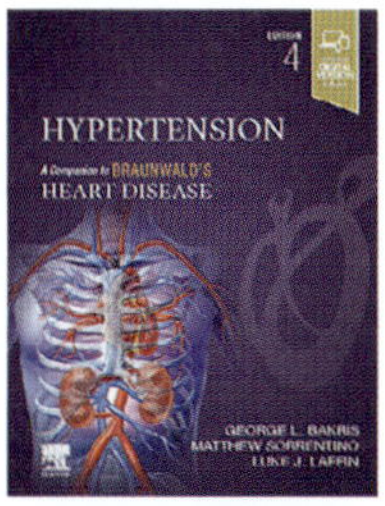

BAKRIS, SORRENTINO, AND LAFFIN
Hypertension

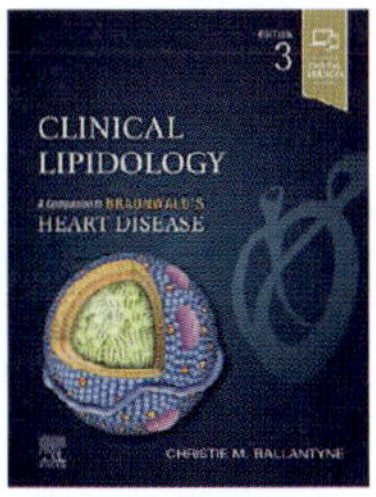

BALLANTYNE
Clinical Lipidology

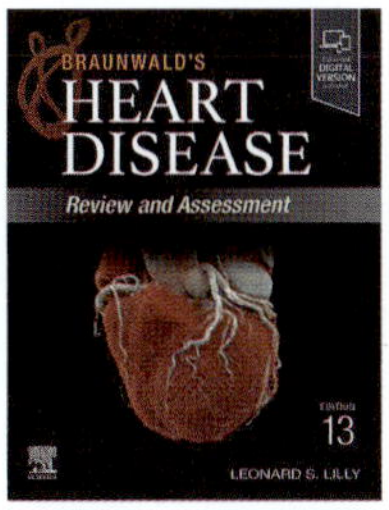

LILLY
Braunwald's Heart Disease Review and Assessment

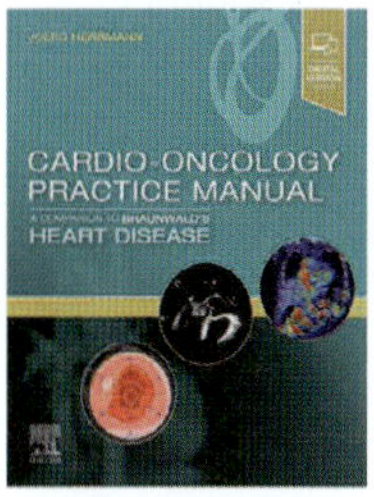

HERRMANN
Cardio-Oncology Practice Manual

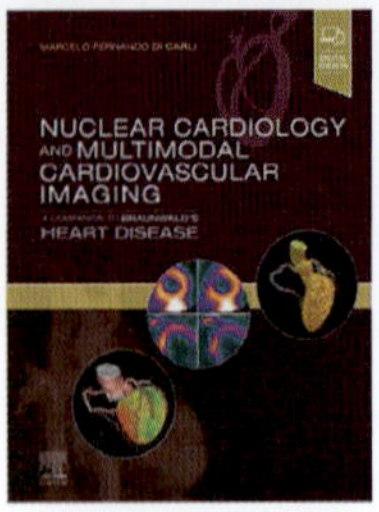

DI CARLI
Nuclear Cardiology and Multimodal Cardiovascular Imaging

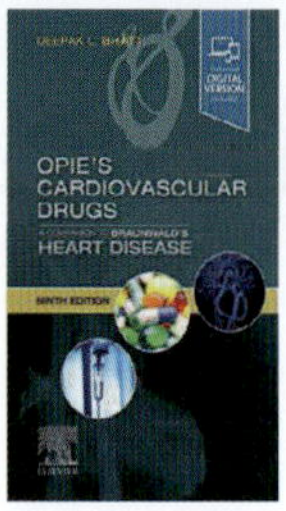

BHATT
Opie's Cardiovascular Drugs

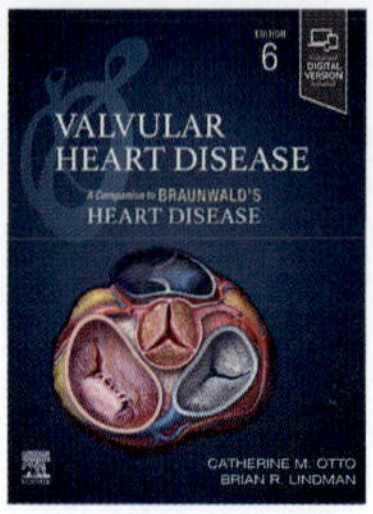

OTTO AND BONOW
Valvular Heart Disease

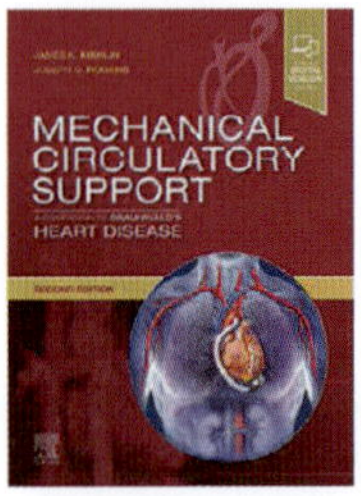

KIRKLIN AND ROGERS
Mechanical Circulatory Support

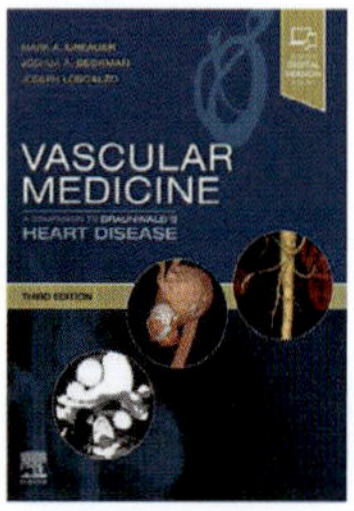

CREAGER
Vascular Medicine

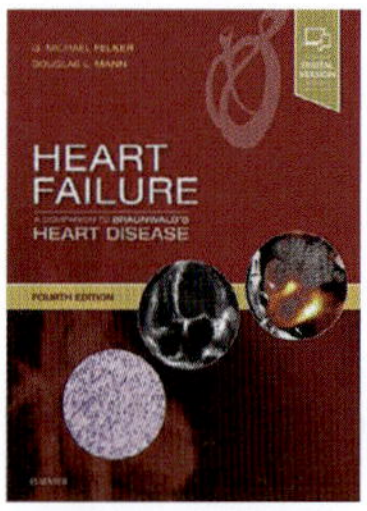

FELKER AND MANN
Heart Failure

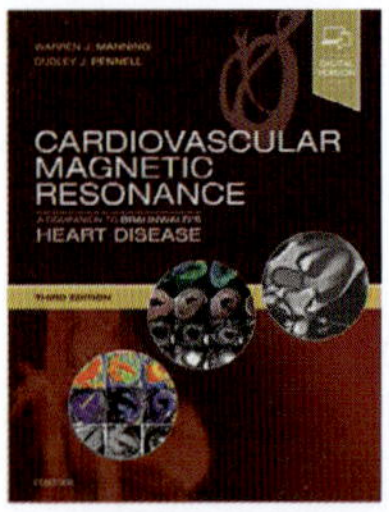

MANNING AND PENNELL
Cardiovascular Magnetic Resonance

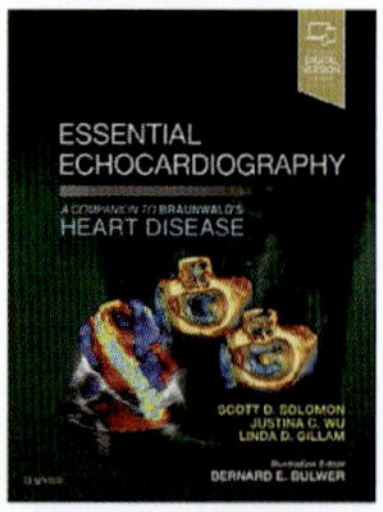

SOLOMON, WU, AND GILLAM
Essential Echocardiography

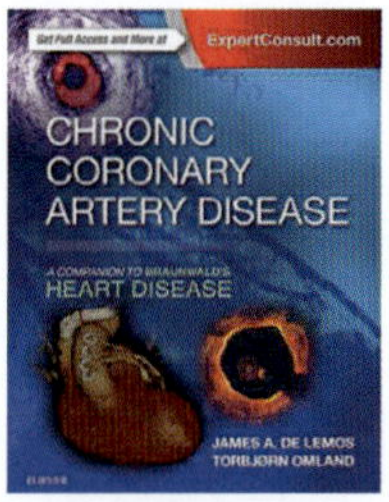

DE LEMOS AND OMLAND
Chronic Coronary Artery Disease

1 Image Acquisition Protocols for Different Types of Cardiac CT

RHANDERSON CARDOSO, ERIC E. WILLIAMSON, AND RON BLANKSTEIN

KEY POINTS

1. Cardiac CT readers should be familiar with the strengths and limitations of cardiac CT relative to other cardiac imaging modalities to guide patient selection and assist referring physicians in selecting the best test to answer the question at hand.
2. Adequate patient selection and patient preparation are essential for obtaining high-quality diagnostic images in cardiac CT.
3. Most cardiac CT indications can be performed with axial acquisition and prospective ECG gating limited to a narrow phase (e.g., 65–80%) of the cardiac cycle to minimize radiation. However, some indications, such as the evaluation of valvular structures, may require a wider phase acquisition window or helical acquisition.
4. Image acquisition parameters and contrast timing will vary for different types of cardiac CT. It is important to tailor the cardiac CT exam based on the clinical question at hand.
5. Delayed imaging after the arterial phase is necessary when assessing for left atrial appendage thrombus.

INTRODUCTION

Cardiac computed tomography (CT) has evolved considerably over the past 2 decades, including marked advances in both hardware and software technology. Recent developments have ranged from scan acquisition and post-processing to image display and interpretation. A few examples of these advances include dual-source scanners, multidetector row systems with increasing numbers of detector elements, iterative reconstruction algorithms, faster workstations, expanded clinical capabilities such as estimating the functional significance on coronary stenoses, and more recently, the use of photon-counting detectors. In parallel, large clinical trials have established the value of cardiac CT in various clinical scenarios, thus expanding the evidence base supporting cardiac CT use in multiple areas of clinical medicine. As a testament to this progress, cardiac CT is now recommended in numerous international guidelines for indications spanning from evaluation of coronary artery disease (CAD) to guiding structural heart disease interventions. Notwithstanding the substantial progress in technology, image quality remains an essential component for the use of cardiac CT in both clinical and research settings. Herein, we review important considerations for patient selection, patient preparation, and imaging protocols for acquisition of high-quality cardiac CT images.

PATIENT SCREENING

Whenever possible, the decision to perform a cardiac CT should be made in the context of shared decision-making between patients and clinicians, while also considering alternative options. A referral to cardiac CT should only be performed if the results are expected to impact management, whether through providing diagnostic or prognostic information. When there is uncertainty, it is important that cardiac CT experts make themselves available to assist in deciding whether cardiac CT will be helpful, and if it is indeed the best modality to answer the clinical question at hand. Thus cardiac CT experts, like all imagers, benefit from training in multimodality imaging so they can serve as "imaging consultants" to guide referring clinicians in selecting the best test among all available options, as well as in determining how to use the test results in making patient management decisions.

There are important contraindications to cardiac CT, which may vary according to the type of exam as well as the available technology. Patient selection for coronary CT angiography (CCTA), for instance, is more rigorous than that of left atrial appendage evaluations, given the need to obtain high-resolution images of the coronary arteries. Severe obesity, heart rate irregularity, inability to tolerate premedications for heart rate control, and small stents are all factors that can impact image quality of CCTA but may be less of an issue for other types of cardiac CT. Further details on patient screening and preparation for CCTA are discussed in Chapter 6, "How to Obtain a High-Quality Coronary CT Angiography."

Other factors, such as hemodynamic instability or inability to cooperate with the study's instructions to remain motionless and perform breath-holding, are contraindications across the spectrum of cardiac CT studies. Pregnancy and contrast-related concerns also apply more broadly across most cardiac CT indications. Notably, all these factors must be considered on a case-by-case basis, as there are circumstances in which the potential benefits of the study may outweigh the risks and/or concerns about image quality (Table 1.1).

Contrast Reactions

Adverse effects of iodinated contrast administration are infrequent and range from mild physiologic reactions to

TABLE 1.1 Contraindications to Cardiac CT

Morbid obesity
Inability to lay flat
Hemodynamic instability
Inability to follow instructions
Inability to perform breath-hold during image acquisition
Pregnancy
Severe renal dysfunction, not on dialysis[a]
Prior anaphylaxis reaction to iodinated contrast media[a]

[a]Applies to contrast-enhanced studies only.
Importantly, there are clinical situations in which benefits of attempting cardiac CT in the presence of a relative contraindication may outweigh potential risks to patient or of having poor image quality. See text for further details.

TABLE 1.2 ACR-recommended Regimens for Premedications in Patients With Prior Allergic Reactions to Iodinated Contrast Media[1]

OUTPATIENT, ELECTIVE	INPATIENT, URGENT
Prednisone 50 mg PO at 13 hours, 7 hours, and 1 hour before contrast administration, with diphenhydramine 50 mg PO or IV 1 hour before contrast administration	Preferred: methylprednisolone 40 mg IV or hydrocortisone 200 mg IV immediately, and then every 4 hours until contrast administration, with diphenhydramine 50 mg IV 1 hour before contrast administration. Typically lasts 4–5 hours.
Methylprednisolone 32 mg PO 12 hours and 2 hours before contrast administration. Diphenhydramine 50 mg may be added, as discussed above.	Dexamethasone 7.5 mg IV immediately and then every 4 hours until contrast administration. Typically lasts 4–5 hours.
If unable to tolerate PO: hydrocortisone 200 mg IV at 13 hours, 7 hours, and 1 hour before contrast administration, with diphenhydramine 50 mg IV 1 hour before contrast administration	Emergency: methylprednisolone 40 mg IV or hydrocortisone 200 mg IV 1 hour before contrast administration plus diphenhydramine 50 mg IV 1 hour before contrast administration.[a]

[a]Regimens <4–5 hours have not been shown to be effective.

life-threatening emergencies. Moderate or severe reactions occur in approximately 0.04% to 0.08% of examinations.[1,2] Unlike classic anaphylactic reactions, the anaphylactoid response to iodinated contrast media does not require prior exposure to contrast. Although institutional policies may vary, patients with severe anaphylactoid reactions to iodinated contrast or moderate to severe breakthrough reactions despite premedication should generally be considered for alternative imaging without the need for iodinated contrast media or, alternatively, be evaluated by an allergy specialist prior to the study if the patient and/or clinical question is not suitable for an alternative imaging modality.

Otherwise, patients with prior allergic reactions to iodinated contrast may be premedicated with a combination of corticosteroids and antihistamines. The exact regimen may vary between institutions. The American College of Radiology recommends a 12- or 13-hour oral regimen for outpatients or inpatients in whom the delay in imaging would not adversely affect treatment, whereas an accelerated intravenous 4- to 5-hour regimen is advised for inpatients in whom care may be adversely impacted by a delay in imaging (Table 1.2).[1]

Unlike anaphylactoid reactions, which can occur independent of dose, nonanaphylactoid reactions are dose dependent. These include cardiac arrhythmias, negative inotropy, pulmonary edema, gastrointestinal reactions, and seizures. Patients with cardiac comorbidities, such as severe aortic stenosis or decompensated heart failure, are particularly susceptible to hemodynamic derangements, although they are still infrequent in this population. The total contrast volume should be minimized in all patients, but particularly in those who are more prone to adverse hemodynamic effects from contrast injection.

Contrast-associated and Contrast-induced Acute Kidney Injury

Contrast-induced acute kidney injury (CI-AKI) typically occurs within 24 to 48 hours of exposure to iodinated contrast media, with an elevation in creatinine and, infrequently, with oliguria. The elevation in creatinine usually peaks at 3 to 5 days after exposure, then returns to baseline within 10 days. The route of contrast administration is a significant risk factor for the incidence of CI-AKI. Intraarterial injections, particularly with manipulation of intraaortic catheters, have a substantially higher rate of CI-AKI than intravenous administration.[3]

The challenge in the literature about the incidence of AKI following intravenous contrast administration has been in the differentiation of true CI-AKI from contrast-associated AKI (CA-AKI), in which contrast administration is temporally, but not causally, related to AKI. Earlier studies were largely performed without control groups, inflating the true incidence of CI-AKI with AKI from other causes. A study with 32,161 patients who had not received contrast within the past 10 days and had daily creatinine measurements over 5 consecutive days found that more than half had an increase of ≥25% in serum creatinine, with more than 40% developing an increase of ≥0.4 mg/dL in serum creatinine.[4]

In fact, controlled studies with propensity matching or multivariable analysis have shown no excess risk of AKI in patients who receive contrast, relative to those who do not, if the baseline estimated glomerular filtration rate (eGFR) is <30 mL/min/1.73 m^2 or with serum creatinine <1.5 mg/dL.[5–7] In those with eGFR <30 mL/min/1.73 m^2, there are conflicting data. Some studies identify contrast use as an independent risk factor for the incidence of AKI in this group, whereas others do not.[5–7]

The decision about administration of iodinated contrast media in patients with an eGFR >30 mL/min/1.73 m^2 who are not on dialysis, or who are on dialysis but not anuric, must be undertaken on a case-by-case basis. Other imaging modalities may be considered if the clinical question can be answered without using iodinated contrast. However, in many circumstances, the benefits of contrast use may outweigh the risks of CI-AKI. Strategies to reduce the risk of CI-AKI include avoiding other nephrotoxic agents, using low-osmolality or iso-osmolality contrast media, and volume expansion with isotonic saline prior to and following administration of iodinated contrast media.[1]

The American College of Radiology recommends assessing renal function prior to intravenous administration of iodinated contrast media in patients with a personal history

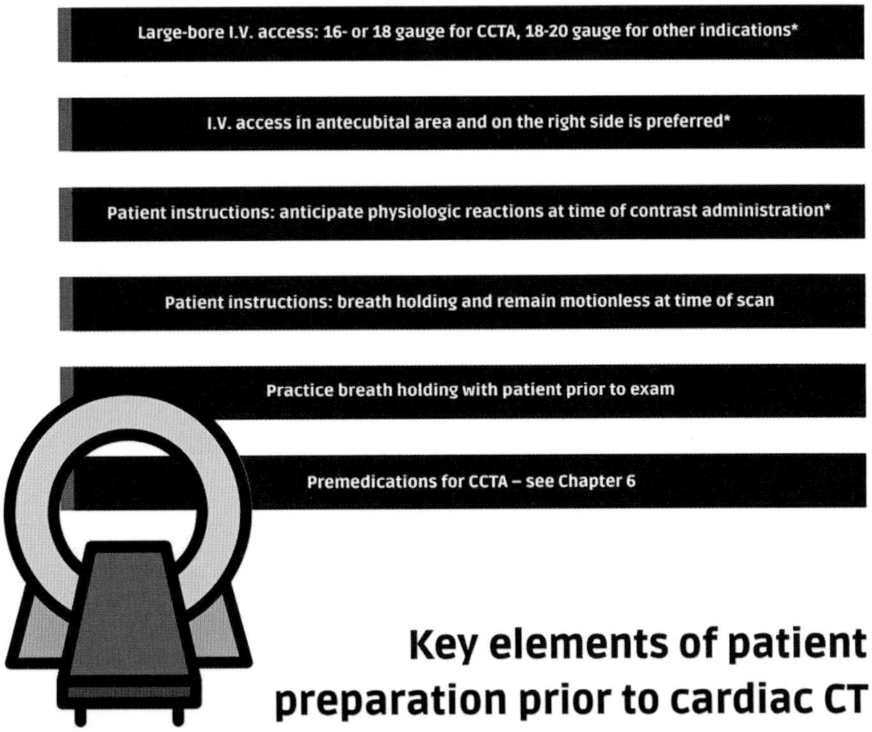

FIG. 1.1 Patient Preparation for Cardiac CT. *Applies to contrast-enhanced studies only. *CCTA*, Coronary computed tomography angiography; *CT*, computed tomography.

of kidney disease, such as those with prior AKI, chronic kidney disease, or albuminuria, as well as in patients taking metformin. In patients without risk factors, evaluation of baseline creatinine is not warranted before administration of iodinated contrast media.

Pregnancy and Lactation

Cardiac CT in pregnant women exposes the fetus to a low dose of radiation, at which no deterministic effects of radiation are expected. However, stochastic effects cannot be excluded.[8] Moreover, there is a potential for neonatal thyroid dysfunction with the administration of iodinated contrast in pregnancy, although the true incidence of this condition is not known.[9] Therefore, whenever possible, alternative imaging modalities without ionizing radiation are preferred. Although institutional policies may differ, the American College of Radiology Practice Parameter for Imaging Pregnant or Potentially Pregnant Adolescents and Women does not require laboratory verification of pregnancy status for chest CTs.[8] In lactating women, it is considered safe to continue breastfeeding after administration of iodinated contrast agents, as the amount of iodine excreted in breast milk and absorbed enterally by the child is considered trivial.[9,10]

PATIENT PREPARATION

Patients undergoing contrast-enhanced cardiac CT should receive a large-bore intravenous access, preferably 16 or 18 gauge, in the antecubital vein. Access in the hand should be avoided due to the higher risk of extravasation, as well as the higher risk of compartment syndrome or tissue injury in the event of an extravasation. The right side is typically preferred due to the possibility of streak artifact related to contrast pooling in the left subclavian vein in the setting of left-sided injections.

Electrocardiographic synchronization (gating) is critical for all cardiac CT examinations. Therefore, after the electrodes are placed on the patient (which should be outside the scan range), the ECG tracing should be reviewed prior to scanning to ensure sufficient voltage on the QRS complex relative to the baseline tracing. If there is low voltage on the QRS and/or increased baseline artifact, tracking of the QRS complexes by the scanner could be jeopardized, and the electrodes should be repositioned until a satisfactory tracing is obtained. In some cases, cleaning the skin to ensure good contact of the electrode with the skin may be helpful; this can be achieved with an alcohol swab as well as with certain commercial skin preparation products.

Patient orientation is another key component of preparation for a successful cardiac CT exam. The patient should be instructed about the importance of breath-holding and remaining motionless during the study. Breath-holding should always be practiced with the patient. The potential for physiologic reactions at the time of contrast injection, such as the sensation of warmth or urinary urge, should be discussed beforehand (Fig. 1.1). Premedication for heart rate control is discussed in Chapter 6 (How to Obtain a High-Quality Coronary CT Angiography) as well as in Chapter 8 (CCTA for Acute Chest Pain: Clinical Indications, Protocols, and Patient Management).

ACQUISITION MODES

Computed tomography utilizes ionizing radiation emitted and absorbed within a rotating gantry. The images

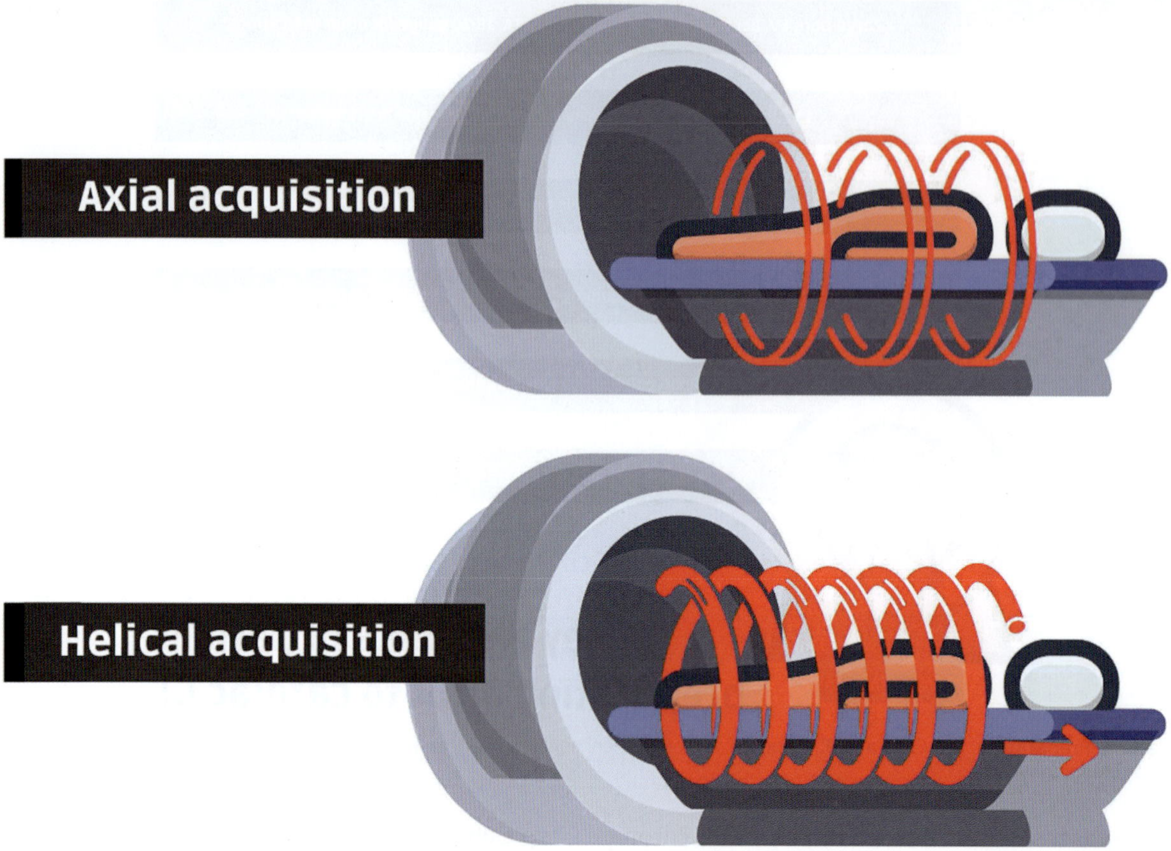

FIG. 1.2 Axial Versus Helical Acquisition. In axial scanning, there is no table movement when the x-ray beam is on, resulting in an axial slice acquisition. The table moves when the x-ray beam is off to allow for coverage along the z-axis. In helical scanning, the table moves continuously while the x-ray beam is on, creating an imaging spiral or helix. (Figure courtesy Ana Vitoria Rocha.)

produced by CT are due to heterogeneous attenuation of x-ray photons according to tissue characteristics. There are two main modes for data acquisition for cardiac CT with respect to the relationship between gantry rotation and patient/table movement. These modes are called axial scanning and helical scanning (Fig. 1.2).

In axial acquisition (also termed "step and shoot" or "sequential mode" by some vendors), data from a particular area of interest are acquired slice by slice during a prespecified portion of the cardiac cycle (e.g., 65–80% of the R-R interval). During data acquisition there is no table movement. The gantry then stops, and the patient/table is moved while the x-ray beam is off. Full coverage of the entire field of view can be achieved in two ways: (1) use of wide-area multidetector system, such as with 320-row scanners that can have up to 16-cm coverage along the z-axis; or (2) use of sequential table movement whereby the table moves to another location along the desired scan range after scanning each volume. This process is done in synchronization with the cardiac cycle so that the same portion of the cardiac cycle is scanned in all volume acquisitions (e.g., 65–80% of the R-R interval). This is called axial acquisition using prospective ECG gating, wherein the QRS complexes detected on the ECG prospectively determine scan initiation and the portion of the cardiac cycle during which images are acquired. The main advantage of axial acquisition is that it is associated with a substantially lower radiation dose; however, the limitations include the potential for misregistration artifacts or, in some scanners, limited number of phases of the cardiac cycle. In general, axial acquisition is almost always preferred when using modern CT scanners due to its lower radiation dose.

Unlike axial acquisition, in helical acquisition (also called spiral acquisition due to the spiral path of the x-ray beam relative to the detector movement) the table moves continuously during the time the x-ray beam is on. This acquisition technique creates a helix of coverage, producing a volumetric scan of the coverage area. To understand helical mode, it is important to review the concept of pitch. Pitch is defined as the distance traveled by the table during a full gantry rotation divided by the collimated width of the detector array (beam width). Beam width is defined as the product of the number of detector rows times the thickness of each slice.

When helical technique is used for cardiac CT, a low pitch (<1), is often employed. With a pitch <1, there is beam overlap, as the table travels less than the beam width, creating redundant data acquisition. These overlapping data are retrospectively assigned to specific phases of the cardiac cycle based on synchronization with the ECG data and are therefore called retrospective ECG gating. The technique of retrospective gating allows flexible reconstructions of scan data, due to beam overlap (as low pitch is associated with oversampling of data) and data acquisition during the entire cardiac cycle. However, this technique can also be associated with high radiation doses for the same reasons. To minimize radiation, ECG-based tube current dose modulation can be implemented with

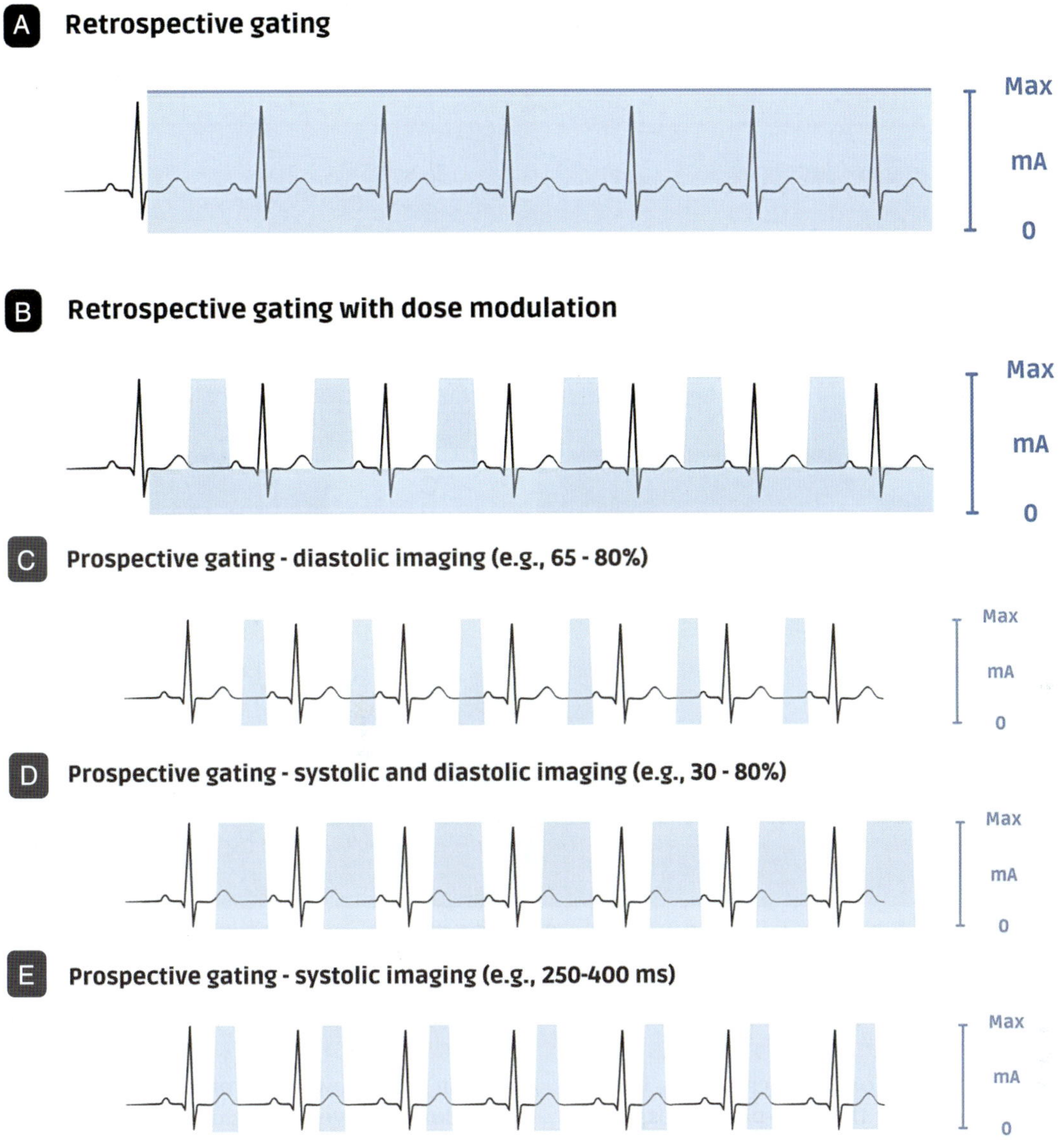

FIG. 1.3 **Retrospective Versus Prospective ECG Gating.** In retrospective gating (A), assignment of QRS position with respect to each image being reconstructed from the raw data (phases of each image) is performed after scanning, that is, retrospectively. To minimize radiation, a strategy of dose modulation can be used (B), wherein tube current is decreased in prespecified phases of the cardiac cycle, such as in systole. In prospective gating, the QRS complexes are tracked and the timing (relative to the R-R interval) and duration (width of phase acquisition window) of data acquisition is triggered prospectively (C–E). In other words, data are acquired at prespecific phases. Depending on the particular indication and patient heart rate, the prespecified phase may be diastolic only (e.g., 65–80% of the R-R cycle, as shown in C); systolic and diastolic (e.g., 30%–80% as shown in D); or systolic only (e.g., 25%–40% or +250–400 ms from the QRS when defining an absolute interval, as shown in E). (Figure courtesy of Ana Vitoria Rocha.)

retrospective helical scanning, wherein the tube current is decreased at prespecified phases of the cardiac cycle. For coronary artery imaging, the tube current modulation typically occurs during systole (Fig. 1.3).

Occasionally, ECG synchronization can misidentify artifacts or T waves as a QRS complex or, alternatively, fail to identify a particular beat as a QRS complex, particularly if it is premature or has low voltage. This may create a particular type of cardiac motion artifact in which the incorrect segment of the R-R interval is used for reconstruction, which may result in absence of data for a given segment (Fig. 1.4). Many scanners have algorithms to avoid and delay scanning if a premature beat is detected or to open the phase acquisition window if the R-R interval is irregular. However, these algorithms are not perfect as an arrhythmia can occur after a scanner has started acquiring data. When performing helical scanning with retrospective ECG gating (and in some cases of axial acquisition with a wide phase acquisition window), it may be possible to perform ECG editing, where synchronizations can be added, eliminated, or moved to align more accurately with the QRS (Fig. 1.4). In prospective ECG gating, this may not always be possible, because ECG synchronization triggered the image acquisition itself. If a prospective ECG gating acquisition is uninterpretable due to a gating error, the alternative is often to repeat the examination. This underscores the importance of verifying optimal ECG gating *before* image acquisition, with enough voltage on the QRS complexes and minimization of artifacts.

Alternatively, helical scanning can also be performed with high-pitch, prospective ECG triggering. Just like in helical scanning with retrospective ECG gating, the table

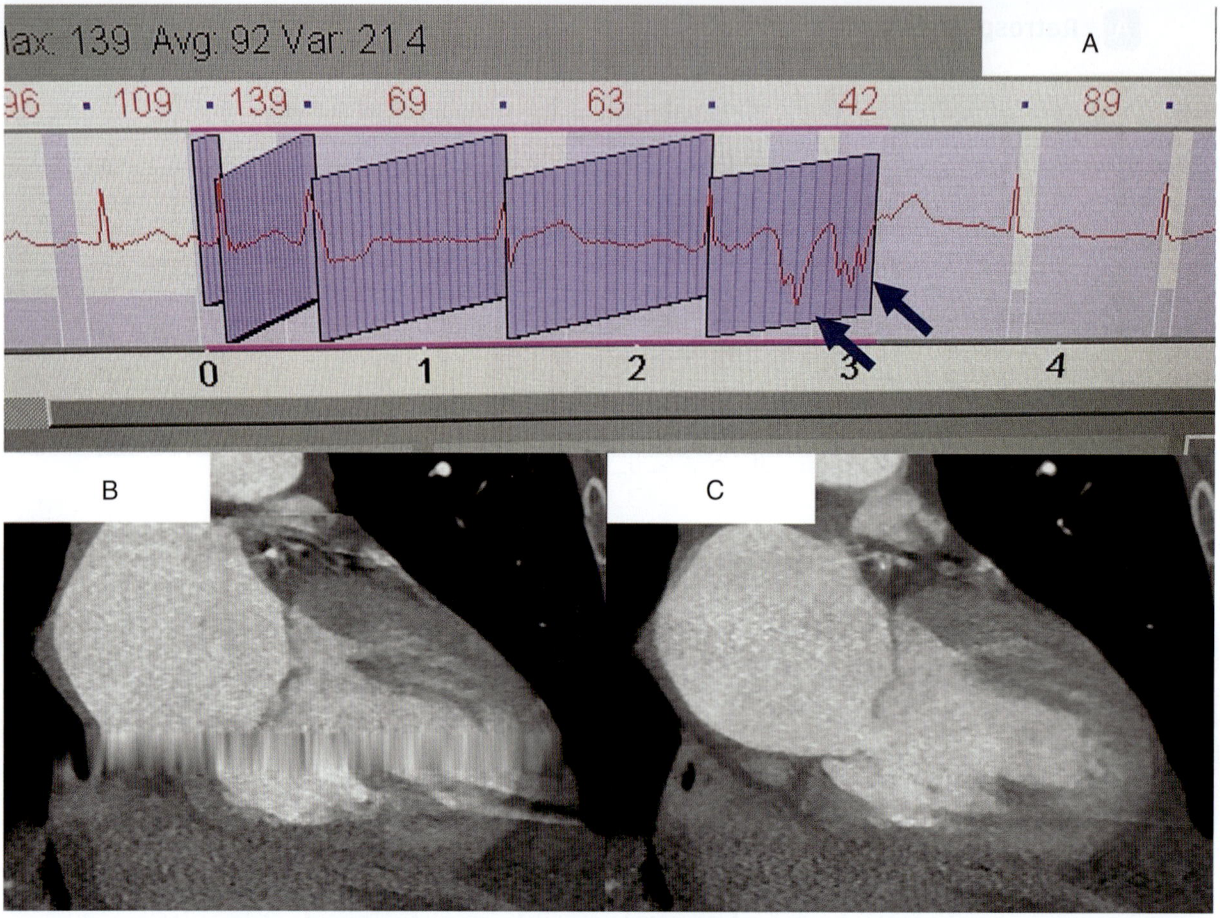

FIG. 1.4 **Helical Acquisition With Retrospective ECG Gating Allows for ECG Editing.** This cardiac CT performed for aortic valve evaluation was acquired in a helical mode with retrospective ECG gating, without dose modulation. There was significant motion artifact due to two artifactual waveforms that had originally been considered QRS complexes (Fig. 1.4A and 1.4B). These were corrected with manual ECG editing, only available in retrospective ECG gating. Fig. 1.4C demonstrates the reconstructed cardiac CT images after ECG editing, now with substantial improvement of the artifact.

moves while x-ray imaging is ongoing, creating a helix of data acquisition. However, in the high-pitch prospective ECG acquisition mode, there is no overlap of data acquisition. On the contrary, high pitch indicates that the distance traveled by the table in a full gantry rotation is greater than the beam width, which would create gaps in image acquisition. Therefore this mode of scanning can only be performed in a dual-source system, with simultaneous data acquisition from the two detectors. When using this mode, the acquired data are just enough to reconstruct a narrow window of the cardiac cycle (e.g., 65% of the R-R interval). Therefore the scan must be exactly timed to image at the phase of interest, which explains why this mode is triggered prospectively. In other words, ECG synchronization determines exactly when scanning will occur.

The main advantages of high-pitch, prospective ECG acquisition are (1) reduction in radiation dose, especially relative to helical scanning with retrospective ECG gating, and (2) eliminating the risk of misregistration artifacts between different datasets that are obtained and then merged during axial scanning with prospective ECG gating. However, because only one phase is available, this mode can only be performed in two circumstances. The first circumstance is in coronary CTA studies, where excellent image quality is expected and data can be obtained in only one phase. This would generally require a regular heart rhythm with a low heart rate, as well as nonobese patients who do not have significant coronary calcifications. Second, when imaging structures for which cardiac motion is less of a problem, such as the aorta. In the latter, any phase should be sufficient to minimize motion and produce adequate image quality. Therefore helical scanning with high pitch becomes an attractive option in such cases when it is available.

CONTRAST INJECTION AND IMAGE TRIGGERING

A sufficient contrast-to-noise ratio is required for diagnostic image quality in contrast-enhanced cardiac CT, with opacification of at least 250 to 300 Hounsfield units (HU) in the structures of interest. To achieve this, contrast media should have a high iodine concentration (270–400 mg of iodine/mL), injected at a high rate, typically of 5 to 7 mL/s for coronary CTA and 4 to 6 mL/s for other indications.[10] The total contrast volume is the product of the total duration of injection (seconds) and the rate of injection (mL/s), wherein the total duration of injection should reflect the scan time plus a few extra seconds. One potential formula for calculating the total volume of injection for coronary CTA is as follows: (estimated scan duration + 4 seconds) × flow rate.

TABLE 1.3 Bolus Tracking Versus Test Bolus Methods for Triggering Image Acquisition

	BOLUS TRACKING	TEST BOLUS
Technique	Real time imaging of contrast arrival	Test run for calculating time from injection to peak contrast opacification
Total contrast	Less volume	More volume
Number of contrast injections	1	2
Total scan time	Shorter	Longer
Test run to simulate compliance with patient instructions and test IV	No	Yes
Risk of failure (see text for examples)	Higher	Lower

To achieve optimal image quality, image acquisition should be timed to take place during peak contrast enhancement in the structure(s) of interest. A fixed time delay from contrast injection to triggering of scan initiation is not adequate, given that the time from injection to peak enhancement may vary substantially between different patients based on caliber and location of IV access, cardiac output, vascular anatomy, and so on. There are two techniques for selecting the ideal time to initiate scanning after contrast injection: bolus tracking and test bolus.

In bolus tracking, the entire volume of contrast for the study is injected, and attenuation is measured sequentially in a prespecified region of interest (ROI), such as the left atrium or the aorta. When attenuation in this ROI reaches a prespecified threshold, that is, attenuation of 100 HU, the scanner triggers breath-holding instructions for the patient followed by initiation of image acquisition.

When using a test bolus, only a small volume of contrast (e.g., 10 mL) is injected initially. Attenuation is measured sequentially in a specific location, such as the ascending aorta. A curve of attenuation of an ROI versus time since injection is then analyzed, which allows for quantification of time from injection to peak contrast enhancement. Therefore, when the full volume of contrast is subsequently injected, the time to peak enhancement is already known for that patient, thereby allowing for precise timing of scan acquisition. Although the test bolus requires two separate injections, with a slightly higher total contrast volume and time for scanning, there is an advantage in testing other aspects of the test, beyond peak enhancement itself. For instance, the first injection, with a low contrast volume, allows a test of the IV access, as well as patient understanding and ability to follow instructions, which are key components to obtain a high-quality image (Table 1.3).

The test bolus method may also be preferred in cases with unusually low cardiac output or abnormal anatomy, such as persistent left-sided superior vena cava (SVC) or other congenital heart disease. In such cases, peak enhancement at the ROI may be very delayed, and bolus tracking may not adequately trigger the scan. Even when the scan is triggered based on the ROI threshold, the short delay from breath-hold commands to scanning may not be enough to achieve peak enhancement. When either of these situations occurs with bolus tracking, the full volume of contrast was already injected, without sufficient contrast opacification, and possibly, a nondiagnostic cardiac CT result. The only alternative would be to reinject a full volume of contrast.

Regarding the type of iodinated contrast media, either iso-osmolar or low-osmolar agents may be used. The IsoCOR randomized trial showed no difference between an iso-osmolar contrast agent (iodixanol 270) and a low-osmolar agent (iopromide 300) in terms of coronary opacification or image quality when the rate of injection and total contrast volume were adjusted for the iodine concentration.[11] The sensation of heat discomfort was slightly less common with the iso-osmolar agent (72% versus 86%); however, this did not translate into a significant difference in heart rate or rhythm.

A saline chaser is typically used to follow the contrast bolus in all contrast-enhanced cardiac CT protocols. The chaser serves two purposes: first, the peak enhancement will be higher because the chaser pushes excess contrast through the inflow veins to maintain a "tighter" column of contrast; second, the chaser dilutes contrast in the systemic veins and right-sided chambers, which reduces streak artifact. This biphasic injection (contrast, then saline) may be substituted in certain protocols by a triphasic scheme, in which there are three distinct phases of injection, as will be discussed in the section for right-sided opacification.

CARDIAC CT PROTOCOLS

The cardiac CT exam starts with acquisition of scout images of the chest for accurate prescription of the scan range. It is important to tailor the scan range to the study being performed. For most indications, coverage should begin approximately 1 to 2 cm below the level of the tracheal bifurcation (i.e., at the area of the main pulmonary artery) and end below the diaphragm, just beyond the inferior wall, for a typical total scan range of 12 to 15 cm. Special circumstances that require a more cephalad scan range include patients with a history of coronary artery bypass grafting, when imaging of the entire course of the internal mammary artery is desired, as well as simultaneous acquisition of CT angiography of the ascending thoracic aorta and/or arch (Fig. 1.5).

Coronary Artery Calcium Score

The coronary artery calcium score (CAC) was initially derived from electron beam CT, acquiring images at 80% of the R-R interval, with 3-mm slice thickness and 130-KVp

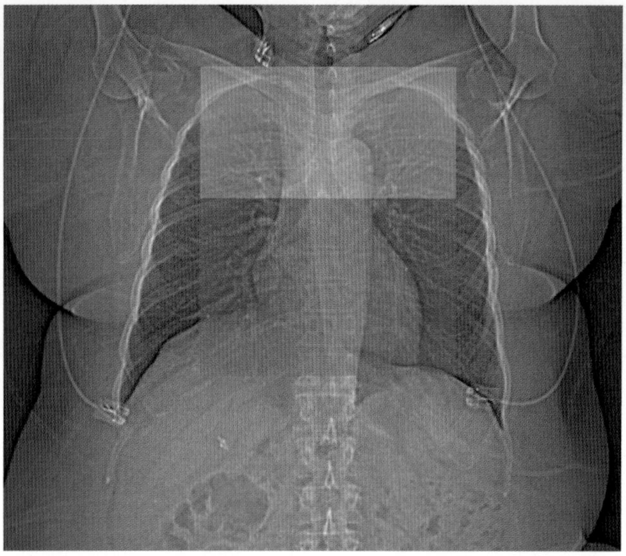

FIG. 1.5 Scout Topogram. Typical field of view used for full cardiac coverage is highlighted in *blue*. In patients with a history of coronary artery bypass grafting, in whom an internal mammary artery was used, the scan range is extended cranially (*gray*).

tube voltage. However, electron beam CT was not ideal for performing CCTA due to poor signal-to-noise ratio and limited spatial resolution.[12] Hence, CAC score has been adapted to multidetector CT, with some modifications, including 120-KVp tube voltage and variable tube current according to the patient's body habitus. Quantification of CAC is performed with the Agatston score, a sum of the individual area-density product of all calcified coronary artery plaques. The method applies a minimum threshold of 1 mm^2 for area and 130 HU for density to consider a lesion as calcified plaque. To determine plaque density, each pixel is weighted by a factor of 1 through 4 based on maximal CT attenuation: 1 for 130 to 199 HU; 2 for 200 to 299 HU; 3 for 300 to 399 HU; and 4 for ≥400 HU.[13]

Because intravenous contrast injection is not needed for CAC assessment, the test does not require any significant patient preparation other than breath-holding instructions. Screening of patients prior to testing includes, most importantly, making sure that the indication for CAC testing is appropriate. Patients with established coronary artery disease (CAD), including prior infarction, coronary revascularization, or anatomic evidence of known CAD (e.g., prior catheterization, nongated chest CT with severe coronary calcifications), are not ideal candidates for CAC testing, as quantification of CAC would not be expected to inform clinical decision-making.

CAC scanning is typically performed with axial acquisition and prospective ECG triggering. As previously discussed, coverage of the full cardiac field of view can be performed within one axial acquisition in systems with a wide-area detector, such as 320-row scanners, or, alternatively, with sequential table movement.

CAC does not usually require rate-controlling agents, such as metoprolol or ivabradine, as quantification of CAC is less susceptible to image degradation from faster heart rates. However, CAC is not completely immune to motion artifact. At faster heart rates (e.g., >75 bpm), there can be significant variability in CAC quantification between different manufactures, particularly for high mass lesions.[14] Therefore, although CAC scanning is typically performed in diastole, consideration should be given to scanning in late systole (e.g., 40% of the R-R interval) if the heart rate is elevated above 75 bpm (or a similar threshold), particularly in scanners with worse temporal resolution. Images may be acquired with thin slices (0.5–0.6 mm for modern scanners); however, reconstruction of images should be performed at 2.5- to 3-mm slice thickness for CAC quantification.[15]

Recently, there has been debate in the cardiac CT field discussing newer techniques for CAC quantification. Despite the strengths and decades-old validation of the Agatston score, advances in CT technology and further research have uncovered novel ways to perform CAC quantification, which may include advantages of improving risk stratification and/or reducing radiation dose. For instance, the Agatston score assigns higher value to higher-density plaques; however, there is actually an inverse association between calcium density and incident coronary events.[16] Similarly, the distribution of CAC adds substantial value to risk prediction beyond the Agatston score.[17] See Chapter 3 (Coronary Artery Calcium Testing: Indications and Patient Management) for further detail.

These concepts for novel strategies in risk stratification with CAC may have an impact on the optimal method to perform image acquisition, reconstruction, and post-processing. For example, the use of thinner slices (i.e., 0.5-mm thickness) may improve sensitivity for detecting smaller calcified lesions, with direct implications for patient management if there is a more accurate discrimination between patients with CAC >0 versus no CAC. Similarly, the threshold of 130 HU in the Agatston score could be revised to include calcified plaques with lower density, given that scanners have improved, and image noise is reduced as compared with older technology. Selective reduction in the tube voltage on CAC testing to 80 or 100 KVp would significantly reduce the radiation dose, while still maintaining adequate image quality for most patients, although with some overestimation of CAC score compared with current standards.[13] Finally, a prospectively triggered helical high-pitch acquisition could lower radiation dose for CAC testing significantly, below 0.5 mSv.[18] In general, these strategies would require some form of recalibration of the calcium score in order to keep it similar to the score derived by current techniques.[13,18] Given the low radiation dose of CAC scoring as it currently stands (1–2 mSv) and the robust validation of the Agatston score, there has been no consensus on if and how to modify the current CAC method.

Whether CAC score should be obtained at the time of CCTA is a matter of controversy. There are several arguments in favor of routinely adding a noncontrast acquisition for computation of CAC prior to CCTA. First, in patients without established CAD, CAC provides a robust, well-validated method for risk stratification. Second, identification of significant CAC in patients without previously known coronary calcifications may lead to a modification in scanning parameters, particularly a higher tube voltage to achieve better image quality. Third, in the presence of extensive coronary artery calcifications, there is a higher probability of having nondiagnostic segments on the CCTA, in which case, and depending on available technology,

TABLE 1.4 Pros and Cons of Adding Routine Coronary Artery Calcium Score to Coronary Computed Tomography Angiography (CCTA) in Patients Without Established Coronary Artery Disease

PROS	CONS
CAC scoring provides a quantitative and validated method for estimating plaque burden and for ASCVD risk stratification	CAD burden can be estimated using other techniques (as recommended by CAD RADS 2.0), which incorporate both calcified and noncalcified plaque
May identify small calcified lesions that can be missed during contrast-enhanced CCTA (especially if low kV used)	CCTA unlikely to miss plaque. In rare cases that calcified plaque not seen by CCTA, the median calcium score was 1[21]
May inform scan acquisition parameters (i.e., kV, phase acquisition window), if significant CAC is present	Adds 1–2 mSv in radiation (not trivial given overall low dose of CCTA when using contemporary scanners), as well as increased time for image acquisition and interpretation
In some practices, CAC testing may result in cancellation of the CCTA if extensive CAC is present	In many centers, there is no particular threshold of CAC above which CCTA would be contraindicated

ASCVD, Atherosclerotic cardiovascular disease; *CAC*, coronary artery calcium score; *CCTA*, coronary CT angiography; *CAD RADS 2.0*, Coronary Artery Disease – Reporting and Data System.

consideration might be given to an alternative imaging modality instead of proceeding with CCTA (Table 1.4).[19]

However, there are important counterarguments to this approach. First, radiation doses from CAC scoring are in the range of 1 to 2 mSv. Current CT technology with adequate heart rate control, diastolic-only imaging, axial scanning, and prospective ECG triggering has allowed for CCTA to be performed with excellent image quality at a similar dose, ranging from 1 to 4 mSv.[20] Therefore, although the total radiation dose would still be low overall, adding CAC to modern-day CCTA may result in nearly doubling of the total radiation dose as compared with CCTA alone.

In addition, there is no definitive cutoff for CAC at which point CCTA might be nondiagnostic. In a study with 119 patients with a median CAC score of 1616 AU, 726 segments with stenosis ≥25% were analyzed by CCTA and invasive coronary angiography within 90 days. CCTA still maintained a high negative predictive value for the diagnosis of obstructive CAD, defined as stenosis >70%. On per-vessel analysis and per-patient analyses, the negative predictive value was 93% and 92%, respectively.[22]

Finally, there is a more practical matter to the workflow of cardiac CT that hinders the usefulness of routine CAC prior to CCTA acquisition. Cancelling CCTA in lieu of alternative testing based on an elevated CAC score would require real-time interpretation of CAC by a CT reader at the scanner, which may not be practical at many sites. Moreover, cancelling the CCTA with the patient already on the table would most often be done without a discussion with referring providers.

Given all these issues, and without a high probability that CCTA would not be diagnostic, it may not be prudent nor feasible to cancel CCTA based on CAC results at the time of CCTA. This is not to say that the presence and amount of CAC on prior CAC testing or noncardiac chest CTs shouldn't be used to guide patient candidacy for CCTA. On the contrary, CCTA protocoling should routinely involve evaluation of CAC from prior studies, as well as conversations with referring providers, when needed, to select the best imaging technique for each patient.

Left Atrium and Left Atrial Appendage Evaluations

There is an increasing demand for cardiac CT for evaluation of the left atrium and left atrial appendage due to the growing prevalence of atrial fibrillation and more frequent indication of atrial fibrillation–related procedures, including cardioversions, catheter ablation, and left atrial appendage occlusion devices. Cardiac CT has excellent accuracy for confirming or excluding the presence of a left atrial appendage thrombus. In a metaanalysis of 27 studies, with nearly 7000 patients, the sensitivity and specificity of cardiac CT with delayed imaging was 98% and 100%, respectively, compared with transesophageal echocardiogram.[23]

When the CT is performed for planning of percutaneous left atrial appendage occlusion, it is useful if patients are scanned in a nonfasting state and remain well hydrated, due to significant variability in left atrial appendage (LAA) size according to cardiac preload.[24]

The preferred cardiac CT acquisition modes to image the left atrium or left atrial appendage are either (1) axial scanning with prospective ECG gating or (2) high-pitch helical scanning with prospective ECG gating. Helical scanning with retrospective ECG gating should be avoided due to the higher radiation dose unless there is a concomitant indication that requires a helical retrospective acquisition, such as the evaluation of cardiac or valvular function.

Cardiac motion is less of a problem for the left atrium as compared with the coronary arteries. Thus strict heart rate control and a wide acquisition window are not necessary. However, if the heart rate is too high, image quality for left atrial appendage evaluation may be degraded, especially because these patients often have an irregular rhythm due to atrial fibrillation. The exact heart rate threshold beyond which cardiac CT will be nondiagnostic for imaging the left atrial appendage is variable, depending on the temporal resolution of each scanner. Imaging sites should be aware of their own scanner limitations and plan the mode and phase of acquisition accordingly.

An expert recommendation statement on cardiac CT for planning transcatheter left atrial appendage occlusion suggested using a 30% to 60% acquisition window.[25] When the goal is not necessarily to measure the left atrial appendage, but rather to exclude thrombus, an even narrower window of diastolic-only or systolic-only images can be obtained. In scanners with good temporal resolution and in patients with a well-controlled heart rate (e.g., <70 bpm), scanning may be performed using diastolic

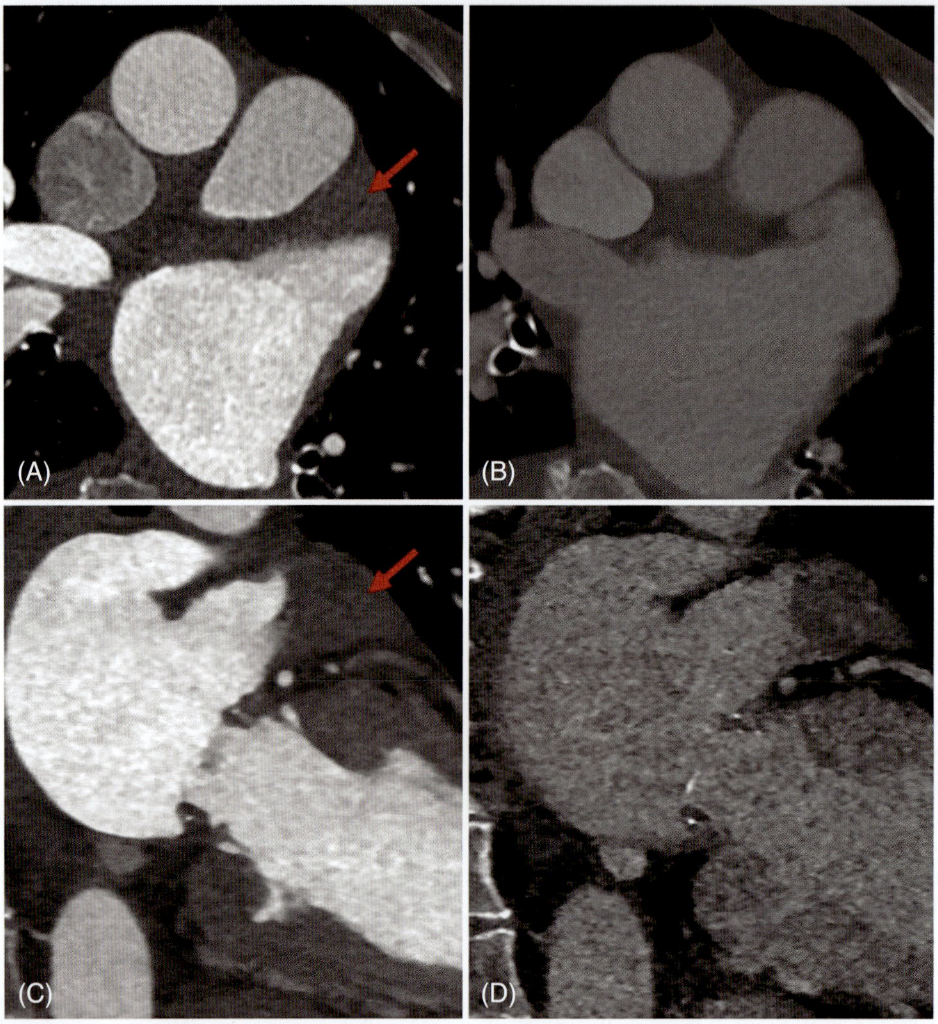

FIG. 1.6 Imaging of the Left Atrial Appendage. (A) and (C) show arterial phase imaging of two different patients, both with a filling defect at the tip of the left atrial appendage (*red arrows*). In the patient from (A), delayed imaging at 45 seconds after contrast injection demonstrated complete opacification of the left atrial appendage (B), indicative of no thrombus. In the patient from (C), the filling defect persisted on delayed imaging (D), indicative of a left atrial appendage thrombus.

images, at 70% to 80% of RR interval. If the heart rhythm is irregular or tachycardiac, scanning in systole may be preferred, at 250 to 400 ms after R-wave or 30% to 40% of the R-R interval, for example. A simpler approach, which automates the process and minimizes chances of protocoling errors, would be to scan all patients for left atrial or left atrial appendage indications in late systole, regardless of the heart rate. The availability of having several phases may be helpful in cases where there are motion artifacts, although these are usually less problematic when evaluating the left atrial appendage.

The most frequently used contrast injection protocol for imaging the LAA is a biphasic protocol, with a total contrast volume of approximately 50 to 70 mL, injected at a rate of 5 mL/s, followed by a saline chaser of 50 mL. As previously discussed, triggering can occur with a test bolus or bolus tracking method. If a bolus tracking method is used, the ROI can be placed in the left atrium, ascending aorta, or descending aorta, with a threshold between 80 and 130 HU. Tube current and peak voltage can be selected automatically with software available by different vendors, with the latter ranging between 70 and 120 kVp.[26] Images are acquired (and reconstructed) at the thinnest slice thickness available for the cardiac CT scanner, ranging from 0.5 to 0.75 mm.

In cardiac CT for evaluation of the left atrial appendage, it is necessary to perform delayed imaging to differentiate thrombus from late filling of the appendage in the setting of slow flow. The second acquisition is performed after a delay of approximately 45 to 60 seconds from the first scan, using a single cardiac phase. Filling defects seen on early and delayed images are consistent with LAA thrombus, whereas filling defects seen only in the arterial phase represent stasis of blood flow, without thrombus (Fig. 1.6). Some have also suggested scanning in prone position for the early and delayed imaging acquisition, with excellent accuracy relative to echocardiography.[27]

Of note, when cardiac CT is performed for measurements of the left atrial appendage, such as prior to percutaneous closure of the appendage, *sequential* axial imaging may lead to misregistration artifacts at the ostium of the left atrial appendage. Therefore, in scanners without full coverage in one axial scan, quality control must be performed immediately at the end of the study to ensure that there is no significant misregistration artifact that may preclude accurate measurements.

Cardiac CT for Left-sided Valvular Indications

The protocol for cardiac CT when imaging for left-sided valves follows certain principles, whether the indication is for (1) procedural planning, such as transcatheter aortic or mitral therapies; (2) structural evaluation of prosthetic valves for thrombus, leaflet thickening, or pannus; or (3) evaluation of suspected endocarditis or infectious complications of native or prosthetic valves.

First, these scans are most commonly performed as helical (or spiral) acquisitions with retrospective ECG gating to allow multiphase imaging and to avoid misregistration artifact from axial scanning. Misregistration artifacts that run through the valve of interest have the potential to make the scan nondiagnostic. Another advantage of retrospective ECG gating is the possibility to perform ECG editing, as previously discussed, if there are gating issues. Axial scanning with prospective ECG gating may be performed for valvular indications when cardiac CT is performed in scanners capable of opening the phase acquisition window to allow for full RR interval coverage. In such cases, there may be advantages to scanners that can acquire the data in one heartbeat with axial scanning, as this eliminates the possibility of misregistration artifacts. High-pitch helical scanning is not appropriate for scanning of heart valves because single-phase acquisition is insufficient in these indications.

Second, when evaluating valvular structures, it is important to scan with a wide window of acquisition throughout the cardiac cycle. Systolic and diastolic images are needed for assessment of leaflet mobility and thickness, annular dimensions, and vegetations. In fact, most valve cases are performed with acquisition throughout the full cardiac cycle (0–99% of the R-R interval). To reduce or limit radiation, other strategies can be used, such as iterative reconstruction, minimizing the scan range, or using dose modulation. The latter, however, should be used selectively. Good image quality with sufficient current should be maintained throughout the target window of acquisition.

Third, a high tube voltage is warranted in the evaluation of prosthetic valves to minimize streak artifacts from metal or other prosthetic material. It is particularly important to pay close attention to this parameter because automatic selection of peak tube voltage by software available in different vendors may default to low energy in patients with small or normal weight and body mass index.

Fourth, in patients with prosthetic material in whom there is a suspicion for pseudoaneurysm, abscess, or other structural valve deterioration, it is helpful to also acquire noncontrast images. This serves the purpose of differentiating contrast from calcification or prosthetic material, including suture pledgets adjacent to vascular structures. Structures that are highly attenuating on both arterial-phase and noncontrast images are prosthetic or postsurgical in nature, whereas those that have soft-tissue attenuation on noncontrast images but are hyperattenuating on arterial-phase images represent true contrast enhancement. In addition, whenever there is a concern for prosthetic valve infection, it may be helpful to perform a delayed-phase CT, at 70 to 90 seconds after injection, to identify late enhancement of granulation tissue, as seen in abscesses. When a triple-phase cardiac CT is needed for a comprehensive valvular evaluation (noncontrast, arterial, and delayed), the nonenhanced and the delayed image acquisition should be performed in a single phase of the cardiac cycle. The limitation of this triple-phase protocol is the high radiation dose. Faure et al. reported a mean total radiation dose of 8.3 ± 3.0 mSv with this protocol, albeit with prospective axial scanning in the arterial phase, centered at the valve of interest to minimize the risk of misregistration artifact and dose modulation beyond 500 ms after the R wave, both of which may limit image quality when assessing for infectious complications of prosthetic heart valves.[28]

Finally, it may be important to assess the thoracic, abdominal, and pelvic vascular anatomy when cardiac CT is performed for preprocedural planning of transcatheter valve interventions, such as transcatheter aortic valve replacement (see Chapter 19, Cardiac Computed Tomography for Transcatheter Aortic Valve Replacement). In these instances, CTA of the chest, abdomen, and pelvis can be performed as a helical, non-ECG-gated acquisition, following the ECG-gated cardiac acquisition. The vascular CTA does not need to be gated because information on the aortic root would already have been acquired during the gated portion of the examination. The total contrast volume in these cases needs to account for the longer duration of the scan. The Expert Consensus Statement on Transcatheter Aortic Valve Implantation from the Society of Cardiovascular Computed Tomography recommends a contrast volume of 50 to 100 mL, injected at 4 to 6 ml/s.[29]

Right-sided Opacification

When contrast-enhanced cardiac CT is performed for standard left-sided indications, such as coronary CTA or left atrial appendage assessment, the typical volume of contrast injected (~50–80 mL) is only enough to opacify left-sided structures. In other words, under normal hemodynamic conditions, when images are acquired, contrast has often already moved beyond the right-sided structures, which are then unopacified. In some cases, it may be helpful to have a small amount of contrast in right side of the heart to evaluate the size of the right-sided chambers. However, there are also advantages to having most (or all) of the contrast in the left side, as under such conditions differences in attenuation between left- and right-sided enhancement may assist in the detection of, often incidental, left-to-right shunts (Fig. 1.7).[30]

Cardiac CT may also be indicated for evaluation of right-sided structures, such as prosthetic tricuspid or pulmonic valves, endocarditis, right ventricular volumetric or functional assessment, or planning for percutaneous valvular interventions (see Chapter 20 Use of Cardiac Computed Tomography in Structural Heart Disease Interventions). In these cases, one potential way to image the right-sided structures is simply to inject a higher volume of contrast (and often also while using a lower contrast injection rate), so that when images are acquired there is still contrast on the right-sided chambers (e.g., 100 mL).[31] However, this may create a problem of flow-related artifacts, also called mixing artifact, wherein there is mixing of contrast-enhanced

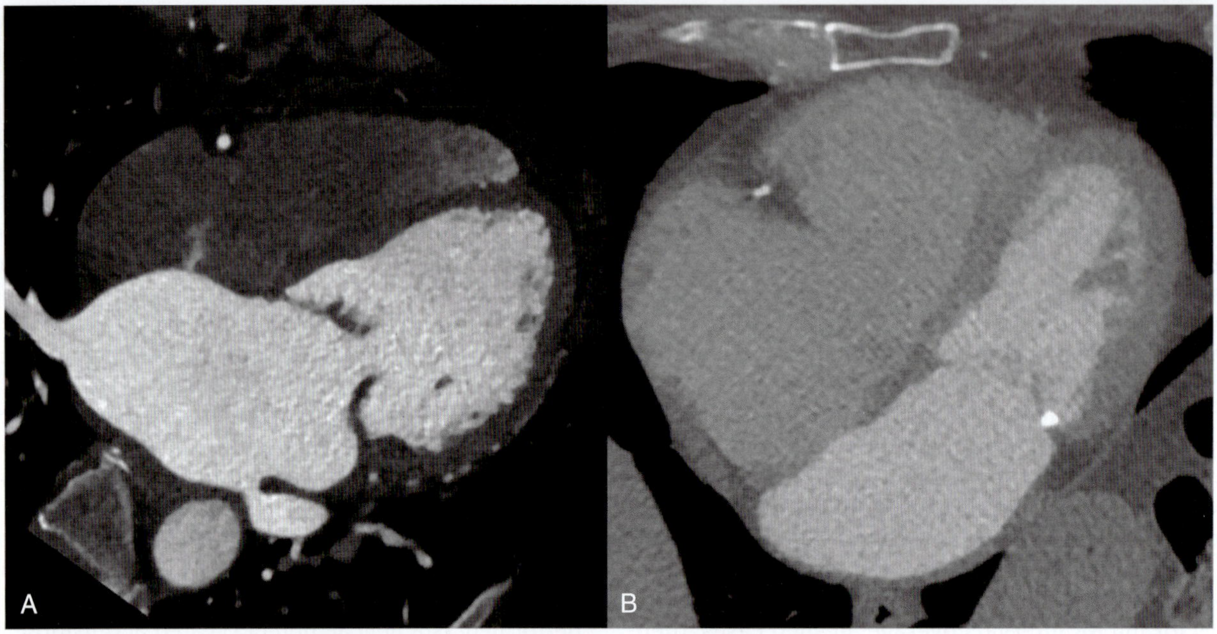

FIG. 1.7 **Cardiac CT for Left- or Right-sided Indications.** Under normal hemodynamic conditions, when cardiac CT is performed for left-sided indications (e.g., coronary, left atrial appendage assessment), with injection of 50 to 75 mL of iodinated contrast media, followed by a saline chaser, there may be no significant contrast opacification on the right-sided chambers by the time images are acquired. In (A), a patent foramen ovale is seen, with left-to-right shunting, facilitated by the substantial difference in contrast opacification between left- and right-sided chambers. Right-sided opacification can be obtained by injecting a larger volume of contrast (e.g., 100 mL) or performing a triphasic acquisition. (B) shows a cardiac CT obtained with a triphasic injection protocol, with a contrast-saline mix favoring contrast in the first phase, followed by a contrast-saline mix favoring saline on the second phase, followed by a saline chaser (third phase).

blood (typically from superior vena cava) with unenhanced blood (usually from inferior vena cava). This approach also can lead to contrast pooling in the systemic veins and right atrium, causing streak and beam-hardening artifacts, despite the use of a saline chaser.

An alternative approach for right-sided opacification is to use a triphasic protocol: first, predominantly contrast (either only contrast or a saline–contrast mix that favors contrast); second, a saline–contrast mix that favors saline; and third, a saline chaser.[32] This protocol typically reduces flow-related artifact from mixing of contrast in the right atrium while still allowing adequate opacification of the right ventricle. For example, phase 1 with 60 mL of 70%/30% at 5 mL/second, phase 2 with 60 mL of 30%/70% at 5 mL/second, and phase 3 with 20 mL of saline chaser at 5 mL/second (Fig. 1.7B).

Ventricular Function

Cardiac CT is also a robust imaging technique for the assessment of right and left ventricular systolic function and may be used for this indication as an alternative to echocardiography or cardiac magnetic resonance imaging when these imaging modalities are limited, for example, due to obesity, poor echocardiographic windows, claustrophobia, and implanted devices.

The most important factor for assessment of ventricular function is to obtain full coverage of the ventricle and to include the entire cardiac cycle, which can be performed with a helical acquisition with retrospective ECG gating, or with axial scanning and prospective ECG gating with 0% to 99% coverage of the R-R interval. As discussed previously, axial scanning can be performed on scanners with wide coverage (up to 320-row, 16-cm coverage) using a single beat acquisition, or with sequential table movement in scanners with smaller coverage along the z-axis. Misregistration artifacts with axial acquisition are less of a problem for evaluating ventricular function. If there are no other concomitant indications, such as valvular or coronary assessment, low-tube voltage can be used, as image noise is less of a concern for differentiating the myocardium from contrast-opacified chambers. Similarly, dose modulation can be used to reduce radiation. If assessment of the right ventricular function is needed, then techniques for right heart opacification should be utilized, as reported in the previous section.[33]

Myocardial Perfusion and Scar

Cardiac CT with stress perfusion has the potential to improve the overall accuracy and specificity of cardiac CT for identification of hemodynamically significant coronary stenoses, with a similar diagnostic accuracy for stress-induced myocardial perfusion defect as single-photon emission computed tomography (SPECT).[34,35] See Chapter 15 (Myocardial Perfusion Imaging Using Stress CT) for further detail.

Stress perfusion in cardiac CT is performed with pharmacologic vasodilators. There are two approaches for cardiac CT perfusion imaging: static and dynamic. In static imaging, a single image is acquired, ideally at peak contrast enhancement. This allows for qualitative evaluation of perfusion in the different myocardial segments. Dynamic perfusion with CT is analogous to dynamic perfusion imaging with positron emission tomography (PET) or magnetic resonance

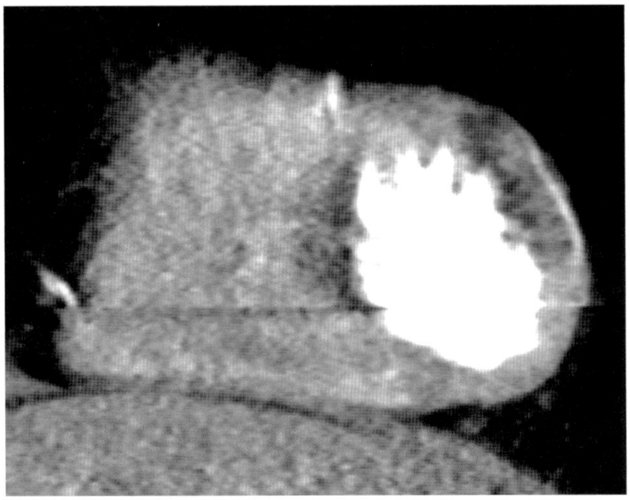

FIG. 1.8 **Cardiac CT Perfusion.** Cardiac CT acquisition in axial mode with sequential scanning may lead to differential contrast opacification of different myocardial segments, simulating a perfusion defect. In this example, images were initiated while myocardial enhancement was increasing, such that more caudal segment (which was acquired last) has a higher contrast opacification than the more cranial and midventricular segment (which were acquired first).

imaging (MRI), with repeated image acquisition throughout the first pass of contrast, which allows for the creation of time attenuation curves and quantification of perfusion in relative or absolute values.

The standard contraindications for vasodilator stress testing also apply to stress CT perfusion and are covered in Chapter 15.[36]

The order in which stress and rest perfusion images are obtained may vary according to institutional preference and/or pretest probability. In those with significant coronary artery calcifications or established CAD, stress perfusion imaging is recommended first. If there is no evidence of a regional perfusion defect, rest images may be aborted. In contrast, in those with low-to-intermediate pretest probability, with no known CAD, it may be preferable to start with rest images. If there is no plaque or only mild/minimal stenoses, then stress perfusion may not be needed. The downside of this approach is potential contamination of delayed contrast from the rest scan, which may persist in the stress scan. If both scans are performed (rest and stress), a 10- to 20-minute delay is needed, regardless of the order of scans, for contrast to wash out of the myocardium before the second scan.[36]

Importantly, stress perfusion must be obtained under peak vasodilator effect of the pharmacologic agent. For regadenoson, this occurs between 1 to 4 minutes after injection. Dipyridamole and adenosine are given as infusions, with average peak vasodilation occurring approximately 6.5 minutes and 1 to 2 minutes after starting the infusion for each of these agents, respectively.[37]

Static stress perfusion images can be performed with helical scanning and retrospective ECG gating or with axial acquisition and prospective ECG gating. The latter should be avoided for stress perfusion in scanners that require sequential table movement (limited axial coverage). The pause in scanning needed for table movement between acquisition of different volumes leads to different myocardial attenuation in each of the axial volumes, which may create a false appearance of a perfusion defect (Fig. 1.8).

In scanners with full coverage (320-slice systems), there is no need for sequential table movement. If a helical scan is used, tube current modulation can be used to limit radiation, with peak current focused in mid-diastole, late systole, or both (e.g., 40–80% of the R-R interval). A multiphase acquisition is preferred, as motion, beam hardening, and other artifacts tend to be variable across different phases of the cardiac cycle, and imagers will need to select the best phase for interpretation. Total contrast volume should be approximately 60 to 70 mL, with a flow rate of 5 to 6 mL/s. The scan can be triggered by bolus tracking or test bolus, with relative advantages and disadvantages as previously discussed.[36,38]

Dynamic stress perfusion follows a similar principle; however, the difference from static CT perfusion is that multiple images are acquired during peak vasodilatation, at multiple different time points during a 20- to 30-second breath-hold and first-pass perfusion. This can be performed with full coverage (single-beat acquisition) or with high-pitch helical scanning, which requires repeat back-and-forth table movement. Dynamic CT perfusion is associated with higher radiation exposure (from repeated scanning) and may require a longer breath-hold time.[39]

In patients with replacement fibrosis and myocardial scar, iodinated contrast media is retained in the extracellular space, similar to how gadolinium is retained in the extracellular space in late gadolinium enhancement (LGE) imaging. Indeed, late iodine enhancement (LIE) has accurate detection and localization of myocardial scar in patients with cardiomyopathies, when compared with LGE.[40] The most important parameters are (1) sufficient volume of overall contrast administration, ranging from 100 to 140 mL; and (2) delayed imaging, at 7 to 10 minutes.

Acquisition of the delayed images can be in axial mode, with prospective ECG triggering, at a single phase (typically in diastole) using a narrow acquisition window to minimize radiation exposure. Focal iodine accumulation is better appreciated on low-voltage acquisition; therefore images can be acquired either with (1) low-voltage, single-energy, at low kVp (80 or 100 kVp); (2) single-source dual-energy with rapid kilovolt peak switching; or (3) dual-source systems with dual energy.[40–42] Table 1.5 summarizes key elements of cardiac CT protocols.

CONCLUSIONS

Cardiac CT has undergone substantial technological advances over recent years and is now used for the evaluation of multiple cardiovascular conditions. Optimal use of cardiac CT, such that it is helpful to clinicians and guides patient care, starts with meticulous patient screening and preparation. Cardiac CT teams should make every effort to instruct patients on what to expect and what to do at the time of image acquisition, including practicing breath-holding. Finally, protocols for cardiac CT differ significantly based on the indication, scanner used, and the anatomy being evaluated. It is important that CT experts become familiar with the protocols for different indications, including nuances that may be particular to specific scanners.

TABLE 1.5 Key Elements of Different Cardiac CT Protocols

PROTOCOL	KEY ELEMENTS
Coronary artery calcium score	Noncontrast; 120 KVp; 2.5- to 3-mm slice thickness
Left atrium and left atrial appendage	50–75 mL at ~5 mL/s; systolic-only or diastolic-only imaging, depending on heart rate and scanner; axial mode with prospective ECG gating is preferred; delayed imaging at 45–60 seconds to evaluate for thrombus versus slow flow
Left-sided valvular evaluation	50–100 mL, injected at 4–6 mL/s; helical mode or axial scanning with coverage; of full R-R interval; if prosthetic material is present, consider high-tube voltage (e.g., 120 kVp) and noncontrast images; delayed phase at 70–90 seconds is recommended if concern for infection/abscess
Right-sided indications	Strategies to opacify right-sided chambers (in addition to the left) include 100 mL at 5 mL/s or a triphasic injection protocol, such as, for example phase 1 with 60 mL of 70%/30% at 5 mL/seconds, phase 2 with 60 mL of 30%/70% at 5 mL/second, and phase 3 with 20 mL of saline chaser at 5 mL/seconds
Ventricular function	Full coverage of the ventricles and scanning of the entire RR cycle is needed; if helical mode with retrospective ECG gating is performed, may use dose modulation to minimize radiation. If right ventricular assessment is needed, opacification of right-sided chambers should be performed as well.
Myocardial perfusion	Performed with pharmacologic vasodilator; static or dynamic images may be obtained; may be performed as a stress-first or rest-first perfusion study. If stress first, rest may be aborted if no evidence of perfusion defect at stress. If rest first, stress may be aborted if no evidence of significant plaque or stenoses.
Myocardial scar (late iodine enhancement)	Volume of iodinate contrast media 100–140 mL; perform delayed imaging at 7–10 minutes from contrast administration; single-phase is sufficient; include low energy (80–100 kVp) acquisition.

Cardiac CT protocols for coronary CT angiography and cardiac masses will be discussed in dedicated chapters.

REFERENCES

1. ACR Committee on Drugs and Contrast Media. ACR Manual on Contrast Media. https://www.acr.org/Clinical-Resources/Contrast-Manual.
2. Mortelé KJ, Oliva M-R, Ondategui S, Ros PR, Silverman SG. Universal use of nonionic iodinated contrast medium for CT: evaluation of safety in a large urban teaching hospital. *AJR Am J Roentgenol*. 2005;184:31–34.
3. Wichmann JL, Katzberg RW, Litwin SE, et al. Contrast-induced nephropathy. *Circulation*. 2015;132:1931–1936.
4. Newhouse JH, Kho D, Rao QA, Starren J. Frequency of serum creatinine changes in the absence of iodinated contrast material: implications for studies of contrast nephrotoxicity. *AJR Am J Roentgenol*. 2008;191:376–382.
5. Davenport MS, Khalatbari S, Cohan RH, Dillman JR, Myles JD, Ellis JH. Contrast material-induced nephrotoxicity and intravenous low-osmolality iodinated contrast material: risk stratification by using estimated glomerular filtration rate. *Radiology*. 2013;268:719–728.
6. Davenport MS, Khalatbari S, Dillman JR, Cohan RH, Caoili EM, Ellis JH. Contrast material-induced nephrotoxicity and intravenous low-osmolality iodinated contrast material. *Radiology*. 2013;267:94–105.
7. McDonald JS, McDonald RJ, Carter RE, Katzberg RW, Kallmes DF, Williamson EE. Risk of intravenous contrast material-mediated acute kidney injury: a propensity score-matched study stratified by baseline-estimated glomerular filtration rate. *Radiology*. 2014;271:65–73.
8. Jonnalagadda P. ACR–SPR Practice Parameter for Imaging Pregnant or Potentially Pregnant Adolescents and Women with Ionizing Radiation. https://www.acr.org/-/media/acr/files/practice-parameters/pregnant-pts.pdf.
9. Puac P, Rodríguez A, Vallejo C, Zamora CA, Castillo M. Safety of contrast material use during pregnancy and lactation. *Magn Reson Imaging Clin N Am*. 2017;25:787–797.
10. Abbara S, Blanke P, Maroules CD, et al. SCCT guidelines for the performance and acquisition of coronary computed tomographic angiography: a report of the society of Cardiovascular Computed Tomography Guidelines Committee: endorsed by the North American Society for Cardiovascular Imaging (NASCI). *J Cardiovasc Comput Tomogr*. 2016;10:435–449.
11. Lubbers MM, Kock M, Niezen A, et al. Iodixanol versus iopromide at coronary CT angiography: lumen opacification and effect on heart rhythm-the randomized IsoCOR trial. *Radiology*. 2018;286:71–80.
12. Kulkarni S, Rumberger JA, Jha S. Electron beam CT: a historical review. *AJR Am J Roentgenol*. 2021;216:1222–1228.
13. Blaha MJ, Mortensen MB, Kianoush S, Tota-Maharaj R, Cainzos-Achirica M. Coronary artery calcium scoring: is it time for a change in methodology? *JACC Cardiovasc Imaging*. 2017;10:923–937.
14. van der Werf NR, Willemink MJ, Willems TP, Vliegenthart R, Greuter MJW, Leiner T. Influence of heart rate on coronary calcium scores: a multi-manufacturer phantom study. *Int J Cardiovasc Imaging*. 2018;34:959–966.
15. Rutten A, Krul SPJ, Meijs MFL, de Vos AM, Cramer M-JM, Prokop M. Variability of coronary calcium scores throughout the cardiac cycle: implications for the appropriate use of electrocardiogram-dose modulation with retrospectively gated computed tomography. *Invest Radiol*. 2008;43:187–194.
16. Criqui MH, Denenberg JO, Ix JH, et al. Calcium density of coronary artery plaque and risk of incident cardiovascular events. *JAMA*. 2014;311:271–278.
17. Blaha MJ, Budoff MJ, Tota-Maharaj R, et al. Improving the CAC score by addition of regional measures of calcium distribution: multi-ethnic study of atherosclerosis. *JACC Cardiovasc Imaging*. 2016;9:1407–1416.
18. Marwan M, Mettin C, Pflederer T, et al. Very low-dose coronary artery calcium scanning with high-pitch spiral acquisition mode: comparison between 120-kV and 100-kV tube voltage protocols. *J Cardiovasc Comput Tomogr*. 2013;7:32–38.
19. Park MJ, Jung JI, Choi Y-S, et al. Coronary CT angiography in patients with high calcium score: evaluation of plaque characteristics and diagnostic accuracy. *Int J Cardiovasc Imaging*. 2011;27(Suppl 1):43–51.
20. Williams MC, Stewart C, Weir NW, Newby DE. Using radiation safely in cardiology: what imagers need to know. *Heart*. 2019;105:798–806.
21. Baliyan V, Scholtz J-E, Kordbacheh H, Hedgire S, Ghoshhajra BB. False-negative low tube voltage coronary CT angiography: high intravascular attenuation at coronary CT angiography can mask calcified plaques. *Radiol Cardiothorac Imaging*. 2019;1:e190039.
22. Kwan AC, Gransar H, Tzolos E, et al. The accuracy of coronary CT angiography in patients with coronary calcium score above 1000 Agatston units: comparison with quantitative coronary angiography. *J Cardiovasc Comput Tomogr*. 2021;15:412–418.
23. Yu S, Zhang H, Li H. Cardiac computed tomography versus transesophageal echocardiography for the detection of left atrial appendage thrombus: a systemic review and meta-analysis. *J Am Heart Assoc*. 2021;10:e022505.
24. Spencer RJ, DeJong P, Fahmy P, et al. Changes in left atrial appendage dimensions following volume loading during percutaneous left atrial appendage closure. *JACC Cardiovasc Interv*. 2015;8:1935–1941.
25. Korsholm K, Berti S, Iriart X, et al. Expert recommendations on cardiac computed tomography for planning transcatheter left atrial appendage occlusion. *JACC Cardiovasc Interv*. 2020;13:277–292.
26. Merzan D, Nowik P, Poludniowski G, Bujila R. Evaluating the impact of scan settings on automatic tube current modulation in CT using a novel phantom. *Br J Radiol*. 2017;90:20160308.
27. Nakamura R, Oda A, Tachibana S, et al. Prone-position computed tomography in the late phase for detecting intracardiac thrombi in the left atrial appendage before catheter ablation for atrial fibrillation. *J Cardiovasc Electrophysiol*. 2021;32:1803–1811.
28. Faure ME, Swart LE, Dijkshoorn ML, et al. Advanced CT acquisition protocol with a third-generation dual-source CT scanner and iterative reconstruction technique for comprehensive prosthetic heart valve assessment. *Eur Radiol*. 2018;28:2159–2168.
29. Blanke P, Weir-McCall JR, Achenbach S, et al. Computed tomography imaging in the context of transcatheter aortic valve implantation (TAVI)/transcatheter aortic valve replacement (TAVR): an expert consensus document of the Society of Cardiovascular Computed Tomography. *J Cardiovasc Comput Tomogr*. 2019;13:1–20.
30. Williamson EE, Kirsch J, Araoz PA, et al. ECG-gated cardiac CT angiography using 64-MDCT for detection of patent foramen ovale. *AJR Am J Roentgenol*. 2008;190:929–933.
31. Guo Y, Yang Z, Shao H, Deng W, Ning G, Dong Z. Right ventricular dysfunction and dilatation in patients with mitral regurgitation: analysis using ECG-gated multidetector row computed tomography. *Int J Cardiol*. 2013;167:1585–1590.
32. Ahn Y, Koo HJ, Kang J-W, Yang DH. Tricuspid valve imaging and right ventricular function analysis using cardiac CT and MRI. *Korean J Radiol*. 2021;22:1946–1963.
33. Te Riele ASJM, Tandri H, Sanborn DM, Bluemke DA. Noninvasive multimodality imaging in ARVD/C. *JACC Cardiovasc Imaging*. 2015;8:597–611.
34. Blankstein R, Shturman LD, Rogers IS, et al. Adenosine-induced stress myocardial perfusion imaging using dual-source cardiac computed tomography. *J Am Coll Cardiol*. 2009;54:1072–1084.
35. Narula J, Chandrashekhar Y, Ahmadi A, et al. SCCT 2021 expert consensus document on coronary computed tomographic angiography: a report of the Society of Cardiovascular Computed Tomography. *J Cardiovasc Comput Tomogr*. 2021;15:192–217.

36. Patel AR, Bamberg F, Branch K, et al. Society of cardiovascular computed tomography expert consensus document on myocardial computed tomography perfusion imaging. *J Cardiovasc Comput Tomogr*. 2020;14:87–100.
37. Henzlova MJ, Duvall WL, Einstein AJ, Travin MI, Verberne HJ. ASNC imaging guidelines for SPECT nuclear cardiology procedures: stress, protocols, and tracers. *J Nucl Cardiol*. 2016;23:606–639.
38. Cury RC, Kitt TM, Feaheny K, et al. A randomized, multicenter, multivendor study of myocardial perfusion imaging with regadenoson CT perfusion vs single photon emission CT. *J Cardiovasc Comput Tomogr*. 2015;9:103–112.e2.
39. Branch KR, Haley RD, Bittencourt MS, Patel AR, Hulten E, Blankstein R. Myocardial computed tomography perfusion. *Cardiovasc Diagn Ther*. 2017;7:452–462.
40. Ohta Y, Kitao S, Yunaga H, et al. Myocardial delayed enhancement CT for the evaluation of heart failure: comparison to MRI. *Radiology*. 2018;288: 682–691.
41. Sinitsyn V. Cardiac dual-energy CT with late iodine enhancement as an alternative to late gadolinium enhancement MRI. *Radiology*. 2018;288: 692–693.
42. Palmisano A, Vignale D, Benedetti G, Del Maschio A, De Cobelli F, Esposito A. Late iodine enhancement cardiac computed tomography for detection of myocardial scars: impact of experience in the clinical practice. *Radiol med*. 2020;125:128–136.

2 Advances in Hardware and Reconstruction Techniques for Cardiac CT

ROOSHA PARIKH AND OMAR K. KHALIQUE

KEY POINTS

1. Recent advances in cardiac CT include dual-source CT, which improves temporal resolution, and better detectors that enable better spatial resolution.
2. Photon-counting detector CT is a cutting-edge advance that significantly improves spatial resolution and limits calcium blooming artifacts.
3. Photon-counting detector CT allows for improved image quality in the presence of coronary stents, heavy coronary calcifications, and low-contrast volume exams.

RECENT ADVANCES IN CARDIAC CT HARDWARE

Numerous advances in CT hardware have helped revolutionize the field of cardiac CT. Increased gantry rotation speed and multidetector technology have allowed the growth and expansion of high spatial and temporal resolution cardiac CT. In addition, improved coverage along the z-axis has enabled whole heart scanning in a single heartbeat. For example, the time required for one rotation of an x-ray tube is reduced by decreasing the gantry rotation time and effectively halved by adding a second x-ray tube and detector system, which is the basis of dual-source CT. This allows faster data acquisition at a specific point of the R-R interval and a reduction in motion artifacts. In some scanner systems, the patient can be moved rapidly through the z-axis to cover the whole heart in a single acquisition.[1] Accordingly, when dual-source CT is used, the temporal resolution can be as low as 66 to 75 ms.

Technical advances in multidetector computed tomography have increased the number of detector rows on the z-axis, and now up to 16-cm wide-area-coverage CT scanners have enabled volumetric scanning of the entire heart in a single acquisition.[2] The advantages of these techniques are that the x-ray tube is only on for a small amount of time and alleviates misregistration artifacts and stair-step artifacts, as the entire image is acquired in one sequence.[1,2] However, due to the size of the gantry and the use of a single-source system, most such scanners have a temporal resolution that is typically greater than 100 ms.

There are several software-based algorithms that will correct motion and other artifacts during image reconstruction. While this has allowed for good-quality cardiac CT despite faster heart rates and arrhythmias such as atrial fibrillation, rigorous heart rate control is still imperative and important for keeping the effective radiation dose as low as possible.

With dual-energy computed tomography (DECT), the different energy spectrum x-ray beams can be used for differentiating materials with similar attenuation at a specific energy. In contrast to single-energy CT systems, the use of dual-energy systems may deliver images with enhanced diagnostic performance due to higher contrast-to-noise ratio (CNR) and decreased beam-hardening artifacts.[3] There are now various commercially available DECT technologies, including two x-ray sources and two detectors, a single source adept to fast switching between two energy levels, a specialized detector adept to acquiring high- and low-energy datasets, and a filter splitting the beam into high- and low-energy beams at the output. Sequential acquisition at different tube voltages is another approach.[3]

INTRODUCTION TO PHOTON-COUNTING DETECTOR CT

Photon-counting detector (PCD) CT is an emergent technology that has led to continued innovation and progress in diagnostic imaging. It was approved by the US Food and Drug Administration for clinical use in September 2021 after over a decade of preclinical testing and analysis.

Traditional CT scanners have conventional energy-integrating detectors (EID) that utilize the principle of x-ray scintillation, meaning that when an x-ray hits the detector, they first generate a light signal before converting that light into an electric signal. In contrast, PCDs do not require the intermediate step of generating light. Instead, they directly convert x-ray photons to an electric signal that is used to create an image.

A PCD is made from a semiconducting material such as cadmium telluride (CdTe), cadmium zinc telluride (CZT), or other materials such as silicon or gallium arsenide that allows for the direct conversion of the x-ray photon to an electrical signal to create an image. Most of the photon-counting CT systems capable of patient scanning described in the literature use CdTe-based detectors[4] (Fig. 2.1).

The many photons that pass through a patient's body and reach the detector can be counted individually, creating a more accurate signal to generate images. There is also an energy dependence of PCD when x-rays impact, as low-energy x-rays produce small amounts of charge and high-energy x-rays produce a higher charge. Another difference of PCD from conventional detectors is that with the elimination of the intermediate step of generating light we can measure each individual x-ray and therefore their individual energies. In addition, a low-energy threshold is set to remove electronic noise, as photons that have an energy below this level are not counted. Once above this threshold, all photons receive uniform weighting irrespective of their

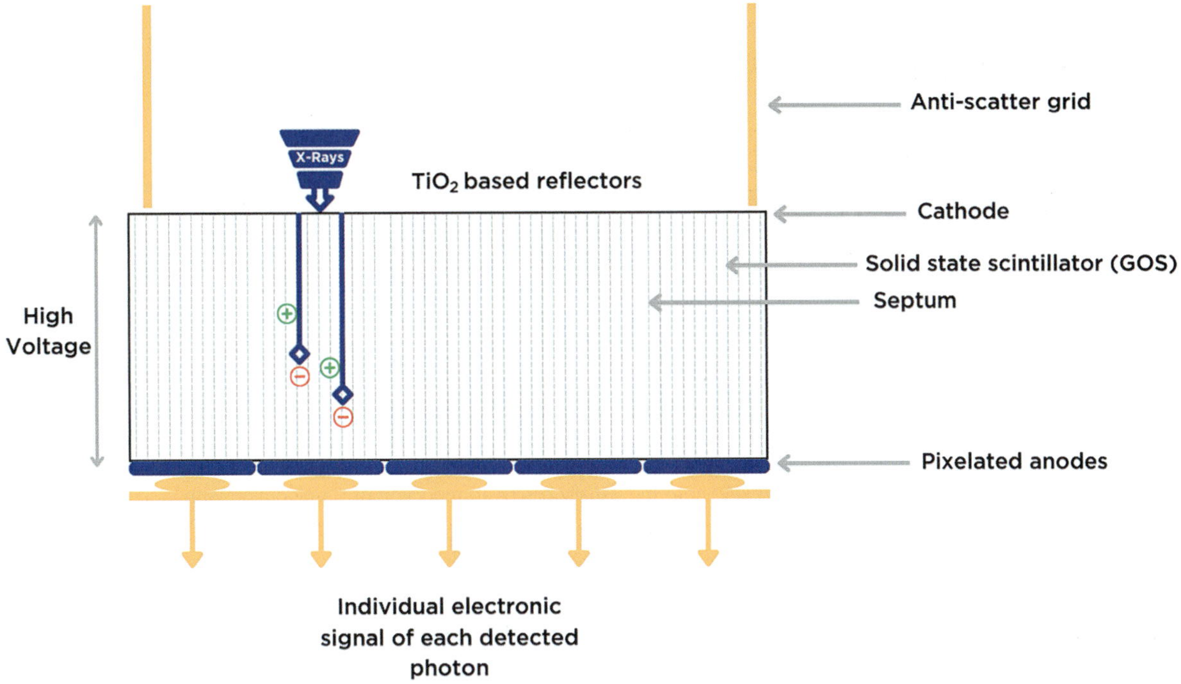

FIG. 2.1 Schematic Representation of a Photon-counting Detector.

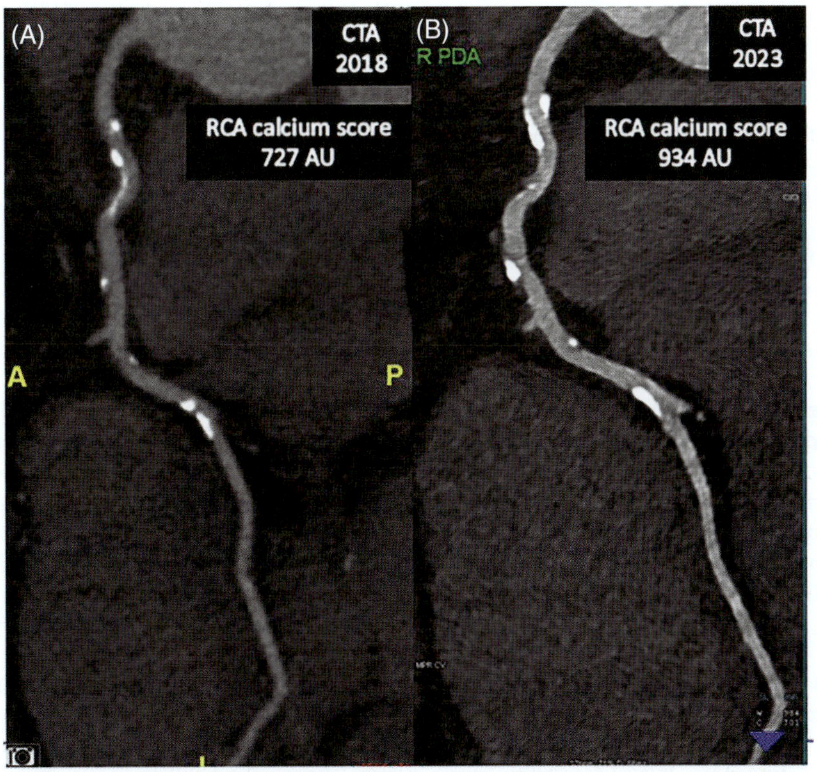

FIG. 2.2 Coronary CT angiography showing right coronary artery of a 69-year-old patient on a clinical wide area detector scanner and single rotation acquisition (0.5-mm slice thickness, 44 bpm) (A), followed by a subsequent scan 5 years later on a photon-counting detector CT scanned in ultra-high-resolution mode (0.2-mm slice thickness, BV44, QIR3, 37 bpm) (B).

energy, therefore improving the image contrast (Fig. 2.2). Photon signals in the low- and high-energy bins are then combined in a similar manner to using dual energy to create virtual monoenergetic (VM) images and other multienergy images that can highlight pathologic diagnostic features. This allows us to have spectral information without any dedicated scan modes or additional technology. Separation of more than two energy bins is possible with the availability of PCD-CT; specific uses are being developed using novel contrast agents in certain scenarios.[5]

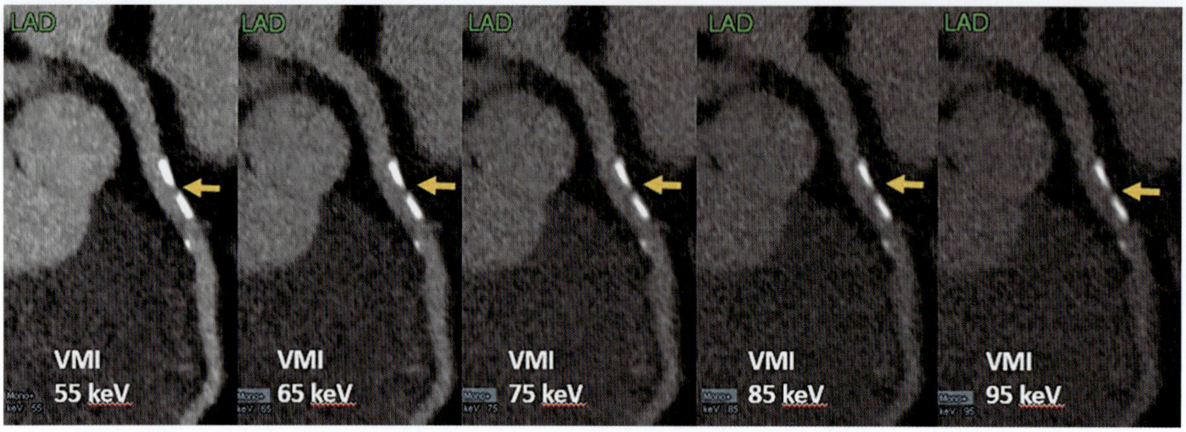

FIG. 2.3 Spectral coronary CT angiography of a 64-year-old patient on a clinical photon-counting detector CT (0.4-mm slice thickness, Qr40, QIR3, 58 bpm). Coronary artery calcium score in the left anterior descending artery (LAD) is 252 Agatston units. Calcified plaque in the LAD (*arrow*). Virtual monoenergetic imaging (VMIs) at 55, 65, 75, 85, and 95 keV: note the visually perceived reduction of Ca blooming with higher keV at the expense of reduced iodine contrast.

There have been prototypes described using silicon as a semiconductor material with a patented "edge-on" positioning. Taking into account the benefits of its purity, abundance, and length, silicon-based, edge-on detectors may allow absence of K-fluorescence and polarization and less sensitivity to pileup and charge sharing. This technology could be a potential contender for future photon-counting CT systems.[6]

Photon-counting CT offers four main technology benefits.

1. **Smaller detector pixels,** which can deliver ultra-high-resolution (UHR) imaging without significant radiation dose penalty and without the need for reflecting septa or comb filters
2. **Lower noise level** by elimination of electronic noise allowing advanced image quality in obese patients and low radiation-dose scans and reproducible and stable CT attenuation values for quantitative CT at low radiation doses
3. **Intrinsic spectral sensitivity** allowing acquisition of dual- or multienergy data at full speed without the need for dedicated scan technologies such as dual-source dual-energy, fast keV switching, or dual-layer detectors
4. **Improved iodine contrast** from equal energy contribution that results in contrast-rich images from increased iodine CNR, potentially reducing the radiation dose

SCAN MODES AND POTENTIAL APPLICATIONS

Virtual monoenergetic imaging (VMI). With VMI, image reconstruction can be fine-tuned to clinical requirements—low-keV VMIs increase image contrast, while high-keV reconstructions reduce blooming of calcified plaques. This allows more accurate assessment compared with window leveling that needs to be performed on conventional CT scanners where noncalcified plaque and calcified plaque simultaneously change characteristics and attenuation (Fig. 2.3). The combined evaluation of high-keV and low-keV VMIs may have a diagnostic impact, with theoretically more accurate assessment of stenosis in the presence of both calcified and noncalcified plaque. The increased iodine CNR in VMIs at low keV may allow a reduction in the amount of contrast agent administered.[7]

Spectral imaging and spectral removal of calcium. A new application based on spectral two-material decomposition makes it possible to selectively detect and differentiate calcium and iodine. With this processing, one can aim to remove calcified plaques from the contrast-filled vessels without reducing the iodine contrast in a virtual noncalcium (VNCa) image. This is important as calcified plaques can appear larger than they actually are due to partial volume effects (blooming), thus leading to overestimation of stenosis (see Chapter 7, Diagnostic Accuracy of CCTA). The VNCa images may enable accurate detection of stenosis by accurately revealing lumen underneath (Fig. 2.4).

Spectral imaging and spectral removal of lumen. In a similar manner, the removal of iodine from contrast-enhanced images while the calcium remains unmodified can allow for virtual noncontrast (VNC) images. This feature may allow quantitative calcium scoring evaluation of both coronary arteries as well as valves to get an approximate estimate of a score (Fig. 2.5). The ability to generate virtual noncontrast CT images from contrast-enhanced CT studies may eliminate the need for a true noncontrast CT examination (e.g., follow-up vascular studies, coronary artery studies with stent and bypass grafts, valve cases), thus reducing total radiation dose.[8]

UHR imaging. With current PCD-CT, a UHR mode can be achieved when using 0.2-mm slice thickness. This results in a minimum detector element size of 0.176×0.151 mm^2 at the isocenter, which allows a maximum spatial in-plane image resolution of 0.11 mm and a maximum through-plane resolution of 0.16 mm. Standard resolution mode uses 0.4-mm slice thickness, resulting from 2×2-UHR subpixels binned together providing a pixel size of 0.352×0.302 mm^2.[9]

Excellent coronary plaque characterization and delineation of the adjacent vessel lumen with no perceived blooming can be achieved with 0.2-mm and 0.1-mm slice thickness and image reconstruction with a sharp kernel (Fig. 2.6). UHR can improve the ability of coronary CT angiography

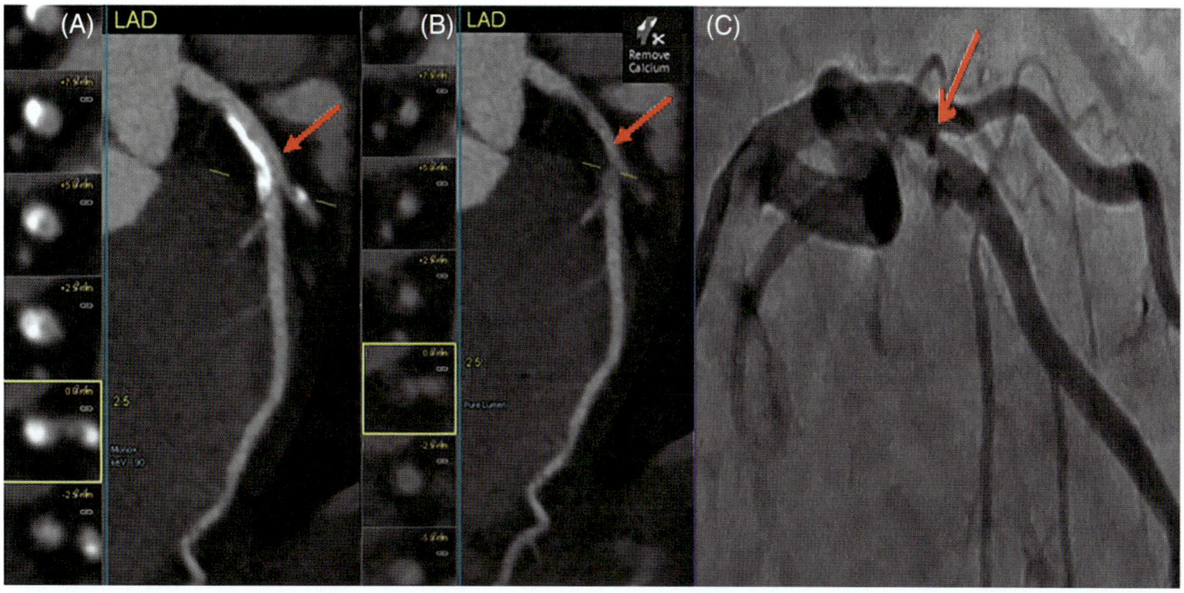

FIG. 2.4 Spectral coronary CT angiography of a 66-year-old patient on a clinical photon-counting detector CT (0.6-mm slice thickness, Qr44, QIR4). Coronary artery calcium score in the left anterior descending artery (LAD) is 426 AU. Calcified plaque in the LAD (*arrow*). (A) Virtual monoenergetic imaging (VMIs) at 90 keV showing moderate to severe stenosis in the proximal LAD. (B) Virtual noncalcium (VNCa) at 90 keV: the calcified plaque is removed from the contrast-filled vessel without reducing the iodine contrast reclassifying to a 50% stenosis. (C) Invasive coronary angiogram confirmed the moderate stenosis (~50%) in the proximal LAD.

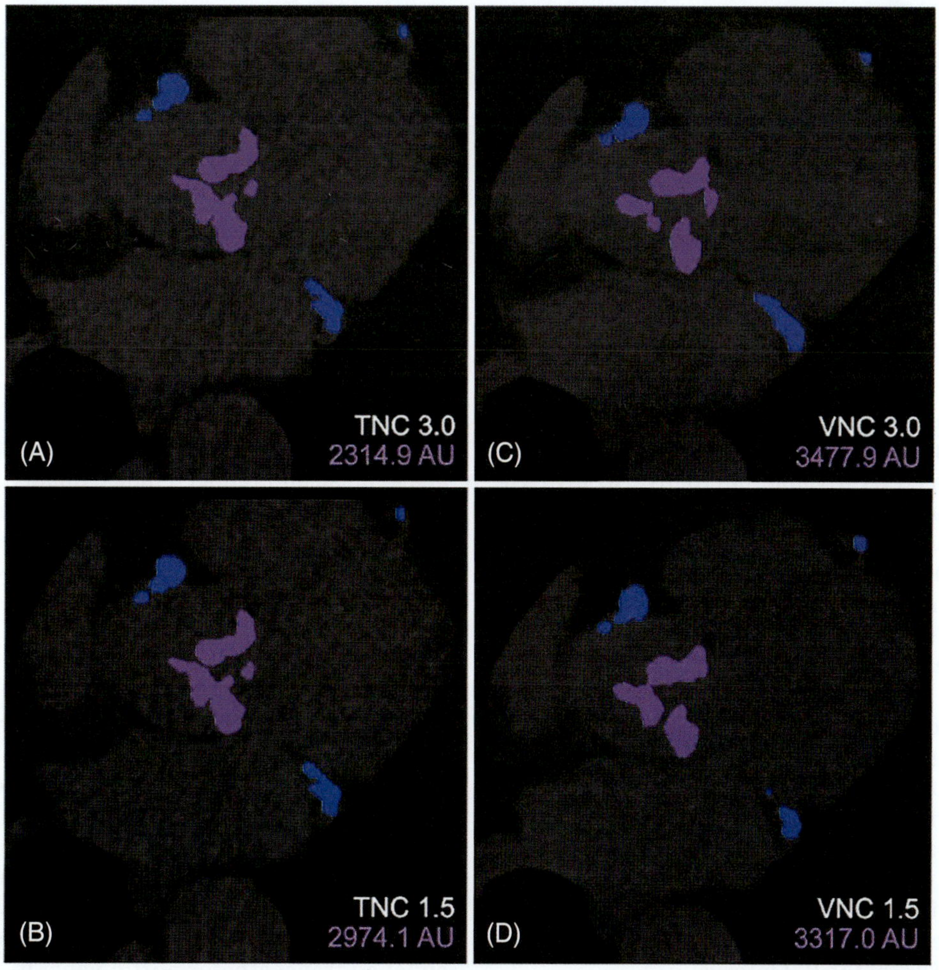

FIG. 2.5 Aortic valve calcium scoring on a clinical photon-counting detector CT. Contours of aortic valve calcium (*purple*) of the same cross section were visualized on (A) true noncalcium (TNC) with 3-mm slice thickness; (B) TNC with 1.5-mm slice thickness; (C) virtual noncontrast (VNC) with 3-mm slice thickness; (D) VNC with 1.5-mm slice thickness. Agatston equivalent values for each study were determined. Differences in calcium scoring were seen both graphically and numerically but allow an approximate estimate of the original value.

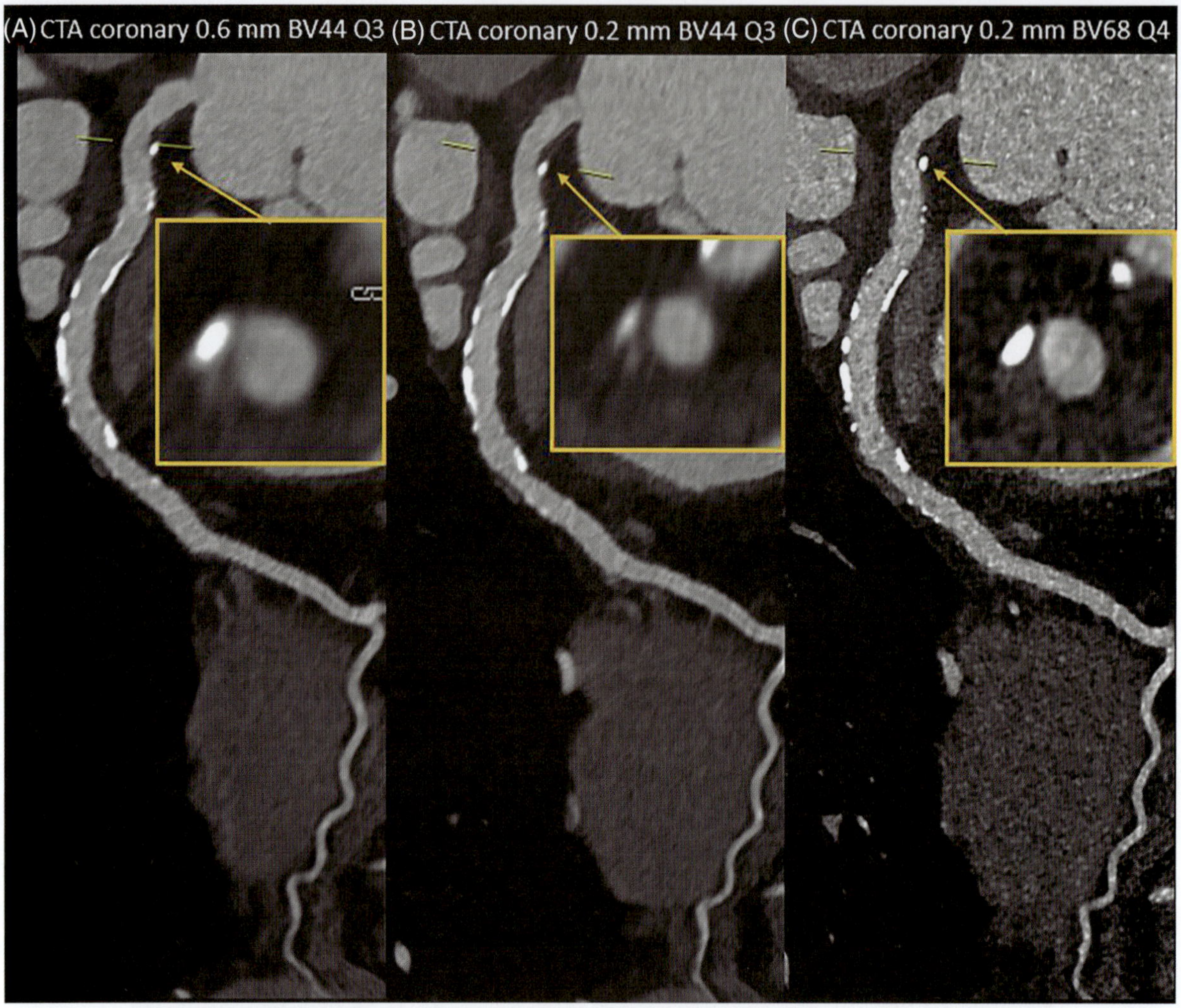

FIG. 2.6 Ultra-high-resolution (UHR) coronary CT angiography (CCTA) of a 75-year-old male patient on a clinical photon-counting detector CT (retrospective ECG gating; 0.2-mm slice thickness, 51 bpm). Coronary artery calcium score of 908 AU, with 515 AU in the left circumflex artery. Proximal left circumflex has noncalcified and calcified plaque with high-risk features causing mild stenosis as shown on cCTA. (A) Standard reference reconstruction (0.6-mm slice, BV44, QIR3). (B) UHR reconstruction (0.2-mm slice, BV44, QIR3). (C) UHR reconstruction (0.2-mm slice, BV68, QIR4). Note the reduced calcium blooming in the sharper kernel reconstruction shown in Panel C.

(CCTA) to detect and characterize plaque as well as more accurately detect stenosis.

CCTA has emerged as a viable alternative to invasive coronary angiography and has demonstrated high diagnostic performance for the detection and exclusion of high-grade anatomic stenoses in native coronary arteries as well as in coronary stents (Fig. 2.7). Calcium blooming and beam hardening from stents is related to the partial volume effect. The presence of heavy calcifications in the native coronary in a stented segment further enhances the metal artifacts and contributes to beam hardening. The use of UHR imaging can help mitigate these challenges, and this acquisition mode can now also utilize spectral imaging and reconstruction options (Figs. 2.8 and 2.9).

UHR scanning can use either a helical or axial image acquisiion mode. In order to minimize misregistration artifacts, a helical acquisition with tube current modulation is most commonly performed, for example using ECG-pulsing window at 30% to 80% of the R-R interval.

The use of sharper kernels leverages the more favorable image quality and can further improve image resolution and reduce artifacts and signal inhomogeneity in the presence of calcium and metal. Very sharp kernels traditionally have been associated with substantially increased image noise and reduced image quality; however, with the improvement in the PCDs over traditional EIDs, the lumen in calcified and stented segments generally exhibits less image noise than would be observed with standard (i.e., non-UHR) techniques.[10–14]

STRUCTURAL HEART PLANNING

PCD CT allows for a detailed depiction of the aortic valve, aortic root, coronary arteries, and potential vascular access routes prior to transcatheter aortic valve replacement procedures. The high-spatial-resolution reconstructions facilitate assessment of hypoattenuating leaflet thickening and leaks for prosthetic valves (Fig. 2.10). The improved spatial resolution and decreased blooming can enhance transcatheter aortic valve in transcatheter aortic valve planning to assess node counting, sealing skirt, risk of coronary obstruction, and sinus sequestration[15] (Fig. 2.11).

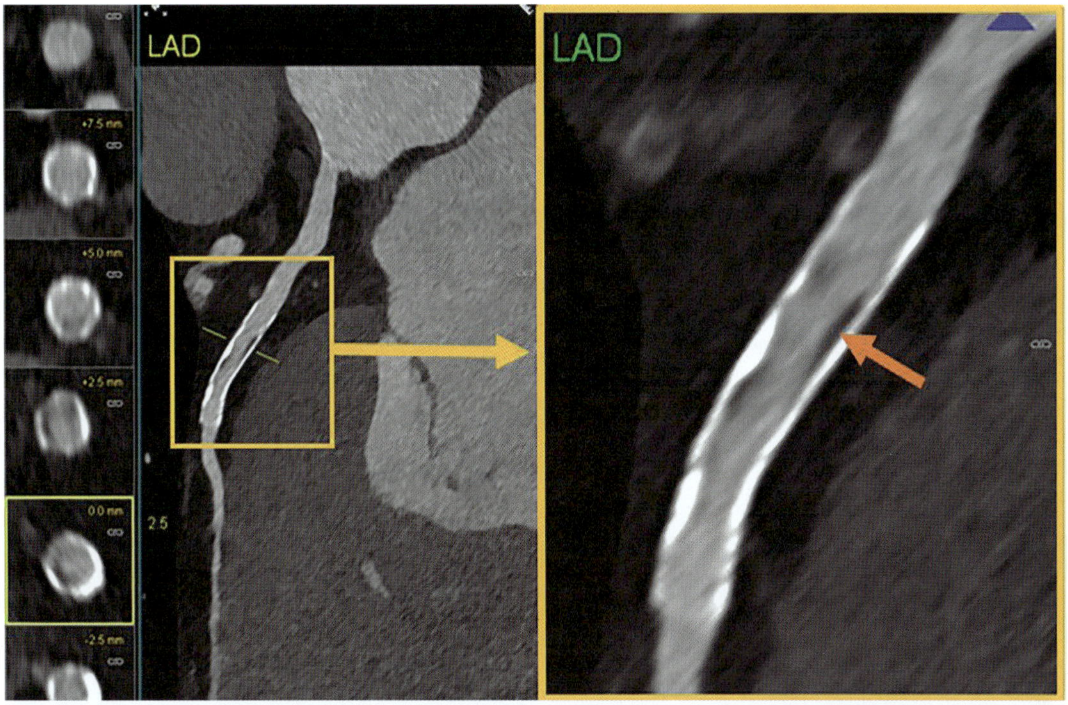

FIG. 2.7 A 3.5 × 24 mm stent in the mid left anterior descending (LAD) artery imaged in ultra-high- resolution (UHR) mode photon-counting detector CT (retrospective ECG gating) with 0.2-mm slice thickness. Stent is patent as seen in the UHR reconstruction (0.2-mm slice, BV44, QIR3). The *orange arrow* shows mild neo-intimal hyperplasia and mild in-stent restenosis.

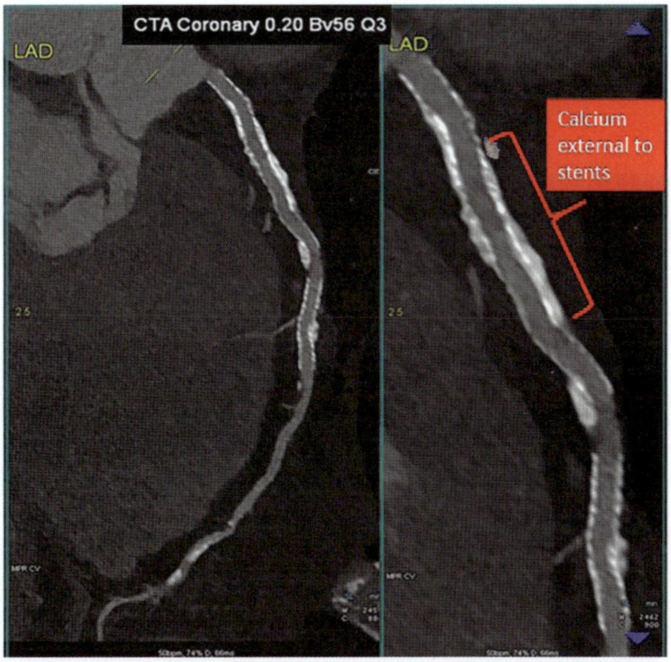

FIG. 2.8 Ultra-high-resolution (UHR) coronary CT angiography of an 83-year-old male patient on a clinical photon-counting detector CT (retrospective ECG gating; 0.2-mm slice thickness, 50 bpm) with three stents in the left anterior descending artery. UHR reconstruction (0.2-mm slice thickness, BV56, QIR3). Note the calcium external to the stents.

RADIATION DOSE

Although the radiation dose of CCTA with PCD-CT at standard resolution is often comparable to dose-optimized examinations with conventional CT, higher radiation dose has been reported for UHR examinations. Higher spatial resolution in UHR examinations is associated with higher radiation dose because it employs smaller detectors, and because helical acquisition is most commonly used. While axial acquisitioin mode can help decrease the radiation dose, the scan time is longer when using this approach, and thus there is potential for more misregistration artifacts. However, the diagnostic advantage from the UHR examination should be considered as well, and the radiation dose can be further optimized by

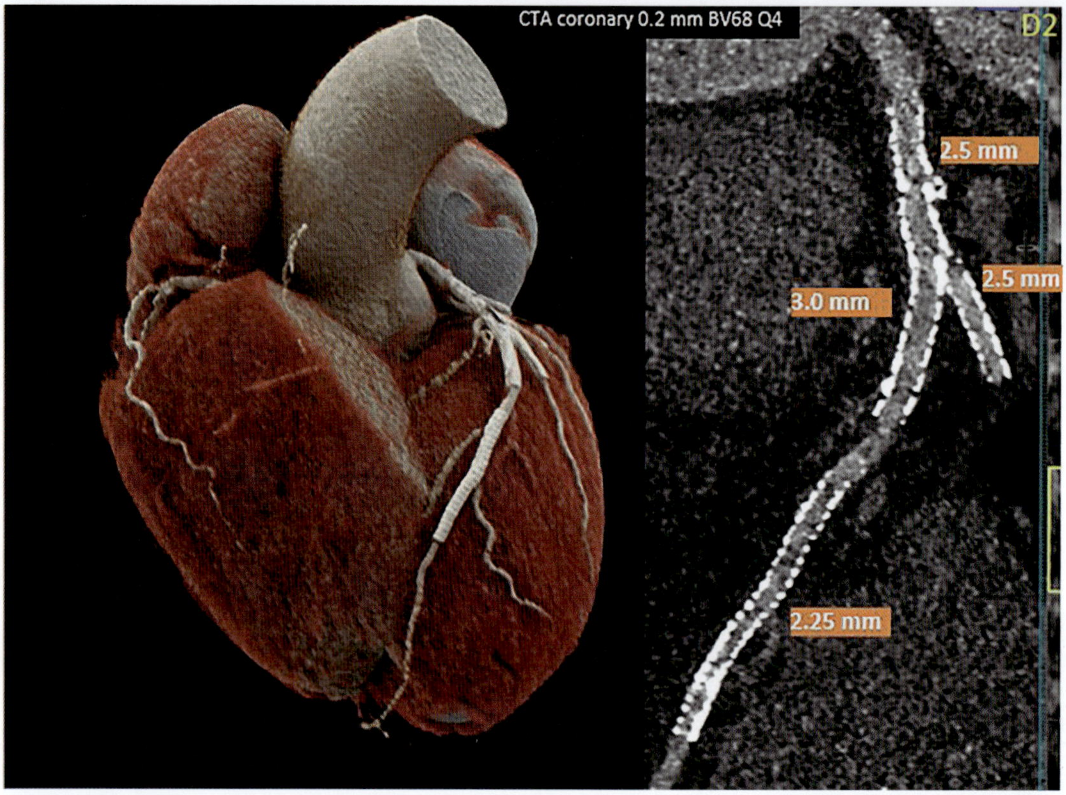

FIG. 2.9 Ultra-high-resolution (UHR) coronary CT angiography of a 57-year-old patient on a photon-counting detector CT (retrospective ECG gating; 0.2-mm slice thickness, 56 bpm) with two stents in the left anterior descending artery and two bifurcation stents of the first and second diagonal arteries. UHR reconstruction (0.2-mm slice thickness, 1024 × 1024 matrix sharp kernel BV68, QIR4). The bifurcation technique of the stents can be well appreciated on these images. The stent sizes are: proximal to mid left anterior descending artery (LAD) 3.0 × 38 mm, distal LAD 2.25 × 28 mm, first diagonal 2.5 × 23 mm, and second diagonal 2.5 × 23 mm.

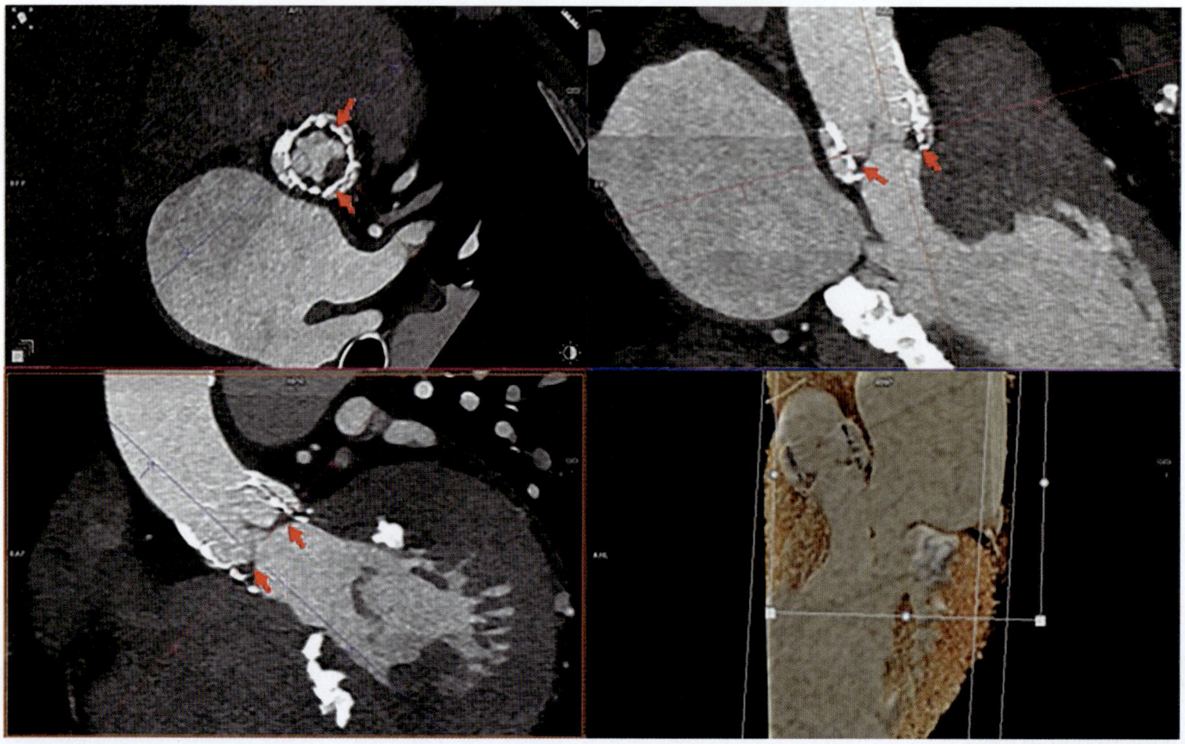

FIG. 2.10 Ultra-high resolution (UHR) postprocedure prosthetic valve imaging of an 82-year-old female patient who is status post transcatheter aortic valve replacement (TAVR) with peak transaortic gradients increasing from 30 mm Hg to 47 mm Hg on transthoracic echocardiogram on a photon-counting detector CT (retrospective ECG gating with dose modulation; 0.2-mm slice thickness, 52 bpm) with balloon expandable TAVR valve in aortic position. UHR reconstruction (0.2-mm slice thickness, BV56, QIR3). Note the hypoattenuated leaflet thickening (HALT) shown by the *red arrows*, involving all three leaflets and maximally the left leaflet. The bottom right image is a cinematic 3D volume–rendered image.

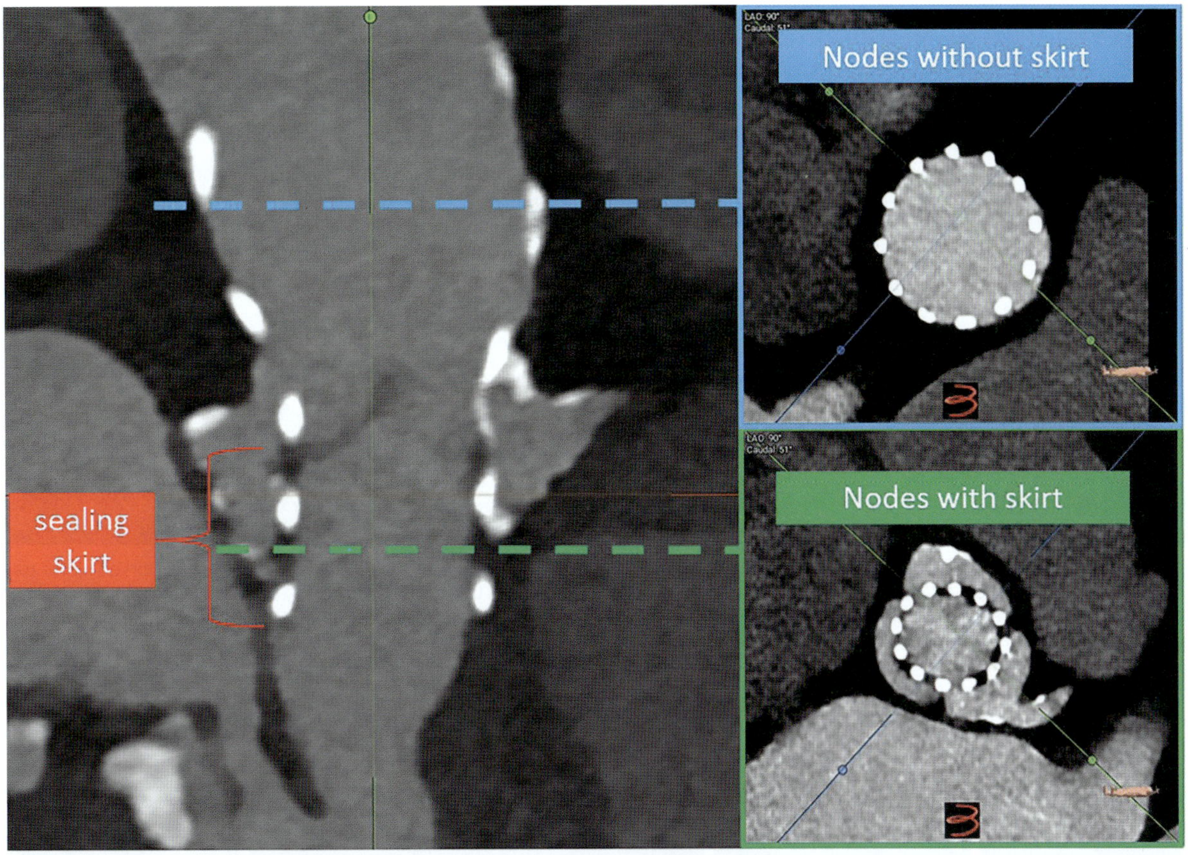

FIG. 2.11 Photon-counting detector CT imaging of a patient who is status post self-expanding transcatheter aortic valve replacement (TAVR) being evaluated for TAV in TAV with the valve's nodes clearly visualized to help with node counting and visualization of the sealing skirt at different node levels.

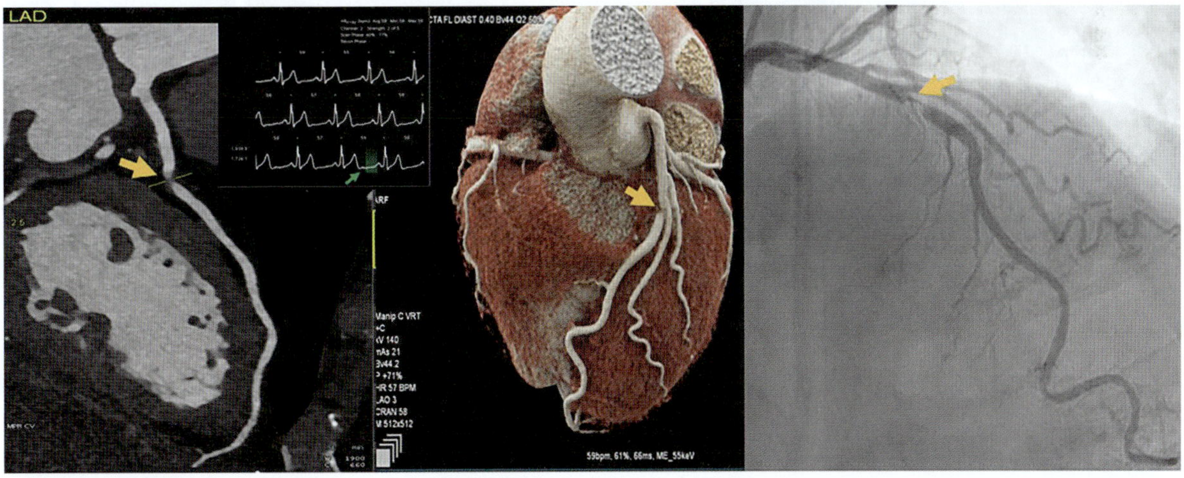

FIG. 2.12 Ultra-fast, low-dose, high-pitch coronary CT angiography (CCTA) of an 83-year-old patient on a clinical photon-counting detector CT; 0.4-mm slice thickness, BV44, QIR2, 57 bpm). Coronary artery calcium score of 35 AU with calcium all in the left anterior descending artery (LAD). Noncalcified plaque in the LAD with severe stenosis (*yellow arrow*) on cCTA that is confirmed on invasive coronary angiogram. This technique enables acquisition of the entire heart within a single cardiac cycle using a time window of approximately 250 ms (*green arrow*) with very low doses of radiation dose of <1.0 mSv.

dose modulation and optimal heart rate control. With current technology of PCD-CT combined with ultra-fast, high-pitch, low-radiation dose, studies are possible by acquisition of the entire heart in a single cardiac cycle[10,12,16] (Fig. 2.12). This approach can result in very low radiaion doses (<1 mSv)

CONTRAST MEDIA

As previously described, the imaging benefits brought by spectral imaging and reduced electronic noise also allows improved iodine signal with a potential reduction of the

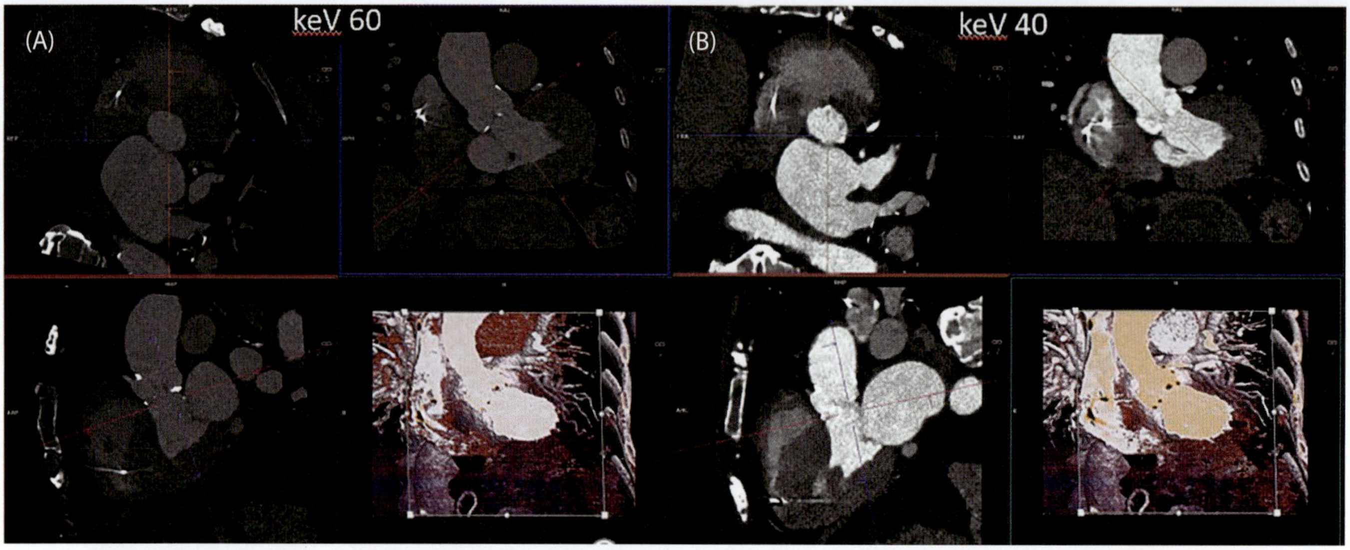

FIG. 2.13 Spectral coronary CT angiography of an 86-year-old patient with severe aortic stenosis and acute kidney injury being worked up for transcatheter aortic valve replacement (TAVR) on a clinical photon-counting detector CT (0.4-mm slice thickness, Qr40, QIR3) with low dose of iodinated contrast and total contrast dose of 45 mL (patient's weight 176 lb, BMI 29 kg/m^2, BSA 1.9). (A) Original image: virtual monoenergetic imaging (VMIs) at 60 keV. (B) Post processing VMIs at 40 keV: the lower energy may allow for a reduction in contrast media and provides diagnostic attenuation and objective image quality for accurate TAVR planning measurements.

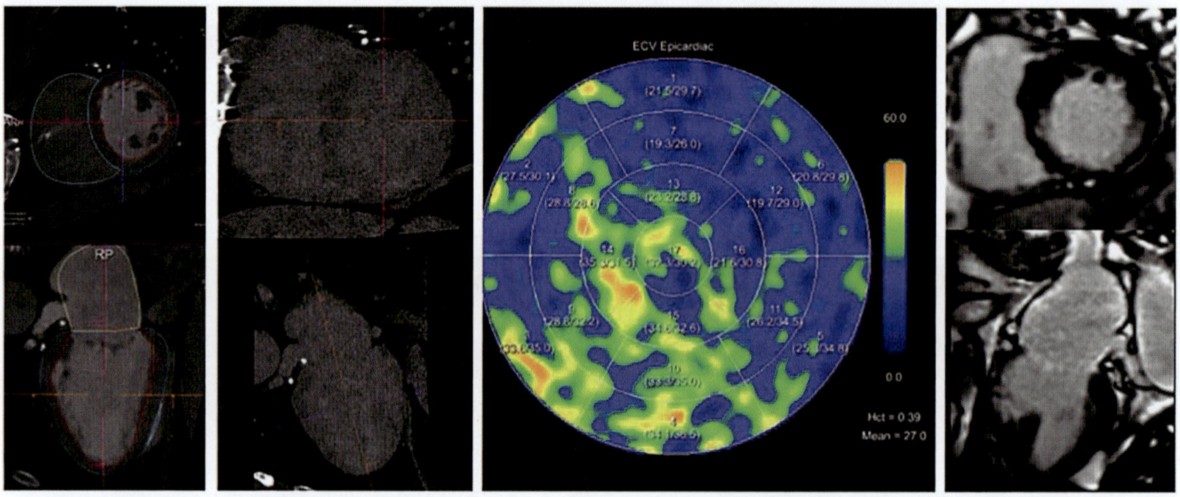

FIG. 2.14 Spectral coronary CT angiography with a late enhancement CT scan and quantification of extracellular volume (ECV) of myocardium in a 70-year-old patient from the delayed contrast scan performed at 5 minutes to demonstrate tissue characterization and elevated ECV CT values observed in the basal to mid inferior, inferoseptal, inferolateral myocardium. Findings were confirmed by cardiac MRI with scar pattern in the same areas of elevated ECV.

use of contrast media, which remains an important consideration for patients suffering from chronic kidney disease.[9] A reduction in contrast media concentration of 50% could obtain diagnostic attenuation and objective image quality for CCTA imaging. This can be used in cases of low-contrast dose for transcatheter aortic valve replacement or other structural planning cases (Fig. 2.13).

Future Direction. Tissue characterization and myocardial fibrosis can be assessed with spectral data. Currently, cardiac magnetic resonance imaging (MRI) using late gadolinium enhancement has been the standard for tissue characterization and quantification of extracellular volume (ECV) of myocardium. Recently, cardiac CT has also been shown as a good alternate method for tissue characterization and ECV assessment. The spectral capabilities of PCD-CT may allow for novel data processing techniques directly from the iodine contrast images and the delayed contrast scan and with a shorter acquisition time[17] (Fig. 2.14). The spectral capability allows this assessment to be performed without a noncontrast image.[18]

For cardiac and coronary CT angiography (CTA), the biggest current advantage of PCD-CT over conventional CT

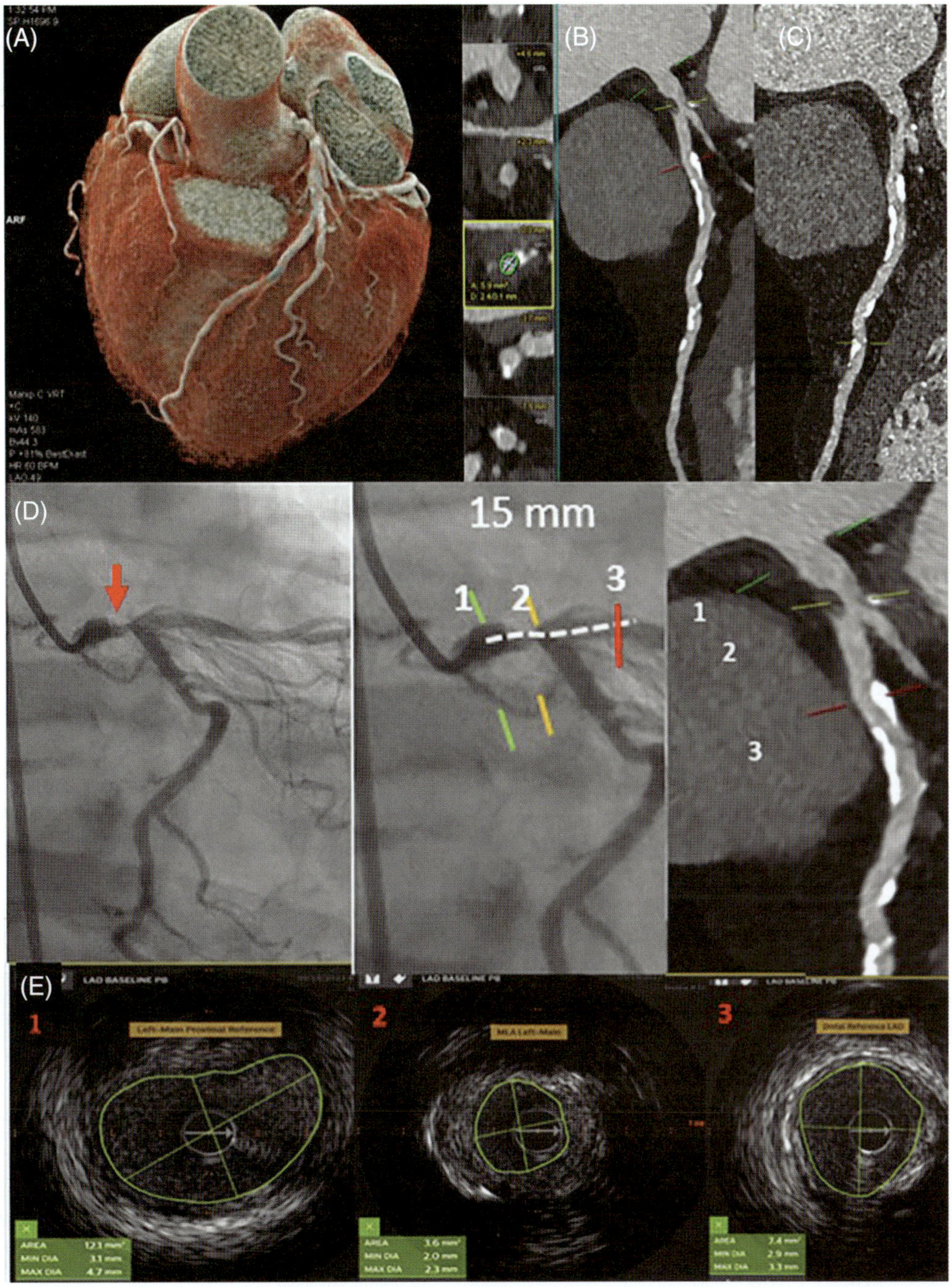

FIG. 2.15 Ultra-high-resolution (UHR) coronary CT angiography (CCTA) of a 70-year-old male patient on a clinical photon-counting detector CT (retrospective ECG gating; 0.2-mm slice thickness, 60 bpm). Coronary artery calcium score of 1135 AU, with 10 AU in the left main and 515 AU in the left anterior descending artery. Distal left main had predominantly noncalcified plaque with severe stenosis as shown on CCTA (*red arrow*). (A) Cinematic volume rendering technique (VRT) of the heart with coronary calcification highlighted. (B) UHR multiplanar reformation (MPR) reconstruction of left main and left anterior descending artery (LAD) (0.2-mm slice, BV44, QIR3). (C) UHR MPR reconstruction of left main and LAD in sharp kernels (0.2-mm slice, BV68, QIR4). Note the reduced calcium blooming in the sharper kernel reconstruction of C. (D) Invasive coronary angiogram confirming the severe left main stenosis (*red arrow*). (E) Intravascular ultrasound (IVUS) at level 1 proximal to the reference stenosis, level 2 set as reference at maximal left main stenosis that confirmed a minimal luminal area of 3.6 mm^2 by IVUS, and level 3 distal to the reference stenosis in the proximal LAD.

appears to be the acquisition of UHR data, with the potential to expand the scope of coronary CTA. Preliminary data suggest UHR CCTA may replace many cases of diagnostic ICA, including in patients with severe calcifications and with prior stent implantation. Thus PCD-CT has the potential to offer CT for patients who previously did not qualify for such testing, thereby providing an option that is safer than invasive testing (Fig. 2.15) Ultra-high-definition CT may improve plaque characterization (see Chapter 11, Approaches to Plaque Imaging by CCTA) as well as visualization of the coronary arteries in patients with coronary stents (see Chapter 10, Evaluation of Coronary Stents and Bypass Grafts).

Acquisition parameters	
KV	Tube voltage for spectral imaging uses either 120 kV or 140 kV. Increased kV allows wider spectral differentiation
MA	Determined by machine and will vary by individual scanner algorithm
Dose modulation	Decreasing the tube current during specific phases of the cardiac cycle during helical acquisition to decrease radiation exposure to the patient
Slice thickness	This describes the size of the collimator detector component and how thick or thin each slice of series can be. May be as low as 0.2 mm in ultra-high resolution scanning or 0.4–0.6 mm or greater in regular scanning mode
Slice interval	Determines overlap in slices. Overlapped slice interval may provide increased signal but should be balanced against increased amount of data and images
Field of view (FOV)	200 × 200 mm^2 or 150 × 150 mm^2
Image quality (IQ) level	An algorithm can be used to select the tube current-time product by balancing the required image quality and image noise
Reconstruction parameters	
Slice thickness	This can be reconstructed to any thickness at or above the minimum collimation
Kernels	Convolution filters refers to the process used to modify the frequency contents of projection data prior to back projection during image reconstruction in a CT scanner that are usually standard, smooth, and sharp. With higher kernel sharpness, SNR and CNR continuously decrease, whereas image noise and vessel sharpness increase.[19] Smooth kernels are used for soft tissue and sharp kernels for calcium or stents.
Quantum reconstruction (QIR)	Reconstruction kernel at different strength levels of QIR (QIR-1 to QIR-4) or QIR off. These help improve image quality and reduce noise. Combination of high iteration with sharp kernel can balance the benefits of sharp kernel with acceptable image noise.
Matrix size	Matrix size of 512 × 512 pixels, 1024 × 1024 pixels

REFERENCES

1. Heseltine TD, Murray SW, Ruzsics B, Fisher M. Latest advances in cardiac CT. *Eur Cardiol*. 2020;15:1–7. https://doi.org/10.15420/ecr.2019.14.2.
2. Kang EJ. Clinical applications of wide-detector CT scanners for cardiothoracic imaging: an update. *Korean J Radiol*. 2019;20(12):1583–1596. https://doi.org/10.3348/kjr.2019.0327.
3. Borges AP, Antunes C, Curvo-Semedo L. Pros and cons of dual-energy CT systems: "one does not fit all. *Tomography*. 2023;9(1):195–216. https://doi.org/10.3390/tomography9010017.
4. Leng S, Bruesewitz M, Tao S, et al. Photon-counting detector CT: system design and clinical applications of an emerging technology. *Radiographics*. 2019;39(3):729–743. https://doi.org/10.1148/rg.2019180115.
5. Jacobsen MC, Thrower SL, Ger RB, et al. Multi-energy computed tomography and material quantification: current barriers and opportunities for advancement. *Med Phys*. 2020;47(8):3752–3771. https://doi.org/10.1002/mp.14241.
6. da Silva J, Grönberg F, Cederström B, et al. Resolution characterization of a silicon-based, photon-counting computed tomography prototype capable of patient scanning. *J Med Imaging (Bellingham)*. 2019;6(4):043502. https://doi.org/10.1117/1.JMI.6.4.043502.
7. Flohr T, Schmidt B, Ulzheimer S, Alkadhi H. Cardiac imaging with photon counting CT. *Br J Radiol*. 2023;96(1152):20230407. https://doi.org/10.1259/bjr.20230407.
8. Mergen V, Ghouse S, Sartoretti T, et al. Cardiac virtual noncontrast images for calcium quantification with photon-counting detector CT. *Radiol Cardiothorac Imaging*. 2023;5(3):e220307. https://doi.org/10.1148/ryct.220307.
9. Sartoretti T, Wildberger JE, Flohr T, Alkadhi H. Photon-counting detector CT: early clinical experience review. *Br J Radiol*. 2023;96(1147):20220544.
10. Fix Martinez M, Klein L, Maier J, et al. Potential radiation dose reduction in clinical photon-counting CT by the small pixel effect: ultra-high resolution (UHR) acquisitions reconstructed to standard resolution. *Eur Radiol*. 2023;34(7):4484–4491.
11. Stein T, Taron J, Verloh N, et al. Photon-counting computed tomography of coronary and peripheral artery stents: a phantom study. *Sci Rep*. 2023;13(1):14806. https://doi.org/10.1038/s41598-023-41854-3.
12. Michael AE, Schoenbeck D, Becker-Assmann J, et al. Coronary stent imaging in photon counting computed tomography: optimization of reconstruction kernels in a phantom. *Eur J Radiol*. 2023;166:110983. https://doi.org/10.1016/j.ejrad.2023.110983.
13. Hagar MT, Soschynski M, Saffar R, et al. Accuracy of ultrahigh-resolution photon-counting CT for detecting coronary artery disease in a high-risk population. *Radiology*. 2023;307(5):e223305. https://doi.org/10.1148/radiol.223305.
14. Mergen V, Sartoretti T, Baer-Beck M, et al. Ultra-high-resolution coronary CT angiography with photon-counting detector CT: feasibility and image characterization. *Invest Radiol*. 2022;57(12):780–788. https://doi.org/10.1097/RLI.0000000000000897.
15. van der Bie J, Sharma SP, van Straten M, et al. Photon-counting detector CT in patients pre- and post-transcatheter aortic valve replacement. *Radiol Cardiothorac Imaging*. 2023;5(2):e220318. https://doi.org/10.1148/ryct.220318 Erratum in: Radiol Cardiothorac Imaging. 2023;5(6):e239002.
16. Rotkopf LT, Froelich MF, Riffel P, et al. Influence of heart rate and heart rate variability on the feasibility of ultra-fast, high-pitch coronary photon-counting computed tomography angiography. *Int J Cardiovasc Imaging*. 2023;39(5):1065–1073. https://doi.org/10.1007/s10554-023-02808-y.
17. Mergen V, Sartoretti T, Klotz E, et al. Extracellular volume quantification with cardiac late enhancement scanning using dual-source photon-counting detector CT. *Invest Radiol*. 2022;57(6):406–411. https://doi.org/10.1097/RLI.0000000000000851.
18. Cundari G, Galea N, Mergen V, Alkadhi H, Eberhard M. Myocardial extracellular volume quantification with computed tomography-current status and future outlook. *Insights Imaging*. 2023;14(1):156. https://doi.org/10.1186/s13244-023-01506-6.
19. Reference Yang Y, Fink N, Emrich T, et al. Optimization of kernel type and sharpness level improves objective and subjective image quality for high-pitch photon counting coronary CT angiography. *Diagnostics (Basel)*. 2023;13(11):1937. https://doi.org/10.3390/diagnostics13111937.

3 Coronary Artery Calcium Scanning: Indications and Patient Management

JELANI K. GRANT, ROGER S. BLUMENTHAL, KHURRAM NASIR, AND MICHAEL J. BLAHA

INTRODUCTION

Atherosclerotic cardiovascular disease (ASCVD) is the leading cause of mortality in the United States.[1] Despite the availability of the Pooled Cohort Equations (PCE) and other risk prediction tools such as the newer Predicting Risk of cardiovascular disease EVENTs (PREVENT) equation, one-third of US adults with a history of clinical ASCVD are unaware of their elevated risk prior to their first ASCVD event.[2] Thus there remains a need to identify patients at the highest risk for future ASCVD events in order to institute appropriate prevention and risk-mitigating therapies. Imaging tools to detect subclinical atherosclerosis remain the most powerful tools to improve risk prediction in apparently healthy adults, and cardiac computed tomography is the modality best suited for risk prediction at the general population level.

In everyday clinical practice, despite their drawbacks, the first step in risk assessment involves the use of traditional risk prediction tools, such as the PCE or the PREVENT equations, to estimate the 10-year risk of an ASCVD or total cardiovascular event and assess candidacy for lipid-lowering therapy. Based on the 2018 American Heart Association (AHA)/American College of Cardiology (ACC)/Multisociety Blood Cholesterol Guideline,[3] for borderline- and intermediate-risk primary prevention patients (i.e., 5–20% 10-year risk using the PCE or PREVENT calculators), a clinician-patient discussion about the benefits, risks, costs, and goals of preventive therapy is supported. At this stage, other risk-enhancing factors can be considered such as a family history of ASCVD or an elevated lipoprotein(a) level. When the initiation of statin therapy remains uncertain from the perspective of either the patient or the treating clinician, coronary artery calcium (CAC) scoring is a recommended next step.[4]

CAC is uniquely well positioned for everyday use in the outpatient setting for risk prediction in otherwise healthy adults. CAC quantification can be performed on any modern multidetector CT scanner with cardiac gating software. CAC scans are fast (~10 minutes of room time), low radiation (~1 mSv), inexpensive (~$50–$200), and do not require the injection of iodinated contrast. Scans can be interpreted in about 2 minutes, with few common interpretation errors, and results are in the form of a single number that is well understood by most patients. CAC scans are performed using a single common protocol all around the world.

Based on the growing body of evidence, recent major guidelines including the NLA (National Lipid Association) Scientific Statement,[5] 2019 ACC/AHA Primary Prevention Risk Assessment Special Report,[6] the 2016 SCCT/STR (Society of Cardiac Computed Tomography/Society of Thoracic Radiology) guideline,[7] and the 2021 AHA/ACC/Multisociety guideline for the evaluation and diagnosis of chest pain[8] endorse the use of CAC scoring to aid in shared decision-making across a range of clinical scenarios. Among other potential indications, CAC scoring is also useful for evaluating low-risk patients with stable chest pain, the risk versus benefit of aspirin use for primary prevention, baseline ASCVD risk prior to coronary CT angiography (CCTA) or as part of the nuclear stress imaging protocol, and aortic valve calcification (AVC) in uncertain aortic stenosis.

In this chapter, we discuss the biology of coronary artery calcification, fundamentals of CAC measurement, comparison with coronary CT angiography, and foundational studies solidifying the role of CAC in advanced risk prediction. Then we turn to clinical CAC interpretation and its role in risk management, including the evolving role of repeat CAC scans to document CAC progression. Next, we talk about other issues surrounding CAC, including interpretation from nongated chest CTs, interpretation of concomitant extra-coronary calcification, and use in multimodality imaging protocols. Finally, we close with a discussion of future directions including ongoing CAC clinical trials, the role of artificial intelligence (AI) in CAC interpretation, and future directions in radiomics or so-called "calciumomics."

THE BIOLOGY OF CAC

The three most common types of vascular calcification include infantile calcification, medial Mönckeberg arterial calcification, and intimal calcification, the latter of which is most directly indicative of atherosclerosis.[9] Decades ago, vascular calcification was thought to be consistent with aging, and the development of coronary artery calcification a passive, degenerative process. However, coronary artery calcification is now recognized as an active pathologic process, the mechanisms by which can be slowed by treating the underlying drivers of atherosclerotic plaque progression. The temporal evolution of atherosclerotic plaque formation includes adaptive intimal thickening, lipid accumulation, inflammation as represented by infiltration by macrophages and T lymphocytes with the development of fatty streaks, and fibroatheroma formation with calcium aggregation.[10,11] Ectopic bone production, a common feature of a middle-aged type IV atheroma, is the basis for coronary artery calcification.[12]

The presence of coronary calcium is generally limited to the subintimal space (i.e., not typically affected by medial calcification), and based on early pathologic work, it is thought to be essentially pathognomonic of atherosclerosis. The total amount of calcium is directly related to the total burden of atherosclerosis in a log-linear relationship. However, even when coronary calcification is severely elevated, it does not necessarily indicate obstructive coronary artery disease (CAD). As such coronary calcification is good marker of total plaque burden but a relatively poor marker of obstructive coronary artery disease.

Traditional CAC scanning protocols identify calcium-containing fibroatheromas as "coronary calcification,"[13] with areas of 1.03 to 1.37 mm^2 represented by 3 to 4 contiguous pixels within a total plaque area of 5 mm^2; however, microcalcifications present in the earliest plaques may not be identified with standard CAC scans and traditional scoring algorithms. As such, traditional CAC testing protocols identify plaque at an early stage, although not at its earliest stages when calcium deposits are small and not sufficiently dense to be detected.[14] By its nature, CAC scans cannot detect noncalcified plaque, albeit the proportion of patients with exclusively noncalcified plaque is small.

Early studies from the 1960s onward used chest radiography, fluoroscopy,[15] or digital subtraction fluoroscopy[16] to demonstrate the potential value of CAC in predicting future coronary events.[17] However, the first electron bean CT (EBCT) and then multidetector CT scanners allowed for greater detection, localization, and quantification of CAC.[18] By 2000 it was known that identifying subclinical atherosclerosis by CAC scanning was superior to all available serum biomarkers or other imaging modalities (e.g., carotid intima-media thickness and carotid plaque burden) for future ASCVD risk assessment.[19,20] However, it has taken decades to move from understanding the biology of coronary calcification to developing imaging tools with adequate temporal and spatial resolution to image calcification, to deployment in everyday clinical practice.

THE FUNDAMENTALS OF CAC MEASUREMENT AND QUANTIFICATION

The introduction of EBCT scanners allowed for quantification of CAC due to higher temporal resolution and reduced motion artifact. The original Agatston score was derived on an EBCT scanner; for a time, EBCT scanners proliferated as clinicians first learned the power of the CAC score. However, modern multidetector CT (MDCT) scanners enhanced spatial resolution and, more importantly, improved early limitations in temporal resolution, and have now completely replaced EBCT in contemporary practice.

The standard acquisition protocol involves axial MDCT performed with prospective electrocardiographic gating in diastole (60–80% of R-R interval on EKG), using a narrow cardiac field of view, 120 kVp tube voltage, and a tube current (mA) varied according to the patient's body weight. The scan range is from below the carina to the base of the heart, approximately 1 cm above and below the coronary arteries, and is performed during a prolonged breath hold. Reconstruction parameters include a slice thickness of 3 mm in the axial soft-tissue window. The Agatston CAC score then defines calcification as contiguous voxels of high attenuation, >130 Hounsfield units (HU), and an area ≥1 mm^2.

The Agatston score of a single calcified coronary lesion is derived as the product of the total plaque area multiplied by a weighting factor based on the peak attenuation of the plaque calcium (from 130 to >400 Hounsfield units). The final Agatston CAC score is determined by adding up the individual scores of all calcified lesions (realizing that a single large plaque could show up on multiple CT slices).[21,22] CAC measurements usually are reported for each of the coronary arteries and as a composite score for the entire image. The final CAC score can be interpreted in two ways: as the absolute score with predetermined CAC risk groups (i.e., 0, 1–99, 100–299, 300–1000, >1000) or as a percentile adjusted for age, sex, and race/ethnicity using databases such as the Multi-Ethnic Study of Atherosclerosis (MESA), a prospective multiethnic cohort study of the prevalence of subclinical cardiovascular disease in the United States.

Two additional CAC scoring methods exist, the volume score and mass score; however, both are less commonly employed because they are so highly correlated with the Agatston score.[23] The volume score estimates the volume of calcified plaque by considering the plaque area and section thickness, ignoring lesion attenuation. The mass score, a measurement of a mineral mass of calcium hydroxyapatite in milligrams, is calculated on the basis of plaque volume, plaque attenuation, and a calibration factor in which the attenuation of water is considered.

Coronary calcifications can be seen on nongated chest CT scans as well, although it is more susceptible to motion artifact. More recently, nongated CT scans have been leveraged to provide CAC measurements by both semiquantitative (visual assessment, i.e., the Coronary Artery Calcium Data and Reporting System [CAC-DRS] score)[24] and quantitative CAC (approximate Agatston scores) methods.

As noted above, CAC scoring is widely available, rapid (<1 second on many modern scanners, <10 minutes room time), highly reproducible, and does not require contrast use and therefore prep time.[25] The median radiation exposure for this procedure with modern testing equipment is approximately 0.5 to 1 mSv, similar to a screening mammogram (Table 3.1).[26,27] Public awareness of CAC scoring has been increasing over time, driven in part by wider endorsement in national guidelines.

CAC VERSUS CORONARY CT ANGIOGRAPHY

In comparison to the assessment of CAC alone, CCTA requires the administration of intravenous contrast to visualize noncalcified plaque and estimate the severity of luminal stenoses and lower heart rates (~60 beats per minute) to avoid

TABLE 3.1 **Typical Effective Doses of Common Radiation Exposures in Health Care**

TEST	EFFECTIVE RADIATION DOSE (MSV)
Coronary artery calcium scoring	0.6–1.5
Coronary CT angiography	3–5
Nongated CT of the chest	5–7
Nuclear stress testing	7–8
Cardiac catheterization	2.5–10
Average US national background radiation per year	3
Screening mammogram	0.5

cardiac motion artifacts. Thus, in patients with iodine allergy, severe kidney dysfunction, or inability to lower the heart rate, CCTA may be contraindicated. Further, situations such as arrhythmias (i.e., atrial fibrillation) may result in unacceptable imaging quality.[28] Although image acquisition by CAC is standard across centers, CCTA acquisition differs by scanner type, technician expertise, and higher interreader variability.

Although both CAC and CCTA assess the extent of plaque burden, CCTA provides the added benefit of visualizing non-calcified plaque. In the absence of coronary calcification by CAC measurement (i.e., CAC = 0) noncalcified plaque is identified in 5% to 16% of cases.[29,30] Although the visualization of noncalcified plaque may theoretically improve risk prediction models beyond that of CAC only, most benefit is seen in symptomatic patients with CAD.[31] In a study of 576 symptomatic participants, the prevalence of obstructive CAD (stenosis >50% by coronary angiography) was 3.4% and 3.9% in low-risk and intermediate-risk participants, respectively.[32] These findings support the use of CAC scoring as an effective gatekeeper to further testing in low-risk patients.[32] For asymptomatic patients, CCTA information has not been shown to result in improved treatment allocation and does not provide additional predictive information for all-cause mortality beyond the assessment of CAC.[33] As such, there is no strong evidence for routine use of CCTA in the primary prevention setting.

CAC scoring may be performed prior to CCTA scans to assist with planning, performance, and interpretation. Although different centers use various cutoffs (CAC >600 or >1000 AU), the presence of extensive coronary calcification on CAC scoring may inhibit the precise assessment of coronary stenoses on CCTA and, in some cases, may help decide if full-contrast CCTA study should still be performed. Furthermore, in addition to traditional cardiac risk factors, knowledge of the CAC score is helpful in assessing the pretest probability of CAD when interpreting the CCTA images.

POPULATION-BASED CAC COHORT STUDIES

In the early 2000s, single-center studies found that CAC measurement may be a strong predictor of future ASCVD risk. The South Bay Heart Watch Study[34] showed the presence of moderate CAC in intermediate-risk patients using the Framingham risk score allowed them to be reclassified to high risk. In 2005, the St. Francis Heart Study[35] compared patients with CAC = 0 to CAC >400 and found a much higher future ASCVD risk with the addition of CAC to the Framingham risk score. MESA[36] was a prospective US multicenter cohort sample of 6814 persons between the ages of 45 and 84 years old (see Table 3.2), and the HNR (Heinz Nixdorf Recall)[37] study included randomly selected participants between the ages of 45 and 74 years old from the general population from three West German cities.

On the basis of similar designs and study protocols, the results of the MESA and HNR studies demonstrated that despite differences in risk factor profiles, CAC scores were similar and age and sex distributions were comparable; in addition, CAC was a strong predictor of ASCVD events in both studies. The Rotterdam study[38] prospectively evaluated 7983 persons at least 55 years of age (mean age: 71.1 ± 5.7 years old) in Rotterdam, Netherlands. Despite differences in the baseline population compared to MESA and HNR, the distribution of CAC and its ability to predict future ASCVD was similar.

The Framingham Heart Study[39] also demonstrated that additional information from MDCT, such as the number of

TABLE 3.2 **Comparison of Selected Major Prospective Observational Cohorts Studying the Coronary Artery Calcium Score: Baseline Characteristics**

	MESA	HNR	ROTTERDAM	FHS	CARDIA	CAC CONSORTIUM	ARIC
Year CAC Study Started	2000–2002	2000–2003	1997–2000	2002–2005	2000–2001	1991–2010	2018–2019
Type of CT scan performed	EBCT and MDCT	EBCT	EBCT	MDCT	EBCT and MDCT	EBCT (93%) and MDCT	MDCT
Number of Participants	6814	4487	2063	3238	3043	66,636	2217
Age range of participants, years (mean)	45–84 (62.2 ± 10.2)	45–74 (59 ± 8)	≥55 (71.1 ± 5.7)	Men >35, women >40 (49 ± 10.9)	32–46 (40.3 ± 3.6)	45–79 (54 ± 11)	age >75
Women, %	53	53	57	54	55	33	60
Percentage with CAC >0 at baseline	Men 52–70%, women 35–45%	Men 82%, women 55%	91% overall	Men 40.5%, women 20.6%	89.8%	45%	90%

ARIC, Atherosclerosis Risk in Communities; *CARDIA*, Coronary Artery Risk Development in Young Adults; *FHS*, Framingham Heart Study; *HNR*, Heinz Nixdorf Recall; *MESA*, Multi-Ethnic Study of Atherosclerosis.

coronary arteries and the presence of CAC in the proximal dominant coronary arteries, were associated with major CAD events. The Jackson Heart Study was a prospective cohort study that investigated CAC in African American individuals from three counties surrounding Jackson, Mississipi.[40] The CARDIA (Coronary Artery Risk Development in Young Adults)[41] was the first prospective cohort to include data on CAC in young patients (32 to 46 years old), demonstrating the presence of CAC (CAC >0) is not uncommon in young patients. The CAC Consortium[42] (2016) was another cohort study that included four US sites (Cedars-Sinai Medical Center and Harbor-UCLA Medical Center [California], PrevaHealth Wellness Diagnostic Center [Ohio], and Minneapolis Heart Institute [Minnesota]) with the main objective of determining the cause of death.

The ARIC (Atherosclerosis Risk in Communities)[43] study is an ongoing cohort of 15,792 individuals, aged 45 to 64 years old, who were initially enrolled between 1987 and 1989 from four US communities and underwent CAC scoring at visit 7 (February 2018 to December 2019). One study from the ARIC cohort demonstrated that CAC is a strong predictor of short-term risk of myocardial infarction and heart failure in those >75 years of age.[44]

RACE, GENDER, AND AGE DIFFERENCES IN CAC MEASUREMENT

One limitation of current ASCVD risk prediction tools such as the PCE is its applicability in racial/ethnic minority groups. We acknowledge that race is a social construct, and the use of CAC testing may help overcome this impediment. Racial/ethnic differences in the presence of CAC have been demonstrated in the MESA cohort,[36] with Black and Hispanic patients having a lower CAC prevalence and burden when compared to White patients (race-based prevalence with Agatston score >0: White 70.4%, Black 52.1%, Hispanic 56.5%, and Chinese 59.2%). Yet after adjusting for atherosclerotic burden, a study using the CAC Consortium[45] reported higher cardiovascular mortality in Black and Hispanic patients when compared with White patients. Similar findings were reported in later studies using the MESA cohort.[46]

This disparity may largely be explained by disparities in socioeconomic status and healthcare utilization between racial/ethnic groups. Using data from the MASALA (Mediators of Atherosclerosis in South Asians Living in America) study,[47] South Asian persons have similarly high CAC prevalence when compared with White patients and should be classified as "Caucasian"[5] when using the MESA CAC reference tool. Despite these racial/ethnic differences, the CAC score is independently associated with ASCVD events, regardless of race, including in Hispanic and Asian persons, who are not represented in the PCE. As such, institutions reporting CAC scores should report both the absolute Agatston CAC score and the race-based CAC percentiles.[5]

CAC is present earlier in men when compared with women, as shown in a comparison study of the MESA and HNR[37] cohorts, as well as the Framingham Heart Study (FHS)[39] (MESA 52–70% male versus 35–5% female, HNR 82% versus 55% and FHS 40.5% versus 20.6%).

Like the PCE, age is a strong risk factor for development of CAC and future ASCVD events. Current guidelines recommend consideration of CAC measurement in middle- to older-aged adults (40 to 79 years old); however, there is increasing interest in CAC as a clinical decision-making tool to identify young adults (<45 years old) at elevated risk or older patients (>75 years old) in whom statin therapy can be withheld when CAC = 0. Although the absolute CAC score is the best predictor of 5- to 10-year ASCVD event risk, the age, sex, and race/ethnicity-based CAC score percentile, derived from the MESA cohort, is the best predictor of relative risk and of lifetime risk trajectory and should be used to estimate lifetime treatment benefit.

THE ROLE OF CAC MEASUREMENT IN THE CLINICAL DECISION-MAKING FOR PRIMARY ASCVD PREVENTION

The most robust evidence for the use of CAC scoring (Fig. 3.1), a Class IIa recommendation, is in adults, 40 to 75 years of age, with LDL-C 70 to 189 mg/dL and intermediate-risk (10-year ASCVD of 7.5–19.9%), or in selected patients at borderline risk (5.0–7.4% 10-year risk).[6] Patients with a CAC score of 0, in the absence of diabetes, current cigarette smoking, or a strong family history of premature ASCVD, are reclassified to low 10-year ASVD risk (<7.5%), suggesting that drug therapy may be of more limited value over the next 5 to 7 years. Those with a score of 100 or more (or at the 75th percentile or higher) are reclassified as high risk and have event rates in the range where the benefit of statin therapy would likely exceed any potential for harm. When the score is 1 to 99, a clinician-patient discussion on the utility of statin use is generally advised, but statin therapy is favored.

Depending on age, reclassification is modest for those patients with a score between 1 and 99, but they remain in a statin benefit group, so clinical judgment and patient preferences should guide decision-making. A study of 4758 MESA participants who were followed over 10.3 years evaluated the implications of the absence of CAC in reclassifying patients from a risk stratum in which statins were recommended to one in which they were not.[48] Among 41% of participants who were recommended moderate- to high-intensity statins based on the PCE had no detectable CAC, and only 4.9% experienced an ASCVD event over 10 years. Furthermore, in those considered for statins (10-year risk of 5% to 7.5%), the absence of CAC was noted in a much larger proportion (57%), with an extremely low 10-year ASCVD risk of 1.5%. The findings of this study suggest that the decision to start statin therapy in the borderline- to intermediate-risk group may essentially be a "coin toss," as approximately half of the borderline-intermediate-risk patients can be reclassified to low risk (CAC = 0) and statin therapy deferred.[49]

Despite the known benefits of statins, discontinuation is common in clinical practice[50] and is associated with adverse consequences.[51] An algorithm that incorporates CAC scoring into clinical decision-making about statin reinitiation in statin-intolerant patients has been proposed. The algorithm (Fig. 3.2) provides a practical approach to the use

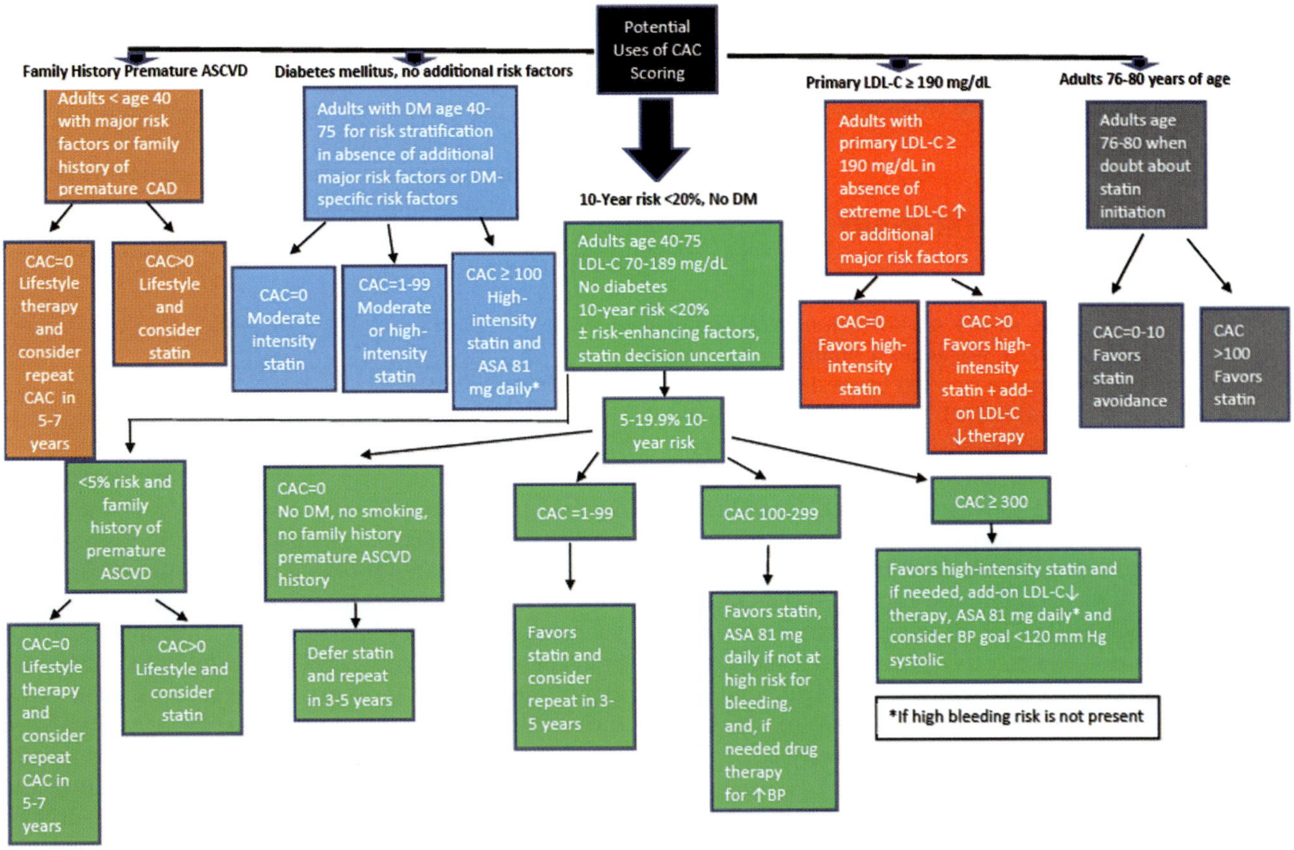

FIG. 3.1 Potential uses of coronary artery calcium scoring according to the 2021 National Lipid Association Scientific Statement.[5]

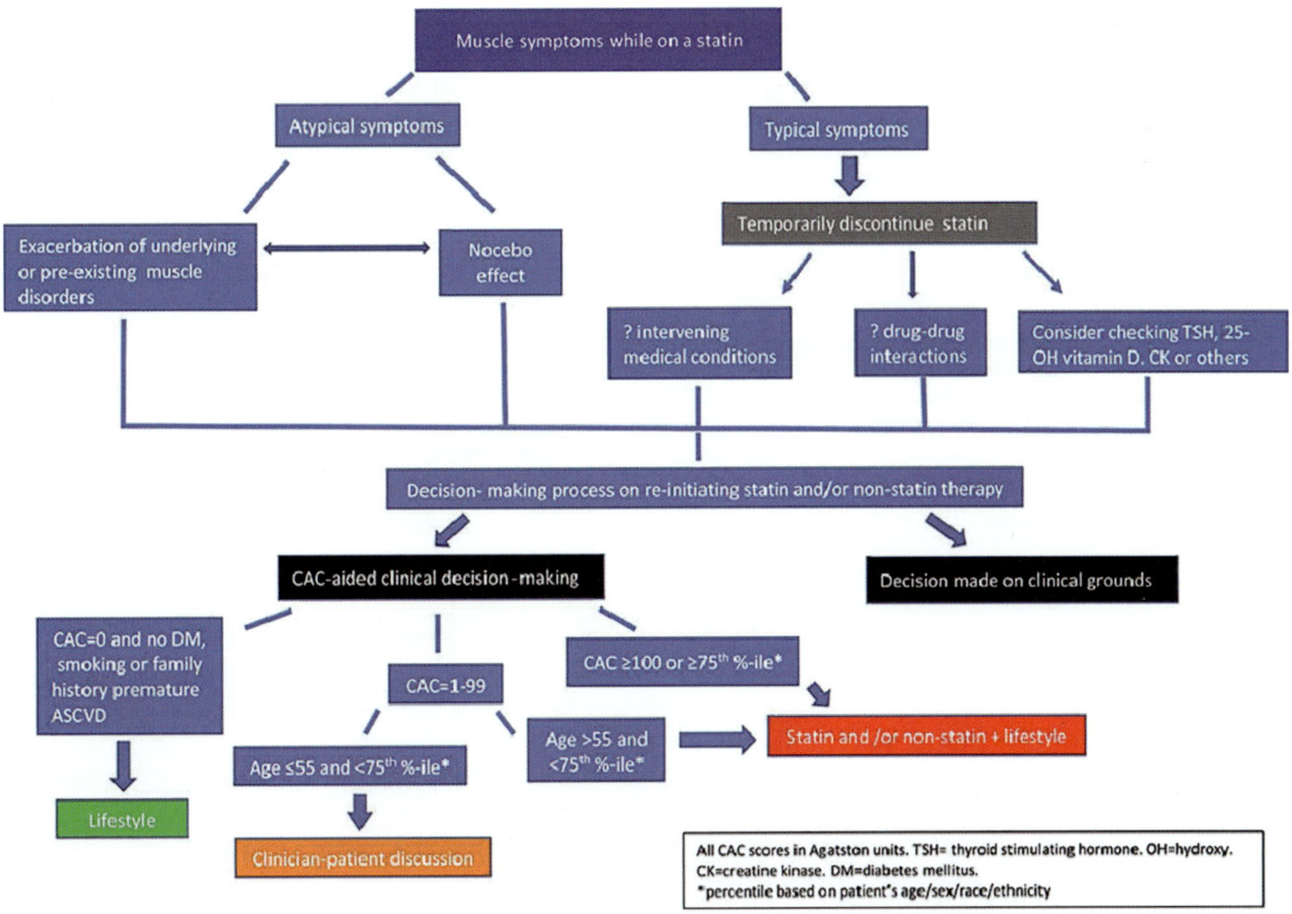

FIG. 3.2 A practical algorithm describing the use of coronary artery calcium scoring to aid in clinical decision-making in patients with statin-attributed side effects.[52]

of this technology in such primary prevention patients.[52] Statin therapy is generally well-tolerated by patients when rechallenged, and the use of CAC scoring is an additive tool to aid in clinical decision-making when managing statin intolerance.

THE PROGRESSION OF CORONARY ARTERY CALCIFICATION

CAC generally progresses slowly on an exponential scale, at approximately 10% to 25% per year. A change in CAC of >20% per year or an increase to >300 in adults at 3 years is indicative of accelerated ASCVD progression, and these patients may benefit from aggressive lipid-lowering therapies.[5] A CAC score of 0 is the single strongest negative predictor for developing a cardiovascular event,[53] the clinical significance of which is to reclassify ASCVD risk in those at borderline and intermediate ASCVD risk. The natural progression of CAC is such that the estimated time period for 25% conversion to CAC >0 for low-, intermediate-, and high–ASCVD risk patients is 6 to 7 years, 4 to 5 years, and 3 years, respectively.[54,55] In those with a CAC score of 0, the 2021 NLA Scientific Statement[5] recommends repeat CAC scoring in 3 to 7 years dependent upon baseline ASCVD risk:

- 5 to 7 years for low-risk patients
- 3 to 5 years for borderline to intermediate risk
- 3 years for those at high risk

It is very unlikely that retesting more frequently than the recommended intervals will miss progression to a high CAC score.

Statins are associated with slower progression of overall coronary atherosclerosis volume, reduced progression of noncalcified plaque, and a reduction of high-risk plaque features.[56] Paradoxically, however, statins modestly increase coronary plaque calcification while simultaneously reducing future ASCVD events.[56,57] The beneficial procalcific effects of statins are thought to be mediated through the stabilization of the fibrous cap of atherosclerotic lesions[58] via the induction of microcalcification. A very low proportion of plaques containing microcalcification rupture, and by rendering plaque microcalcifications more confluent and denser, statins reduce vessel wall stress, contributing to plaque stability.[58] Therefore, in clinical practice for those patients whose baseline CAC scores are ≥ 100, CAC progression cannot be used to measure the efficacy of statin therapy.[5]

THE COMMUNICATION OF CAC-BASED ATHEROSCLEROTIC CARDIOVASCULAR DISEASE RISK

Several tools are currently available for communicating CAC-based risk (Fig. 3.3A). First, the MESA Risk Score Calculator is a validated tool that uses traditional risk factors with/without the CAC score to estimate an individual's 10-year risk of coronary heart disease. This online calculator is available at https://www.mesa-nhlbi.org/CACReference.aspx.[59] Next, the CAC score reference web tool, utilizing the MESA database (US population) for age 45 to 84, provides the probability of nonzero calcium, and the 25th, 50th, 75th, and 90th percentiles for age, sex, and race/ethnicity.[60] Patient-specific age, sex, and race/ethnicity-based CAC score percentiles can be derived from the calculator by inputting a given CAC score. Similar CAC scoring calculators exist for Western European, Asian, and Brazilian populations.

Lastly, the coronary age calculator is easy to use and translates the MESA coronary heart disease risk estimates into biological age language. The coronary age[61] for an individual is the age at which an average healthy individual would have an equivalent estimated coronary heart disease (CHD) risk as that calculated for the index individual either with or without the CAC score available. The use of these scoring tools is best illustrated using the examples below.

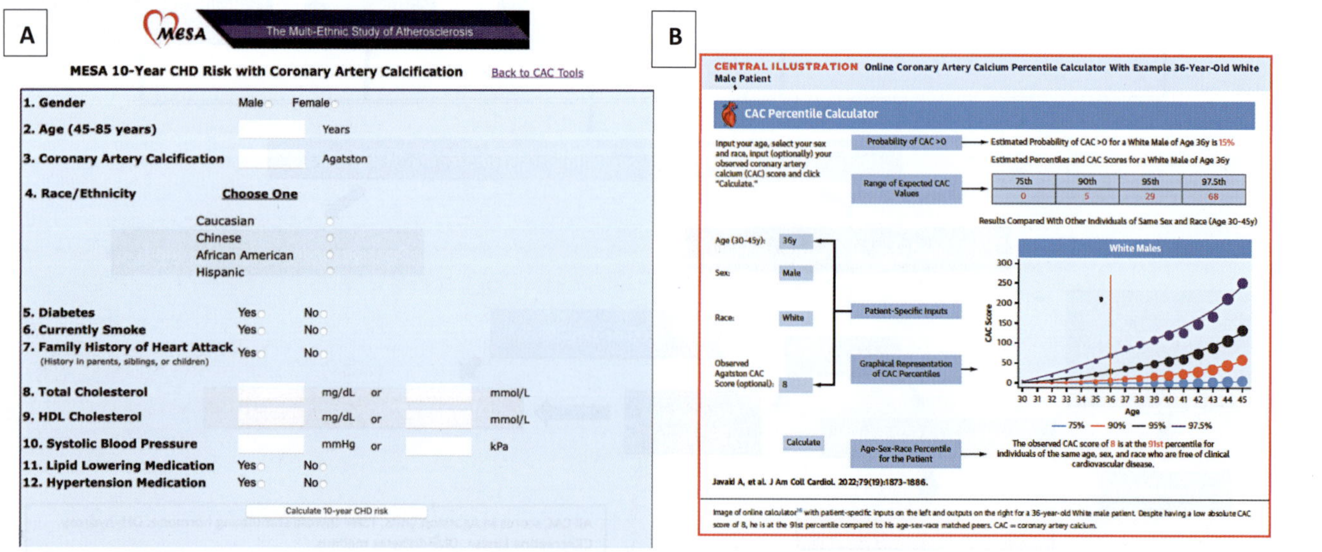

FIG. 3.3 (A) An example of the MESA Risk Score Calculator and the CAC score reference web tool is available online at: https://www.mesa-nhlbi.org/CACReference.aspx.[59,60] (B) Image of the online calculator with patient-specific inputs on the left and outputs on the right.[63] This calculator is available at: https://www.cac-tools.com.

EXAMPLE 1

A 55-year-old White male with total cholesterol of 225 mg/dL, high-density lipoprotein cholesterol of 60 mg/dL, systolic blood pressure of 139 mm Hg, a family history of premature coronary heart disease, and a CAC score of 300.

- Using the PCE, he has a 10-year ASCVD risk score of 7%
- Using the MESA calculator, he has a 10-year Coronary Heart Disease (CHD) risk score of 14% once accounting for his CAC score
- Using the coronary age calculator, without including his CAC score, his coronary age is 61 years old
- Using the coronary age calculator, including his CAC score, his coronary age is 77 years old

EXAMPLE 2

A 55-year-old White male with total cholesterol of 225 mg/dL, high-density lipoprotein cholesterol of 60 mg/dL, systolic blood pressure of 139 mm Hg, a family history of premature coronary heart disease, and a CAC score of 0.

- Using the PCE, he has a 10-year ASCVD risk score of 7%
- Using the MESA calculator, he has a 10-year CHD risk score of 3% once accounting for his CAC score
- Using the coronary age calculator, without including his CAC score, his coronary age is 61 years old
- Using the coronary age calculator, including his CAC score, his coronary age is 42 years old

From the examples above, the inclusion of CAC scores differentiated 10-year risk and arterial age upward for example 1, and downward for example 2. These tools may be more easily understandable to patients and assist in risk reporting during the clinician-patient discussion.

There are limitations of the current CAC-based risk estimators. As the calculators were developed using the MESA cohort, the applicable age ranges and racial representation are limited to those from MESA. This includes patients between the ages of 45 and 84 years old and racial/ethnic groups including Caucasian, Chinese American, African American, or Hispanic patients only.

CAC SCORING IN YOUNGER PATIENTS

Risk estimation remains challenging yet vitally important in patients at the extremes of age, particularly in the case of young adults <40 years old, to identify and reduce long-term risk. The presence of any CAC in young adults is associated with elevated fatal and nonfatal CAD risk.[62]

The largest study of CAC in US young adults to date harmonized three datasets—CARDIA, the CAC Consortium, and the Walter Reed Cohort—to study CAC in 19,725 asymptomatic individuals aged 30 to 45 years without known atherosclerotic cardiovascular disease.[63] The authors determined the probability of CAC >0 and propose a calculator to determine age-sex-race percentiles for US adults aged 30 to 45 years. The overall prevalence of CAC >0 was 21%. The presence of any CAC (CAC >0) placed the following groups at >90th percentile: all females, White males at age 34 years, and Black males at age 37 years.

The presence of any CAC in this age group is abnormal, and utilizing CAC percentiles provides a method to compare how high a CAC score is in an individual relative to his or her age-sex-race matched peers. The interactive percentile calculator for age 30 to 45 is shown in Fig. 3.3B and is available at https://www.cac-tools.com. The 2021 NLA Guideline[5] expanded the population of individuals eligible for CAC scanning to select adults aged <40 years with a family history of premature ASCVD or multiple ASCVD risk factors.

CAC TO INFORM RISK VERSUS BENEFIT DISCUSSION OF ASPIRIN FOR PRIMARY PREVENTION

The evidence supporting aspirin use for the secondary prevention of ASCVD is robust. However, in recent years for older adults, the risk versus benefit ratio continues to favor avoiding aspirin therapy for primary ASCVD prevention.[64–66] In lieu of the shifting paradigm, the US Preventive Services Task Force (USPSTF) changed its recommendations to advise against initiating low-dose aspirin in any adults 60 years or older (Grade D).[67] Furthermore, the USPSTF downgraded aspirin for primary prevention in adults aged 40 to 59 years to Grade C.

In the absence of high bleeding risk, CAC scoring may be a useful tool to further delineate patients in whom the benefits of aspirin for primary prevention outweigh the risks (Fig. 3.4).[68–70] Participants with CAC ≥100 have a lower estimated number needed to treat (NNT) compared to the number needed to harm (NNH), showing anticipated benefit from aspirin. However, when CAC = 0, the 5-year NNH is lower than the NNT (567 vs. 1190), indicating net harm from aspirin. As such, the benefits of aspirin use for primary prevention appear to outweigh the bleeding risks only in patients with CAC >100 without high bleeding risk.

CAC IN THE MANAGEMENT OF OBESITY AND DIABETES MELLITUS

A study of patients with metabolic syndrome and diabetes mellitus enrolled in the MESA study suggested that future ASCVD risk in patients with diabetes can be further delineated using CAC scoring.[71] Patients with CAC = 0 had an ASCVD risk of 8.2%, whereas those with CAC >0 had significantly higher ASCVD risk (e.g., CAC 1–99 10-year risk was 15%, and CAC >100 10-year risk was >20%). Further studies have supported these findings[72] and shown that CAC scoring predicts ASCVD events independent of standard risk factors in both type 1 and type 2 diabetes, and as such, may help identify patients at higher ASCVD risk who may benefit from more aggressive primary prevention therapies.[5,73] Similar results have been shown for patients with obesity without diabetes.[74]

In cases where access to and the allocation of ASCVD risk-reducing cardiometabolic agents (GLP-1 agonists and SGLT-2 inhibitors) is limited by cost, for example, ideal candidates who may accrue the most benefit can be identified by CAC scoring (e.g., those with CAC >100).[75]

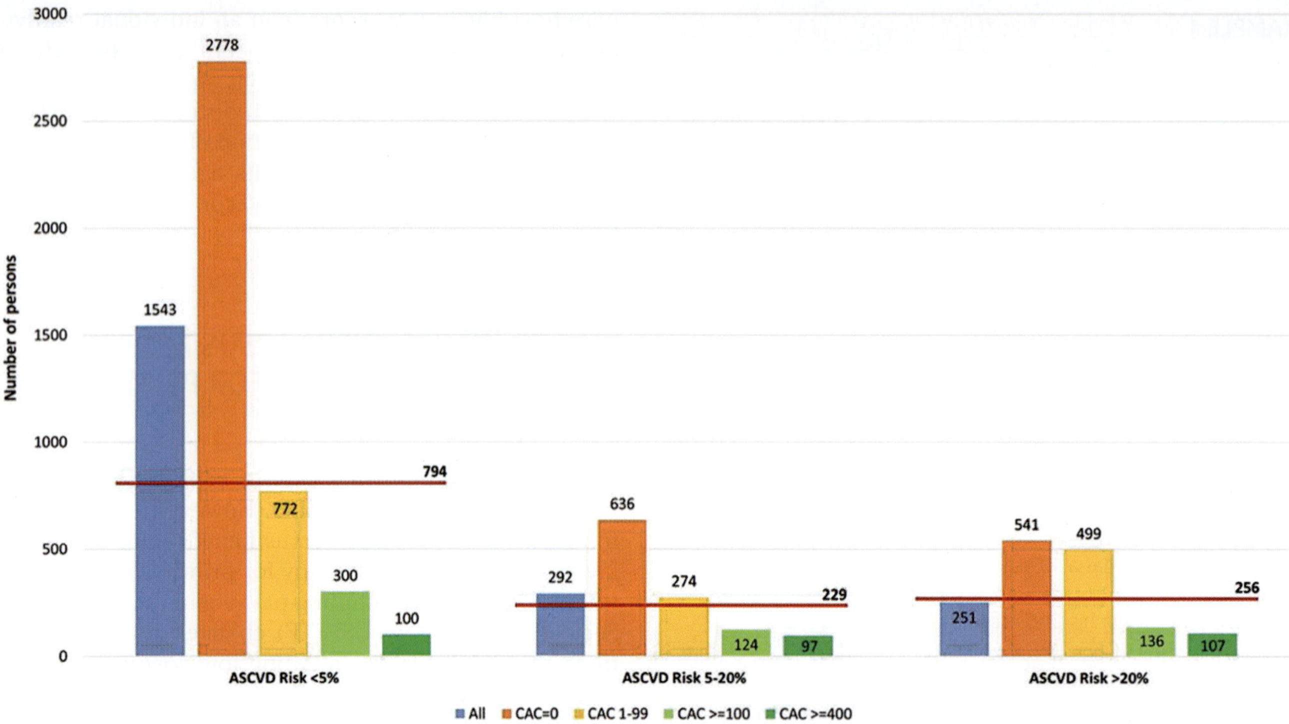

FIG. 3.4 Number needed to treat with low-dose aspirin during 5 years to prevent one cardiovascular disease event and number needed to cause a major bleeding event by baseline coronary artery calcium score.[69] The red horizontal lines represent the number needed to harm threshold for each atherosclerotic cardiovascular disease risk stratum. When the bars are below the red line, there is anticipated benefit to aspirin therapy.

CAC TO INFORM USE OF NONSTATIN THERAPIES

In the 2022 ACC Expert Decision Consensus Pathway (ECDP) on nonstatin therapy, CAC >100 should guide initiation of high-intensity statin therapy. In patients who have a <50% LDL-C reduction from baseline or on-treatment LDL-C ≥70 mg/dL, it is recommended to consider the addition of ezetimibe to maximally tolerated statins. Those patients with CAC ≥1000 constitute a unique population at substantially higher risk for ASCVD events and mortality. Two studies, one using data from the MESA cohort[76] and the other using data from the CAC Consortium population,[77] reported that a CAC score ≥1000 was associated with similar annualized major adverse cardiovascular event (MACE) (3.4 per 100 person-years) and ASCVD death rates (0.8% per year), rates that are similar to those observed in the placebo group of the FOURIER (Further Cardiovascular Outcomes Research with PCSK9 Inhibition in Subjects with Elevated Risk) trial[78] (Fig. 3.5).

Although lipid-lowering therapy for secondary prevention is generally more aggressive, the findings of these studies demonstrate that some primary prevention individuals, particularly those with CAC ≥1000, may carry a higher risk profile and warrant more aggressive management. As such, in the 2022 ACC ECDP on nonstatin use, in adults with CAC scores ≥1000, it is reasonable to use high-intensity statin therapy, and if necessary, guideline-based add-on LDL-C-lowering therapies (ezetimibe and consideration of PCSK9-inhibitors[79]) to achieve a >50% reduction in LDL-C, and optimally an LDL-C <70 mg/dL.[5]

CAC IN HYPERTENSION

Increased CAC is associated with worse cardiovascular outcomes in patients with hypertension and allows for personalized systolic blood pressure goals. One study demonstrated enhanced cardiovascular risk stratification using CAC among 16,167 adults in the CAC Consortium with hypertension who met the inclusion criteria for the SPRINT (Systolic Blood Pressure Intervention Trial) trial.[80] Furthermore, a CAC score of 220 (confidence range, 165–270) was associated with equivalent cardiovascular disease mortality rate to that observed in SPRINT (a trial that showed the benefit of tight blood pressure control).

The results of a second study[81] provided insight into the use of CAC to guide therapeutic decisions for treatment of early blood pressure elevation. This study included 3733 participants from MESA with a systolic blood pressure between 120 and 179 mm Hg. The most striking finding was that persons with CAC = 0 in both the prehypertension (120–139 mm Hg) and mild hypertension (140–159 mm Hg) systolic blood pressure categories had low 10-year event rates (<7.5 per 1000 person-years). Individuals with CAC ≥100 were estimated to benefit from more aggressive blood pressure lowering (systolic blood pressure <120 mm Hg), with risk stratification most notable in those with early (Stage 1) hypertension.

CAC IN LOW-RISK STABLE CHEST PAIN

The 2021 AHA/ACC/Multi-society Guideline for the Evaluation and Diagnosis of Chest Pain[82] placed particular

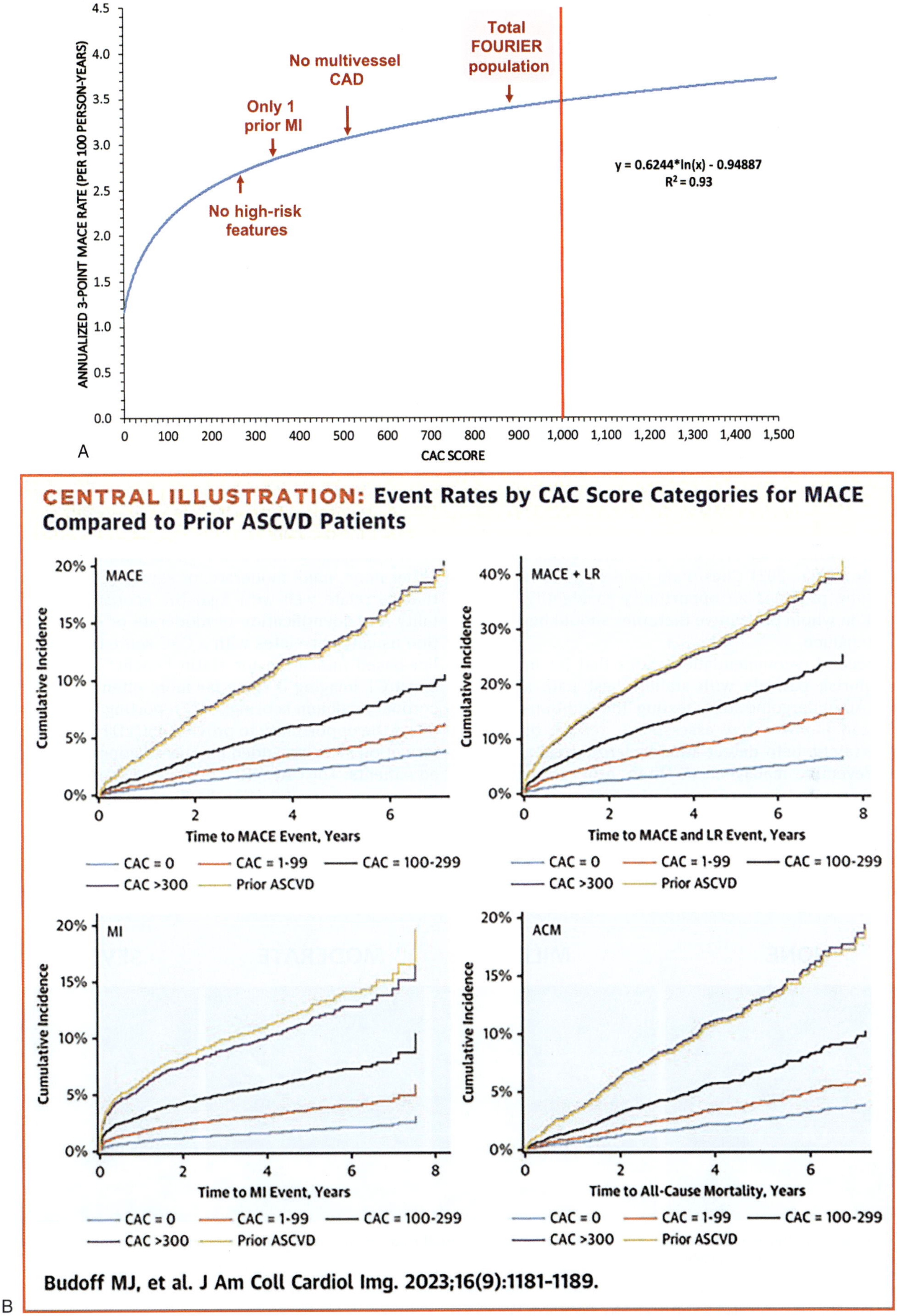

FIG. 3.5 (A) Coronary artery calcium (CAC) identifies secondary prevention risk. At a CAC score ≥1000, the annualized 3-point major adverse cardiovascular event (MACE) rate (per 100 person-years) is similar to that of the placebo group in the FOURIER population.[76] (B) CAC identifies secondary prevention risk. Patients with CAC >300 have event rates comparable to those with established atherosclerotic cardiovascular disease.[109]

importance on preventive care in those with nonobstructive disease.[83] Two main recommendations, both Class IIa, endorse the use of CAC scoring. First, for low-risk patients with stable chest pain and no known CAD, the guideline states that CAC testing can be used to identify patients who have a low likelihood of obstructive CAD in whom further testing can be deferred.

The PROMISE trial[31] enrolled 10,003 symptomatic outpatients without diagnosed CAD whose physicians believed that nonurgent, noninvasive cardiovascular testing was necessary for the evaluation of suspected CAD. Of 1457 symptomatic patients with a CAC of zero, only 22 (1.5%) had ≥50% stenosis and only 7 (0.5%) had >70% stenosis by CCTA. Furthermore, among seven studies with 3924 symptomatic patients with a CAC of zero, the pooled incidence of cardiovascular events was 1.8% over a mean follow-up ranging from 17 to 84 months.[84]

A metaanalysis comprising 13 studies including 12,376 patients with acute chest pain undergoing simultaneous CAC and CCTA assessment demonstrated that the absence of CAC was associated with a very low prevalence of obstructive CAD (for CAC = 0, negative predictive value: 98% [95% CI: 0.96–99]), a low prevalence of nonobstructive CAD (13% [95% CI: 0.10–0.16]), and a low annualized risk of major adverse cardiac events (0.8% overall event rate).[85] The 2021 Chest Pain Guideline[83] noted that CAC testing provides an opportunity to identify those with CAC in whom preventive therapies should be initiated or intensified.

The second recommendation states that for intermediate-high-risk patients with stable chest pain and no known CAD undergoing stress testing, the addition of CAC testing can improve risk assessment, reduce diagnostic uncertainty, help detect atherosclerotic plaque, and guide preventive management. Often, a negative stress test is interpreted as the absence of coronary artery disease; however, more than half of middle-aged to older patients with normal stress myocardial perfusion imaging have a CAC score ≥100.[86] CAC scoring identifies subclinical atherosclerosis, provides a quantitative assessment of atherosclerotic plaque burden, and may identify intermediate-high-risk patients with stable chest pain and a negative stress test in whom preventive therapies can be initiated or intensified.

CORONARY ARTERY CALCIFICATION ON NONCONTRAST NONGATED CHEST CT

Although quantitative CAC scoring is performed using ECG gating, the finding of coronary calcification on nongated chest CT scans done for noncardiac indications also provides prognostic information that may be useful in statin and other preventive therapy decision-making. The SCCT and the STR recommend reporting qualitative interpretation of CAC on all noncontrast chest CT scans (Class I recommendation).[7,87] Both Agatston scoring and manually calculated ordinal scoring for CAC on nongated chest CT studies correlate well with gated cardiac CT scores, provide high interreader correlation, and predict mortality,[88] but are time consuming.

The fastest method is the visual estimation of CAC as either none, mild, moderate, or severe (Fig. 3.6), findings that correlate well with Agatston scores and with mortality. The identification of moderate or severe calcification usually correlates with a CAC score of >100, a guideline-based indication for statin benefit.[6] As noncontrast chest CT imaging is done far more often than dedicated coronary calcium scoring, CAC reporting on such studies offers the opportunity to provide ASCVD risk reduction information in an expanded number of appropriately selected patients. The CAC-DRS[22] provides a standardized method for communicating CAC findings on all noncontrast CT scans (Table 3.3).

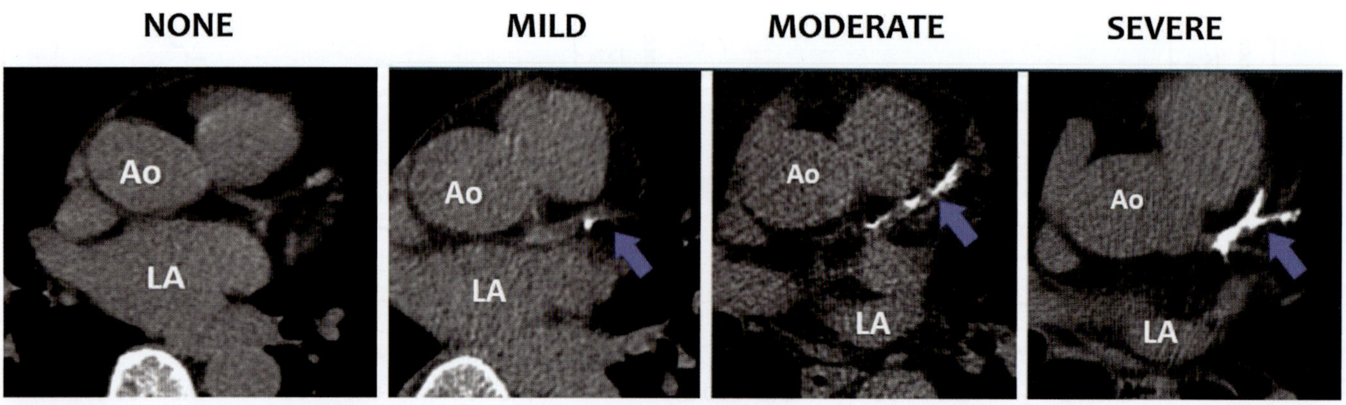

FIG. 3.6 Reporting of incidental coronary artery calcification by the visual reassessment method on noncontrast CT scans of the chest. The *arrow* represents areas of coronary calcifications.
Ao, Aorta; *LA*, left atrium.
None: no coronary calcification visualized (CAC-DRS 0).
Mild: isolated flecks of calcification within a coronary segment (CAC-DRS V1).
Moderate: more calcification than can be considered mild, but less than the description of severe (CAC-DRS V2).
Severe: continuous calcification within a coronary segment (CAC-DRS V3).

TABLE 3.3 CAC-DRS Category-Determined Risk Classifications and Treatment Recommendations[22]

CAC SCORE	CAC SCORING METHOD		RISK	TREATMENT RECOMMENDATION
	AGATSTON (A SCORING)	VISUAL (V SCORING)		
CAC-DRS 0	0	None	Very low	Statin generally not recommended[a]
CAC-DRS 1	1–99	Mild	Mildly increased	Moderate intensity statin
CAC-DRS 2	100–299	Moderate	Moderately increased	Moderate- to high-intensity statin and aspirin 81 mg
CAC-DRS 3	>300	Severe	Moderately to severely increased	High-intensity statin and aspirin 81 mg

[a]Excluding familial hypercholesterolemia

CAC, Coronary artery calcium; *CAC-DRS*, Coronary Artery Calcium Data and Reporting System.

Modifiers are available; the first describes the scoring method used (A = Agatston or V = visual estimation), and the second indicates the number of vessels with CAC (N = 1 to 4). For example, visually severe CAC afflicting the left anterior descending, left circumflex, and right coronary artery would be CAC-DRS V3/N3.

CORONARY ARTERY CALCIFICATION IN SINGLE-PHOTON EMISSION COMPUTED TOMOGRAPHY (SPECT) AND POSITRON EMISSION TOMOGRAPHIC (PET) MYOCARDIAL PERFUSION IMAGING (MPI)

A major limitation of SPECT and PET MPI testing is the possibility of false-positive perfusion defects caused by soft tissue attenuating structures, such as the diaphragm and breasts.[89] Cameras that incorporate multidetector row CT scanners have been introduced at the time of MPI to perform attenuation correction and decrease the possibility of unnecessary downstream testing.[90] CAC scoring can be obtained from the CT component of these hybrid scanners without increasing radiation exposure. CAC scores obtained from the attenuation scans acquired at the time of perfusion imaging are highly predictive of risk, including in patients for whom there is no evidence of myocardial ischemia.[91,92]

A study of 492 patients from three centers reported high accuracy and reproducibility of the visual estimation of CAC (93% agreement within one scoring category) in patients who underwent both PET/SPECT MPI with CT attenuation correction and a dedicated CAC score examination.[93] These findings are corroborated in further studies.[94] CT attenuation scans done with SPECT/PET scans should be routinely assessed for visually estimated CAC that can affect clinical decision-making in terms of treatment with antiplatelet and lipid-lowering agents in patients without known flow-limiting coronary disease.

EXTRA-CORONARY CALCIFICATIONS: AORTIC VALVE CALCIFICATION AND THORACIC AORTA CALCIFICATION

Calcium scoring of the aortic valve can also be performed using the Agatston method (Fig. 3.7).[95] As with the Agatston score for CAC, a threshold of 130 HU is used to detect areas of calcium. In asymptomatic patients, the AVC score is the best predictor of long-term incidence of severe aortic stenosis.[96]

Although the first-line, gold-standard tool for assessing aortic stenosis severity remains echocardiography, the measurement of AVC can be useful in assessing aortic stenosis severity in patients for whom echocardiography is inconclusive and the true severity of disease remains in doubt. According to the 2020 ACC/AHA Guideline for the Management of Valvular Heart Disease,[97] AVC measurement can be used in low-flow, low-gradient severe aortic stenosis as an alternative to dobutamine stress echocardiography, to identify true severe aortic stenosis. The sex-specific AVC thresholds to identify severe aortic stenosis are >1300 in women and >2000 in men.

Pitfalls in the analysis of AVC include the challenge of excluding calcium from the left ventricular outflow tract, aortic sinus, coronary arteries, and mitral annulus when obtaining the AVC Agatston score. As such, it is of value to visualize the aortic valve in multiple planes, including the aortic annular plane, to confidently identify the valvular calcium to be included.

Thoracic aortic calcification (TAC) can be readily detected on routine CAC scans and is highly predictive of stroke and total mortality. As opposed to CAC, which appears first in men, TAC may occur first in women with higher TAC burden relative to CAC burden. The total number of extracoronary sites afflicted with calcification is a strong predictor of total mortality.[98]

COST EFFECTIVENESS—A NEED FOR WIDER COVERAGE OF CORONARY ARTERY CALCIFICATION SCORING

The most significant barrier to more widespread implementation of CAC scoring is that the test has limited coverage by most insurance carriers and is therefore most often a cash-pay test. Although the cost of obtaining a CAC scoring examination is variable, it is available in most locations for $50 to $200.[99] When comparing the use of CAC scoring to the "treat all with statin therapy" approach to guide shared clinical decision-making, CAC scoring is cost effective and affords a reasonable option to risk stratify as well as facilitate shared decision-making without any significant downstream adverse outcomes, loss of quality of life, and/or increased costs.[100] For example, approximately 50% of patients at borderline to intermediate risk have a CAC score of zero and can be reclassified to low risk with a decision to defer statin

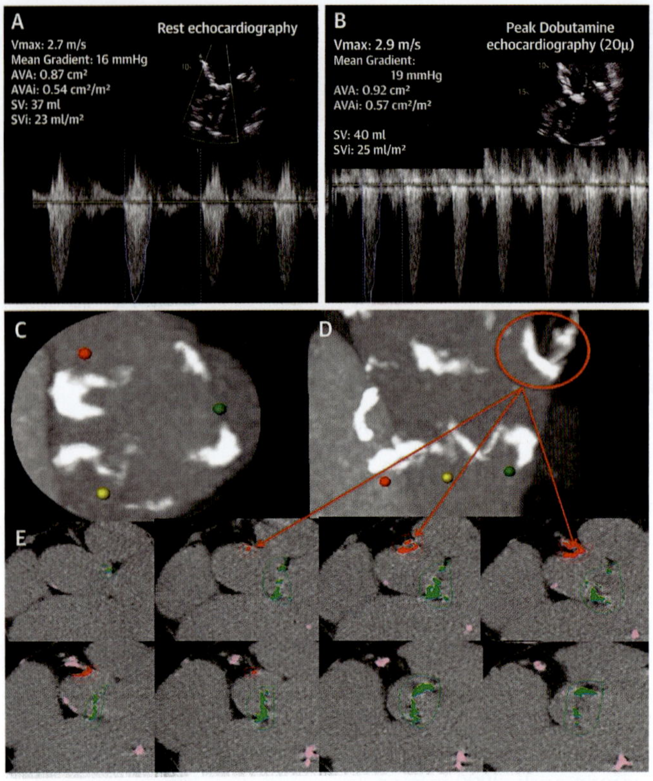

FIG. 3.7 Evaluation of low-flow aortic stenosis patient with aorta and coronary calcification.[97] In (A), the resting echocardiogram shows the evaluation of a patient with low-flow low-gradient aortic stenosis and decreased ejection fraction. In (B), the peak dobutamine stress echocardiogram at 20 µg/min shows poor contractile reserve (SVi: 25 ml/m²) and no change in gradient/velocity. Owing to the lack of increase in flow, the dobutamine stress echocardiography is inconclusive regarding the aortic stenosis severity. Noncontrast CT showing (C) "en face" view of aortic valve leaflets (maximum intensity projection image) with calcification of the base of the trileaflet valve and (D) aortic outflow tract orientation, demonstrating calcification in the right coronary artery ostium and adjacent aortic sinus wall. The measurement of aortic valve calcification (AVC) *(green)* was performed on (E) axial multiplanar reformat images from left ventricular outflow tract to aortic direction and demonstrated a nonsevere aortic stenosis (AVC: 1553 AU). The inclusion of sinus/coronary calcification *(red)* in the AVC would have inappropriately graded the stenosis as severe (AVC + sinus/coronary calcification: 2059 AU). Indeed, any calcium that appears in close proximity to the right coronary ostium on axial views is not valvular calcium because the right and left aortic valve leaflets are never visualized on the same slice. *AU*, Arbitrary unit; *AVA*, aortic valve area; *AVC*, aortic valve calcification; *AVAi*, indexed aortic valve area; *LVOT*, left ventricular outflow tract; *SV*, stroke volume; *SVi*, stroke volume indexed to body surface area; V_{max}, peak aortic jet velocity.

therapy for 3 to 5 years.[48] At present, insurance coverage for CAC scoring is increasing but still limited.

CAC MEASUREMENT IN CLINICAL TRIALS

Early CAC trials, including the St. Francis Heart Study[101] and EISNER Trial,[102] showed modest differences in ASCVD event rates (with statin therapy in the setting of high CAC) and downstream risk factors (as a result of behavior change following CAC); however, both studies were limited by small sample sizes and were underpowered to detect differences in event rates. Further limitations to conducting CAC trials included the high cost associated with such trials, exposure to ionizing radiation, the potential for incidental findings (8% of cardiac CTs) leading to inappropriate downstream testing, and the ethical challenge of withholding primary prevention therapies from patients with extensive CAC randomized to placebo.[103] As such, in 2019, the National Heart, Lung, and Blood Institute (NHLBI) organized a workshop and concluded that additional evidence to support the current guideline-based CAC recommendations for middle-aged adults is very likely to come from ongoing trials.[104]

Since then, the DANCAVAS (Five-Year Outcomes of the Danish Cardiovascular Screening) trial[105] evaluated all-cause mortality, MACE, and cost effectiveness from a societal perspective related to comprehensive cardiovascular screening (including CAC scoring) among men 65 to 74 years of age in Denmark. The trial showed that randomization to cardiac CT led to an 11% decreased risk of all-cause mortality in men <70 years old (HR 0.89; 95% CI 0.83–0.96), no increase in downstream revascularization (HR 0.93; 95% CI 0.85–1.02), and that the approach was cost effective from a societal perspective. However, DANCANVAS utilized various ASCVD screening tools and, when interpreted in its entirety, these measures did not decrease all-cause mortality (HR 0.95, 95% CI 0.90 to 1.00, $p = 0.06$). A limitation of the study was the lack of enrollment of women.

CorCal (Effectiveness of a Proactive Cardiovascular Primary Prevention Strategy, With or Without the Use of Coronary Calcium Screening, in Preventing Future Major Adverse Cardiac Events; NCT03439267) is an ongoing US-based trial, expected to end in May 2026, assessing the effectiveness of a proactive cardiovascular primary prevention strategy, with or without CAC screening. The ROBINSCA (Risk Or Benefit IN Screening for CArdiovascular Diseases) trial[106] is a Dutch population-based study that aims to establish whether CAC imaging in asymptomatic individuals followed by preventive treatment will reduce CHD-related mortality and morbidity by at least 15% compared with traditional risk factor assessment after 5 years of follow-up.

PREVENTABLE is an ongoing trial randomizing approximately 15,000 patients over the age of 75 to atorvastatin 40 mg daily versus placebo. Embedded in PREVENTABLE is a blinded CAC score in approximately 6000 patients that will be used at the end of the study to determine which older patients might benefit the most from statin therapy.

FUTURE DIRECTIONS

In the near future, we anticipate major advancement in the use of deep machine learning models in contemporary practice, for detecting and informing CAC-based strategies.[104] The NOTIFY-1 Project (Incidental Coronary Artery Calcium: Opportunistic Screening of Prior Non-gated Chest CTs to Improve Statin Rates)[107] was a randomized quality improvement project of 2113 patients in the Stanford healthcare system. The objective was to evaluate the impact of notifying clinicians and patients of incidental CAC on prior clinical nongated chest CT. Patient and clinician notification of incidental CAC led to a significant increase in statin prescriptions within 6 months (51.2% in the notification arm vs. 6.9% with usual care, $P < .001$). A larger outcomes-driven NOTIFY trial is planned.

The use of deep machine learning models on noncardiac CT scans of the chest provides an opportunity to leverage imaging data that already exists with standardized and relatively faster reporting times. Deep Machine Learning (DML) models also show promise in identifying new features of calcified lesions on CAC scans that predict ASCVD risk (lesion shape, voxel attenuation heterogeneity, etc). As a particular application of the emerging field of radiomics, these patterns in coronary calcification not readily captured by the human eye are referred to as "calciumomics."

Lastly, the implementation of preexisting CAC scores in clinical databases, incidental CAC on nongated CT scans, and high CAC as a screening tool for enrollment in RCTs facilitates the assessment of high-quality evidence of efficacy for novel add-on therapies and informing a cost-effective, high-value prevention of ASCVD in highest-risk asymptomatic individuals.[108]

CONCLUSION

CAC scanning remains a simple but powerful tool with great relevance to modern practice despite its development in 1990. Contemporary guidelines endorse the use of CAC scoring, in conjunction with the PCE or PREVENT risk estimators, to restratify risk and further determine primary prevention therapies in borderline and intermediate-ASCVD-risk patients who are uncertain about their true risk and are unclear as to whether to begin pharmacologic preventive therapies. Primary prevention decisions that can be readily guided by CAC include those regarding statin therapy, LDL-C goals, nonstatin therapy, aspirin, blood pressure goals, and cardiometabolic therapies.

More recently, further guideline-supported indications for the use of CAC scoring have emerged and include: (1) identifying patients with a low likelihood of obstructive CAD use in low-risk patients presenting with stable CAD, (2) enhancing risk assessment in intermediate-high-risk patients undergoing stress testing, (3) delineating risk in younger patients and older patients, (4) informing management of statin-associated muscle symptoms, (5) predicting long-term risk of aortic stenosis and assessing aortic stenosis severity in patients with low-flow low-gradient severe aortic stenosis by echocardiography, and (6) incidental detection and appraisal of CAC severity on routine nongated chest CTs.

Future randomized trials including CorCal, ROBINSCA, and CAC PREVENTABLE are on the horizon with results expected in the next 1 to 5 years. We expect the field of CAC scanning to undergo a significant revolution in the era of deep machine learning, which can automate CAC interpretation and perhaps inform the development of a new CAC score to replace the traditional Agatston score.

REFERENCES

1. Tsao CW, Aday AW, Almarzooq ZI, et al. Heart disease and stroke statistics—2022 update: a report from the American Heart Association. 2022;145(8):e153-e639. https://doi.org/10.1161/CIR.0000000000001052.
2. Patel N, Bhargava A, Kalra R, et al. Trends in lipid, lipoproteins, and statin use among U.S. adults: impact of 2013 cholesterol guidelines. *J Am Coll Cardiol.* 2019;74(20):2525–2528. https://doi.org/10.1016/j.jacc.2019.09.026.
3. Grundy SM, Stone NJ, Bailey AL, et al. 2018 AHA/ACC/AACVPR/AAPA/ABC/ACPM/ADA/AGS/APhA/ASPC/NLA/PCNA guideline on the management of blood cholesterol: a report of the American College of Cardiology/American Heart Association Task Force on clinical practice guidelines. *Circulation.* 2019;139(25):e1082–e1143. https://doi.org/10.1161/CIR.0000000000000625.
4. Whelton SP, Blaha MJ. Coronary artery calcium: from risk prediction to treatment allocation and clinical trials. *Heart.* 2023;109(22):1714–1721. https://doi.org/10.1136/heartjnl-2022-321711.
5. Orringer CE, Blaha MJ, Blankstein R, et al. The National Lipid Association scientific statement on coronary artery calcium scoring to guide preventive strategies for ASCVD risk reduction. *J Clin Lipidol.* 2021;15(1):33–60. https://doi.org/10.1016/j.jacl.2020.12.005.
6. Lloyd-Jones DM, Braun LT, Ndumele CE, et al. Use of risk assessment tools to guide decision-making in the primary prevention of atherosclerotic cardiovascular disease: a special report from the American Heart Association and American College of Cardiology. *J Am Coll Cardiol.* 2019;73(24):3153–3167. https://doi.org/10.1016/j.jacc.2018.11.005.
7. Hecht HS, Cronin P, Blaha MJ, et al. 2016 SCCT/STR guidelines for coronary artery calcium scoring of noncontrast noncardiac chest CT scans: a report of the Society of Cardiovascular Computed Tomography and Society of Thoracic Radiology. *J Cardiovasc Comput Tomogr.* 2017;11(1):74–84. https://doi.org/10.1016/j.jcct.2016.11.003.
8. Gulati M, Levy PD, Mukherjee D, et al. 2021 AHA/ACC/ASE/CHEST/SAEM/SCCT/SCMR guideline for the evaluation and diagnosis of chest pain: a report of the American College of Cardiology/American Heart Association Joint Committee on clinical practice guidelines. *Circulation.* 2021;144(22):e368–e454. https://doi.org/10.1161/cir.0000000000001029.
9. Otsuka F, Sakakura K, Yahagi K, Joner M, Virmani R. Has our understanding of calcification in human coronary atherosclerosis progressed? *Arterioscler Thromb Vasc Biol.* 2014;34(4):724–736. https://doi.org/10.1161/ATVBAHA.113.302642.
10. Stary HC, Chandler AB, Dinsmore RE, et al. A definition of advanced types of atherosclerotic lesions and a histological classification of atherosclerosis. A report from the Committee on Vascular Lesions of the Council on Arteriosclerosis, American Heart Association. *Arterioscler Thromb Vasc Biol.* 1995;15(9):1512–1531. https://doi.org/10.1161/01.atv.15.9.1512.
11. Stary HC, Chandler AB, Glagov S, et al. A definition of initial, fatty streak, and intermediate lesions of atherosclerosis. A report from the Committee on Vascular Lesions of the Council on Arteriosclerosis, American Heart Association. *Circulation.* 1994;89(5):2462–2478. https://doi.org/10.1161/01.cir.89.5.2462.
12. Tintut Y, Alfonso Z, Saini T, et al. Multilineage potential of cells from the artery wall. *Circulation.* 2003;108(20):2505–2510. https://doi.org/10.1161/01.CIR.0000096485.64373.C5.
13. Sandfort V, Lima JAC, Bluemke DA. Noninvasive imaging of atherosclerotic plaque progression. *Cir Cardiovasc Imaging.* 2015;8(7):e003316. https://doi.org/10.1161/CIRCIMAGING.115.003316.
14. Rumberger JA, Simons DB, Fitzpatrick LA, Sheedy PF, Schwartz RS. Coronary artery calcium area by electron-beam computed tomography and coronary atherosclerotic plaque area. A histopathologic correlative study. *Circulation.* 1995;92(8):2157–2162. https://doi.org/10.1161/01.cir.92.8.2157.
15. Bartel AG, Chen JT, Peter RH, Behar VS, Kong Y, Lester RG. The significance of coronary calcification detected by fluoroscopy. A report of 360 patients. *Circulation.* 1974;49(6):1247–1253. https://doi.org/10.1161/01.CIR.49.6.1247.
16. Detrano R, Markovic D, Simpfendorfer C, et al. Digital subtraction fluoroscopy: a new method of detecting coronary calcifications with improved sensitivity for the prediction of coronary disease. *Circulation.* 1985;71(4):725–732. https://doi.org/10.1161/01.CIR.71.4.725.
17. Margolis JR, Chen JT, Kong Y, Peter RH, Behar VS, Kisslo JA. The diagnostic and prognostic significance of coronary artery calcification. A report of 800 cases. 1980;137(3):609-616. https://doi.org/10.1148/radiology.137.3.7444045
18. Mao SS, Pal RS, McKay CR, et al. Comparison of coronary artery calcium scores between electron beam computed tomography and 64-multidetector computed tomographic scanner. *J Comput Assist Tomogr.* 2009;33(2):175–178. https://doi.org/10.1097/RCT.0b013e31817579ee.
19. Yeboah J, Young R, McClelland RL, et al. Utility of nontraditional risk markers in atherosclerotic cardiovascular disease risk assessment. *J Am Coll Cardiol.* 2016;67(2):139–147. https://doi.org/10.1016/j.jacc.2015.10.058.
20. Goff DC, Lloyd-Jones DM, Bennett G, et al. 2013 ACC/AHA guideline on the assessment of cardiovascular risk: a report of the American College of Cardiology/American Heart Association Task Force on practice guidelines. *J Am Coll Cardiol.* 2014;63(25, Part B):2935–2959. https://doi.org/10.1016/j.jacc.2013.11.005.
21. McClelland RL, Chung H, Detrano R, Post W, Kronmal RA. Distribution of coronary artery calcium by race, gender, and age. 2006;113(1):30-37. https://doi.org/10.1161/CIRCULATIONAHA.105.580696
22. Hecht HS, Blaha MJ, Kazerooni EA, et al. CAC-DRS: coronary artery calcium data and reporting system. An expert consensus document of the Society of Cardiovascular Computed Tomography (SCCT). *J Cardiovasc Comput Tomogr.* 2018;12(3):185–191. https://doi.org/10.1016/j.jcct.2018.03.008.
23. Gupta A, Bera K, Kikano E, et al. Coronary artery calcium scoring: current status and future directions. *Radiographics.* 2022;42(4):947–967. https://doi.org/10.1148/rg.210122.
24. Chiles C, Duan F, Gladish GW, et al. Association of coronary artery calcification and mortality in the national lung screening trial: a comparison of three scoring methods. *Radiology.* 2015;276(1):82–90. https://doi.org/10.1148/radiol.15142062.

25. Orringer CE, Maki KC. HOPE for rational statin allocation for primary prevention: a coronary artery calcium picture is worth 1000 words. *Mayo Clin Proc*. 2020;95(8):1740–1749. https://doi.org/10.1016/j.mayocp.2020.01.016.
26. Messenger B, Li D, Nasir K, Carr JJ, Blankstein R, Budoff MJ. Coronary calcium scans and radiation exposure in the multi-ethnic study of atherosclerosis. *Int J Cardiovasc Imaging*. 2016;32(3):525–529. https://doi.org/10.1007/s10554-015-0799-3.
27. Patel AA, Fine J, Naghavi M, Budoff MJ. Radiation exposure and coronary artery calcium scans in the society for heart attack prevention and eradication cohort. *Int J Cardiovasc Imaging*. 2019;35(1):179–183. https://doi.org/10.1007/s10554-018-1431-0.
28. Mortensen MB, Blaha MJ. Is there a role of coronary CTA in primary prevention? Current state and future directions. *Curr Atheroscler Rep*. 2021;23(8):44. https://doi.org/10.1007/s11883-021-00943-2.
29. Nasir K, Cainzos-Achirica M, Valero-Elizondo J, et al. Coronary atherosclerosis in an asymptomatic U.S. population. *JACC Cardiovasc Imaging*. 2022;15(9):1604–1618. https://doi.org/10.1016/j.jcmg.2022.03.010.
30. Bergström G, Persson M, Adiels M, et al. Prevalence of subclinical coronary artery atherosclerosis in the general population. *Circulation*. 2021;144(12):916–929. https://doi.org/10.1161/circulationaha.121.055340.
31. Douglas PS, Hoffmann U, Patel MR, et al. Outcomes of anatomical versus functional testing for coronary artery disease. *N Engl J Med*. 2015;372(14):1291–1300. https://doi.org/10.1056/NEJMoa1415516.
32. van Werkhoven JM, de Boer SM, Schuijf JD, et al. Impact of clinical presentation and pretest likelihood on the relation between calcium score and computed tomographic coronary angiography. *Am J Cardiol*. 2010;106(12):1675–1679. https://doi.org/10.1016/j.amjcard.2010.08.014.
33. Cho I, Al'Aref SJ, Berger A, et al. Prognostic value of coronary computed tomographic angiography findings in asymptomatic individuals: a 6-year follow-up from the prospective multicentre international CONFIRM study. *Eur Heart J*. 2018;39(11):934–941. https://doi.org/10.1093/eurheartj/ehx774.
34. Greenland P, LaBree L, Azen SP, Doherty TM, Detrano RC. Coronary artery calcium score combined with Framingham score for risk prediction in asymptomatic individuals. *JAMA*. 2004;291(2):210–215. https://doi.org/10.1001/jama.291.2.210.
35. Arad Y, Goodman KJ, Roth M, Newstein D, Guerci AD. Coronary calcification, coronary disease risk factors, C-reactive protein, and atherosclerotic cardiovascular disease events: the St. Francis heart study. *J Am Coll Cardiol*. 2005;46(1):158–165. https://doi.org/10.1016/j.jacc.2005.02.088.
36. Bild DE, Detrano R, Peterson D, et al. Ethnic differences in coronary calcification. *Circulation*. 2005;111(10):1313–1320. https://doi.org/10.1161/01.CIR.0000157730.94423.4B.
37. Erbel R, Delaney JAC, Lehmann N, et al. Signs of subclinical coronary atherosclerosis in relation to risk factor distribution in the Multi-Ethnic Study of Atherosclerosis (MESA) and the Heinz Nixdorf Recall Study (HNR). *Eur Heart J*. 2008;29(22):2782–2791. https://doi.org/10.1093/eurheartj/ehn439.
38. Hofman A, Brusselle GGO, Murad SD, et al. The Rotterdam study: 2016 objectives and design update. *Eur J Epidemiol*. 2015;30(8):661–708. https://doi.org/10.1007/s10654-015-0082-x.
39. Ferencik M, Pencina KM, Liu T, et al. Coronary artery calcium distribution is an independent predictor of incident major coronary heart disease events. *Circ Cardiovasc Imaging*. 2017;10(10):e006592. https://doi.org/10.1161/CIRCIMAGING.117.006592.
40. Cruz DE, Tahir UA, Hu J, et al. Metabolomic analysis of Coronary heart disease in an African American Cohort from the Jackson Heart study. *JAMA Cardiol*. 2022;7(2):184–194. https://doi.org/10.1001/jamacardio.2021.4925.
41. Okwuosa TM, Greenland P, Ning H, Liu K, Lloyd-Jones DM. Yield of screening for coronary artery calcium in early middle-age adults based on the 10-year framingham risk score: the CARDIA study. *JACC Cardiovasc Imaging*. 2012;5(9):923–930. https://doi.org/10.1016/j.jcmg.2012.01.022.
42. Blaha MJ, Whelton SP, Al Rifai M, et al. Rationale and design of the coronary artery calcium consortium: a multicenter cohort study. *J Cardiovasc Comput Tomogr*. 2017;11(1):54–61. https://doi.org/10.1016/j.jcct.2016.11.004.
43. Williams O. The Atherosclerosis Risk in Communities (ARIC) study-design and objectives. *Am J Epidemiol*. 1989;129(4):687–702.
44. Mok Y, Honda Y, Wang FM, et al. Coronary artery calcification and one-year cardiovascular disease incidence in the 75-and-older population: the ARIC study. *Circ Cardiovasc Imaging*. 2023;16(6):e015026. https://doi.org/10.1161/circimaging.122.015026.
45. Orimoloye OA, Budoff MJ, Dardari ZA, et al. Race/ethnicity and the prognostic implications of coronary artery calcium for All-cause and cardiovascular disease mortality: the coronary artery calcium consortium. *J Am Heart Assoc*. 2018;7(20):e010471. https://doi.org/10.1161/JAHA.118.010471.
46. Nasir K, Shaw LJ, Liu ST, et al. Ethnic differences in the prognostic value of coronary artery calcification for all-cause mortality. *J Am Coll Cardiol*. 2007;50(10):953–960. https://doi.org/10.1016/j.jacc.2007.03.066.
47. Kanaya AM, Kandula NR, Ewing SK, et al. Comparing coronary artery calcium among U.S. South Asians with four racial/ethnic groups: the MASALA and MESA studies. *Atherosclerosis*. 2014;234(1):102–107. https://doi.org/10.1016/j.atherosclerosis.2014.02.017.
48. Nasir K, Bittencourt MS, Blaha MJ, et al. Implications of coronary artery calcium testing among statin candidates according to American College of Cardiology/American Heart Association cholesterol management guidelines: MESA (Multi-Ethnic Study of Atherosclerosis). *J Am Coll Cardiol*. 2015;66(15):1657–1668. https://doi.org/10.1016/j.jacc.2015.07.066.
49. Grant JK, Orringer CE. Coronary and extra-coronary subclinical atherosclerosis to guide lipid-lowering therapy. *Curr Atheroscler Rep*. 2023;25(12):911–920. https://doi.org/10.1007/s11883-023-01161-8.
50. Bytyçi I, Penson PE, Mikhailidis DP, et al. Prevalence of statin intolerance: a meta-analysis. *Eur Heart J*. 2022;43(34):3213–3223. https://doi.org/10.1093/eurheartj/ehac015.
51. Serban MC, Colantonio LD, Manthripragada AD, et al. Statin intolerance and risk of coronary heart events and all-cause mortality following myocardial infarction. *J Am Coll Cardiol*. 2017;69(11):1386–1395. https://doi.org/10.1016/j.jacc.2016.12.036.
52. Orringer CE, Blaha MJ, Stone NJ. Coronary artery calcium scoring in patients with statin associated muscle symptoms: prescribing statins for those most likely to benefit. *J Clin Lipidol*. 2021;15(6):782–788. https://doi.org/10.1016/j.jacl.2021.09.052.
53. Shareghi S, Ahmadi N, Young E, Gopal A, Liu ST, Budoff MJ. Prognostic significance of zero coronary calcium scores on cardiac computed tomography. *J Cardiovasc Comput Tomogr*. 2007;1(3):155–159. https://doi.org/10.1016/j.jcct.2007.10.001.
54. Dzaye O, Dardari ZA, Cainzos-Achirica M, et al. Incidence of new coronary calcification: time to conversion from CAC = 0. *J Am Coll Cardiol*. 2020;75(13):1610–1613. https://doi.org/10.1016/j.jacc.2020.01.047.
55. Dzaye O, Dardari ZA, Cainzos-Achirica M, et al. Warranty period of a calcium score of zero: comprehensive analysis from MESA. *JACC Cardiovasc Imaging*. 2021;14(5):990–1002. https://doi.org/10.1016/j.jcmg.2020.06.048.
56. Lee S-E, Chang H-J, Sung JM, et al. Effects of statins on coronary atherosclerotic plaques: the PARADIGM study. *JACC Cardiovasc Imaging*. 2018;11(10):1475–1484. https://doi.org/10.1016/j.jcmg.2018.04.015.
57. Puri R, Nicholls SJ, Shao M, et al. Impact of statins on serial coronary calcification during atheroma progression and regression. *J Am Coll Cardiol*. 2015;65(13):1273–1282. https://doi.org/10.1016/j.jacc.2015.01.036.
58. Maldonado N, Kelly-Arnold A, Vengrenyuk Y, et al. A mechanistic analysis of the role of microcalcifications in atherosclerotic plaque stability: potential implications for plaque rupture. *Am J Physiol Heart Circ Physiol*. 2012;303(5):H619–H628. https://doi.org/10.1152/ajpheart.00036.2012.
59. McClelland RL, Jorgensen NW, Budoff M, et al. 10-year coronary heart disease risk prediction using coronary artery calcium and traditional risk factors: derivation in the MESA (Multi-Ethnic study of atherosclerosis) with validation in the HNR (Heinz Nixdorf Recall) study and the DHS (Dallas heart study). *J Am Coll Cardiol*. 2015;66(15):1643–1653. https://doi.org/10.1016/j.jacc.2015.08.035.
60. McClelland RL, Chung H, Detrano R, Post W, Kronmal RA. Distribution of coronary artery calcium by race, gender, and age: results from the Multi-Ethnic Study of Atherosclerosis (MESA). *Circulation*. 2006;113(1):30–37. https://doi.org/10.1161/circulationaha.105.580696.
61. Blaha MJ, Naazie IN, Cainzos-Achirica M, et al. Derivation of a coronary age calculator using traditional risk factors and coronary artery calcium: the multi-ethnic study of atherosclerosis. *J Am Heart Assoc*. 2021;10(6):e019351. https://doi.org/10.1161/JAHA.120.019351.
62. Carr JJ, Jacobs Jr DR, Terry JG, et al. Association of coronary artery calcium in adults aged 32 to 46 years with incident coronary heart disease and death. *JAMA Cardiol*. 2017;2(4):391–399. https://doi.org/10.1001/jamacardio.2016.5493.
63. Javaid A, Dardari Zeina A, Mitchell Joshua D, et al. Distribution of coronary artery calcium by age, sex, and race among patients 30–45 years old. *J Am Coll Cardiol*. 2022;79(19):1873–1886 & CAC percentile calculator. https://doi.org/10.1056/NEJMoa1804988.
64. Bowman L, Mafham M, Wallendszus K, et al. Effects of aspirin for primary prevention in persons with diabetes mellitus. *N Engl J Med*. 2018;379(16):1529–1539. https://doi.org/10.1056/NEJMoa1804988.
65. Gaziano JM, Brotons C, Coppolecchia R, et al. Use of aspirin to reduce risk of initial vascular events in patients at moderate risk of cardiovascular disease (ARRIVE): a randomised, double-blind, placebo-controlled trial. *Lancet*. 2018;392(10152):1036–1046. https://doi.org/10.1016/s0140-6736(18)31924-x.
66. McNeil JJ, Woods RL, Nelson MR, et al. Effect of aspirin on disability-free survival in the healthy elderly. *N Engl J Med*. 2018;379(16):1499–1508. https://doi.org/10.1056/NEJMoa1800722.
67. Lloyd-Jones DM. USPSTF report on aspirin for primary prevention. *JAMA Cardiol*. 2022;7(7):667–669. https://doi.org/10.1001/jamacardio.2022.0935.
68. Arnett DK, Blumenthal RS, Albert MA, et al. 2019 ACC/AHA guideline on the primary prevention of cardiovascular disease: executive summary: a report of the American College of Cardiology/American Heart Association Task Force on clinical practice guidelines. *Circulation*. 2019;140(11):e563–e595. https://doi.org/10.1161/CIR.0000000000000677.
69. Cainzos-Achirica M, Miedema MD, McEvoy JW, et al. Coronary artery calcium for personalized allocation of aspirin in primary prevention of cardiovascular disease in 2019. *Circulation*. 2020;141(19):1541–1553. https://doi.org/10.1161/CIRCULATIONAHA.119.045010.
70. Ajufo E, Ayers CR, Vigen R, et al. Value of coronary artery calcium scanning in association with the net benefit of aspirin in primary prevention of atherosclerotic cardiovascular disease. *JAMA Cardiol*. 2021;6(2):179–187. https://doi.org/10.1001/jamacardio.2020.4939.
71. Malik S, Zhao Y, Budoff M, et al. Coronary artery calcium score for long-term risk classification in individuals with type 2 diabetes and metabolic syndrome from the Multi-Ethnic study of atherosclerosis. *JAMA Cardiol*. 2017;2(12):1332–1340. https://doi.org/10.1001/jamacardio.2017.4191.

72. Valenti V, Hartaigh Bó, Cho I, et al. Absence of coronary artery calcium identifies asymptomatic diabetic individuals at low near-term but not long-term risk of mortality. *Circ Cardiovasc Imaging*. 2016;9(2):e003528. https://doi.org/10.1161/CIRCIMAGING.115.003528.
73. Lloyd-Jones DM, Morris PB, Ballantyne CM, et al. 2017 focused update of the 2016 ACC expert consensus decision pathway on the role of non-statin therapies for LDL-cholesterol lowering in the management of atherosclerotic cardiovascular disease risk. *J Am Coll Cardiol*. 2017;70(14):1785–1822. https://doi.org/10.1016/j.jacc.2017.07.745.
74. Boakye E, Grandhi GR, Dardari Z, et al. Cardiovascular risk stratification among individuals with obesity: the Coronary artery calcium consortium. *Obesity*. 2023;31(9):2240–2248. https://doi.org/10.1002/oby.23832.
75. Cainzos-Achirica M, Patel Kershaw V, Quispe R, et al. Coronary artery calcium for the allocation of GLP-1RA for primary prevention of atherosclerotic cardiovascular disease. *JACC Cardiovasc Imaging*. 2021;14(7):1470–1472. https://doi.org/10.1016/j.jcmg.2020.12.024.
76. Peng AW, Dardari ZA, Blumenthal RS, et al. Very high coronary artery calcium (≥1000) and association with cardiovascular disease events, non–cardiovascular disease outcomes, and mortality. *Circulation*. 2021;143(16):1571–1583. https://doi.org/10.1161/CIRCULATIONAHA.120.050545.
77. Peng AW, Mirbolouk M, Orimoloye OA, et al. Long-term all-cause and cause-specific mortality in asymptomatic patients with CAC ≥1,000: results from the CAC consortium. *JACC Cardiovasc Imaging*. 2020;13(1, Part 1):83–93. https://doi.org/10.1016/j.jcmg.2019.02.005.
78. Sabatine MS, Giugliano RP, Keech AC, et al. Evolocumab and clinical outcomes in patients with cardiovascular disease. *N Engl J Med*. 2017;376(18):1713–1722. https://doi.org/10.1056/NEJMoa1615664.
79. Cainzos-Achirica M, Quispe R, Mszar R, et al. Coronary artery calcium score to refine the use of PCSK9i in asymptomatic individuals: a Multicohort study. *J Am Heart Assoc*. 2022;11(16):e025737. https://doi.org/10.1161/jaha.122.025737.
80. Uddin SMI, Mirbolouk M, Kianoush S, et al. Role of coronary artery calcium for stratifying cardiovascular risk in adults with hypertension. *Hypertension*. 2019;73(5):983–989. https://doi.org/10.1161/hypertensionaha.118.12266.
81. McEvoy JW, Martin SS, Dardari ZA, et al. Coronary artery calcium to guide a personalized risk-based approach to initiation and intensification of antihypertensive therapy. *Circulation*. 2017;135(2):153–165. https://doi.org/10.1161/circulationaha.116.025471.
82. Gulati M, Levy PD, Mukherjee D, et al. 2021 AHA/ACC/ASE/CHEST/SAEM/SCCT/SCMR guideline for the evaluation and diagnosis of chest pain: a report of the American College of Cardiology/American Heart Association Joint Committee on clinical practice guidelines. *Circulation*. 2021;144(22):e368–e454. https://doi.org/10.1161/CIR.0000000000001029.
83. Cardoso R, Shaw LJ, Blumenthal RS, et al. Preventive cardiology advances in the 2021 AHA/ACC chest pain guideline. *Am J Prev Cardiol*. 2022;11:100365. https://doi.org/10.1016/j.ajpc.2022.100365.
84. Sarwar A, Shaw LJ, Shapiro MD, et al. Diagnostic and prognostic value of absence of coronary artery calcification. *JACC Cardiovasc Imaging*. 2009;2(6):675–688. https://doi.org/10.1016/j.jcmg.2008.12.031.
85. Agha AM, Pacor J, Grandhi GR, et al. The prognostic value of CAC zero among individuals presenting with chest pain: a meta-analysis. *JACC Cardiovasc Imaging*. 2022;15(10):1745–1757. https://doi.org/10.1016/j.jcmg.2022.03.031.
86. Berman DS, Wong ND, Gransar H, et al. Relationship between stress-induced myocardial ischemia and atherosclerosis measured by coronary calcium tomography. *J Am Coll Cardiol*. 2004;44(4):923–930. https://doi.org/10.1016/j.jacc.2004.06.042.
87. Munden RF, Carter BW, Chiles C, et al. Managing incidental findings on thoracic CT: mediastinal and cardiovascular findings. A white paper of the ACR Incidental Findings Committee. *J Am Coll Radiol*. 2018;15(8):1087–1096. https://doi.org/10.1016/j.jacr.2018.04.029.
88. Hughes-Austin JM, Dominguez 3rd A, Allison MA, et al. Relationship of coronary calcium on standard chest CT scans with mortality. *JACC Cardiovasc Imaging*. 2016;9(2):152–159. https://doi.org/10.1016/j.jcmg.2015.06.030.
89. Garcia EV. SPECT attenuation correction: an essential tool to realize nuclear cardiology's manifest destiny. *J Nucl Cardiol*. 2007;14(1):16–24. https://doi.org/10.1016/j.nuclcard.2006.12.144.
90. O'Connor MK, Kemp B, Anstett F, et al. A multicenter evaluation of commercial attenuation compensation techniques in cardiac SPECT using phantom models. *J Nucl Cardiol*. 2002;9(4):361–376. https://doi.org/10.1067/mnc.2002.122676.
91. Chang SM, Nabi F, Xu J, et al. The coronary artery calcium score and stress myocardial perfusion imaging provide independent and complementary prediction of cardiac risk. *J Am Coll Cardiol*. 2009;54(20):1872–1882. https://doi.org/10.1016/j.jacc.2009.05.071.
92. Engbers EM, Timmer JR, Ottervanger JP, Mouden M, Knollema S, Jager PL. Prognostic value of coronary artery calcium scoring in addition to single-photon emission computed tomographic myocardial perfusion imaging in symptomatic patients. *Circ Cardiovasc Imaging*. 2016;9(5):e003966. https://doi.org/10.1161/CIRCIMAGING.115.003966.
93. Einstein AJ, Johnson LL, Bokhari S, et al. Agreement of visual estimation of coronary artery calcium from low-dose CT attenuation correction scans in hybrid PET/CT and SPECT/CT with standard agatston score. *J Am Coll Cardiol*. 2010;56(23):1914–1921. https://doi.org/10.1016/j.jacc.2010.05.057.
94. Mouden M, Jager PL, van Dalen JA, van Dijk JD. Added value of coronary artery calcium score in the reporting of SPECT versus PET myocardial perfusion imaging. *J Nucl Cardiol*. 2022;29(5):2448–2456. https://doi.org/10.1007/s12350-021-02789-2.
95. Pawade T, Sheth T, Guzzetti E, Dweck MR, Clavel M-A. Why and how to measure aortic valve calcification in patients with aortic stenosis. *JACC Cardiovasc Imaging*. 2019;12(9):1835–1848. https://doi.org/10.1016/j.jcmg.2019.01.045.
96. Whelton SP, Jha K, Dardari Z, et al. Prevalence of aortic valve calcium and the long-term risk of incident severe aortic stenosis. *JACC Cardiovasc Imaging*. 2024;17(1):31–42. https://doi.org/10.1016/j.jcmg.2023.02.018.
97. Otto CM, Nishimura RA, Bonow RO, et al. 2020 ACC/AHA guideline for the management of patients with valvular heart disease: a report of the American College of Cardiology/American Heart Association Joint Committee on clinical practice guidelines. *J Am Coll Cardiol*. 2021;77(4):e25–e197. https://doi.org/10.1016/j.jacc.2020.11.018.
98. Tison GH, Guo M, Blaha MJ, et al. Multisite extracoronary calcification indicates increased risk of coronary heart disease and all-cause mortality: the Multi-Ethnic study of atherosclerosis. *J Cardiovasc Comput Tomogr*. 2015;9(5):406–414. https://doi.org/10.1016/j.jcct.2015.03.012.
99. Nasir K, Bittencourt MS, Blaha MJ, et al. Implications of coronary artery calcium testing among statin candidates according to American College of Cardiology/American Heart Association cholesterol management guidelines MESA (Multi-Ethnic study of atherosclerosis). *J Am Coll Cardiol*. 2015;66(15):1657–1668. https://doi.org/10.1016/j.jacc.2015.07.066.
100. Hong Jonathan C, Blankstein R, Shaw Leslee J, et al. Implications of coronary artery calcium testing for treatment decisions among statin candidates according to the ACC/AHA cholesterol management guidelines. *JACC Cardiovasc Imaging*. 2017;10(8):938–952. https://doi.org/10.1016/j.jcmg.2017.04.014.
101. Arad Y, Spadaro LA, Roth M, Newstein D, Guerci AD. Treatment of asymptomatic adults with elevated coronary calcium scores with atorvastatin, vitamin C, and vitamin E: the St. Francis heart study randomized clinical trial. *J Am Coll Cardiol*. 2005;46(1):166–172. https://doi.org/10.1016/j.jacc.2005.02.089.
102. Rozanski A, Gransar H, Shaw LJ, et al. Impact of coronary artery calcium scanning on coronary risk factors and downstream testing: the EISNER (Early Identification of Subclinical Atherosclerosis by Noninvasive Imaging Research) prospective randomized trial. *J Am Coll Cardiol*. 2011;57(15):1622–1632. https://doi.org/10.1016/j.jacc.2011.01.019.
103. McEvoy JW, Martin SS, Blaha MJ, et al. The case for and against a coronary artery calcium trial: means, motive, and opportunity. *JACC Cardiovasc Imaging*. 2016;9(8):994–1002. https://doi.org/10.1016/j.jcmg.2016.03.012.
104. Greenland P, Michos Erin D, Redmond N, et al. Primary prevention trial designs using coronary imaging. *JACC Cardiovasc Imaging*. 2021;14(7):1454–1465. https://doi.org/10.1016/j.jcmg.2020.06.042.
105. Lindholt JS, Søgaard R, Rasmussen LM, et al. Five-year outcomes of the danish cardiovascular screening (DANCAVAS) trial. *N Engl J Med*. 2022;387(15):1385–1394. https://doi.org/10.1056/NEJMoa2208681.
106. Vonder M, van der Aalst CM, Vliegenthart R, et al. Coronary artery calcium imaging in the ROBINSCA trial: rationale, design, and technical background. *Acad Radiol*. 2018;25(1):118–128. https://doi.org/10.1016/j.acra.2017.07.010.
107. Sandhu AT, Rodriguez F, Ngo S, et al. Incidental coronary artery calcium: opportunistic screening of prior non-gated chest CTs to improve statin rates (NOTIFY-1 project). *Circulation*. 2023;147(9):703–714. https://doi.org/10.1161/CIRCULATIONAHA.122.062746.
108. Cainzos-Achirica M, Anugula D, Mszar R, et al. Rationale and pathways forward in the implementation of coronary artery calcium-based enrichment of randomized trials. *Am Heart J*. 2022;243:54–65. https://doi.org/10.1016/j.ahj.2021.09.006.
109. Budoff MJ, Kinninger A, Gransar H, et al. When does a calcium score equate to secondary prevention? Insights from the Multinational CONFIRM registry. *JACC Cardiovasc Imaging*. 2023;16(9):1181–1189. https://doi.org/10.1016/j.jcmg.2023.03.008.

4 Coronary Computed Tomography Angiography for Primary Prevention

DAVID E. NEWBY AND MATTHEW J. BUDOFF

KEY POINTS

- Based on expert opinion, primary prevention of cardiovascular disease is currently guided by cardiovascular risk scores, but this approach can lead to substantial under- and overtreatment.
- Coronary computed tomography angiography provides a noninvasive method of screening for the presence of coronary artery disease.
- Coronary computed tomography angiography has the potential to improve compliance with medication and promote uptake of positive lifestyle choices to improve clinical outcomes, but this has yet to be established.

INTRODUCTION

Cardiovascular disease is the commonest cause of death worldwide. The World Health Organization (WHO) estimates that nearly 18 million people die from cardiovascular disease each year. Since 1990, more people have died from cardiovascular disease than any other cause. Importantly, more than 75% of these deaths occur in low- or middle-income countries, and over 85% are attributable to myocardial infarction or stroke.

For the majority of people, acute fatal or nonfatal myocardial infarction is the first manifestation of coronary heart disease. The absence of antecedent symptoms means that there is little opportunity to intervene or to prevent the occurrence of these fatal or nonfatal coronary heart disease events. This has led to the concept of primary prevention of coronary heart disease. Primary prevention is restricted to people who have no symptoms or clinical manifestations of coronary heart disease and is often targeted at modifying lifestyle and risk factors with the aim of preventing or delaying the onset of coronary heart disease. Secondary prevention refers to people who have already developed angina or had a myocardial infarction, and the focus is to prevent recurrent events and to decrease coronary heart disease mortality. This distinction is, however, becoming increasingly less clear, especially with the more widespread use of coronary computed tomography angiography. In particular, identification of coronary artery disease by coronary computed tomography angiography in patients either without symptoms or symptoms that are not attributable to coronary heart disease does lead to the question of whether they should be considered for primary or secondary prevention. Some have argued that coronary computed tomography angiography has demonstrated that such people have preexisting and established coronary heart disease, whereas others have maintained that a qualifying clinical event is still required before they should be considered for secondary prevention. This nuance does have implications for the interpretation and application of current primary and secondary prevention guidelines, although these recommendations were established prior to the widespread use of coronary computed tomography angiography. It will be interesting to see whether the distinction between primary and secondary prevention continues to add value with more widespread screening for coronary heart disease and whether we should now use the term *prevention* without further qualification.

PRIMARY PREVENTION GUIDELINES

Population

Current primary prevention guidelines do not recommend unselected population cardiovascular risk assessment but opportunistic or systematic assessments in people over 40 years with at least one cardiovascular risk factor. North American guidelines (American College of Cardiology/American Heart Association Guideline, 2019) restrict this to individuals aged below 75 years, whereas the National Institute of Health and Care Excellence guidelines have an age limit of 85 years[1] and the European guidelines (European Society of Cardiology Guideline, 2019) do not have an upper age limit. Younger people (20 to 39 years) can be considered for assessment of cardiovascular risk, but this is not routinely recommended.

Cardiovascular Risk Scores

Given the absence of symptoms for most patients who develop cardiovascular disease, cardiovascular risk scores were developed to identify those at greatest risk of a clinical event. This provides a logical basis upon which to guide cardiovascular risk factor management and to initiate targeted preventive therapies in those at greatest risk rather than treat the entire population. They are based on known cardiovascular risk factors although many do not incorporate all risk factors, such as family history, social deprivation, or inflammatory disorders. The thresholds for treatment are also debated, but over time, treatment thresholds have declined and commonly have moved to around a 10% 10-year risk of a cardiovascular event. However, despite the near universal adoption of these guidelines and cardiovascular risk scores, there are a number of significant problems associated with their use.

The dominance of age for risk prediction is important. The incidence of cardiovascular disease is very dependent on age and so risk scores tend to overtreat older patients and undertreat younger patients. Indeed, most patients who suffer a myocardial infarction below the age of 50 years would not have qualified for preventive therapies prior to the event.[2] Conversely, nearly all males over the age of 60 years would qualify for preventive therapy irrespective of the presence of a cardiovascular risk factor.[3] Ultimately, the performance of risk scores is modest with an overall accuracy or c-statistic of around 0.75.[4] Moreover, risk scores need constant updating due to the changing incidence of population-level cardiovascular events as well as the need for its calibration to the population to which it is being applied.[5] Cardiovascular risk scores often perform less well in underserved and ethnically diverse populations.

The implementation and acceptability of cardiovascular risk scores needs to be considered. Most cardiovascular risk scores require healthcare resource through medical consultation and clinical biochemistry assessments of risk factor profiles. This can generate considerable cost and resource requirements when systematic cardiovascular risk assessments are employed at a population level. For the individual patient, understanding and engagement with an estimated 10-year or lifetime cardiovascular risk can be challenging. Indeed, over two-thirds of patients who have an estimated risk above recommended treatment thresholds decline the use of preventive therapies.[3] Moreover, in those who are prescribed medication, only approximately half of individuals adhere to, and persist with, long-term prescriptions of these therapies.[6]

Cardiovascular risks scores have a grade 1 recommendation in both North American and European guidelines.[7,8] However, the level of evidence is grade C consistent with the fact that risk-based assessments have little evidence to support their use and guideline recommendations are based on modeling and empirical expert consensus. Indeed, a Cochrane systematic review of nearly 100,000 participants concluded that cardiovascular disease risk scores may have little or no effect on cardiovascular disease events compared with usual care (event rates of 5.4% versus 5.3%; relative risk 1.01, 95% CI 0.95–1.08).[9] This begs the question of whether there is more we can do to improve our approach to cardiovascular risk assessments and whether an approach of screening for the disease would be more appropriate given the high prevalence of coronary heart disease in the general population.

Screening for Heart Disease

The rationale for screening for heart disease should follow the same concepts as screening for other diseases that are deadly, treatable, and prevalent. Atherosclerotic heart disease is a perfect example that meets criteria for screening. It has a long incubation period, an easily identifiable early-stage lesion (coronary atherosclerotic plaque), and clinical responses to treatment once the lesion is identified. We routinely screen for other diseases, such as breast and colon cancer, yet at least 10-fold more die from coronary heart disease and stroke each year than these other diseases.[10] Coronary heart disease is a preventable disease and kills 600,000 people a year in the United States, and the rates of coronary heart disease are rising. The concept of prevention consists of periodic screening, and that is entirely possible with coronary artery calcium scoring and coronary computed tomography angiography. Recent guidelines issued by the American Cancer Society recommend screening for colon cancer beginning at age 45 years and repeating the procedure every 5 to 10 years, dependent upon individual cancer risk and findings at colonoscopy. Yet guidelines for routine use of coronary computed tomography angiography to screen for early heart disease do not yet exist.

Computed Tomography Coronary Artery Calcium Scores

The scan to determine the coronary artery calcium score is a low-radiation, noninvasive, and proven test for detecting and quantifying calcific coronary atherosclerosis. It is widely adapted by multiple societies and its use is endorsed by guidelines to better inform primary prevention treatment strategies in asymptomatic adults.[11] The development of coronary artery calcium starts at a relatively early stage of atherosclerosis and can be detected before luminal encroachment begins, with clinical data going back to the early 1990s.[12] Once identified, numerous preventive therapies can be applied, including lifestyle and drug therapies that have been shown to reduce cardiovascular events. The concept of prevention depends on reducing cardiac risk factors whose therapies can be intensified once arterial atherosclerotic plaque is identified. The 2018 American College of Cardiology/American Heart Association guidelines on the management of blood cholesterol endorsed the coronary artery calcium score as a tiebreaker in the decision to withhold, postpone, or initiate statin therapy for adults at intermediate or borderline risk of atherosclerotic cardiovascular disease.

Studies involving the coronary artery calcium scan have shown that knowledge of elevated coronary artery calcium or a score of 0 would facilitate the initiation of and long-term adherence to statins if the patient is at high risk or deferral if they are at low risk. Data from the Multi-Ethnic Study of Atherosclerosis (MESA) cohort of 5185 people were used to conclude that adding the coronary artery calcium score to the risk estimator resulted in a better prediction of atherosclerotic cardiovascular disease events.[13]

Shortcomings of Current Approaches

The risk scores used for the prediction of cardiovascular events can overestimate[14] or underestimate[15] atherosclerotic cardiovascular disease risk for certain subgroups. Thus the 2019 American College of Cardiology/American Heart Association Guideline on the Primary Prevention of Cardiovascular Disease advocates for the use of use additional risk-enhancing factors (family history of premature atherosclerotic cardiovascular disease, chronic kidney disease, chronic inflammatory conditions, etc.) to guide decisions about preventive interventions for borderline- or intermediate-risk adults. However, the value of preventive therapy may remain uncertain in this group, and some patients may be reluctant to take medical therapy without objective evidence of increased atherosclerotic cardiovascular disease risk. At the same time, the majority of atherosclerotic cardiovascular disease events occur in patients who would have otherwise been considered intermediate risk.[16] Coronary artery calcium score and coronary computed tomography angiography have emerged with a goal to improve risk prediction and potentially guide therapy in the individual patient.

Using global risk assessment tools, which are population based, ignores individual variabilities and susceptibilities to disease, duration of disease, and leads to misclassification. Traditional risk factor assessment does not fully account for the coronary risk and, in some cohorts, underestimates the prediction of risk even in patients with established risk factors for atherosclerosis. Many individuals still suffer events in the absence of established risk factors for atherosclerosis.[17] Conversely, large recent studies have demonstrated that traditional risk factors and risk assessment tools can overestimate risk in many healthier populations. The American College of Cardiology/American Heart Association Pooled Risk equation was evaluated in a large cohort of patients and demonstrated overestimation of risk (approximately fourfold higher estimated risk than observed risk) across multiple risk categories and sociodemographic subgroups. Rana et al.[18] evaluated 307,591 eligible adults without diabetes over 5 years and calculated their risk (expected) and compared it to observed events. In each predicted risk category, observed 5-year event rates were substantially lower than predicted. Similar atherosclerotic cardiovascular disease risk overestimation and poor calibration were observed in racial, ethnic, sex, and socioeconomic subgroups and among patients receiving statins. They concluded that "in a large, contemporary 'real-world' population, the American College of Cardiology/American Heart Association Pooled Cohort Risk Equation substantially overestimated actual 5-year risk in adults without diabetes, overall and across sociodemographic subgroups."

In 2009, the landmark trials by Blaha et al.[19] and Sarwar et al.[20] provided the first glimpse into the potential value of the absence of coronary artery calcium score for "de-risking" otherwise at-risk individuals. This concept was coined as the "power of zero" and is firmly supported by the fact that the absence of coronary artery calcium score is the strongest negative risk marker in clinical practice, identifying patients at very low 10-year risk. Consequently, recent American College of Cardiology/American Heart Association guidelines[11] recommended coronary artery calcium score scoring to aid in the decision-making regarding statin or aspirin initiation in borderline- or intermediate-risk patients for whom the indication to recommend therapy is unclear. The Jackson Heart study has suggested that this assessment-guided strategy using coronary artery calcium score of 0 is cost-effective as compared to initiating statin therapy in all intermediate-risk adults.[21]

Although coronary artery calcium demonstrates improvements in calibration and risk assessment and allows for personalized or individualized risk assessment, it also has significant limitations. Calcification of the coronaries represents the tip of the iceberg, and many studies have demonstrated that the calcium score correlates well with histology, autopsy, and angiographic disease burdens. Higher levels of coronary artery calcium score parallel the total coronary atheroma burden. However, coronary artery calcium score only represents one facet of atherosclerosis, and noncalcified plaque, low-attenuation plaque, and fibrous plaque are not visible on a coronary artery calcium score scan. The progression of coronary atherosclerosis, and its clinical implications, are better tracked on coronary computed tomography angiography, as coronary artery calcium score cannot assess changes in noncalcified plaque and conversion of noncalcified and high-risk plaque to calcified plaque. Further, statins increase coronary artery calcium score scores while decreasing cardiovascular events, demonstrating that regression or stabilization of plaque and changes in plaque morphology cannot be visualized by this method. The presence and location of noncalcified plaque, stenosis, and high-risk plaque features, visible on coronary computed tomography angiography, adds prognostic value and has clinical implications for the initiation and intensity of preventive therapies.

Coronary artery calcium score has many strengths, including it can be performed rapidly, in a reproducible fashion with minimal radiation exposure, and without the need for intravenous contrast and at a low cost. However, it is not without limitations. Its use for ruling out coronary artery disease has been challenged in the past. In the Multi-Ethnic Study of Atherosclerosis, up to a third of total events occurred in patients with a coronary artery calcium score zero, and in the coronary artery calcium score consortium cohort, 43% of cardiovascular deaths occurred in participants without evidence of coronary calcium. In the recent Miami Heart Study (MiHEART), 2359 middle-aged and predominantly low-risk (74% in atherosclerotic cardiovascular disease risk <5%) asymptomatic individuals were evaluated with coronary artery calcium score and coronary computed tomography angiography. The prevalence of any coronary plaque on coronary computed tomography angiography was 16% among those with coronary artery calcium score of 0. Furthermore, in this group, 0.8% had stenosis ≥50%, 0.1% stenosis ≥70%, and 2.3% high-risk plaque features.[22] Similar findings were observed in the Swedish CArdioPulmonary bioImage Study (SCAPIS), a nationwide open-access population-based cohort of 30,154 men and women. Of the 25,182 participants without known coronary heart disease, 6% to 9% of those with a zero calcium score had evidence of atherosclerosis with only 0.4% having obstructive coronary artery disease.[23]

Another potential limitation of coronary artery calcium score is the presence of subtle calcified plaque below the score threshold, which, even when minimal, is associated with increased adverse cardiovascular outcomes. Although modern imaging technology has advanced, the Agatston scoring method has remained unchanged since its introduction, and consideration of a change in coronary artery calcium score scoring methodology has been recommended. Lately, it has been proposed that smaller and less dense calcified plaques below the conventional detection threshold can be identified by eliminating the size threshold and reducing the Hounsfield units (HU) threshold to ≥120.[24]

CORONARY COMPUTED TOMOGRAPHY ANGIOGRAPHY

Evaluation of Coronary Artery Disease

Coronary computed tomography angiography is the noninvasive test of choice for the identification of coronary artery disease in patients with stable chest pain symptoms.[25–27] Its use is associated with a twofold improvement in diagnostic certainty[28] and, in individual patient data meta-analysis, has a very high degree of accuracy for the diagnosis of obstructive coronary artery disease.[29] This improved diagnostic certainty leads to alterations in drug therapies and rates of coronary revascularization that translate into a substantial reduction in 5-year rates of coronary heart disease death or myocardial infarction.[28,30] Moreover, in comparison to invasive coronary angiography, coronary computed tomography angiography is quicker and associated with lower rates of procedural complications, unnecessary invasive angiography, and coronary revascularization.[31] This leads to a reduction in overall costs without increasing radiation exposure.[31,32,33]

The benefits of coronary computed tomography angiography in patients with acute chest pain are less marked, but its use has been associated with shorter hospitalizations and lower costs in low-risk populations[34,35] and avoidance of invasive coronary angiography and downstream testing in those with intermediate-risk chest pain.[36,37] The latter appears to be mediated through the identification of normal coronary arteries.

Asymptomatic Populations

The use of coronary computed tomography angiography in asymptomatic individuals is not currently recommended in national or international guidelines. This reflects the lack of evidence to demonstrate whether this is an appropriate or effective strategy. There is also a suggestion from observational studies that abnormal coronary computed tomography angiography findings in asymptomatic individuals are associated with modest increases in the use of secondary testing and coronary revascularization that were applied outside of evidence-based guidelines and potentially of questionable value.[38] So why would it have a role in primary prevention of coronary heart disease?

In the Scottish Computed Tomography of the HEART (SCOT-HEART) trial, the added benefit of coronary computed tomography angiography was assessed in patients with stable chest pain referred to the cardiology clinic.[28] Diagnosis, treatment, and management was changed in approximately one in four patients, and this ultimately led to an approximately 40% reduction in the subsequent rates of coronary heart disease death or nonfatal myocardial infarction.[30] The final diagnosis of angina due to coronary heart disease was made in a third of trial participants, although there was a tendency for coronary computed tomography angiography to reclassify more people as not having angina due to coronary artery disease. Intriguingly, 5-year coronary event rates were much lower in participants who underwent coronary computed tomography angiography and had been clinically classified as not having angina due to coronary artery disease (Fig. 4.1).[39] This likely reflects better diagnostic reclassification but also the detection of incidental asymptomatic coronary atherosclerosis and its treatment with lifestyle interventions and preventive therapies.

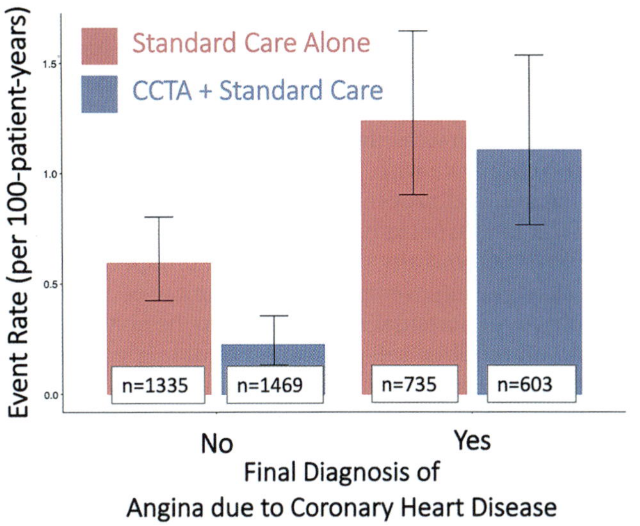

FIG. 4.1 Coronary event (coronary heart disease death or nonfatal myocardial infarction) rates in 4146 patients with (*right panel*) or without (*left panel*) angina due to coronary heart disease. Coronary computed tomography angiography (CCTA) reclassified more patients as not having angina due to coronary artery disease than standard of care alone, but event rates were reduced by nearly two-thirds in those who underwent coronary computed tomography angiography (incidence rate: 0.23 [95% CI 0.13–0.35] vs. 0.59 [95% CI 0.42–0.80] per 100 patient-years respectively; $P<.001$). (Data from Adamson et al.[39].)

Two-thirds or more of patients with stable chest pain referred for a cardiology opinion do not have angina due to coronary artery disease,[28,40] and yet this population accounts for a third of all subsequent fatal or nonfatal myocardial infarctions.[40] Many of these patients have cardiovascular risk factors, and the referral for a cardiology opinion is usually to confirm that despite cardiovascular risk factors, the patient does not have angina due to coronary artery disease. While symptomatic with chest pain, these patients often have transient symptoms attributable to musculoskeletal or gastrointestinal causes and are arguably similar to asymptomatic patients with cardiovascular risk factors. These patients are at increased likelihood of having subclinical coronary atherosclerosis albeit without symptoms of angina. Moreover, in the SCOT-HEART trial, patients who presented with nonanginal chest pain and a normal electrocardiogram had greater proportional reductions in coronary events than those with possible angina.[39] Again, this is consistent with the identification and treatment of previously unrecognized coronary atherosclerosis with lifestyle interventions and preventive therapies.

These data strongly suggest that, for the optimal prevention of coronary heart disease events, we may need to take a screening approach to detect coronary atherosclerosis. Indeed, given the poor uptake of preventive interventions based on risk scores, screening for coronary atherosclerosis may provide a more compelling argument that patients can more readily understand. Rather than a concept of probabilistic risk of whether individuals may or may not suffer a future coronary event, the identification and direct confirmation of the early disease process may provide a more compelling and complete understanding for the patient. Indeed, there is evidence that confirming the presence of atherosclerosis through imaging of carotid plaques or coronary artery calcification improves the acceptability of, and compliance with, lifestyle interventions, risk factor modification, and preventative therapy use.[41,42] Strong motivation is key, especially in individuals who have full and active lives without any symptoms. The prospect of unwelcome lifestyle interventions and initiation of preventive therapies with potential side effects may be challenging to accept and requires self-motivation to obtain potential future long-term benefits.

Normal Coronary Arteries

The documentation of normal coronary arteries is highly valued by patients, especially when they have risk factors, family history, or chest pain symptoms of uncertain etiology. Indeed, in patients with stable chest pain, the demonstration of normal coronary arteries and the cessation of preventive therapy is associated with marked improvements in quality of life.[43] It is likely that the same may apply to asymptomatic individuals at increased cardiovascular risk, although this has yet to be established. Of course, there is the concern that confirmation of normal coronary arteries may encourage poor compliance with lifestyle advice and risk factor modification, and it is unknown how this could impact the future long-term risks of cardiovascular disease. However, in the medium term, patients with normal coronary arteries have a very low risk of coronary events.[44,45]

Asymptomatic Nonobstructive Coronary Artery Disease

In patients who suffer an acute myocardial infarction, the culprit atherosclerotic plaque is nonobstructive (<70% stenosis) in the majority (~80%) of cases. This has been a consistent finding in both postmortem studies and serial coronary angiography studies. This has been further confirmed by large clinical trials of coronary computed tomography angiography. In both the Prospective Multicenter Imaging Study for Evaluation of Chest Pain (PROMISE) and SCOT-HEART trials,[44,45] most coronary events occurred in patients with nonobstructive coronary artery disease. Therefore the identification and treatment of nonobstructive disease is going to provide the greatest opportunity to prevent coronary heart disease events. Coronary computed tomography angiography is the most sensitive noninvasive method of detecting nonobstructive disease and is superior to even invasive coronary angiography in identifying coronary atherosclerotic plaque.[31]

Asymptomatic Obstructive Coronary Artery Disease

The presence and extent of obstructive coronary artery disease is a strong prognostic predictor of outcome that has been the cornerstone of modern cardiology practice. However, the burden of disease is not synonymous with the functional consequences of disease. For the latter, this is important for symptom management. Patients with angina due to obstructive coronary artery disease gain symptomatic benefit from antianginal therapy and coronary revascularization. We should not confuse symptom benefit from prognostic benefit. Randomized controlled trials have consistently demonstrated that coronary revascularization does not prevent 5-year rates of recurrent coronary events.[46,47] Although these trials were performed in symptomatic populations, it highlights that for patients without symptoms, there is no clear mandate to undertake coronary revascularization because this is unlikely to change outcome with perhaps the exception of coronary artery bypass surgery for left main stem disease (Fig. 4.2) or severe proximal three-vessel coronary artery disease.

Previous studies have suggested that obstructive disease identified on coronary computed tomography angiography does lead to an increase in functional testing and coronary revascularization.[38,48] However, the rationale for such testing and intervention is uncertain and perhaps reflects the lack of evidence base. Given that no symptom benefit will be obtained, and the absence of prognostic benefits, functional testing and coronary revascularization is not indicated except for left main stem disease or severe proximal three-vessel coronary artery disease. The focus of treatment should therefore be on preventive therapies of aspirin and statin as well as consideration for renin-angiotensin system inhibitor therapy, especially in those with hypertension, diabetes mellitus, or signs of left ventricular dysfunction.[25,26,49]

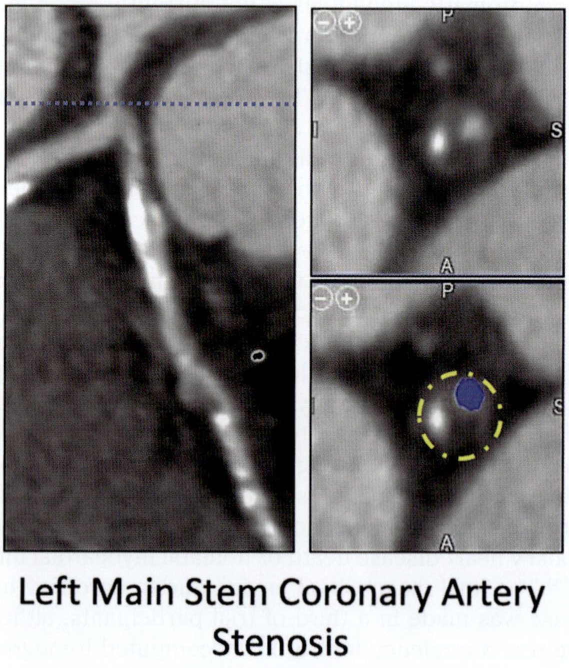

FIG. 4.2 Severe left main stem stenosis in a 60-year-old asymptomatic individual with no cardiovascular risk factors who underwent coronary artery bypass graft surgery. *Blue dashed line* shows cross-section for images in lefthand panels. Right hand panels shows coronary lumen (*blue*) within coronary artery (*dashed yellow circle*) consistent with 80% to 90% stenosis.

Plaque Burden Versus Stenosis

Whilst the number of vessels with obstructive coronary artery disease has been seen as the gold standard of assessing risk, this is increasingly being called in to question. Patients with obstructive disease often have a greater overall burden of disease, and the associations of risk may be more to do with extent or burden of disease rather than the severity of a focal stenosis.

In a regional audit of nearly 25,000 patients from Denmark, the risk of major adverse cardiac events was higher in those with obstructive coronary artery disease than those without, but when adjusting for the degree of plaque burden, this was no longer the case.[50] Furthermore, in the Copenhagen General Population Study, nearly 10,000 people over the age of 40 years underwent a coronary computed tomography angiogram. This demonstrated that although obstructive disease was associated with a marked increase in the risk of myocardial infarction, it was the extent of disease that predicted death or myocardial infarction, and this was independent of the extent of obstructive disease.[51]

Randomized Controlled Trials of Computed Tomography Angiography in Asymptomatic Individuals

To date, there has been only one randomized controlled trial to be completed in asymptomatic individuals: the FACTOR-64 trial.[52] This trial was conducted in nearly 1000 people with diabetes mellitus who were felt to be at high risk. Subjects were randomized to standard of care plus coronary computed tomography angiography or standard of care alone. After 4 years of follow-up, there was no effect on clinical outcome: primary endpoint of all-cause death, nonfatal myocardial infarction, or unstable angina. However, the primary event rate was very low at approximately 1% per year and, at baseline, there was a very high use of statin therapy (>70%), and the average low-density lipoprotein concentration was already below 90 mg/dL. At the end of trial conduct, there were no differences in risk factor management (blood pressure, glycemic control, or triglycerides) except a very small difference in statin prescribing (3% higher) and low-density lipoprotein cholesterol concentrations (2 mg/dL lower) in patients undergoing coronary computed tomography angiography. Thus, in this extremely well treated population, there was little scope for coronary computed tomography angiography to guide major changes in patient treatments or risk factor management, and perhaps it was unsurprising that clinical outcomes were unaffected. The use of coronary computed tomography angiography in asymptomatic individuals thus remains unproven.

Limitations

Coronary computed tomography angiography has a number of limitations when applied to an asymptomatic population that should be acknowledged. This technique is associated with substantial healthcare resource, cost, and technical expertise. It is also associated with exposure to ionizing radiation, although modern protocols and scanners have reduced the overall effect radiation dose to 2 to 4 mSv. Incidental findings are common and require follow-up, although some represent important occult clinical disease, the detection of which can be advantageous to the patient.[53] Finally, there are the adverse consequences of highlighting the presence of coronary artery disease to asymptomatic individuals and the anxiety and quality-of-life impact this may provoke.[43] However, such issues are also pertinent to the application of risk scores and the future risk of ill health and cardiovascular disease.

FUTURE DIRECTIONS

Trials in Primary Prevention

Reflecting the increasing interest in this area, there are several ongoing and emerging clinical trials that are assessing the clinical value of cardiac computed tomography in asymptomatic individuals (Table 4.1). These trials have been

TABLE 4.1 Current Randomised Controlled Trials of Coronary Computed Tomography Angiography in Asymptomatic Individuals

TRIAL ACRONYM	SAMPLE SIZE	RANDOMIZATION	INCLUSION CRITERIA	RECRUITMENT SITES	RECRUITMENT COMMENCEMENT	DURATION OF FOLLOW-UP	PRIMARY ENDPOINT	TRIAL REGISTRATION
SCOT-HEART 2 Trial	6000	1:1 CTCA vs. standard of care	40 to 70 years At least one cardiovascular risk factor or age over 60 years	100 to 200 Scottish primary care practices	January 2020	5 years	Coronary heart disease death or nonfatal myocardial infarction	NCT03920176
RESPECT	15000	1:1 CTCA vs. standard of care	40 to 70 years At least one cardiovascular risk factor	Nanjing, China	July 2022	5 years	Cardiac death, myocardial infarction, angina, or emergency coronary revascularization	NCT05431309
DANE-HEART	6000	1:1 CTCA vs. standard of care	40 to 70 years At least one cardiovascular risk factor or age over 60 years	Copenhagen, Denmark	January 2023	5 years	Coronary heart disease death or nonfatal myocardial infarction	TBC

initiated in the last few years and are not expected to report for at least 5 years. Further insights are anticipated soon from the Dutch Risk Or Benefit IN Screening for CArdiovascular disease (ROBINSCA) trial that is assessing the value of computed tomography calcium scoring in population screening approaches.[54] Early indications suggest that a coronary artery calcium score–based approach results in a third fewer individuals being prescribed preventive therapies compared to those assessed with a cardiovascular risk score–based approach.[55] This underscores the marked tendency of cardiovascular risk scores to overtreat a substantial number of individuals who do not have coronary artery disease.

Recent primary prevention trials of antiplatelet therapy have highlighted that beneficial reductions in atherothrombotic events are counterbalanced by the increased hazard of major bleeding events.[56] This has led to a reluctance to prescribe antiplatelet therapy for the primary prevention of atherosclerotic cardiovascular disease. However, because risk scores overestimate risk, many of the individuals treated with antiplatelet therapy do not have underlying atherosclerotic disease, and they will have the hazards without the potential to benefit from such therapy. A screening approach with coronary computed tomography angiogram avoids this imbalance and hence would allow a more targeted approach that may allow for the benefits to outweigh the small hazard of major bleeding. It would also allow for the more targeted application of additional interventions, such as the addition of proprotein convertase subtilisin/kexin type 9 inhibitors, to be used in addition to statin therapy. This could be graded according to the burden of plaque disease present.

Assessment of Novel Therapies

The emergence of a noninvasive imaging modality, such as coronary computed tomography angiography, now not only permits quantification of plaque burden but also allows for further distinction of plaque components and identification of vulnerable plaques. Application of these findings continues to extend the prospect of coronary computed tomography angiography in evaluation and management of atherosclerotic coronary artery disease in clinical practice. Coronary computed tomography angiography is especially effective in quantitative and qualitative plaque assessment and is now considered in many studies to be the imaging modality of choice in monitoring changes in coronary plaque. It has been used in many clinical trials that have demonstrated the benefits of several therapeutic agents and has excellent correlation with previously used invasive imaging modalities. As compared with intravenous ultrasound and other invasive techniques, it is safer, easier, less cumbersome, and dramatically less costly for coronary plaque analysis.[57] Similar to the effects of statins on coronary computed tomography angiography–identified atherosclerosis, other salutary medical therapies also slow plaque progression, including icosapent ethyl[58] and colchicine.[59] Multiple large prospective randomized multicenter coronary computed tomography angiography trials are ongoing, studying the effect of antiinflammatory, hypoglycemic, proprotein convertase subtilisin/kexin type 9, and statin therapies on atherosclerosis.

Given low achievable radiation and high reproducibility, coronary computed tomography angiography now not only permits quantification of plaque burden but also allows for further distinction of plaque components and identification of vulnerable plaques. Application of these findings continue to extend the prospect of coronary computed tomography angiography in the evaluation and management of atherosclerotic coronary artery disease in clinical practice. Quantifying plaque serially may help guide therapy, leading to intensification of treatments in those persons who are exhibiting significant progression of atherosclerosis.

Evolution of Risk Prediction

Advanced plaque metrics, such as evaluating for low-attenuation plaque, and accurate measures of plaque burden are now being used to classify and to quantify atherosclerotic plaque burden, far beyond the calcium score. The ability of automated measurements, which can be done in seconds with automated computer programs, makes this an attractive method to quantify plaque burden at one time point and then be able to follow atherosclerosis over time. In addition to plaque burden and specific measures of atherosclerosis, vascular inflammation has been long identified as a main driver for the initiation and propagation of atherosclerosis. Inflammatory cells play an integral role in the mechanism of plaque injury and rupture. Improvements in computed tomographic imaging and interpretation have matured its use into a noninvasive imaging modality capable of advanced anatomical assessment, including better understanding of plaque burden, fat density, and identification of high-risk markers, such as peri-coronary fat density and high-risk plaque. The enticement of adding incremental measures that afford additional risk stratification to coronary computed tomography angiography and coronary artery calcium score testing without additional imaging or participant burden has great appeal for risk prediction, to maximize the utility of coronary computed tomography angiography.

PLAQUE CHARACTERIZATION

Much work is going into automated methods to characterize coronary plaque. Over the past 3 decades, efforts changed from purely demonstrating its performance to quantify coronary luminal stenosis when compared to invasive angiographic reference, to a measure of plaque quantity, such as using coronary artery calcium score and other quantitative measures. More recently, there has been a shift toward evaluating the clinical utility of atherosclerotic plaque characteristics to identify at-risk patients. In a landmark study by Motoyama et al.[60] of 1059 patients undergoing coronary computed tomography angiography, positive arterial remodeling and low-attenuation plaques, defined as lesions with <30 Hounsfield units on coronary computed tomography angiography, were strong predictors of acute coronary syndromes. The importance of these atherosclerotic plaque characteristics was underscored by the fact that all patients experiencing acute coronary syndromes after coronary computed tomography angiography did not possess any luminal stenosis >75% at the time of coronary computed tomography angiography. This is consistent with prior work demonstrating that most lesions that are responsible for acute myocardial infarction are not high-grade stenosis severity prior to the event.

A more recent study, Hell et al.,[61] presented long-term results of patients undergoing coronary computed tomography angiography followed for future cardiac death. A total of 2748 patients without prior known coronary artery disease underwent coronary computed tomography angiography, with 32 patients experiencing cardiac death at a mean follow-up of 3.2 years. Coronary computed tomography angiograms were analyzed by semi-automated software for a number of coronary atherosclerotic plaque findings, including total plaque volume, stenosis severity, noncalcified plaque volume, low-attenuation plaque volume, calcified plaque volume, and contrast density differences between the proximal and distal portion of the vessels. When adjusted by the extent of coronary artery disease, these atherosclerotic plaque characteristics were strong predictors of cardiac death. Total, noncalcified, and low-attenuation plaque volumes conferred a more than twofold increase in the hazards of experiencing cardiac death. These atherosclerotic plaque characteristic metrics were more predictive than stenosis severity ≥50% or ≥70%, neither of which effectively predicted cardiac death. Finding predictors of events in persons without obstructive disease may be even more insightful in asymptomatic persons, who are much more likely to only have nonobstructive disease prior to an event. New automated software is becoming available that can quantify plaque in minutes, making this a potentially clinically useful tool.

PERICORONARY ADIPOSE TISSUE

Pericoronary fat beds adjacent to the proximal coronary arteries are metabolically active and give rise to inflammatory mediators that are pro-atherogenic including adipokines, macrophages, and lymphocytes. The concept is that inflammation within the pericoronary adipose tissue increases tissue density, and this gradient or density can be measured without additional scanning.

In the Cardiovascular RISk Prediction using Computed Tomography (CRISP-CT) study,[62] prospective outcome data from two independent cohorts of consecutive patients undergoing coronary computed tomography angiography in Erlangen, Germany (derivation cohort) and Cleveland, Ohio, USA (validation cohort) were evaluated. Pericoronary adipose tissue attenuation mapping was performed around the three major coronary arteries, and the proximal right coronary artery was used as a marker of coronary inflammation. After adjustment for age, sex, cardiovascular risk factors, modified Duke coronary artery disease index, and tube voltage, they found incremental and independent predictive value for all-cause and cardiac mortality. After multivariable analysis, there was independent risk with a the hazard ratio of 2.15 (95% CI 1.33–3.48; $P = .017$) in the derivation cohort and 2.06 (95% CI 1.50–2.83; $P < .0001$) in the validation cohort. Pericoronary fat attenuation index improved risk discrimination in both cohorts, leading to significant reclassification for all-cause and cardiac mortality.

The investigators of CRISP-CT concluded that the pericoronary fat attenuation index enhances cardiac risk prediction and stratification over and above current state of-the-art assessment in coronary computed tomography angiography by providing a quantitative measure of coronary inflammation. High pericoronary fat attenuation index values (cutoff ≥–70.1 HU) were an indicator of increased cardiac mortality and, therefore, could guide early targeted primary prevention in patients. This unique biomarker of vascular inflammation has great potential to add major predictive value. The full potential and further validation of this marker is still lacking, but this opens the door to great incremental information, coupling, for the first time, inflammation and atherosclerosis burden with coronary computed tomography angiography.

RADIOMICS

The current interpretation of coronary computed tomography angiography images mainly depends on subjective and qualitative analysis. Radiomics uses advanced image analysis to extract large amounts of quantitative information from digital images, which often is not otherwise distinguishable to the human eye.

The current applications of radiomics in cardiac computed tomography mainly involve research into coronary plaques, pericoronary adipose tissue, and plaque quantification. The goal is to assist the identification of vulnerable plaques or patients, improve cardiac risk prediction and stratification, discriminate myocardial pathology, and offer new prospects to personalize cardiovascular medicine. The mined data can be used to establish undiscovered correlations between imaging features and clinical end points. To date, some proof-of-concept studies have demonstrated the feasibility and diagnostic performance of cardiac computed tomography radiomics analysis. Although research into radiomics began only recently, several studies point to its potential clinical value in assessing future cardiac risk and guiding prevention and treatment strategies. Cardiac computed tomography radiomics has a lot to offer to patients and physicians with potential to define cardiac disease phenotypes on imaging with higher precision.

CONCLUSIONS

Large-scale prospective studies have demonstrated the prognostic importance of computed tomography plaque quantification including coronary artery calcium score, coronary artery stenosis, and atherosclerotic plaque characteristics. A myriad of other potential markers of risk, including epicardial fat, aortic wall, valve calcification, and cardiac chamber sizes, all potentially add both diagnostic and prognostic value to coronary computed tomography angiography. The utility of coronary computed tomography angiography in asymptomatic persons remains to be established but shows great promise. Until validated, coronary artery calcium score continues to be the primary test in this asymptomatic population for the near future at least. Along with advancements in cardiac computed tomography imaging, radiomics may provide more precise phenotyping of cardiovascular disease for patients and doctors, which can improve diagnostic, prognostic, and therapeutic decision-making in the future.

REFERENCES

1. National Institute for Health and Care Excellence, NICE Clinical Guideline 95 [CG181]. *Cardiovascular Disease: Risk Assessment and Reduction, Including Lipid Modification*. London: NICE; 2014.
2. Singh A, Collins BL, Gupta A, et al. Cardiovascular risk and statin eligibility of young adults after an MI: partners YOUNG-MI registry. *J Am Coll Cardiol*. 2018;71:292–302.
3. Ueda P, Lung TW, Clarke P, Danaei G. Application of the 2014 NICE cholesterol guidelines in the English population: a cross-sectional analysis. *Br J Gen Pract*. 2017;67:e598–e608.
4. Grammer TB, Dressel A, Gergei I, et al. Cardiovascular risk algorithms in primary care: results from the DETECT study. *Sci Rep*. 2019;9:1101.
5. Genders TS, Steyerberg EW, Hunink MG, et al. Prediction model to estimate presence of coronary artery disease: retrospective pooled analysis of existing cohorts. *BMJ*. 2012;344:e3485.
6. Hope HF, Binkley GM, Fenton S, Kitas GD, Verstappen SMM, Symmons DPM. Systematic review of the predictors of statin adherence for the primary prevention of cardiovascular disease. *PLoS ONE*. 2019;14:e0201196.
7. Arnett DK, Blumenthal RS, Albert MA, et al. 2019 American College of Cardiology/American Heart Association Guideline on the Primary Prevention of Cardiovascular Disease: executive summary: a report of the American College of Cardiology/American Heart Association Task Force on Clinical Practice Guidelines. *J Am Coll Cardiol*. 2019;74:1376–1414.
8. Visseren FLJ, Mach F, Smulders YM, et al. 2021 ESC Guidelines on cardiovascular disease prevention in clinical practice. *Eur J Prev Cardiol*. 2022;29:5–115.
9. Karmali KN, Persell SD, Perel P, Lloyd-Jones DM, Berendsen MA, Huffman MD. Risk scoring for the primary prevention of cardiovascular disease. *Cochrane Database Syst Rev*. 2017;3:CD006887.
10. De Goma EM, Karlsberg RP, Judelson DR, Budoff MJ. The underappreciated impact of heart disease. *Womens Health Issues*. 2010;20:299–303.
11. Grundy SM, Stone NJ Guideline Writing Committee for the 2018 Cholesterol Guidelines. 2018 Cholesterol Clinical Practice Guidelines: Synopsis of the 2018 American Heart Association/American College of Cardiology/Multisociety Cholesterol Guideline. *Ann Intern Med*. 2019;170(11):779–783. doi:10.7326/M19-0365.
12. Budoff MJ, Georgiou D, Brody AS, et al. Ultrafast computed tomography as a diagnostic modality in the detection of coronary artery disease: a multicenter study. *Circulation*. 1996;93:898–904.
13. McClelland RL, Jorgensen NW, Budoff M, et al. 10-year coronary heart disease risk prediction using coronary artery calcium and traditional risk factors. *J Am Coll Cardiol*. 2015;66:1643–1653.
14. Wolfson J, Vock DM, Bandyopadhyay S, et al. Use and customization of risk scores for predicting cardiovascular events using electronic health record data. *J Am Heart Assoc*. 2017;6:e003670.
15. Muntner P, Colantonio LD, Cushman M, et al. Validation of the atherosclerotic cardiovascular disease Pooled Cohort risk equations. *JAMA*. 2014;311:1406–1415.
16. Yeboah J, Young R, McClelland RL, et al. Utility of nontraditional risk markers in atherosclerotic cardiovascular disease risk assessment. *J Am Coll Cardiol*. 2016;67:139–147.
17. Budoff MJ. Screening for ischemic heart disease with cardiac CT: current recommendations. *Scientifica (Cairo)*. 2012;2012:812046.
18. Rana JS, Tabada GH, Solomon MD, et al. Accuracy of the atherosclerotic cardiovascular risk equation in a large contemporary, multiethnic population. *J Am Coll Cardiol*. 2016;67(18):2118–2130. doi:10.1016/j.jacc.2016.02.055.
19. Blaha M, Budoff MJ, Shaw LJ, et al. Absence of coronary artery calcification and all-cause mortality. *JACC Cardiovasc Imaging*. 2009;2:692–700.
20. Sarwar A, Shaw L, Shapiro M, et al. Diagnostic and prognostic value of absence of coronary artery calcification. *JACC Cardiovasc Imaging*. 2009;2:675–688.
21. Spahillari A, Zhu J, Ferket BS, et al. Cost-effectiveness of contemporary statin use guidelines with or without coronary artery calcium assessment in African American individuals. *JAMA Cardiol*. 2020;5:871–880.
22. Nasir K, Cainzos-Achirica M, Valero-Elizondo J, et al. Coronary atherosclerosis in an asymptomatic U.S. population. *JACC Cardiovasc Imaging*. 2022;15:1604–1618.
23. Bergström G, Persson M, Adiels M, et al. Prevalence of subclinical coronary artery atherosclerosis in the general population. *Circulation*. 2021;144:916–929.
24. Tzolos E, Han D, Klein E, et al. Detection of small coronary calcifications in patients with Agatston coronary artery calcium score of zero. *J Cardiovasc Comput Tomogr*. 2022;16:150–154.
25. Fihn SD, Gardin JM, Abrams J, et al. 2012 ACCF/AHA/ACP/AATS/PCNA/SCAI/STS Guideline for the diagnosis and management of patients with stable ischemic heart disease: a report of the American College of Cardiology Foundation/American Heart Association Task Force on Practice Guidelines, and the American College of Physicians, American Association for Thoracic Surgery, Preventive Cardiovascular Nurses Association, Society for Cardiovascular Angiography and Interventions, and Society of Thoracic Surgeons. *J Am Coll Cardiol*. 2012;60:e44–e164.
26. Knuuti J, Wijns W, Saraste A, et al. 2019 ESC Guidelines for the diagnosis and management of chronic coronary syndromes. *Eur Heart J*. 2020;41:407–477.
27. National Institute for Health and Care Excellence, NICE Clinical Guideline 95 [CG95]. *Recent-Onset Chest Pain of Suspected Cardiac Origin: Assessment and Diagnosis*. London: NICE; 2016.
28. The Scottish Computed Tomography of the HEART (SCOT-HEART) Trial Investigators; Chief InvestigatorNewby DE. Computed tomography coronary angiography in patients with suspected angina due to coronary heart disease. *Lancet*.. 2015;385:2383–2391.
29. Haase R, Schlattmann P, Andreini D, et al. Diagnosis of obstructive coronary artery disease using computed tomography angiography in patients with stable chest pain depending on clinical probability and in clinically important subgroups: meta-analysis of individual patient data. *Br Med J*. 2019;365:l1945.
30. The Scottish Computed Tomography of the HEART (SCOT-HEART) Trial InvestigatorsNewby DE, Adamson PD, Berry C, et al. Coronary CT angiography and the future risk of myocardial infarction. *N Engl J Med*.. 2018;379:924–933.
31. DISCHARGE Trial Group, Maurovich-Horvat P, Bosserdt M, Kofoed KF, et al. CT or invasive coronary angiography in stable chest pain. *N Engl J Med*. 2022;386:1591–1602.
32. Chang HJ, Lin FY, Gebow D, et al. Selective referral using coronary computed tomography angiography versus direct referral for individuals referred to invasive coronary angiography for suspected CAD: a randomized, controlled, open-label trial. *JACC Cardiovasc Imaging*. 2019;12:1303–1312.
33. Dewey M, Rief M, Martus P, et al. Evaluation of computed tomography in patients with atypical angina or chest pain clinically referred for invasive coronary angiography: randomised controlled trial. *BMJ*. 2016;355:i5441. doi:10.1136/bmj.i5441.
34. Litt HI, Gatsonis C, Snyder B, et al. CT angiography for safe discharge of patients with possible acute coronary syndromes. *N Engl J Med*. 2012;366:1393–1403.
35. Hoffmann U, Truong QA, Schoenfeld DA, et al. Coronary CT angiography versus standard evaluation in acute chest pain. *N Engl J Med*. 2012;367:299–308.
36. Dedic A, Lubbers MM, Schaap J, et al. Coronary CT angiography for suspected ACS in the era of high-sensitivity troponins: randomized multicenter study. *J Am Coll Cardiol*. 2016;67:16–26.
37. Gray AJ, Roobottom C, Smith JE, et al. Early computed tomography coronary angiography in patients with suspected acute coronary syndrome: randomised controlled trial. *BMJ*. 2021;374:n210.
38. McEvoy JW, Blaha MJ, Nasir K, et al. Impact of coronary computed tomographic angiography results on patient and physician behavior in a low-risk population. *Arch Intern Med*. 2011;171:1260–1268.
39. Adamson PD, Hunter A, Williams MC, et al. Diagnostic and prognostic benefits of computed tomography coronary angiography using the 2016 NICE guidance within a randomised trial. *Heart*. 2018;104:207–214.
40. Sekhri N, Feder GS, Junghans C, Hemingway H, Timmis AD. How effective are rapid access chest pain clinics? Prognosis of incident angina and non-cardiac chest pain in 8762 consecutive patients. *Heart*. 2007;93:458–463.
41. Näslund U, Ng N, Lundgren A, et al. Visualization of asymptomatic atherosclerotic disease for optimum cardiovascular prevention (VIPVIZA): a pragmatic, open-label, randomised controlled trial. *Lancet*. 2019;393:133–142.
42. Orakzai RH, Nasir K, Orakzai SH, et al. Effect of patient visualization of coronary calcium by electron beam computed tomography on changes in beneficial lifestyle behaviors. *Am J Cardiol*. 2008;101:999–1002.
43. Williams MC, Hunter A, Shah A, et al. Symptoms and quality of life in patients with suspected angina undergoing CT coronary angiography: a randomised controlled trial. Scottish Computed Tomography of the HEART (SCOT-HEART) Trial Investigators. *Heart*. 2017;103:995–1001.
44. Singh T, Bing R, Dweck MR, et al. Exercise ECG and CT coronary angiography in patients with suspected stable angina pectoris: a post-hoc analysis of the randomised SCOTHEART trial. *JAMA Cardiol*. 2020;5:e201567.
45. Hoffmann U, Ferencik M, Udelson JE, et al. Prognostic value of noninvasive cardiovascular testing in patients with stable chest pain: insights from the PROMISE trial (Prospective Multicenter Imaging Study for Evaluation of Chest Pain). *Circulation*. 2017;135:2320–2332.
46. Boden WE, O'Rourke RA, Teo KK, et al. Optimal medical therapy with or without PCI for stable coronary disease. *N Engl J Med*. 2007;356:1503–1516.
47. Maron DJ, Hochman JS, Reynolds HR, et al. Initial invasive or conservative strategy for stable coronary disease. *N Engl J Med*. 2020;382:1395–1407.
48. Douglas PS, Hoffmann U, Patel MR, et al. Outcomes of anatomical versus functional testing for coronary artery disease. *N Engl J Med*. 2015;372:1291–1300.
49. Bangalore S, Fakheri R, Wandel S, Toklu B, Wandel J, Messerli FH. Renin angiotensin system inhibitors for patients with stable coronary artery disease without heart failure: systematic review and meta-analysis of randomized trials. *BMJ*. 2017;356:j4.
50. Mortensen MB, Dzaye O, Steffensen FH, et al. Impact of plaque burden versus stenosis on ischemic events in patients with coronary atherosclerosis. *J Am Coll Cardiol*. 2020;76:2803–2813.
51. Fuchs A, Kühl JT, Sigvardsen PE, et al. Subclinical coronary atherosclerosis and risk for myocardial infarction in a Danish cohort. *Ann Intern Med*. 2023;176:433–442.

52. Muhlestein JB, Lappé DL, Lima JA, et al. Effect of screening for coronary artery disease using CT angiography on mortality and cardiac events in high-risk patients with diabetes: the FACTOR-64 randomized clinical trial. *JAMA*. 2014;312:2234–2243.
53. Williams MC, Hunter A, Shah ASV, et al. Impact of noncardiac findings in patients undergoing CT coronary angiography: a substudy of the Scottish computed tomography of the heart (SCOT-HEART) trial. *Eur Radiol*. 2018;28:2639–2646.
54. Vonder M, van der Aalst CM, Vliegenthart R, et al. Coronary artery calcium imaging in the ROBINSCA trial: rationale, design, and technical background. *Acad Radiol*. 2018;25:118–128.
55. van der Aalst CM, Denissen SJAM, Vonder M, et al. Screening for cardiovascular disease risk using traditional risk factor assessment or coronary artery calcium scoring: the ROBINSCA trial. *Eur Heart J Cardiovasc Imaging*. 2020;21:1216–1224.
56. ASCEND Study Collaborative GroupBowman L, Mafham M, Wallendszus K, et al. Effects of aspirin for primary prevention in persons with diabetes mellitus. *N Engl J Med*. 2018;379:1529–1539.
57. Rasouli ML, Shavelle DM, French WJ, McKay CR, Budoff MJ. Assessment of coronary plaque morphology by contrast-enhanced computed tomographic angiography: comparison with intravascular ultrasound. *Coronary Artery Disease*. 2006;17:359–364.
58. Budoff MJ, Bhatt DL, Kinninger A, et al. Effect of icosapent ethyl on progression of coronary atherosclerosis in patients with elevated triglycerides on statin therapy: final results of the EVAPORATE trial. *Eur Heart J*. 2020;41:3925–3932.
59. Vaidya K, Arnott C, Martinez G, et al. Colchicine and Plaque Stabilization in Patients with Acute Coronary Syndrome. *JACC Cardiovasc Imaging*. 2019;11:305–316.
60. Motoyama S, Sarai M, Harigaya H, et al. Computed tomographic angiography characteristics of atherosclerotic plaques subsequently resulting in acute coronary syndrome. *J Am Coll Cardiol*. 2009;54:49–57.
61. Hell MM, Motwani M, Otaki Y, et al. Quantitative global plaque characteristics from coronary computed tomography angiography for the prediction of future cardiac mortality during long-term follow-up. *Eur Heart J Cardiovasc Imaging*. 2017;18:1331–1339.
62. Oikonomou EK, Marwan M, Desai MY, et al. Non-invasive detection of coronary inflammation using computed tomography and prediction of residual cardiovascular risk (the CRISP CT study): a post-hoc analysis of prospective outcome data. *Lancet*. 2018;392:929–939.

5 Sex Differences in Coronary Atherosclerosis Atherosclerosis in Women: Underlying Physiology and Sex-specific Differences

LINDSEY R. MITRANI, LESLEE J. SHAW, AND FAY Y. LIN

KEY POINTS

1. Coronary artery calcium scores differ systematically by age and sex.
2. Risk enhancers for coronary artery disease in women include coronary artery calcium scores but also sex-specific risk factors including ovarian disorders, hypertensive and endocrine complications of pregnancy, and a higher prevalence of autoimmune disorders
3. Nonobstructive coronary artery disease and high-risk plaque features are more prognostically important in women compared with men by coronary CT angiography.
4. Conditions including MINOCA, INOCA, and SCAD disproportionately affect women compared with men.

INTRODUCTION

Cardiovascular disease is the leading cause of death in women, accounting for 22% of all deaths.[1] Although atherosclerotic cardiovascular disease (ASCVD) classically presents as a disease affecting older men, a growing body of literature highlights increasing ASCVD in women, affecting 44.4% ≥20 years old, an increase of 25% over the last decade.[2,3] Overall, women present with coronary artery disease (CAD) later in life, with more anginal symptoms and ischemia, with a lesser burden of significant obstructive CAD.[4–6] Acute coronary syndromes in women are more likely to have nonobstructive coronary artery disease and may be more likely to have plaque erosion.[7] Cardiac computed tomography evaluates coronary anatomy and has increasing uptake in use and in recent chest pain guidelines.[8] Coronary computed tomographic angiography (CCTA) may lead to better prognostication and faster diagnosis in women.[9] This chapter will highlight research on sex differences in cardiac CT related with regards to presentation, risk factors, imaging, treatment, and outcomes.

BACKGROUND

Sex and Gender

In this discussion, we use the terminology of sex differences to refer to biological differences, including genetic and ovarian exposures, that distinguish males and females. Female sex hormones influence body and heart size, regulate vasomotor tone, modulate cholesterol regulation, and have a potent effect on inflammation (Fig. 5.1). Gender roles are influenced by societal norms that may differ by culture, race, and ethnicity. Gender behaviors and expectations, for example related to physical activity, may influence cardiovascular risk factors and medical decision-making. Sex differences are related but not identical to gender differences, and the majority of cardiovascular literature does not distinguish the impact of gender separately from sex.

Sex Differences in Coronary Pathology

The three primary mechanisms of coronary thrombosis are plaque rupture, plaque erosion, and rarely, calcified nodule (Fig. 5.2).[10] Plaque rupture occurs with the disruption of the fibrous cap over necrotic core, defined as cholesterol crystals in necrotic debris, abruptly stimulating the formation of contiguous thrombus. The precursor lesion to plaque rupture is a thin cap fibroatheroma, a lesion with a <75-μm fibrous cap overlying a large necrotic core, positive remodeling, and increased plaque burden.[11,12]

Plaque erosion occurs when luminal thrombosis arises without an exposed necrotic core as an inciting event, and the precursor lesion can be a wider range of plaque types.[13] Compared to lesions with plaque rupture, lesions with plaque erosion exhibit lower plaque burden, calcification, and positive remodeling.[14] Men are more prone to plaque rupture as a cause of fatal coronary events (35% in men and 17% in women), whereas women are more prone to plaque erosion (14% in men versus 34% in women).[10] Among autopsy-confirmed atherosclerotic deaths, women had a lower likelihood of obstructive CAD at 63% compared with 77% of men ($P = .002$), despite similar pathologic evidence of myocardial infarction at 38% for women and 45% of men ($P = .18$).[15] Among the entire cohort, 17% of those with myocardial infarction had nonobstructive CAD.[15] These differences in underlying mechanism may explain the difference in acute coronary syndrome with nonobstructive coronary arteries (ACS), with a 15% prevalence among women compared with 8% of men.[7]

Intravascular imaging with intravascular ultrasound (IVUS) and optical coherence tomography (OCT) have identified major pathology correlates in vivo.[16] The Providing Regional Observations to Study Predictors of Events in the Coronary Tree (PROSPECT) study identified high-risk precursors to myocardial infarction culprit lesions by the presence of three major features: lipid-rich plaque by backscatter IVUS, minimal luminal area, and cross-sectional plaque burden.[17] Women had a similar frequency of culprit lesions compared to men but fewer nonculprit lesions and similar plaque burden per lesion.[18] OCT has the advantage over IVUS of fibrous cap visualization to distinguish between plaque erosion and plaque rupture and has identified plaque erosion in approximately one-third of myocardial infarctions. Plaque erosion in vivo, unlike in autopsy, does not exhibit sex differences. Clinically, plaque erosion presents more commonly with non-ST-segment elevation myocardial infarction, among patients who are younger and have fewer traditional cardiovascular risk factors.[19]

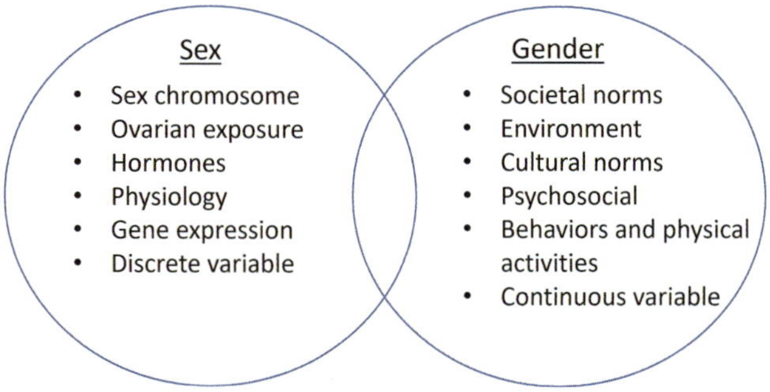

FIG. 5.1 Sex Versus Gender. Sex differences refer to biological, genetic, and physiologic exposure, whereas gender differences relate to societal norms and behaviors.

CORONARY ARTERY CALCIUM SCORING FOR ASYMPTOMATIC WOMEN

Risk stratification based on traditional cardiac risk factors with ASCVD risk score is the prerequisite for primary prevention with lipid-lowering therapy. However, for patients with intermediate levels of risk (ASCVD 10-year risk of 7.5–20%), current guidelines recommend consideration of risk enhancers to improve accuracy of prediction, including CAC score to personalize risk.[20] Additional risk enhancers relevant to women include ovarian and reproductive factors and a higher likelihood of autoimmune disorders (Fig. 5.3). Premature ovarian failure and polycystic ovarian syndrome are both risk factors for major adverse cardiac events (Table 5.1). Complications of pregnancy are an important and neglected part of cardiovascular history: gestational hypertension increases the risk of cardiovascular disease by an odds ratio of 1.7[21]; preeclampsia by threefold[21]; and gestational diabetes increases risk mediated by a 10-fold increase in type 2 diabetes.[22] Women with autoimmune disorders such as rheumatoid arthritis have double to triple the risk of myocardial infarction (MI) and ASCVD mortality, in addition to women with systemic lupus erythematosus, who also have increased risk profile.[23] Coronary calcification on noncontrast CT is a late sign of progressive atherosclerosis. Microcalcification resulting from macrophage apoptosis is a key pathologic finding in necrotic core but is well below the spatial resolution of CT

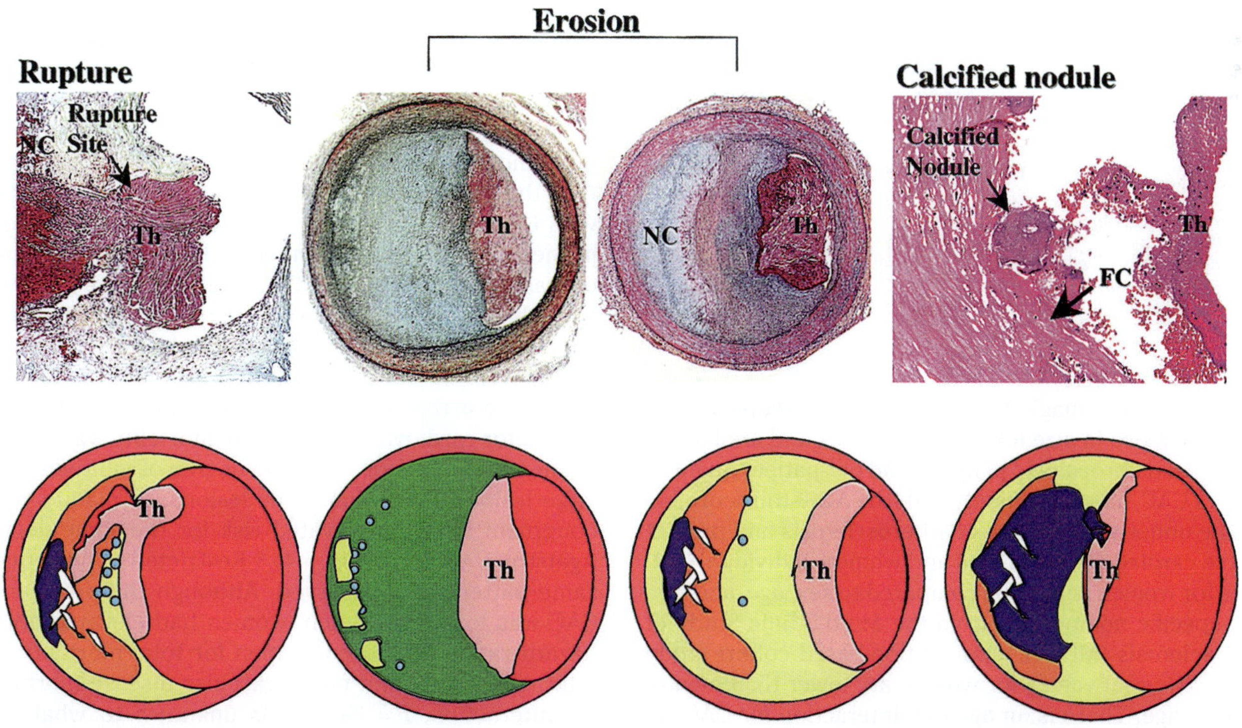

FIG. 5.2 Etiology of Plaque. Atherosclerotic lesions with thrombi can be divided into plaque rupture, plaque erosion, and calcified nodule. Ruptured plaques contain luminal thrombi(Th) overlying a large necrotic core (NC) uncovered by the rupture of a thin fibrous cap(Fc). Plaque erosions contain luminal thrombi over endothelial disruption, without contiguity with NC; underlying lesions are filled with smooth muscle cells and proteoglycans with extracellular lipid pools or necrotic core in the deep intima. Calcified nodules are plaques with luminal thrombi contiguous with calcifications protruding through the fibrous cap. (From Virmani R, Kolodgie FD, Burke AP, Farb A, Schwartz SM. Lessons from sudden coronary death: a comprehensive morphological classification scheme for atherosclerotic lesions. *Arterioscler Thromb Vasc Biol.* 2000;20[5]:1262–1275.)

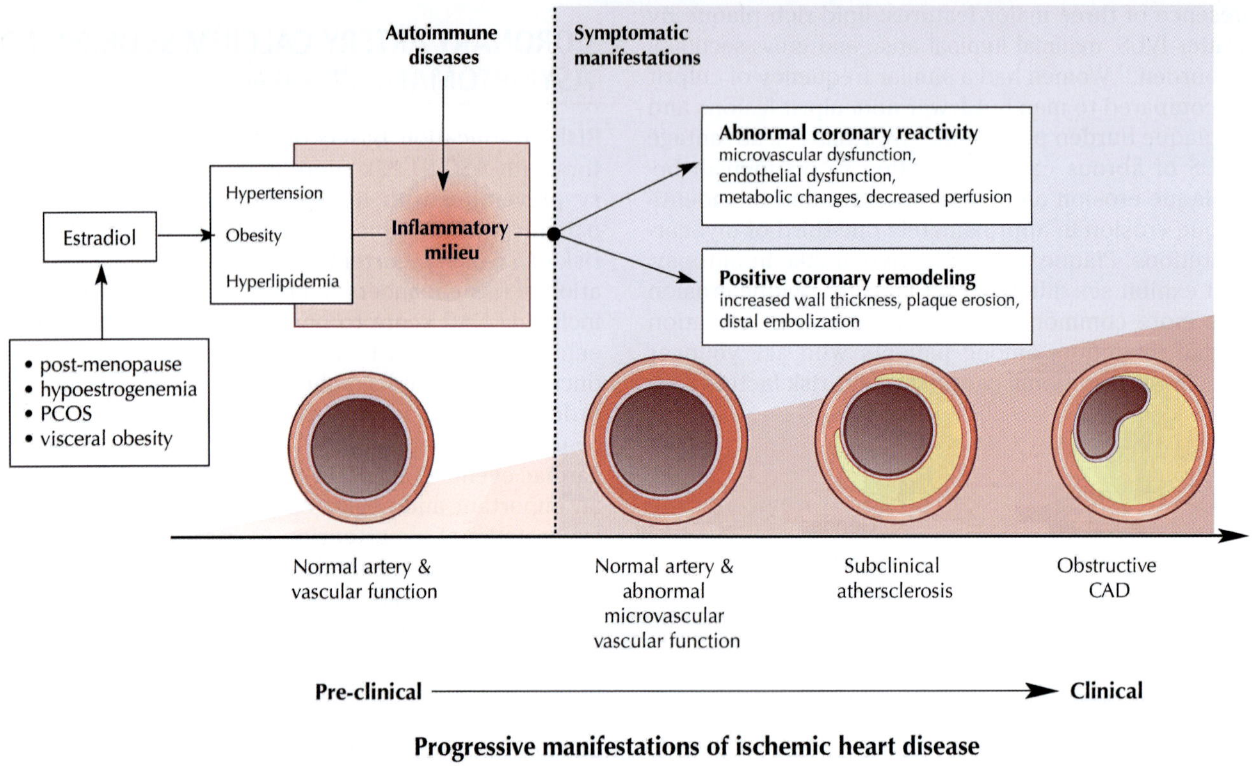

FIG. 5.3 Model of Ischemic Heart Disease in Women. Overarching model of ischemic heart disease in women. *CAD*, Coronary artery disease; *PCOS*, polycystic ovarian syndrome. (From Shaw LJ, Bugiardini R, Merz CN. Women and ischemic heart disease: evolving knowledge. *J Am Coll Cardiol*. 2009;54[17]:1561–1575.)

TABLE 5.1 Risk Factors for Women: Risk Factors Specific to Women for Development of Atherosclerosis

Risk Factors for Atherosclerosis in Women
Premature menopause
Polycystic ovarian syndrome
Gestational hypertension
Preeclampsia
Gestational diabetes
Autoimmune disorders
Visceral obesity
Hypertension

and intravascular imaging techniques. Macroscopic calcifications increase in size for fibroatheromas and are largest for stabilized fibrocalcific plaques, and per-patient quantification of CAC, most commonly with the Agatston score, reflect the underlying volume of atherosclerosis and predict adverse cardiac events in men and women. Individual CAC values for women should be compared to sex, age, and ethnicity-specific nomograms from the Multi-Ethnic Study of Atherosclerosis (MESA), a population-based cohort study of CAC.[24] Normal values for women are lower than men of the same age. There is an age–sex interaction for CAC, as women present with CAC on average 10 years later than men, and 83% to 95% of women below 50 years old have a calcium score of zero.[5,25] Even among octogenarians and nonagenarians, although CAC is near ubiquitous in men, 16% of women had CAC ≤10.[26] In every cohort, CAC = 0 has high negative predictive value for major adverse cardiac events in both men and women. For these reasons, CAC is recommended in current ACC/AHA guidelines as a risk enhancer to spare lipid-lowering therapy for CAC = 0 for women with borderline ASCVD risk of 5% to 7.5% events over 10 years, or to clarify ASCVD risk enhancers notable for women.[27]

Although the prevalence of CAC is lower in women, the outcomes of women for any degree of CAC > 0 are worse than that of men. Women in the long-term CAC Consortium with 6% to 10% 10-year predicted risk, compared to men in the same risk group, tended to be older, with a greater prevalence and extent of CAC, and women with CAC >10 had a higher mortality risk compared to similar men.[28] For any strata of CAC, women had fewer lesions and fewer involved vessels but greater lesion size and higher plaque density to arrive at a similar CAC score, and the relative hazard for cardiovascular disease mortality was higher for women than men for the same degree of multivessel CAC, large lesions, more numerous lesions, or plaque volume, congruent with the elevated risk for the same degree of Agatston CAC score (Fig. 5.4).[25] Restricted to diabetics, the same pattern was observed. Although the prevalence of CAC was lower in women, women had elevated adjusted hazard ratios compared to men for total mortality (p for interaction 0.01) and cardiovascular disease mortality (P for interaction, $P = .04$).[29] It is unknown to what degree worse outcomes for women are attributable to biology or treatment; in emergency department patients with CAC >100 and nonobstructive coronary disease, women were less likely than men to be taking aspirin and statins upon follow-up.[30]

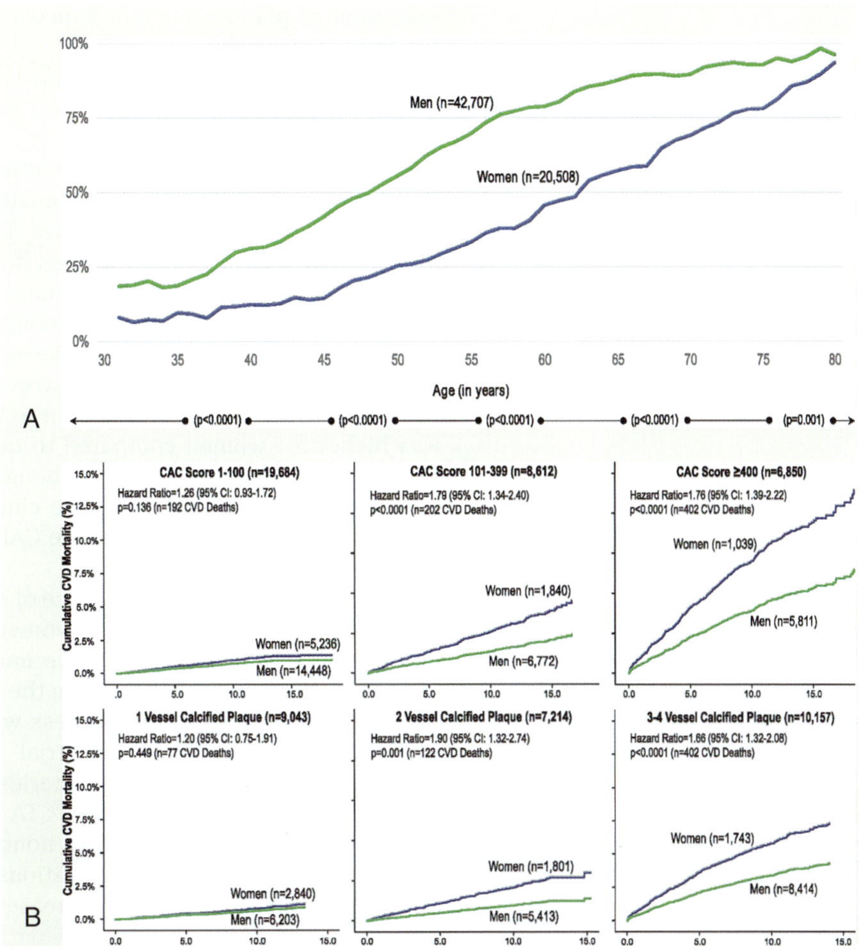

FIG. 5.4 Women have lower coronary artery calcium (CAC) scores compared with men but exhibit higher mortality for high scores and more vessels involved in a retrospective study of long-term cardiovascular mortality from 63,215 patients in the CAC consortium. (A Comparison of detectable coronary artery calcium score >0 across age groups in men and women. CAC exhibits the age–sex interaction of atherosclerosis progression with an inflection in the average CAC score in women at age 46 years old. (B Cardiovascular disease mortality among women and men by CAC score and number of calcified vessels. The presence of coronary artery disease increases cardiovascular disease risk more steeply in women than in men. (From Shaw LJ, Min JK, Nasir K, et al. Sex differences in calcified plaque and long-term cardiovascular mortality: observations from the CAC Consortium. *Eur Heart J.* 2018;39[41]:3727–3735.)

CORONARY CT ANGIOGRAPHY IN SYMPTOMATIC WOMEN

Functional Versus Anatomic Evaluation of Chest Pain

Functional evaluation with stress testing, with or without myocardial imaging, is the mainstay of chest pain evaluation in the United States. However, the Prospective Multicenter Imaging Study for Evaluation of Chest Pain (PROMISE) trial comparing cardiac CT to functional evaluation demonstrated that over 50% of events occurred in patients who did not demonstrate ischemia on the functional study.[31] Additionally, one-third of cardiac events will occur in patients with initially nonobstructive disease on CTA, further identifying patients at risk.[31] When comparing CTA to stress testing, CTA distinguished patients as having mild abnormalities compared with normal in the PROMISE trial (Fig. 5.5).

Functional evaluation has special considerations in women. Women have decreased ability to achieve maximal exercise, and an increased prevalence of obesity, both of which limit the diagnostic accuracy of exercise stress.[32] Breast artifact can limit diagnostic accuracy of single-photon emission computerized tomography (SPECT) and stress echocardiography.[33] In the Calcium Imaging and Selective CT Angiography in Comparison to Functional Testing for Suspected Coronary Artery Disease (CRESCENT) study, both men and women had fewer indeterminate tests with cardiac CT compared with exercise testing (Fig. 5.6).[34] Additionally, women had more frequent negative calcium scores compared with men.

Cardiac CT in Women

Contrast-enhanced CCTA directly visualizes coronary and cardiac anatomy, overcoming many of the challenges of stress testing in women. Cardiac CT scan is currently considered a first-line diagnostic modality in chest pain for intermediate to high-risk women, with a Class IA recommendation.[4] Although the primary application of CCTA has been to evaluate luminal stenoses, CCTA also identifies extraluminal plaque, both calcified and noncalcified. Like CAC = 0, the presence of completely normal coronary arteries by CCTA, with no evidence of nonobstructive

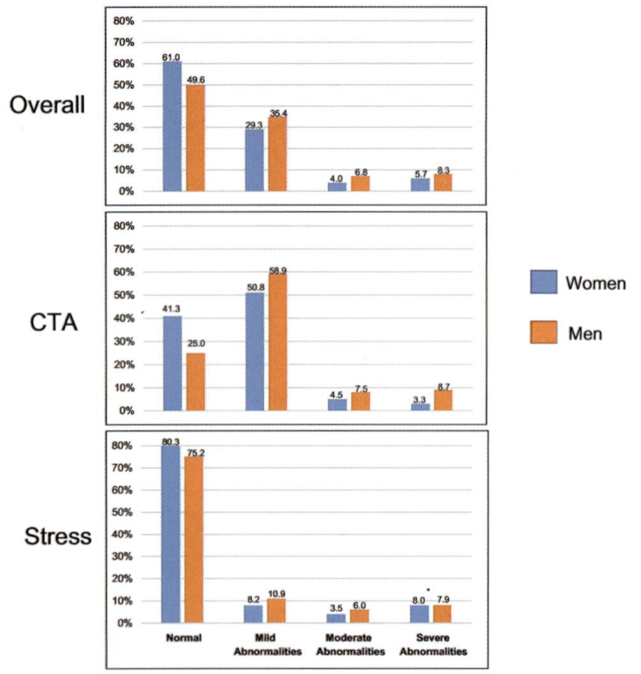

FIG. 5.5 Computed tomography angiography (CTA) identifies increased mild abnormalities for both genders, whereas an increased number of women show normal coronary arteries on CTA compared with men. Sex differences in noninvasive tests in the PROMISE trial examining 8966 patients comparing CTA compared with stress testing (exercise electrocardiogram, stress echocardiography, or stress nuclear). *Represents the only nonstatistically significant comparison. (From Pagidipati NJ, Coles A, Hemal K, et al. Sex differences in management and outcomes of patients with stable symptoms suggestive of coronary artery disease: insights from the PROMISE trial. *Am Heart J.* 2019;208:28–36.)

extraluminal plaque, has a high negative predictive value for cardiac events.[35,36]

Women are more likely to have normal CCTA and less likely to have obstructive CAD than men (Figs. 5.7–5.11).[9,35,36] An age–sex interaction is also evident, and in age <45, female sex is highly protective for any CAD.[37] In the Coronary CT Angiography Evaluation for Clinical Outcomes: An International Multicenter (CONFIRM) Registry, for the same degree of CAD, women have the same elevated risk of major adverse cardiac events as men in 5632 subjects over 5 years, without sex interactions.[38] In the larger CONFIRM cohort of 24,775, all-cause mortality was similarly elevated for every degree of obstructive CAD except for three-vessel coronary disease, where the relative hazard was higher for women compared to men (heart rate 4.21 versus 3.27, $P < .001$).[35] Overall, although the prevalence in men and women are different, the clinical significance of normal coronaries and obstructive CAD is roughly similar in men and women.

However, the clinical significance of nonobstructive coronary artery disease is greater in women than men. Despite less obstructive CAD, women have more frequent angina symptoms than men.[38,39] Patients in the International Study of Comparative Health Effectiveness with Medical and Invasive Approaches (ISCHEMIA) trial who had ischemia with nonobstructive coronary arteries (INOCA) by both noninvasive stress testing and CCTA are fourfold more likely to be female.[40] In addition, nonobstructive disease has important prognostic implications for women. Nonobstructive left main disease increases the risk of major

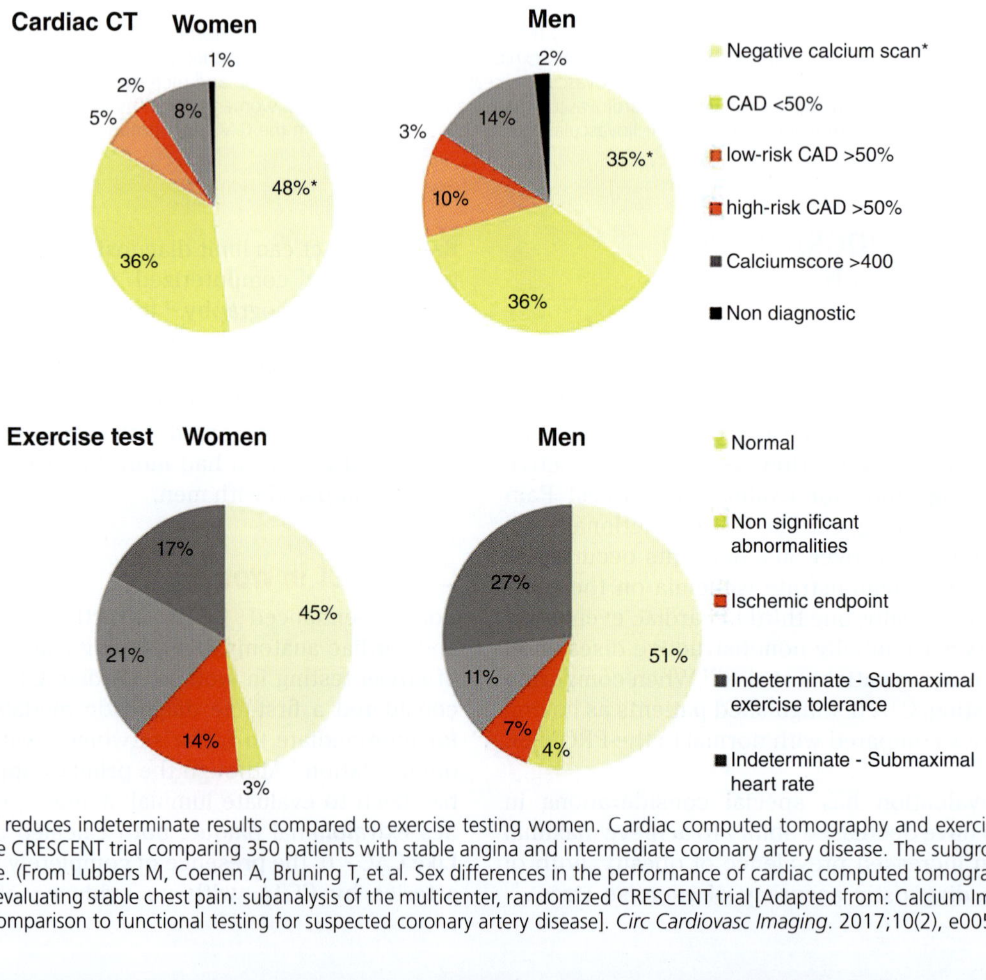

FIG. 5.6 Cardiac CT reduces indeterminate results compared to exercise testing women. Cardiac computed tomography and exercise stress test results stratified by sex in the CRESCENT trial comparing 350 patients with stable angina and intermediate coronary artery disease. The subgroups in men are also included in this figure. (From Lubbers M, Coenen A, Bruning T, et al. Sex differences in the performance of cardiac computed tomography compared with functional testing in evaluating stable chest pain: subanalysis of the multicenter, randomized CRESCENT trial [Adapted from: Calcium Imaging and Selective CT Angiography in comparison to functional testing for suspected coronary artery disease]. *Circ Cardiovasc Imaging.* 2017;10(2), e005295.)

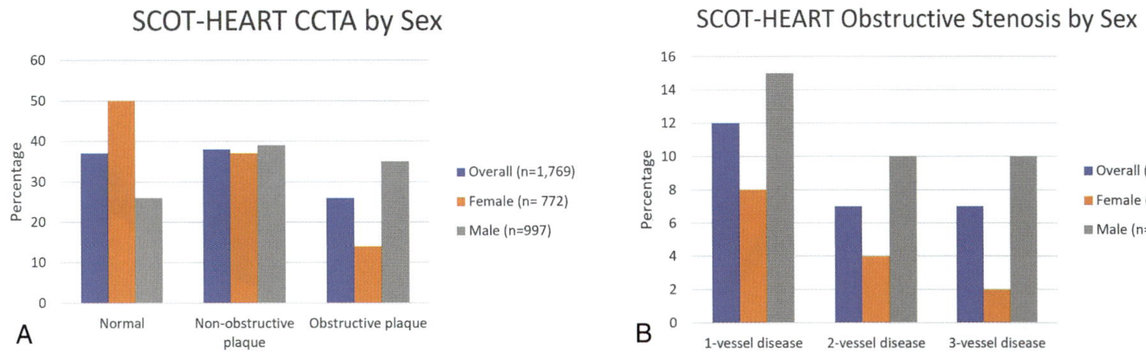

FIG. 5.7 Women have less obstructive plaque, though equal amounts of nonobstructive plaque compared with men. Coronary cardiac tomography visual assessment of (A) obstructive plaque and (B) number of vessels involved comparing by sex in the SCOT-HEART randomized study examining 1769 patients randomized to the use of CT in outpatient cardiology clinic versus standard of care. (Adapted from Williams MC, Kwiecinski J, Doris M, et al. Sex-specific computed tomography coronary plaque characterization and risk of myocardial infarction. *JACC Cardiovasc Imaging*. 2021;14[9]:1804–1814.)

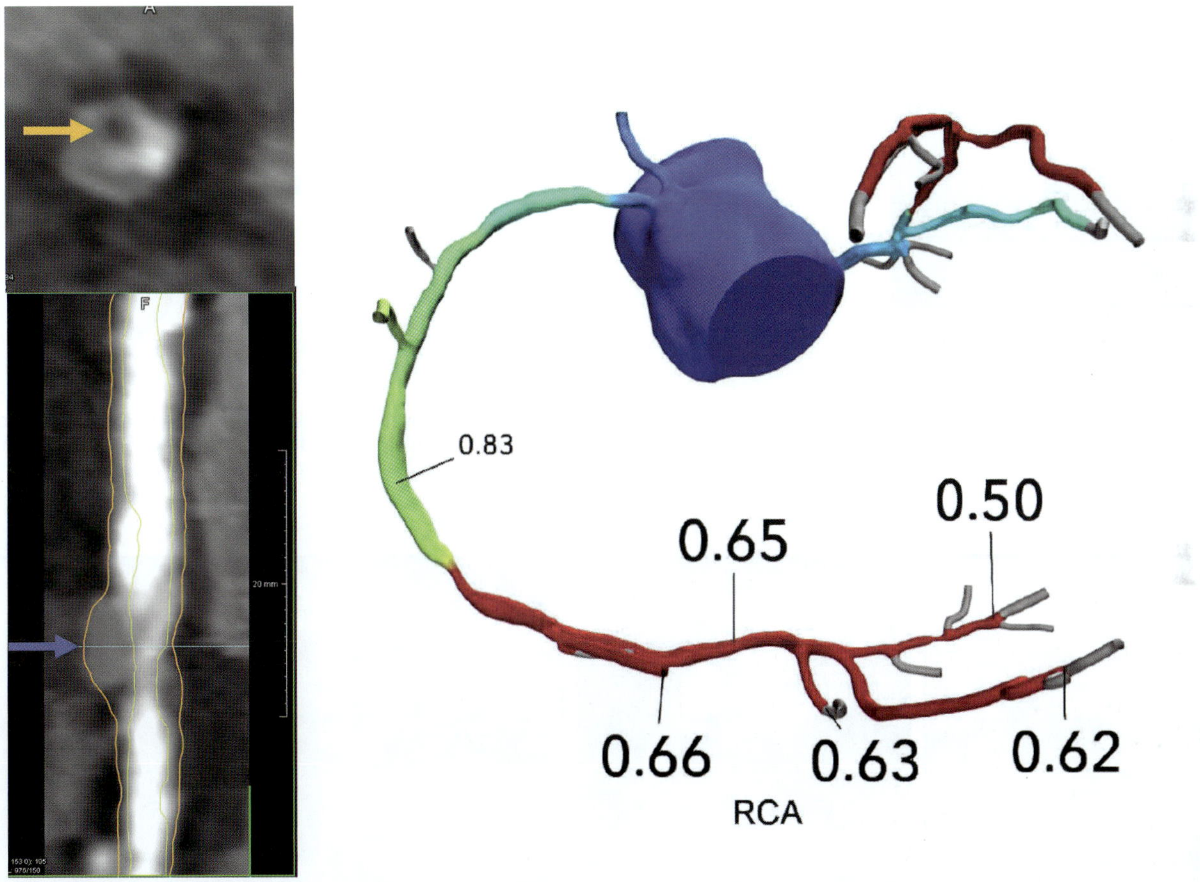

FIG. 5.8 High-risk plaque with low-attenuation plaque and positive remodeling. A 67-year-old woman with peripheral arterial disease and multiple coronary artery disease risk factors presented with typical angina. Coronary computed tomography demonstrated a right coronary artery lesion (*blue arrow*) with low-attenuation plaque (Hounsfield unit 35, *yellow arrow*) with positive remodeling in between extensive calcifications. Both myocardial perfusion imaging and CT-calculated fractional flow reserve were abnormal. The invasive fractional flow reserve was 0.61.

adverse cardiac events in women but not in men ($P = .001$ for interaction), and women with nonobstructive left main disease had a nearly 80% higher risk for events than men with nonobstructive left main disease.[41]

Sex also impacts several high-risk plaque features that can be visualized by CCTA and are associated with thin cap fibroatheroma and incident adverse cardiac events: low-attenuation plaque, positive remodeling, and napkin-ring sign. Like severe stenoses and CAC, high-risk plaque features are less common in women. Among patients in the Incident COroNary Syndromes Identify by Computed Tomography (ICONIC) study who had baseline CCTA before incident myocardial infarction, female subjects had no difference in high-risk plaque features, although they had lower total and low-attenuation plaque volumes.[42] In the Scottish Computed Tomography of the HEART (SCOT-HEART) randomized controlled trial of CCTA compared with standard of care in low- to intermediate-risk patients, high-risk plaque characteristics and plaque burden were decreased among women compared to men overall but similar in those with incident myocardial infarction and low-attenuation plaque predicted incident MI equally in

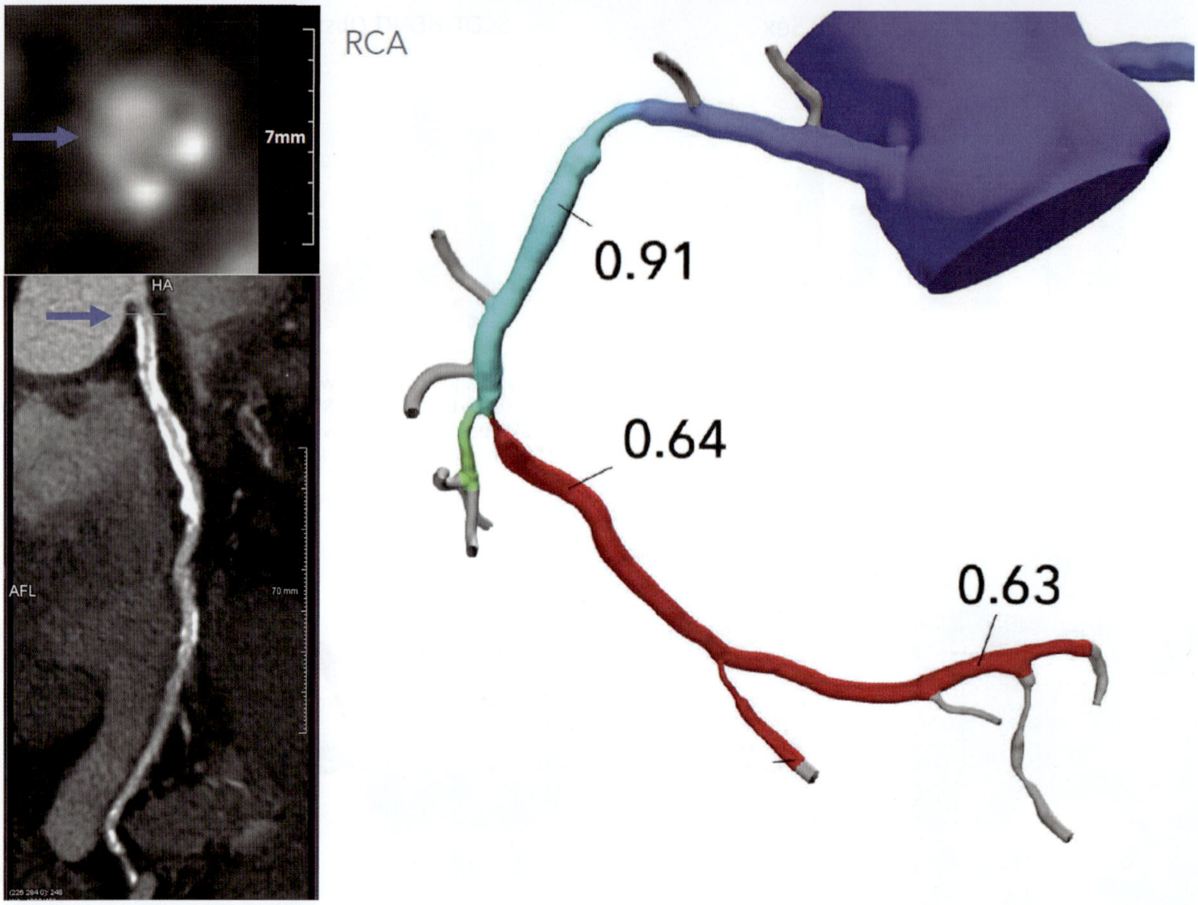

FIG. 5.9 Elderly woman with diffuse atherosclerosis, high plaque burden, and small vessels. A 79-year-old 52-kg woman with prior stroke and diabetes presented with dyspnea on exertion. On coronary computed tomography (CCTA), she had a heavily calcified right coronary artery (RCA) with diffuse disease, high plaque burden, and multiple serial stenoses, with a small lumen diameter even at the most proximal portion (*blue arrow*). The invasive fractional flow reserve was 0.5 distal to the third tandem lesion.

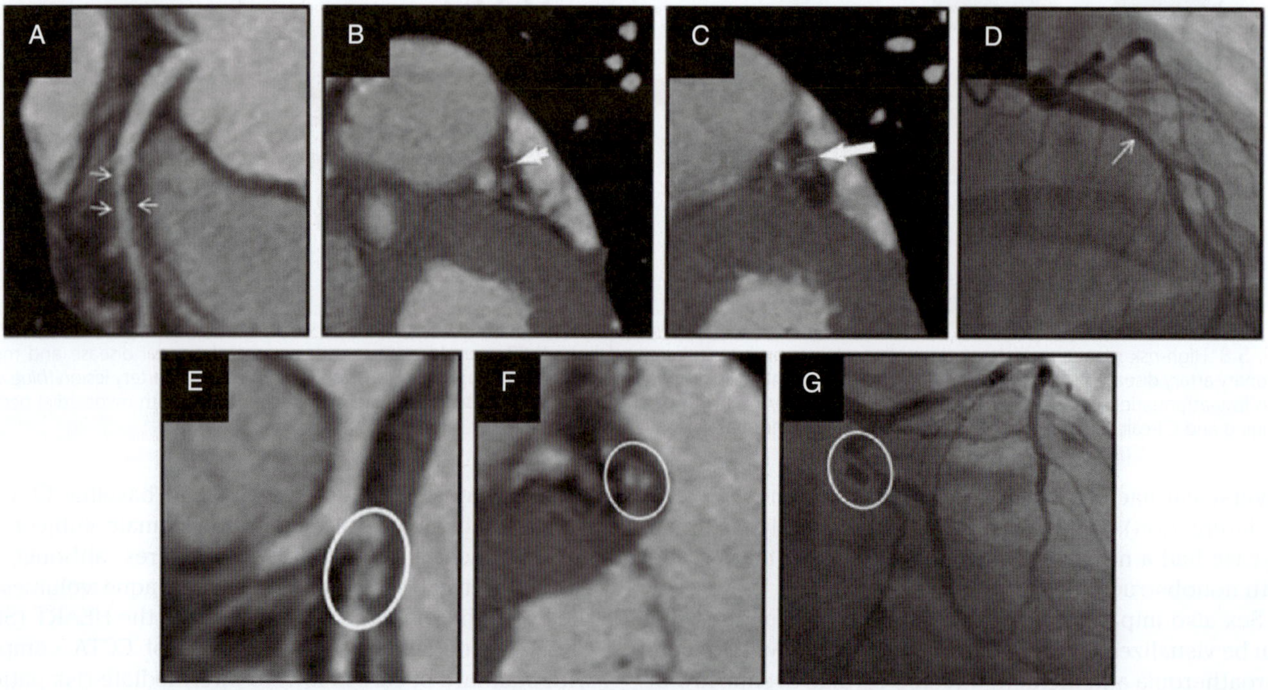

FIG. 5.10 Case Examples of Spontaneous Coronary Artery Dissection. A) CCTA of left anterior descending coronary artery dissection (*arrow*) with long tapered stenosis and intramural hematoma, B and C) epicardial fat stranding, and D) corresponding invasive coronary angiography. E) and F) CCTA of Dissection of left circumflex artery (circled) with G) corresponding invasive coronary angiography. (From Tweet MS, Akhtar NJ, Hayes SN, Best PJ, Gulati R, Araoz PA. Spontaneous coronary artery dissection: acute findings on coronary computed tomography angiography. *Eur Heart J Acute Cardiovasc Care*. 2019;8[5]:467–475.)

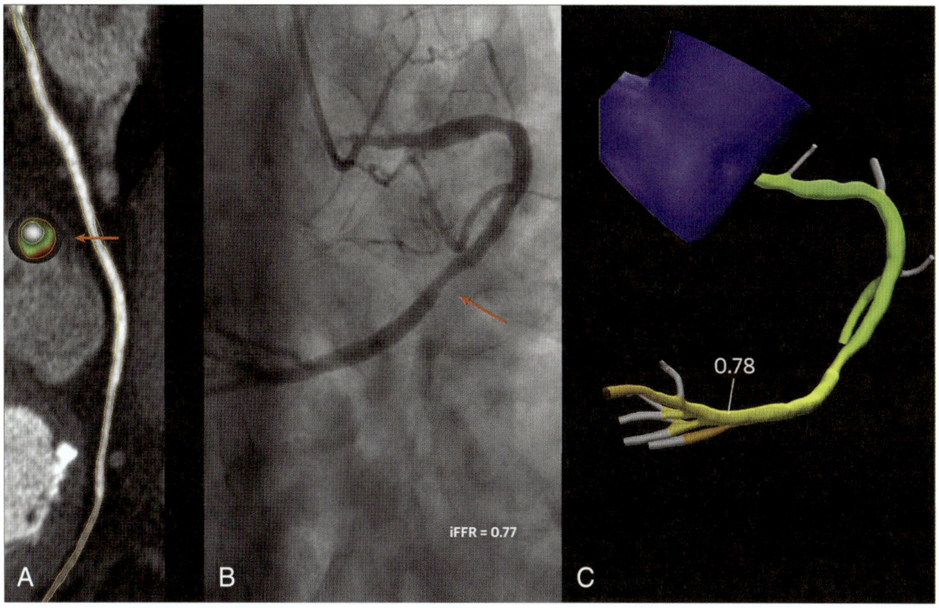

FIG. 5.11 Case example of ischemia with no obstructive coronary arteries (INOCA). A 78-year old-woman with hypertension and diabetes presented with nonexertional chest pain and dyspnea. She had an intermediate positive stress electrocardiogram test. Her coronary computed tomography (CCTA) showed multiple lesions, all <50% stenosis. (A) CCTA of the right coronary artery, *orange arrows* demonstrate the cross-section of the maximal diameter stenosis, *red* shows necrotic core <30 Hounsfield units (HU), *light green* shows fibrofatty plaque 31–130 HU, and dark green shows fibrous plaque 131–350 HU. (B) Invasive coronary angiography (ICA) was nonobstructive and invasive fractional flow reserve (iFFR) measurement was abnormal. (C) Fractional flow reserve computed tomography (FFR-CT) of the right coronary artery (RCA) correlated well with invasive FFR.

TABLE 5.2 Mortality by Degree of Obstruction in Men Versus Women in the CONFIRM Registry Examining 24,775 Patients Undergoing CCTA

	AGE <65 YRS				AGE ≥65 YRS			
	MALE		FEMALE		MALE		FEMALE	
CAD SEVERITY	HR	95% CI	HR	95% CI	HR	95% CI	HR	95% CI
Normal	0.7	0.36–1.36	1	Reference	5.53	2.74–11.2	3.72	1.97–7.02
Nonobstructive	1.65	0.93–2.91	1.59	0.79–3.21	7.79	4.72–12.9	8.08	4.86–13.4
1-vessel disease	2.46	1.26–4.82	2.23	0.95–2.23	10.54	6.13–18.1	8.28	4.60–14.9
2-vessel disease	4.16	1.97–8.82	6.59	2.65–16.3	14.73	8.20–26.5	11.96	6.10–23.5
3-vessel/left main disease	6.8	3.35–13.8	10.59	4.50–24.9	16.25	9.38–28.2	18.68	10.0–34.7

CCTA, coronary computed tomography; *HR*, heart rate.

From Min JK, Dunning A, et al. Age- and sex-related differences in all-cause mortality risk based on coronary computed tomography angiography findings results from the International Multicenter CONFIRM (coronary CT angiography evaluation for clinical outcomes: an international multicenter registry) of 23,854 patients without known coronary artery disease. *J Am Coll Cardiol*. 2011;58:849–860.

men and women.[43] In contrast, the PROMISE trial demonstrated that high-risk plaque was a stronger predictor of major adverse cardiac events (MACE) in women than men and in patients with nonobstructive than obstructive coronary artery disease.[44] One possible explanation for the discrepancy in sex differences between studies is the higher prevalence of obstructive CAD in ICONIC and SCOT-HEART compared to PROMISE; if nonobstructive disease mediates the relationship between sex and high-risk plaque, then the sex difference will be more evident when nonobstructive disease is more common (Table 5.2).

Quantitative measurements of the coronary tree are affected by body size and sex. Patients with higher body surface area (BSA) have a larger vessel volume and plaque volume, with a 250 mm^3 increase in vessel volume for each 0.1 m^2 increase in BSA.[45] Women have smaller vessel, plaque, and lumen volumes and shorter vessel length than men.[45] Normalization of plaque volume by vessel volume is a way to account for body size and unmeasured arteries due to artifact, and it has been variously termed *percent atheroma volume* (PAV) in the IVUS and CCTA literature and mean plaque burden or percent aggregate plaque volume (%APV) in the CCTA literature. Even after normalization, women have lower PAV compared to men (Tables 5.3 and 5.4). In the Progression of AtheRosclerotic PlAque DetermIned by Computed TomoGraphic Angiography Imaging (PARADIGM) study of serial CCTA, women tended to be older than men, with lower plaque volume, and there was an approximately 9-year delay in women developing total plaque volume compared to men. After multivariate adjust-

TABLE 5.3 ***Women have increased angina and Rose Dyspnea Score compared with men.*** **Angina history for women compared with men in the ISCHEMIA randomized trial examining 5179 patients with moderate to severe ischemia to revascularization versus medical therapy**

WOMEN HAVE INCREASED ANGINA AND ROSE DYSPNEA SCORE COMPARED WITH MEN.			
	RANDOMIZED, NO./TOTAL NO. (%)		
CHARACTERISTIC	WOMEN (N = 1168)	MEN (N = 4011)	*P* VALUE
Angina history			
Baseline Seattle Angina Questionnaire Angina			
Frequency Scale			
Median (IQR)	80 (70–100)	90 (70-100)	<.001
Daily angina (0–30)	33/1156 (2.9)	83/3954 (2.1)	
Weekly angina (31–60)	249/1156 (21.5)	746/3954 (18.9)	
Monthly angina (61–99)	565/1156 (48.9)	1678/3954 (42.4)	<.001
No angina in past month (100)	309/1156 (26.7)	1447/3954 (36.6)	
Participant has ever had angina	1068/1168 (91.4)	3573/4011 (89.1)	.02
Angina began or became more frequent over the past 3 mo	329/1064 (30.9)	1026/3564 (28.8)	.18
Dyspnea status over the past month[a]			
None	670/1168 (57.4)	2493/4011 (62.2)	
NYHA class I	178/1168 (15.2)	821/4011 (20.5)	<.001
NYHA class II	320/1168 (27.4)	697/4011 (17.4)	
Rose Dyspnea Score			
0	304/1115 (27.3)	1508/3785 (39.8)	
1	381/1115 (34.2)	1358/3785 (35.9)	
2	204/1115 (18.3)	553/3785 (14.6)	<.001
3	106/1115 (9.5)	240/3785 (6.3)	
4	120/1115 (10.8)	126/3785 (3.3)	

[a]There were no randomized participants in NYHA classes III-IV.

CCTA, Coronary computed tomography angiography, *CMR*, stress cardiac magnetic resonance imaging, *IQR*, interquartile range; *LAD*, left anterior descending coronary artery, *LCx*, left circumflex coronary artery; *LM*, left main; *NYHA*, New York Heart Association; *RCA*, right coronary artery.

From Reynolds HR, Shaw LJ, Min JK, et al. Association of sex with severity of coronary artery disease, ischemia, and symptom burden in patients with moderate or severe ischemia: secondary analysis of the ISCHEMIA randomized clinical trial. *JAMA Cardiol*. 2020;5(7):773–786.

TABLE 5.4 **Effect of sex on plaque burden comparing men versus women in the PARADIGM study examining 1479 patients with suspected coronary atherosclerosis with serial CCTA >2 years apart**

WOMEN HAVE SMALLER PERCENT ATHEROMA VOLUME, CORRECTING FOR SMALLER VESSEL VOLUME AND LENGTH.			
	MALE (N = 864)	FEMALE (N = 615)	*P* VALUE
CCTA			
PV, mm^3	61.4 (10.0–155.1)	29.6 (0.0–102.5)	<.001
PAV, %	2.8 (0.44–7.4)	1.5 (0.0–5.7)	<.001
Vessel volume, mm^3	2428 ± 1066	2075 ± 922	<.001
Vessel length, mm	404 ± 123	384 ± 123	<.001
BSA, m^2	1.90 ± 0.19	1.69 ± 0.17	<.001

BSA, body surface area; *CCTA*, coronary computed tomography angiography; *PAV*, percent atheroma volume; *PV*, plaque volume.

From van Rosendael AR, Lin FY, Ma X, et al. Percent atheroma volume: optimal variable to report whole-heart atherosclerotic plaque burden with coronary CTA, the PARADIGM study. *J Cardiovasc Comput Tomogr*. 2020;14(5):400–406.

ment, men and women had similar rates of progression for total plaque volume, but female sex was associated with greater calcified but slower noncalcified plaque progression. Women had a lower prevalence of high-risk plaque at baseline and less development of high-risk plaques than men.[46]

CT-CALCULATED FRACTIONAL FLOW RESERVE

CT fractional flow reserve (FFR-CT) uses computational fluid dynamic models to estimate pressures in the coronary artery tree across lesions. In the Assessing Diagnostic Value of Noninvasive FFR-CT in Coronary Care (ADVANCE) registry of 4737 symptomatic patients across 38 international centers, women comprised 34% of all subjects with older age and presented with more atypical symptoms.[47,48] Women had less obstructive CAD by CCTA, lower likelihood of positive FFR-CT ≤0.80 for the same degree of CCTA stenosis, and less referral to invasive coronary angiography (ICA); however, once the FFR-CT was <0.80, referral to in ICA in women was equally likely as in men (55% versus 57%). By ICA, women were slightly less likely to have obstructive CAD (32% versus 25%) and revascularization (31% versus 36%), although once the FFR-CT was ≤0.75, revascularization was similar (42% versus 46%).

EXTRA-CORONARY FINDINGS IN WOMEN

As the purpose of coronary arteries is to efficiently deliver blood flow to the myocardium, the diameter and volume of coronary arteries should be scaled to the myocardial mass. The degree of mismatch between the coronary vessel volume (V) and LV mass (M), or the V/M ratio, can be routinely calculated during estimation of FFR-CT.[49] Patients with low V/M ratio independently predicts FFR <0.80 independent of stenosis and plaque measures.[50] Abnormally low V/M ratio is observed in microvascular angina even with normal FFR-CT.[51] V/M ratio is also significantly lower in diabetics compared to nondiabetics, even in nonobstructive disease.[52,53] The depressed V/M ratios in these conditions, both of which disproportionately affect women, are notable because the ADVANCE registry of FFR-CT showed that symptomatic women normally have an increased, not decreased, V/M ratio. In ADVANCE women had less obstructive CCTA and higher FFR-CT and also a higher estimated FFR-CT for the same degree of stenosis. The sex difference occurs because women have lower coronary vessel volume and disproportionately even lower myocardial mass, resulting in a higher V/M ratio. Because FFR-CT models myocardial demand proportional to myocardial mass, a higher V/M ratio will result in higher estimated FFR-CT for the same degree of stenosis.[47]

A substudy of the Prospective Head-to-Head Comparison of Coronary CT Angiography, Myocardial Perfusion SPECT, PET, and Hybrid Imaging for Diagnosis of Ischemic Heart Disease using Fractional Flow Reserve as Index for Functional Severity of Coronary Stenoses (PACIFIC) cohort observed that patients with V/M ratio below median were more likely to have abnormal hyperemic myocardial blood flow and fractional flow reserve. V/M was not associated with coronary flow reserve (CFR) in PACIFIC, but there may have been reduced power to detect associations of V/M with microvascular angina because (1) there was a trend to abnormal resting myocardial blood flow, so that coronary flow reserve ratio of rest versus hyperemia was unchanged, and (2) the prevalence of macrovascular ischemia was very high, so that there were few patients with purely microvascular angina.[54] In total, these results suggest that some portion of abnormal coronary flow in INOCA is associated with macrovascular ischemia, measured by FFR or FFR-CT; some portion of microvascular angina is attributable to anatomic mismatch between the coronary bed and subtended myocardium, measured by V/M ratio and independent of FFR-CT; and finally, V/M was not associated with coronary flow reserve (CFR) in PACIFIC.

Other noncoronary features observed on CCTA may also display sex differences. Left ventricular (LV) function can be observed in retrospectively gated CCTA, at the cost of higher radiation exposure, and can be used to diagnose reduced ejection fraction. On the other hand, hyperdynamic LV function >65% is more frequent in older women and is associated with increased mortality in women, whereas it is protective in men.[55,56] Epicardial adipose tissue (EAT) exhibits paracrine and inflammatory effects associated with atherosclerosis and atrial fibrillation and is associated with increased cardiometabolic diseases and adverse LV mass and remodeling.[57] Women after menopause or in late perimenopause have greater volumes of heart fat than women before or in early perimenopause independent of age, obesity, and other covariates, and EAT is associated with reduced estradiol.[58]

RADIATION DOSE AND EXPOSURE IN CCTA COMPARED TO OTHER MODALITIES

For any diagnostic test, the risks to a patient for radiation dose exposure must be balanced by the quality and value of information resulting from the test. Radiation dose is an important consideration for women because ionizing radiation is potentially teratogenic in women of childbearing age, and cumulative chest radiation is potentially harmful for breast cancer. Radiation dose reduction strategies should be applied in all women undergoing CT imaging.[59] The average radiation dose for current generation CCTA is 2 to 4 milliSieverts (mSv) for high-pitch helical compared with 0.5 to 7 mSv for prospectively triggered axial imaging. Helical acquisitions with tube current modulation have doses of 6 to 20 mSv and are avoided for routine imaging.[60,61] By way of comparison, the average radiation dose is 11 to 18 for SPECT with dual sestamibi, 4 mSv for Rubidium positron emission tomography (PET), and none for stress exercise ECG, stress echo, and stress perfusion coronary magnetic resonance testing.[61] Radiation dose reduction strategies, which can be achieved by tailoring CCTA scanning protocols by patient heart rate and body habitus, can reduce radiation dose more than 10-fold while achieving similar image quality, and CCTA in women have higher image quality than men.[62] Another strategy for dose reduction is by using CAC >0 to screen subjects to forego CCTA.[34]

The radiation exposure of the upfront nondiagnostic test must be balanced against the exposure from downstream testing, including invasive angiography for false-positive noninvasive tests. In the CRESCENT study, women had decreased need for downstream testing compared to men.[34] In SCOT-HEART, more women were reclassified as not having CAD, resulting in fewer downstream tests and treatments with no prognostic penalty by sex.[9] In PROMISE, women with abnormal noninvasive testing were less likely to have obstructive CAD, resulting in lower referral to angiography than men.[63] False positives by functional testing may explain the greater risk stratification value of CCTA over stress testing in PROMISE.[31] Abnormal CTAs were less common than abnormal stress tests in women, whereas abnormal CTAs were more common than abnormal stress tests in men, so that CCTA may be a more informative risk stratification modality for women.[64] Misclassification for women can occur even earlier in the diagnostic cascade, at the stage of risk scoring; Framingham and Diamond-Forrestor risk scores were predictive of a positive CCTA in men, whereas age, body mass index, and Framingham risk score predicted positive CCTA in women.[36]

Spontaneous Coronary Artery Dissection

Spontaneous coronary artery dissection (SCAD) is an acute coronary event due to the formation of a hematoma leading to separation of the intima from the underlying vessel.[65] SCAD disproportionately affects women with up to 35% of all ACS cases in women ≤50 years old attributed to SCAD.[66] Mechanisms connecting SCAD to a disease predominantly of women implicate sex hormones, affecting women who are nulliparous, pregnant, and after childbirth.[65] Women who present with SCAD during pregnancy face more serious consequences of cardiogenic shock, impaired left ventricular function, and multivessel disease.[65] The utility of CCTA as a diagnostic tool for SCAD remains to be delineated with a variety of imaging findings. One study of 14 patients with SCAD showed abrupt luminal stenosis present 64% of the time, intramural hematoma at 50%, tapered luminal stenosis at 36%, and dissection 14% of the time.[67] Secondary features identified include epicardial fat stranding, coronary artery tortuosity, and coronary bridging.[67] Importantly, hematoma may appear similar on CCTA to noncalcified atherosclerotic plaque, leading to challenges in relying on CCTA for diagnosis. However, due to the elevated risks of iatrogenic coronary dissection and vessel occlusion in invasive angiography of SCAD, there is increased attention on CCTA of SCAD to spare procedural risks.

CONCLUSION

Cardiac CT is an anatomic approach to primary prevention and chest pain evaluation that can be a useful alternative to functional testing in women. Sex differences by CAC and CCTA reflect underlying sex differences in atherosclerosis and coronary pathophysiology. Nonobstructive coronary plaque and subclinical atherosclerosis is particularly important in women. Conditions of particular relevance to women, including INOCA and SCAD, also have unique features by CCTA. Future research will elucidate the clinical role of CT in workup of microvascular angina and features of plaque erosion.

REFERENCES

1. Xu JQ MS, Kochanek KD, Arias E. Deaths: final data for 2019. *Natl Vital Stat Rep*. 2021:70.
2. Virani SS, Alonso A, Aparicio HJ, et al. Heart disease and stroke statistics-2021 update: a report from the American Heart Association. *Circulation*. 2021;143:e254–e743.
3. Roger VL, Go AS, Lloyd-Jones DM, et al. Heart disease and stroke statistics—2011 update: a report from the American Heart Association. *Circulation*. 2011;123:e18–e209.
4. Gulati M, Levy PD, Mukherjee D, et al. 2021 AHA/ACC/ASE/CHEST/SAEM/SCCT/SCMR guideline for the evaluation and diagnosis of chest pain: a report of the American College of Cardiology/American Heart Association Joint Committee on clinical practice guidelines. *Circulation*. 2021;144:e368–e454.
5. Reynolds HR, Bairey Merz CN, Berry C, et al. Coronary arterial function and disease in women with no obstructive coronary arteries. *Circ Res*. 2022;130:529–551.
6. Shaw LJ, Bugiardini R, Merz CN. Women and ischemic heart disease: evolving knowledge. *J Am Coll Cardiol*. 2009;54:1561–1575.
7. Berger JS, Elliott L, Gallup D, et al. Sex differences in mortality following acute coronary syndromes. *JAMA*. 2009;302:874–882.
8. Serruys PW, Hara H, Garg S, et al. Coronary computed tomographic angiography for complete assessment of coronary artery disease: JACC state-of-the-art review. *J Am Coll Cardiol*. 2021;78:713–736.
9. Mangion K, Adamson PD, Williams MC, et al. Sex associations and computed tomography coronary angiography-guided management in patients with stable chest pain. *Eur Heart J*. 2020;41:1337–1345.
10. Virmani R, Kolodgie FD, Burke AP, Farb A, Schwartz SM. Lessons from sudden coronary death: a comprehensive morphological classification scheme for atherosclerotic lesions. *Arterioscler Thromb Vasc Biol*. 2000;20:1262–1275.
11. Virmani R, Burke AP, Farb A, Kolodgie FD. Pathology of the vulnerable plaque. *J Am Coll Cardiol*. 2006;47:C13–C18.
12. Falk E. Pathogenesis of atherosclerosis. *J Am Coll Cardiol*. 2006;47:C7–12.
13. Partida RA, Libby P, Crea F, Jang IK. Plaque erosion: a new in vivo diagnosis and a potential major shift in the management of patients with acute coronary syndromes. *Eur Heart J*. 2018;39:2070–2076.
14. van den Hoogen IJ, Gianni U, Al Hussein Alawamlh O, et al. What atherosclerosis findings can CT see in sudden coronary death: plaque rupture versus plaque erosion. *J Cardiovasc Comput Tomogr*. 2020;14:214–218.
15. Smilowitz NR, Sampson BA, Abrecht CR, Siegfried JS, Hochman JS, HR Reynolds. Women have less severe and extensive coronary atherosclerosis in fatal cases of ischemic heart disease: an autopsy study. *Am Heart J*. 2011;161:681–688.
16. Raber L, Mintz GS, Koskinas KC, et al. Clinical use of intracoronary imaging. Part 1: guidance and optimization of coronary interventions. An expert consensus document of the European Association of Percutaneous Cardiovascular Interventions. *Eur Heart J*. 2018;39:3281–3300.
17. Stone GW, Maehara A, Lansky AJ, et al. A prospective natural-history study of coronary atherosclerosis. *N Engl J Med*. 2011;364:226–235.
18. Lansky AJ, Ng VG, Maehara A, et al. Gender and the extent of coronary atherosclerosis, plaque composition, and clinical outcomes in acute coronary syndromes. *JACC Cardiovasc Imaging*. 2012;5:S62–S72.
19. Kolte D, Yonetsu T, Ye JC, Libby P, Fuster V, Jang IK. Optical coherence tomography of plaque erosion: JACC focus seminar part 2/3. *J Am Coll Cardiol*. 2021;78:1266–1274.
20. Grundy SM, Stone NJ, Bailey AL, et al. 2018 AHA/ACC/AACVPR/AAPA/ABC/ACPM/ADA/AGS/APhA/ASPC/NLA/PCNA guideline on the management of blood cholesterol: executive summary: a report of the American College of Cardiology/American Heart Association Task Force on clinical practice guidelines. *J Am Coll Cardiol*. 2019;73:3168–3209.
21. Grandi SM, Filion KB, Yoon S, et al. Cardiovascular disease-related morbidity and mortality in women with a history of pregnancy complications. *Circulation*. 2019;139:1069–1079.
22. Vounzoulaki E, Khunti K, Abner SC, Tan BK, Davies MJ, Gillies CL. Progression to type 2 diabetes in women with a known history of gestational diabetes: systematic review and meta-analysis. *BMJ*. 2020;369:m1361.
23. Salmon JE, Roman MJ. Subclinical atherosclerosis in rheumatoid arthritis and systemic lupus erythematosus. *Am J Med*. 2008;121:S3–S8.
24. McClelland RL, Chung H, Detrano R, Post W, Kronmal RA. Distribution of coronary artery calcium by race, gender, and age: results from the Multi-Ethnic Study of Atherosclerosis (MESA). *Circulation*. 2006;113:30–37.
25. Shaw LJ, Min JK, Nasir K, et al. Sex differences in calcified plaque and long-term cardiovascular mortality: observations from the CAC Consortium. *Eur Heart J*. 2018;39:3727–3735.
26. Kuller LH, Lopez OL, Mackey RH, Rosano C, Edmundowicz D, Becker JT, Newman AB. Subclinical cardiovascular disease and death, dementia, and coronary heart disease in patients 80+ years. *J Am Coll Cardiol*. 2016;67:1013–1022.
27. Arnett DK, Blumenthal RS, Albert MA, et al. 2019 ACC/AHA guideline on the primary prevention of cardiovascular disease: a report of the American College of Cardiology/American Heart Association Task Force on clinical practice guidelines. *J Am Coll Cardiol*. 2019;74:e177–e232.
28. Kelkar AA, Schultz WM, Khosa F, et al. Long-term prognosis after coronary artery calcium scoring among low-intermediate risk women and men. *Circ Cardiovasc Imaging*. 2016;9:e003742.

29. Wong ND, Cordola Hsu AR, Rozanski A, et al. Sex differences in coronary artery calcium and mortality from coronary heart disease, cardiovascular disease, and all causes in adults with diabetes: the coronary calcium consortium. *Diabetes Care*. 2020;43:2597–2606.
30. Kim BS, Chan N, Hsu G, et al. Sex differences in coronary arterial calcification in symptomatic patients. *Am J Cardiol*. 2021;149:16–20.
31. Hoffmann U, Ferencik M, Udelson JE, et al. Prognostic value of noninvasive cardiovascular testing in patients with stable chest pain: insights from the PROMISE trial (Prospective Multicenter Imaging study for evaluation of chest pain). *Circulation*. 2017;135:2320–2332.
32. Gondoni LA, Liuzzi A, Titon AM, et al. A simple tool to predict exercise capacity of obese patients with ischaemic heart disease. *Heart*. 2006;92:899–904.
33. Kohli P, Gulati M. Exercise stress testing in women: going back to the basics. *Circulation*. 2010;122:2570–2580.
34. Lubbers M, Coenen A, Bruning T, et al. Sex differences in the performance of cardiac computed tomography compared with functional testing in evaluating stable chest pain: subanalysis of the multicenter, randomized CRESCENT trial (Calcium Imaging and selective CT Angiography in Comparison to Functional Testing for Suspected Coronary Artery Disease). *Circ Cardiovasc Imaging*. 2017;10.
35. Min JK, Dunning A, Lin FY, et al. Age- and sex-related differences in all-cause mortality risk based on coronary computed tomography angiography findings results from the International Multicenter CONFIRM (coronary CT angiography evaluation for clinical outcomes: an international multicenter registry) of 23,854 patients without known coronary artery disease. *J Am Coll Cardiol*. 2011;58:849–860.
36. Hemal K, Pagidipati NJ, Coles A, et al. Sex differences in demographics, risk factors, presentation, and noninvasive testing in stable outpatients with suspected coronary artery disease: insights from the PROMISE trial. *JACC Cardiovasc Imaging*. 2016;9:337–346.
37. Otaki Y, Gransar H, Cheng VY, et al. Gender differences in the prevalence, severity, and composition of coronary artery disease in the young: a study of 1635 individuals undergoing coronary CT angiography from the prospective, multinational confirm registry. *Eur Heart J Cardiovasc Imaging*. 2015;16:490–499.
38. Schulman-Marcus J, Hartaigh B, Gransar H, et al. Sex-specific associations between coronary artery plaque extent and risk of major adverse cardiovascular events: the CONFIRM long-term registry. *JACC Cardiovasc Imaging*. 2016;9:364–372.
39. Reynolds HR, Shaw LJ, Min JK, et al. Association of sex with severity of coronary artery disease, ischemia, and symptom burden in patients with moderate or severe ischemia: secondary analysis of the ISCHEMIA randomized clinical trial. *JAMA Cardiol*. 2020;5:773–786.
40. Reynolds HR, Diaz A, Cyr DD, et al. Ischemia with nonobstructive coronary arteries: insights from the ISCHEMIA trial. *JACC Cardiovasc Imaging*. 2022;16(1):63–74.
41. Xie JX, Eshtehardi P, Varghese T, et al. Prognostic significance of nonobstructive left main coronary artery disease in women versus men: long-term outcomes from the CONFIRM (coronary CT angiography evaluation for clinical outcomes: an international multicenter) registry. *Circ Cardiovasc Imaging*. 2017;10:e006246.
42. Conte E, Dwivedi A, Mushtaq S, et al. Age- and sex-related features of atherosclerosis from coronary computed tomography angiography in patients prior to acute coronary syndrome: results from the ICONIC study. *Eur Heart J Cardiovasc Imaging*. 2021;22:24–33.
43. Williams MC, Kwiecinski J, Doris M, et al. Sex-specific computed tomography coronary plaque characterization and risk of myocardial infarction. *JACC Cardiovasc Imaging*. 2021;14:1804–1814.
44. Ferencik M, Mayrhofer T, Bittner DO, et al. Use of high-risk coronary atherosclerotic plaque detection for risk stratification of patients with stable chest pain: a secondary analysis of the PROMISE randomized clinical trial. *JAMA Cardiol*. 2018;3:144–152.
45. van Rosendael AR, Lin FY, Ma X, et al. Percent atheroma volume: optimal variable to report whole-heart atherosclerotic plaque burden with coronary CTA, the PARADIGM study. *J Cardiovasc Comput Tomogr*. 2020;14:400–406.
46. Lee SE, Sung JM, Andreini D, et al. Sex differences in compositional plaque volume progression in patients with coronary artery disease. *JACC Cardiovasc Imaging*. 2020;13:2386–2396.
47. Fairbairn TA, Dobson R, Hurwitz-Koweek L, et al. Sex differences in coronary computed tomography angiography-derived fractional flow reserve: lessons from ADVANCE. *JACC Cardiovasc Imaging*. 2020;13:2576–2587.
48. Patel MR, Norgaard BL, Fairbairn TA, et al. 1-year impact on medical practice and clinical outcomes of FFRCT: the ADVANCE registry. *JACC Cardiovasc Imaging*. 2020;13:97–105.
49. Choi JH, Kim E, Kim HY, Lee SH, Kim SM. Allometric scaling patterns among the human coronary artery tree, myocardial mass, and coronary artery flow. *Physiol Rep*. 2020;8:e14514.
50. Taylor CA, Gaur S, Leipsic J, et al. Effect of the ratio of coronary arterial lumen volume to left ventricle myocardial mass derived from coronary CT angiography on fractional flow reserve. *J Cardiovasc Comput Tomogr*. 2017;11:429–436.
51. Grover R, Leipsic JA, Mooney J, et al. Coronary lumen volume to myocardial mass ratio in primary microvascular angina. *J Cardiovasc Comput Tomogr*. 2017;11:423–428.
52. Kuneman JH, El Mahdiui M, van Rosendael AR, et al. Coronary volume to left ventricular mass ratio in patients with diabetes mellitus. *J Cardiovasc Comput Tomogr*. 2022;16:319–326.
53. Xu H, Sun L, Miao C, Jin Y, Hou Y. Type 2 diabetes mellitus is associated with increased left ventricular mass independent of coronary artery volume. *Clin Radiol*. 2019;74 972 e17-972 e23.
54. van Diemen PA, Schumacher SP, Bom MJ, et al. The association of coronary lumen volume to left ventricle mass ratio with myocardial blood flow and fractional flow reserve. *J Cardiovasc Comput Tomogr*. 2019;13:179–187.
55. Gebhard C, Buechel RR, Stähli BE, et al. Impact of age and sex on left ventricular function determined by coronary computed tomographic angiography: results from the prospective multicentre CONFIRM study. *Eur Heart J Cardiovasc Imaging*. 2017;18:990–1000.
56. Gebhard C, Maredziak M, Messerli M, et al. Increased long-term mortality in women with high left ventricular ejection fraction: data from the CONFIRM (coronary CT angiography evaluation for clinical outcomes: an international multicenter) long-term registry. *Eur Heart J Cardiovasc Imaging*. 2020;21:363–374.
57. Ardissino M, McCracken C, Bard A, et al. Pericardial adiposity is independently linked to adverse cardiovascular phenotypes: a CMR study of 42 598 UK Biobank participants. *Eur Heart J Cardiovasc Imaging*. 2022;23:1471–1481.
58. El Khoudary SR, Shields KJ, Janssen I, et al. Cardiovascular fat, menopause, and sex hormones in women: the SWAN cardiovascular fat ancillary study. *J Clin Endocrinol Metab*. 2015;100:3304–3312.
59. Truong QA, Rinehart S, Abbara S, et al. Coronary computed tomographic imaging in women: an expert consensus statement from the Society of Cardiovascular Computed Tomography. *J Cardiovasc Comput Tomogr*. 2018;12:451–466.
60. Deseive S, Pugliese F, Meave A, et al. Image quality and radiation dose of a prospectively electrocardiography-triggered high-pitch data acquisition strategy for coronary CT angiography: the multicenter, randomized PROTECTION IV study. *J Cardiovasc Comput Tomogr*. 2015;9:278–285.
61. Hirshfeld Jr JW, Ferrari VA, Bengel FM, et al. 2018 ACC/HRS/NASCI/SCAI/SCCT expert consensus document on optimal use of ionizing radiation in cardiovascular imaging-best practices for safety and effectiveness, part 1: radiation physics and radiation biology: a report of the American College of Cardiology Task Force on expert consensus decision pathways. *J Am Coll Cardiol*. 2018;71:2811–2828.
62. Stocker TJ, Nühlen N, Schmermund A, et al. Impact of dose reduction strategies on image quality of coronary CTA in real-world clinical practice: a subanalysis of PROTECTION VI registry data. *AJR Am J Roentgenol*. 2021;217:1344–1352.
63. Pagidipati NJ, Coles A, Hemal K, et al. Sex differences in management and outcomes of patients with stable symptoms suggestive of coronary artery disease: insights from the PROMISE trial. *Am Heart J*. 2019;208:28–36.
64. Pagidipati NJ, Hemal K, Coles A, et al. Sex differences in functional and CT angiography testing in patients with suspected coronary artery disease. *J Am Coll Cardiol*. 2016;67:2607–2616.
65. Hayes SN, Tweet MS, Adlam D, et al. Spontaneous coronary artery dissection: JACC state-of-the-art review. *J Am Coll Cardiol*. 2020;76:961–984.
66. Nakashima T, Noguchi T, Haruta S, et al. Prognostic impact of spontaneous coronary artery dissection in young female patients with acute myocardial infarction: a report from the Angina Pectoris-Myocardial Infarction Multicenter Investigators in Japan. *Int J Cardiol*. 2016;207:341–348.
67. Tweet MS, Akhtar NJ, Hayes SN, Best PJ, Gulati R, Araoz PA. Spontaneous coronary artery dissection: acute findings on coronary computed tomography angiography. *Eur Heart J Acute Cardiovasc Care*. 2019;8:467–475.

6 How to Obtain a High-Quality Coronary CT Angiography

STEPHAN ACHENBACH, MOHAMED MARWAN, AND ALOHA MEAVE GONZÁLEZ

KEY POINTS

- Imaging of the coronary arteries is difficult because of their small dimensions and rapid motion. Coronary CT angiography (CCTA) stretches the temporal and spatial resolution of computed tomography to its very limits. Artifacts caused by motion, partial volume effects, or insufficient contrast enhancement are the most frequent causes of reduced image quality in CCTA.
- If image quality is impacted by artifact, a frequent consequence may be false-positive interpretations regarding the presence of coronary artery stenoses.
- For reliably high image quality with a low likelihood of relevant artifacts, important measures include: Assuring a low heart rate with minimal variability during acquisition; using breathhold commands that guarantee reliable breath-holding, including thorough practice prior to image acquisition; administration of nitrates whenever not contraindicated; and achieving a compact contrast agent bolus with high iodine delivery rate throughout the duration of the scan.

INTRODUCTION

Coronary CT angiography (CCTA) is firmly embedded into clinical practice, and numerous practice guidelines list CCTA as the test of first choice for many patients with suspected coronary artery disease or acute chest pain.[1–5] Typically, the aim of CCTA is to reliably rule out obstructive coronary artery lesions. Frequently, guidelines mandate limiting the use of CCTA to individuals in whom fully diagnostic image quality can be expected, or they list specific patient criteria that make CT an appropriate or less appropriate test in a given individual.[1–4] This is an expression of the fact that fully diagnostic image quality may not be readily achievable in all patients and in all clinical situations, and that degraded image quality has a detrimental effect on the interpretation and reporting accuracy of CCTA. Due to the small dimensions and rapid motion of the coronary arteries, their complex three-dimensional anatomy, and occasionally the presence of severe calcification, the use of computed tomography imaging for coronary visualization stretches the technical capabilities even of high-end CT systems to their very limits. It is therefore necessary to optimize image acquisition protocols and to adapt them to individual patient characteristics. Some of the most important aspects are described in this chapter.

ARTIFACTS AND DETERMINANTS OF IMAGE QUALITY IN CCTA

In many instances, CCTA allows imaging of the coronary artery lumen with high image quality in order to identify or rule out the presence of obstructive coronary artery lesions. "High image quality" refers to datasets that allow visualization of the major coronary vessels and large side branches without interruption of their continuity, with sufficient contrast to separate the coronary lumen from the surrounding tissue and coronary atherosclerotic plaque (both calcified and noncalcified), and without blurring or unsharp borders (see Fig. 6.1). A major factor that will influence image quality is the sharpness of calcified coronary atherosclerotic plaque that is frequently present in the coronary wall, immediately adjacent to the coronary lumen (see Fig. 6.2). Calcified plaque may impact visualization of the coronary lumen and the ability to identify or rule out luminal stenoses in two ways: On one hand, the high density of coronary calcium may lead to partial volume effects (so-called "blooming"). These partial volume effects cause calcified plaques to appear larger in the CT datasets than they actually are because the average density of voxels, which are only partly filled by calcified plaque, is so high that in the reconstructed images, the entire voxel seems to be filled with calcium. Consequently, the artificially high volume taken up by calcified plaques may cause the appearance that they partially obscure the coronary lumen (see Fig. 6.3). On the other hand, any high-density object that moves during the acquisition of the CT image can give rise to image reconstruction artifacts that have a dark, unsharp appearance. This prominently applies to calcified coronary plaque (see Fig. 6.4). Even small, hardly discernible amounts of coronary artery motion during acquisition of the CT dataset may therefore result in low-density artifacts immediately adjacent to calcified coronary plaque. Such artifacts can lead to apparent narrowing or even interruption of coronary lumen continuity and frequently cause false-positive interpretation regarding the presence of coronary artery stenoses (see Figs. 6.5 and 6.6). This is a relatively frequent problem in severely calcified vessel segments (see Fig. 6.7).

The relatively limited temporal resolution of computed tomography is therefore the main factor that limits the image quality of CCTA. It can lead to blurring and unsharp contours of the coronary arteries, and in a more subtle way it can cause artifacts adjacent to calcified coronary plaque as described above. Because the speed of motion of the coronary arteries varies widely during the cardiac cycle,[6–9] reliable synchronization of CT data acquisition or reconstruction to the patient's ECG and appropriate

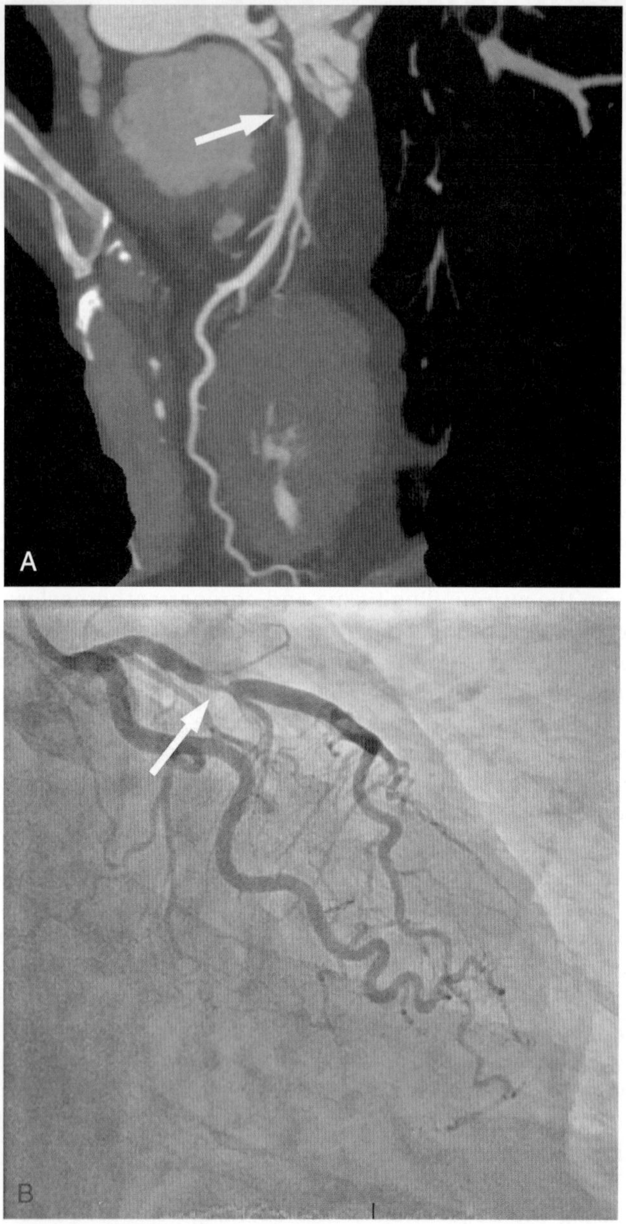

FIG. 6.1 Coronary CT angiography of the left anterior descending coronary artery, showing a high-grade proximal stenosis (*arrow*, A). Corresponding invasive coronary angiogram (B).

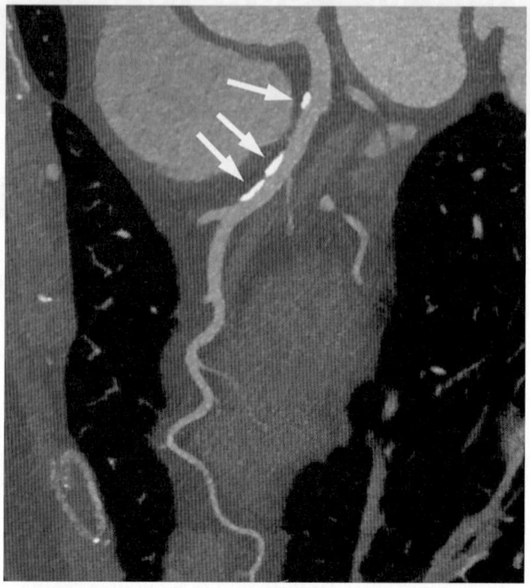

FIG. 6.2 Well-defined visualization of coronary calcification (*arrows*) in a high-quality coronary CT angiography dataset.

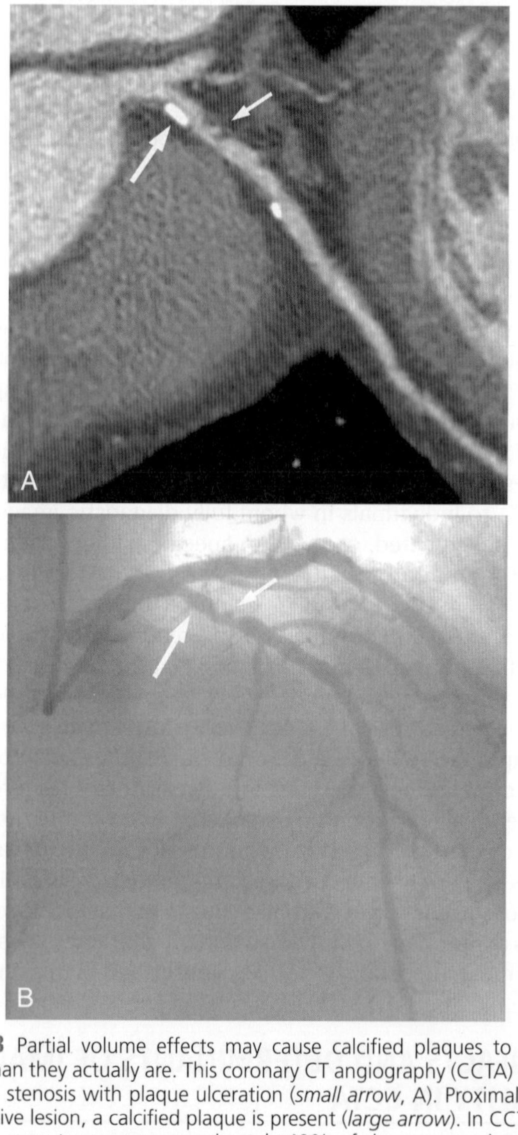

FIG. 6.3 Partial volume effects may cause calcified plaques to appear larger than they actually are. This coronary CT angiography (CCTA) dataset shows a stenosis with plaque ulceration (*small arrow*, A). Proximal to this obstructive lesion, a calcified plaque is present (*large arrow*). In CCTA, this plaque seems to occupy approximately 40% of the coronary lumen just proximal to the ulcerated lesion. Invasive angiography shows a lack of any lumen encroachment at the respective site (B).

selection of a cardiac phase with minimal coronary motion are important prerequisites to obtain high-quality, artifact-free CCTA datasets. Higher heart rates, with faster coronary motion, are associated with a more frequent occurrence of motion-related artifacts and may be associated with lower diagnostic accuracy—in particular, decreased specificity.[10–13] During the cardiac cycle, and especially for patients with lower heart rates, the phase with minimal coronary motion is usually mid-diastole. Atrial contraction during end-systole results in very fast coronary motion. The duration of diastole decreases with increasing heart rate (see Fig. 6.8). Therefore diastolic acquisition is advantageous particularly in patients with low heart rates (e.g., <65 beats/min), whereas imaging at an end-systolic time point may be advantageous in higher heart rates and in patients in whom an irregular heart rate may be present during data acquisition.

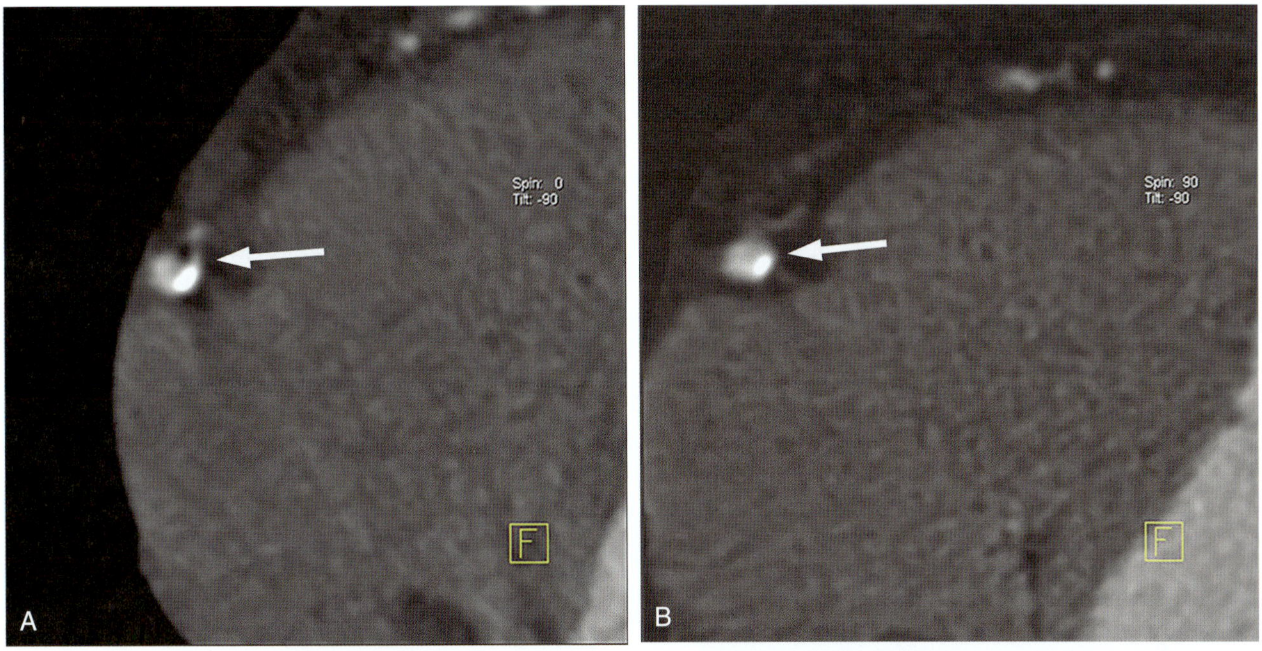

FIG. 6.4 Motion can cause low-density artifact immediately adjacent to calcified plaque (*arrow*, A). Panel B shows the same segment of the right coronary artery reconstructed at a slightly different time instant in the cardiac cycle, with almost complete absence of motion artifact.

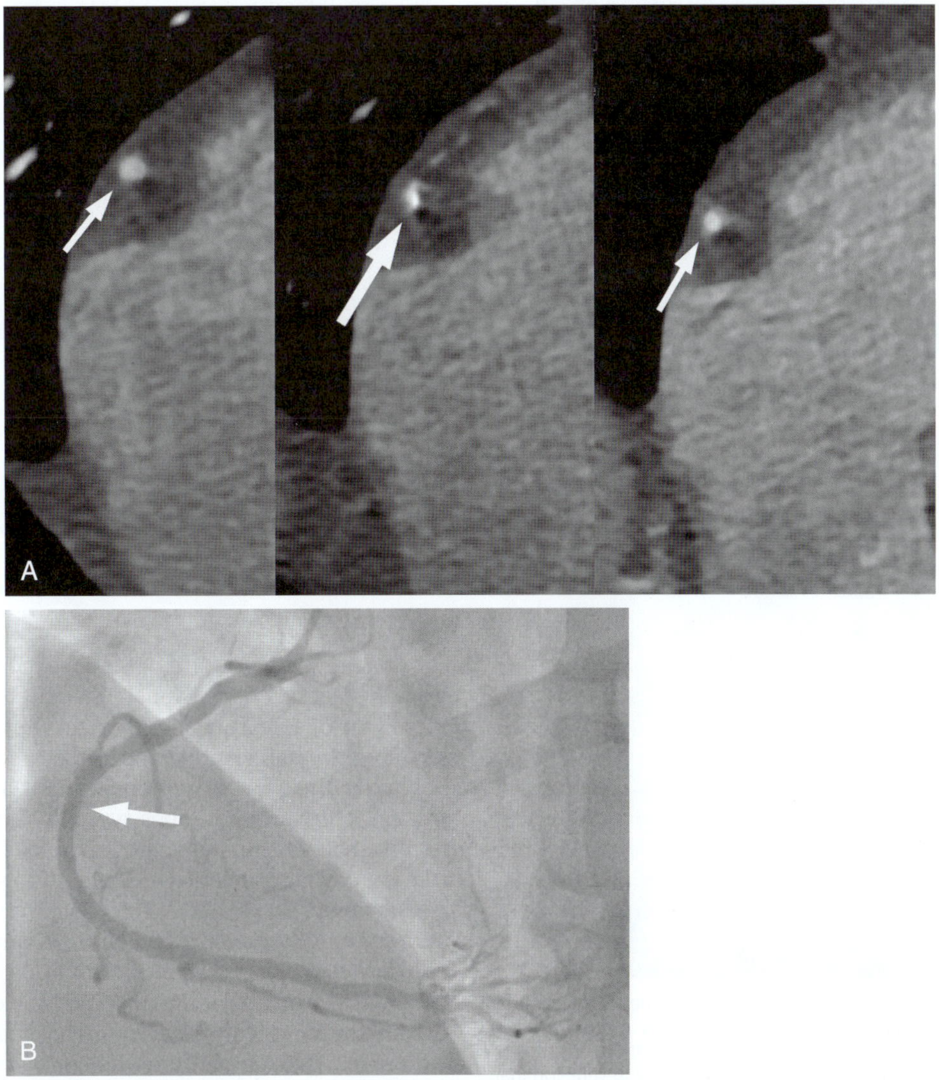

FIG. 6.5 The effect demonstrated in Fig. 6.4 can cause false-positive interpretations of coronary stenoses. Panel A shows three consecutive cross-sections of the right coronary artery (*arrows*), with the impression of a significant lumen reduction (*large arrow*). However, this is caused by low-density artefacts as a consequence of calcium and coronary motion. Invasive angiography demonstrates the absence of any obstructive coronary lesion (B).

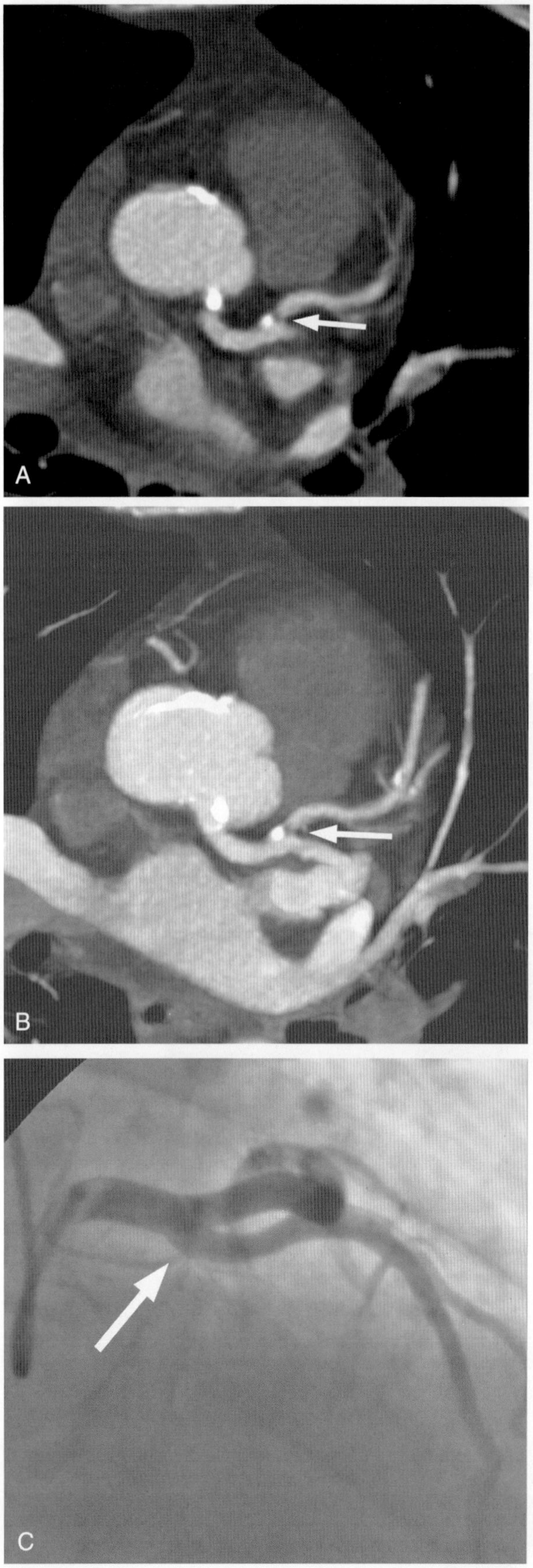

FIG. 6.6 False-positive coronary stenosis as a consequence of motion artifact secondary to coronary calcification. Low-density motion artifact adjacent to a small calcified plaque at the ostium of the left anterior descending coronary artery creates the impression of a severe luminal narrowing (A: multiplanar reconstruction, B: maximum intensity projection, C: invasive coronary angiogram).

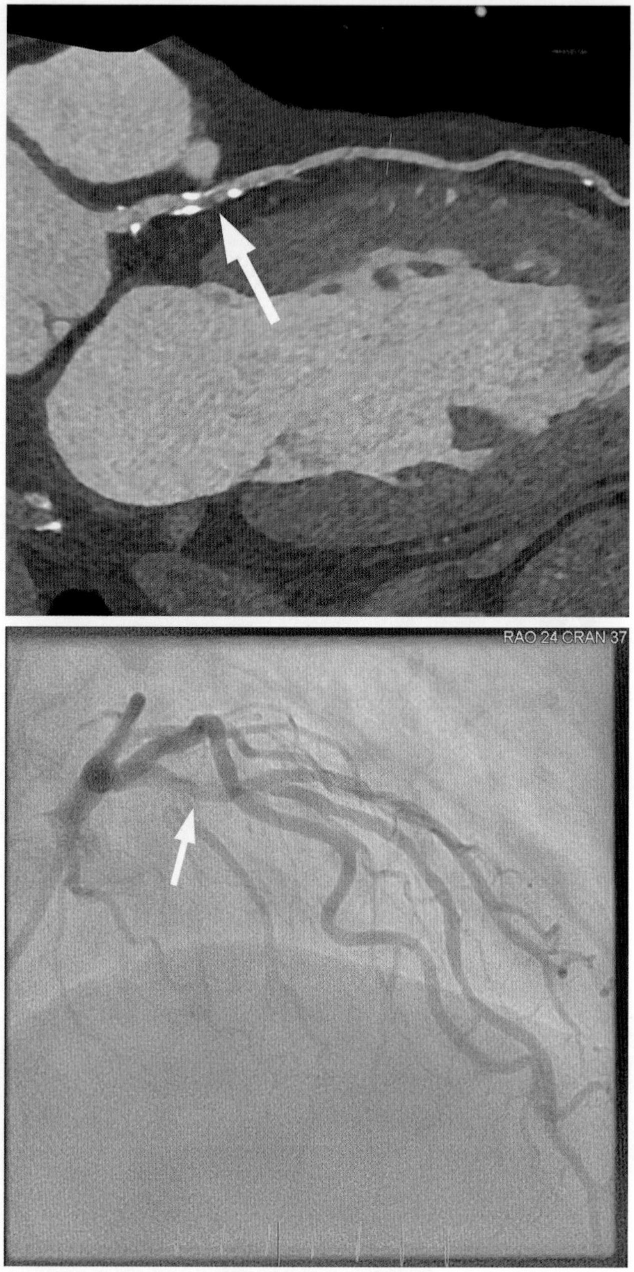

FIG. 6.7 False-positive finding of a coronary stenosis in a calcified segment of the proximal left anterior descending coronary artery (*arrows*).

A further difficulty and potential for image artifacts arises from the fact that data acquisition for CCTA typically requires more than one heart beat. Although CT systems with 320 slices may have sufficiently wide detectors to cover the entire volume of the heart in just one heart beat and without table motion, other scanner types typically require image acquisition over more than one cardiac cycle. This, in turn, means that the coronary arteries are "pieced together" from several consecutive heart beats in the reconstructed image datasets. In order to fully visualize the entire course and all segments of a coronary artery, five or more cardiac cycles may be necessary. It is crucial that the position of all coronary arteries is exactly the same during each cardiac cycle used for imaging. Otherwise, the continuity of the coronary lumen may be interrupted ("misalignment artifact"). This may cause the appearance of a coronary artery stenosis (see Fig. 6.9). Many CT

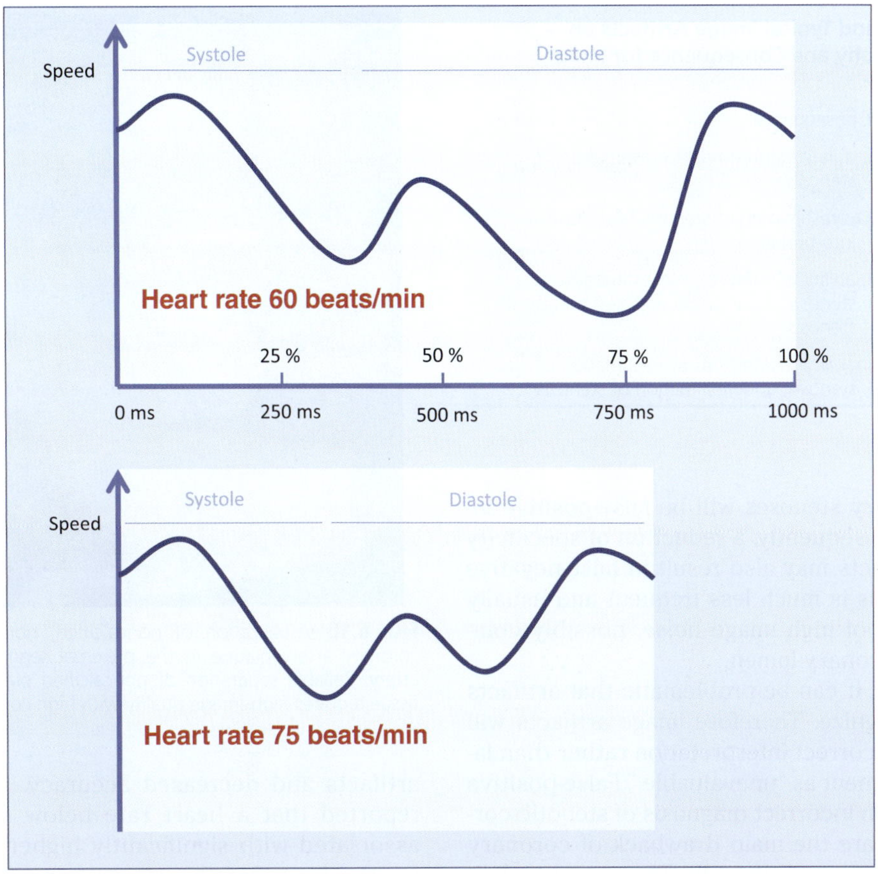

FIG. 6.8 Velocity of coronary motion during the cardiac cycle for low and high heart rates (schematic representation). The duration of the diastolic time window with relatively slow coronary motion decreases with increasing heart rate. For coronary imaging, a diastolic time window is usually optimal if heart rate is low, but systolic imaging may be more appropriate for higher heart rates.

systems use interpolation to reduce misalignment artifacts caused by slightly different positions of a coronary artery during subsequent heart beats[14] This interpolation improves visual image quality but can in turn result in blurring or unsharpness of a coronary artery and potential misinterpretation as luminal narrowing. Reliable ECG synchronization, a constant heart rate during image acquisition (particularly for visualization of the coronary arteries in diastole), and a reliable breathhold are important factors to avoid misalignment artifacts in CCTA.

Finally, any imaging requires sufficient contrast to noise ratio. In CCTA, this means that the difference in x-ray attenuation between the coronary lumen and the surrounding tissue must be sufficiently high and random image noise sufficiently low to allow reliable delineation of the coronary lumen. Image noise is determined by x-ray tube parameters such as tube current and voltage, and one major determinant of luminal x-ray attenuation is the speed and timing of contrast agent delivery. Care must therefore be taken to choose appropriate tube settings and to use suitable protocols for contrast injection.

IMPORTANCE OF IMAGE QUALITY

When imaging artifacts or impaired image quality affect the interpretation of coronary CT angiography datasets, the most frequent consequence regarding the identifica-

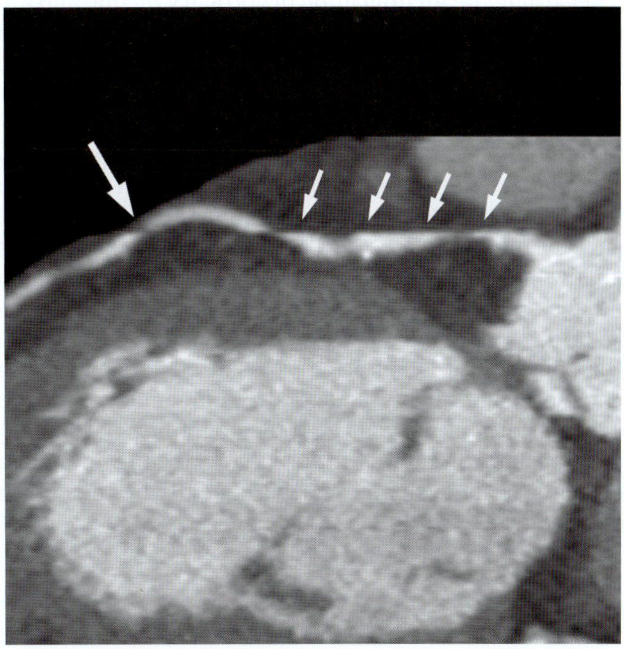

FIG. 6.9 Misalignment artifact. In this multiplanar rendering of a coronary CT angiography dataset showing the proximal and mid-left anterior descending coronary artery in lateral orientation (orthogonal to the axial imaging plane), a misalignment artifact can clearly be identified as a horizontal line that interferes with clear visualization of the proximal left anterior descending coronary artery (*small arrows*). It also causes a short interruption of the lumen continuity in the mid-segment of the left anterior descending coronary artery which might be misinterpreted as stenosis (*large arrow*).

TABLE 6.1 Frequent and Typical Image Artifacts on Coronary CT Angiography and Consequence for Image Interpretation

Artifact	Consequence
Motion artifact	Inability to interpret, overestimation of stenosis
Misalignment artifact	Overestimation of stenosis/false-positive interpretation
Severe calcification	Inability to interpret, overestimation of stenosis, occasionally underestimation of stenosis
High image noise	Inability to interpret, overestimation of stenosis, underestimation of stenosis

tion of coronary artery stenoses will be false-positive interpretations and, consequently, a reduction of specificity (see Table 6.1). Artifacts may also result in false-negative interpretation, but this is much less frequent and usually occurs in the setting of high image noise, possibly combined with a small coronary lumen.

In clinical practice, it can be problematic that artifacts may be hard to recognize. Therefore image artifacts will frequently result in incorrect interpretation rather than labeling a coronary segment as "unevaluable." False-positive interpretations with an incorrect diagnosis of stenotic coronary artery lesions are the main drawback of coronary CT angiography when applied clinically. They may result in unnecessary downstream testing, including invasive procedures, and all efforts must be undertaken to minimize their occurrence.

Regarding the identification of coronary plaque and atherosclerotic plaque burden, the visualization of calcified plaque shows relatively little dependence on image quality. Neither false-negative nor false-positive findings occur to a clinically relevant extent unless there is extreme reduction of image quality, which would be straightforward to recognize. The identification of noncalcified plaque, on the other hand, requires excellent image quality with absence of motion-related artifact as well as high-contrast and low-image noise. Both false-positive and false-negative findings are possible when image quality is impaired (see Fig. 6.10).

In summary, it is important to assure high and fully diagnostic image quality and to strive for minimal artifact when performing coronary CT angiography, particularly since misinterpretation, rather than labeling individual segments as "unevaluable," may frequently be the clinical consequence.

PREDICTORS OF IMAGE QUALITY

Heart Rate and Heart Rate Variability

Based on the types and causes of artifacts outlined above, several factors can be identified that influence image quality and diagnostic accuracy of CCTA. Numerous studies have demonstrated that a high heart rate and heart rate irregularity are associated with an increased risk of

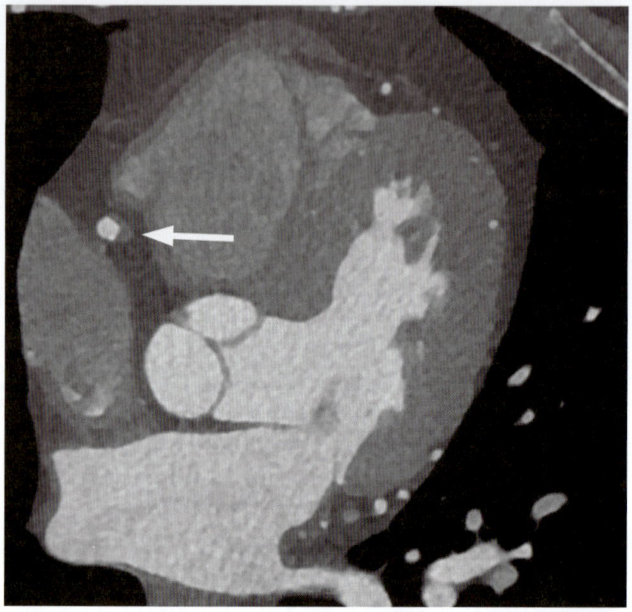

FIG. 6.10 Visualization of noncalcified, nonobstructive atherosclerotic coronary artery plaque in the proximal segment of the right coronary artery. Reliable separation of noncalcified plaque and pericoronary soft tissue requires high-image quality with high contrast and low image noise.

artifacts and decreased accuracy. A large metaanalysis reported that a heart rate below 62 beats/minute was associated with significantly higher diagnostic accuracy for the identification of coronary artery stenoses using CT systems with 64 slices or more.[13] The extent to which heart rate and heart rate variability influence diagnostic accuracy depends on the type of CT system that is used. The dependence of image quality and diagnostic accuracy on having a low heart rate is less pronounced for more modern systems with faster gantry rotation times, or when using a dual-source CT. Some authors, however, do find an influence of heart rate on the accuracy and robustness of image interpretation even for the most modern systems.[10–12,15] It is important to emphasize that low heart rates allow the use of low radiation-dose image acquisition protocols, whereas higher heart rates mandate protocols associated with higher exposure. In fact, registries consistently demonstrate that low heart rate is a predictor of low radiation exposure.[16,17] Current guidelines for image acquisition in CCTA recommend to aim for a heart rate of 60 beats per minute or less, but they leave room for individual decision-making regarding higher target heart rates depending on the scanner generation that is used and the indication for the examination.[18]

Coronary Calcium

The extent of coronary calcifications influence image quality, the likelihood of artifact, and the accuracy of CCTA. There is, however, no prespecified "upper limit" of coronary calcium above which a CCTA examination should not be performed. Even a single calcified plaque can occasionally cause false-positive results (see Fig. 6.6), and even large amounts of calcium do not necessarily render a coronary CT angiography data set unevaluable if

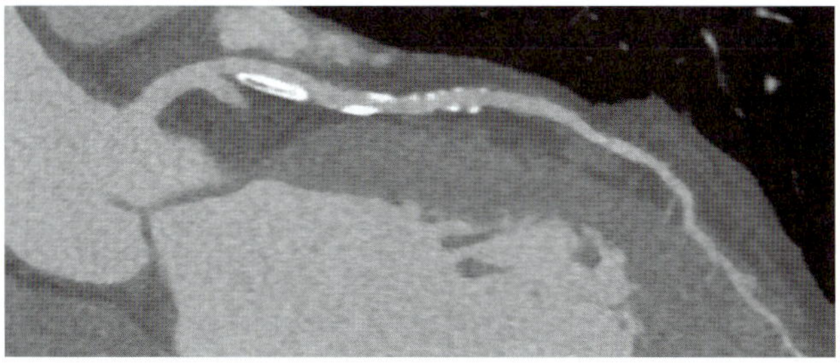

FIG. 6.11 In coronary CT angiography datasets of high quality—with good luminal contrast, low image noise, and absence of motion-induced artifacts—the coronary lumen can remain well visible in spite of the presence of pronounced calcification.

all other parameters are optimal (Fig. 6.11). The decision whether or not to proceed to coronary CT angiography if relatively large amounts of coronary calcium are present must therefore be made on a case-by-case basis and should include considerations such as the indication for the scan and the presence or absence of other factors that may affect image quality, in particular heart rate and body weight.

Body Weight

A higher body weight is associated with higher image noise. Excessively high body weight may substantially degrade image quality. Higher body mass also requires higher radiation exposure to reduce image noise. Neither body weight nor body mass index are ideal predictors of image noise, which is in fact best predicted by the amount of solid body tissue that needs to be penetrated by the x-rays in the area of the heart.[19,20] Again, there is no single threshold for body weight or body mass index above which CCTA should not be considered, and the decision needs to incorporate several factors, including heart rate and heart rate variability, the indication for the scan, and the willingness to accept relatively high radiation exposure.

Contrast Enhancement

Poor contrast enhancement of the coronary lumen negatively affects image quality and interpretability. Therefore high iodine content contrast agent is recommended over low iodine content contrast agent, and high-contrast flow rates are recommended for intravenous injection.[18] Tube voltage (higher iodine contrast for lower tube voltages) and body weight also affect the contrast that is achieved in the coronary artery lumen. Contrast is furthermore affected by coronary artery diameter.

Coronary Artery Diameter

It has been reported that smaller coronary diameters negatively affect image quality and diagnostic accuracy of CCTA.[11] In most cases, the coronary diameter cannot be determined prior to CCTA, but smaller coronary diameters can be assumed in certain individuals, for example, in a person with long-standing diabetes. Also, larger coronary diameters are achieved by premedication using nitrates, which is therefore highly recommended prior to coronary

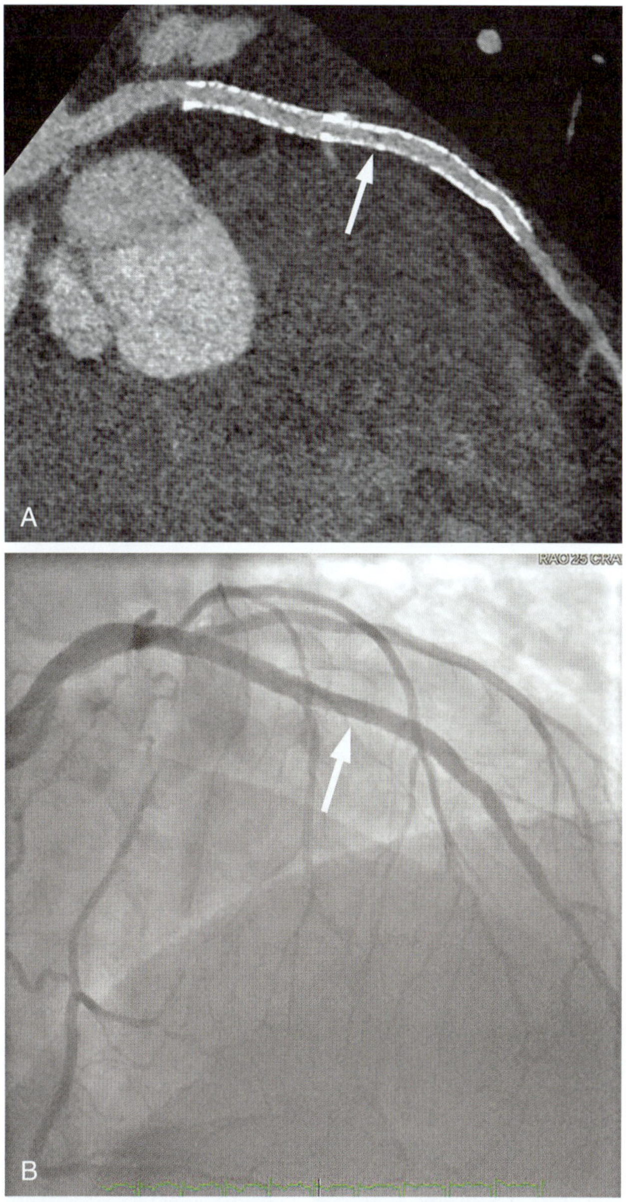

FIG. 6.12 Coronary CT angiography (A) and invasive coronary angiography (B) of the proximal left anterior descending coronary artery in a patient with implanted coronary stents (3.5-mm nominal diameter). Even though no obvious artifacts are present, a short interruption of the continuity of the contrast-enhanced lumen within the stent does not allow to reliably rule out in-stents stenosis by CT (*arrow*).

CT angiography.[18] Of note, nitrates may also have other effects, such as increased coronary flow that may in turn increase intraluminal contrast.

Stents, Sternal Wires, Pacemakers/ICDs, and Other Implants

Metal has very high CT attenuation and may therefore give rise to artifacts, particularly due to partial volume effects and motion. Although the image quality in coronary segments that contain stents can be very high and frequently allow diagnostic assessment, artifacts that mimic the presence of focal or diffuse in-stent stenosis can occur and may be virtually indiscernible from true lumen narrowing (see Fig. 6.12). The likelihood of such

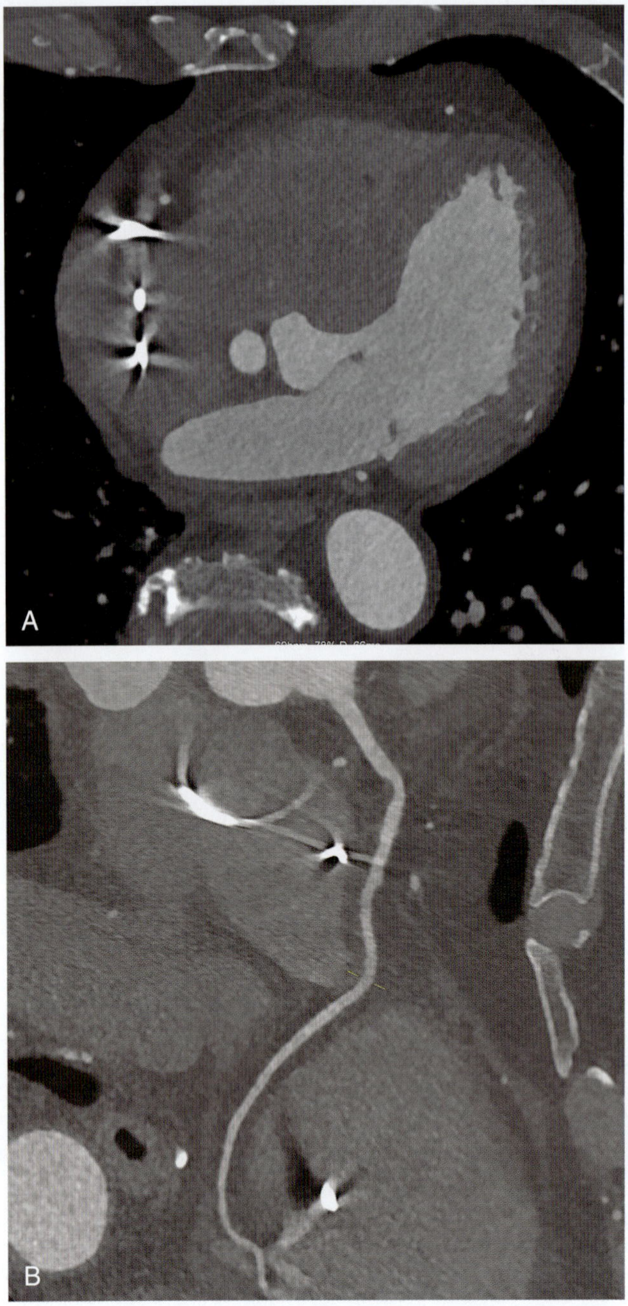

FIG. 6.13 Coronary CT angiography (A, B) in a patient with a dual-chamber pacemaker. The metal electrodes cause typical motion artifacts induced by high-density structures, but these are sufficiently far away from the coronary arteries to not interfere with their interpretation.

artifacts depends on scanner generation, heart rate, image noise, stent diameter, and many other factors, but official guidelines do not currently recommend the routine use of coronary CT angiography in patients with implanted coronary stents.[1–5] Sternal wires after cardiac surgery, newer-generation metal heart valves, as well as pacemakers and implanted cardioverter-defibrillators, may cause substantial artifacts in coronary CT angiography datasets. In the vast majority of cases, however, these artifacts occur in areas that are sufficiently distant to the coronary arteries so that their evaluation is not impaired (see Fig. 6.13). Consequently, they should not usually be considered a contraindication to CCTA. Left ventricular assist devices constitute an exception. They may cause severe metallic artifacts that may affect the left coronary artery so that an individual decision on whether or not to perform coronary CT angiography must be made.

TABLE 6.2 Patient Factors That Are Considered Absolute or Relative Contraindications for the Use of Coronary CT Angiography to Identify the Presence of Coronary Artery Stenoses[1,3]

Inability to remain in supine position or to cooperate with breathhold instructions
Clinical instability (e.g., acute respiratory distress, unstable arrhythmia)
Contraindication to beta blockade in the presence of an elevated heart rate and lack of availability of other medications to achieve target heart rate
Arrhythmia or high heart rate variability
Morbid obesity
Pregnancy or possible pregnancy (according to local protocols)
Allergy to iodinated contrast (according to local protocols)
Impaired renal function (according to local protocols)
Contraindications to nitroglycerin (if indicated)

PERFORMING CCTA

The decision whether CCTA is the appropriate test for a given patient, protocols for patient preparation, and in particular, choice of the image acquisition mode and scan parameters are highly dependent on the type of CT system that is used and on institutional practice. In general, CT systems with 64 or more simultaneously acquired slices are considered acceptable to perform CCTA.[18] As a general concept, scanners with a smaller number of detector rows and scanners with slower gantry rotation require more stringent patient preselection and preparation than more technically advanced systems. However, even for the most modern systems, the likelihood to achieve fully diagnostic images and the ability to use low radiation-dose image acquisition protocols both increase with more careful patient selection and preparation, in particular with more stringent heart rate control.

Patient Selection/Exclusion Criteria

The most frequent indication for CCTA is to rule in or rule out the presence of significant coronary artery stenoses and guide further management in suspected coronary artery disease. Several other tests are available for that same purpose. CCTA should preferentially be taken into consideration when pretest probability is relatively low and when fully diagnostic image quality can be expected. The recent Clinical Practice Guideline for the Evaluation of Chest Pain as well as the 2023 Multimodality Appropriate Use Criteria for the Detection and Risk Assessment of Chronic Coronary Disease[1,3] list several patient criteria that would favor the use of alternative diagnostic approaches over coronary CT angiography (see Table 6.2). Next to contraindications for iodinated contrast agent, the most relevant criteria include elevated heart rate, arrhythmia, severe obesity, and the inability to accurately follow breathhold commands. Also, a previously known very high coronary calcium score and the presence of coronary stents, particularly with diameters of 3.0 mm or less, should be a reason to consider alternative testing.

Patient Preparation

- Patient Instruction and Training

CCTA requires some cooperation of the patient. It is therefore essential for reliably high image quality that all patients are instructed about the image acquisition sequence beforehand. This should include information about the need to remain in supine position with arms raised above the head for a period of several minutes, the harmless nature of temperature sensations that may be induced by contrast injection and, importantly, instruction about the need to accurately follow breathhold commands, and to do so in the same way for each one of the various image acquisition steps.

CCTA images are acquired during deep inspiration and patients should receive specific instructions about the type of breathhold command that will be given. Importantly, test breathholds should be performed using the very same command that will be used for data acquisition. The ideal time for the "test breathholds" is when the patient is placed on the CT table with ECG leads already attached because this allows verification of heart rate and heart rate variability in deep inspiration (which are often substantially different from free breathing) and to make sure that the ECG signal remains stable.

All patient instructions should be given before the initiation of the image acquisition sequence. Operators should abstain from giving additional instructions between the individual acquisitions. This promotes a calm and relaxed atmosphere (conducive to low heart rate) and helps avoid different breathhold maneuvers (such as "particularly deep inspiration") between localizer or other preparatory scans and acquisition of the contrast-enhanced CCTA dataset. Patient cooperation, particularly an accurate and consistent breathhold, is of utmost importance for scan quality. Patient instruction therefore deserves special attention and care.

- Patient Positioning

Patients are positioned supine in the CT scanner, with arms raised above the head. It is important to provide for a convenient way to keep the arms raised during the scan procedure to minimize the likelihood that patients will shift their position. A comfortable support to rest the arms or a handle to hold on to makes it substantially easier for the patient to keep their arms raised without moving. Although it is possible to perform scans with one or both arms placed next to the torso if the patient cannot elevate their arms, this will increase image noise and may cause artifacts.

Table height should be adjusted so that the heart is in the center of gantry rotation to optimize temporal and spatial resolution.

- Premedication

The ideal heart rate and rhythm for CCTA is a regular rhythm of 60 beats per minute or less.[18] CT systems with particularly high temporal resolution may allow a somewhat more lenient approach to heart rate—but even for those systems, image quality becomes more stable and reliable, and the use of low-radiation dose protocols is facilitated when heart rate is low. It is therefore encouraged to strive for target heart rates of 60 beats per minutes or less across all CT acquisition platforms. Beta blockers are considered the first-line approach to achieve heart rate control for the purpose of CCTA. Protocols may include oral beta blockade with immediate release formulations, intravenous injection, or a combination of both. Typical protocols employ the use of 50 to 100 mg metoprolol p.o. 1 hour before the scan and/or single or repeated injection of 5 mg metoprolol, up to a maximum dose of 20 to 25 mg, immediately before scan initiation. Some authors have suggested to start beta blocker medication several days before CT, but this is uncommon practice. Esmolol, a short-acting intravenous beta blocker (e.g., 0.8 mg/kg), has also been proposed and allows for faster return of the heart rate to baseline levels than metoprolol. An alternative oral or intravenous medication is ivabradine. It does not impact blood pressure but is only effective in sinus rhythm and can be given in addition to beta blocker therapy. The typical oral dose to prepare for CCTA is 5 to 15 mg. Because of its slow onset of action, ivabradine medication should be given at least 1 hour or more before CT. It is likely to be more effective if started one or several days before CT.

Coronary dilatation improves image quality for CCTA and has been shown to increase diagnostic accuracy.[18] Unless contraindicated, medication with sublingual nitrates administered as spray or tablets[21] is therefore considered standard for all CCTA examinations that are intended to assess the coronary arteries. Contraindications include aortic valve stenosis and left ventricular outflow tract obstruction, severe hypotension, and active medication with phosphodiesterase inhibitors. Nitrates should be administered at the start of the scan sequence, immediately after the patient has been placed on the scanner bed, because their vasodilatory effect reaches a maximum after several minutes and lasts for only 20 to 30 minutes.

- Intravenous access

Intravenous access for contrast injection must be sufficiently large to allow high flow rates. The preferential venous access for contrast injection in CCTA is via a cubital vein. Central venous injection is not advantageous. It results in very high and inhomogeneous contrast in the superior vena cava and right atrium that may cause streak artifacts that impair coronary evaluation. Forearm positions are possible even though associated with slightly longer contrast transit times. Most institutions will discourage venous access at the back of the hand. Correct position and functioning of the intravenous access has to be assured because contrast extravasation can cause severe tissue damage.

Acquisition Protocols

- Image acquisition mode

The two basic image data acquisition modes for CCTA are spiral/helical acquisition with retrospectively ECG-gated image reconstruction and prospectively ECG-triggered sequential acquisition. Prospectively triggered high-pitch spiral/helical acquisition is a third scan mode but only available on a limited number of CT systems. The selection of scan mode and specific image acquisition parameters is highly dependent on the CT system that is available. It is also influenced by heart rate and heart rate variability. Regarding image quality, and in very general terms, spiral/helical acquisition with retrospective ECG gating allows for high flexibility to choose the ideal phase for image reconstruction, which may help avoid motion artifacts. This flexibility is reduced when ECG-based tube current modulation is used (which in turn substantially lowers radiation exposure). Prospectively ECG-triggered axial or sequential acquisition usually affords relatively low radiation exposure at the expense of limited flexibility concerning the time point of image reconstruction. This flexibility may be increased by widening the phase acquisition window ("padding"), which in turn increases radiation exposure. Concerning the balance between image quality and radiation exposure, a good basic advice is to choose a scan protocol that limits radiation exposure to a narrow time window in mid-diastole for all patients with low and stable heart rates. In patients with heart rates above 60/min to 65/min, the available time window for image reconstruction should include late systole, and flexibility regarding the time point for image reconstruction should be ensured when patients do not have a stable heart rate.

Settings for tube potential ("voltage") and tube current are also determined by scanner specifics. Although 120 kV tube potential has long been considered the standard for CCTA, substantial reductions in dose without compromise of image quality can be achieved by using 100 kV or less. Reducing tube potential to below 120 kV without a substantial compromise in image quality is possible for patients with a body weight below 100 kg and body mass index below 30 kg/m^2.[18]

- Breathhold command

Reliable breath-holding is essential for high-image quality in CCTA. Based on clinical experience, short breathhold commands that are often used for imaging other body regions ("breathe in—hold your breath") are not adequate for CCTA. A long breathhold command sequence ("breathe in—breathe out—breathe in—hold your breath") is highly preferrable. This sequence of breathhold commands should be given extremely slowly (i.e., over 14–20 seconds). A long, slow breathhold command allows patients to easily follow the requested respiratory maneuvers without feeling rushed. It is advisable to record the breathhold command and to use the same recorded command for each step of the image acquisition sequence, including localizer scans. This will ensure that the patient will then hear exactly the same command several times and feel comfortable following it. It is not advisable to encourage a "particularly deep" inspiration for acquisition of the contrast-enhanced dataset. Forced particularly deep inspiration may change venous flow to the heart and may thus impact contrast agent transit time. It may also lead to more caudal diaphragmatic position and mispositioning of the scan volume relative to the heart.

- Coronary calcium scan

The question of whether or not a nonenhanced coronary calcium acquisition should be performed prior to all CCTA acquisitions remains disputed. Unusually and unexpectedly high amounts of coronary calcium might lead to reconsideration whether a contrast-enhanced acquisition is reasonable. Also, the additional acquisition may help confirm or adjust the imaging volume for subsequent CCTA and to identify problems with heart rate or patient breathhold. In most cases, the additional radiation exposure of performing a nonenhanced coronary calcium acquisition may therefore be justified.

- Contrast agent, timing, and contrast injection

Adequate intraluminal contrast enhancement is essential to allow accurate and reliable interpretation of CCTA. Important aspects include iodine concentration, contrast delivery rate, and contrast timing. In general, contrast agents with high iodine concentration are preferred over lower concentration agents, and concentrations between 270 and 400 mg iodine/mL are recommended.[18] Within that range, there seems to be no significant influence of the specific iodine concentration on image quality and diagnostic accuracy. A higher injection rate for lower concentration agents can achieve a similar iodine delivery rate in spite of lower injection pressures and results in identical luminal attenuation.[22] Typical contrast volumes range from 50 to 120 mL. Contrast injection rate is typically 5 to 7 mL/s, and contrast injection should be followed by injection of approximately 50 mL saline at the same flow rate in order to "push" the contrast bolus through the peripheral veins. Instead of a pure saline flush, some investigators prefer a mixture of contrast agent and saline that will enhance visualization of right-sided cardiac structures (see Chapter 1 for further detail).

Contrast injection and data acquisition must be carefully synchronized. This can either be achieved by a separate "test bolus" acquisition to measure the contrast agent transit time (10 mL of contrast agent followed by at least 50 mL of saline, both at the anticipated injection rate for CCTA), or by "bolus tracking" which starts the CCTA acquisition when there is a change in CT attenuation at a pre-specified location (e.g. when contrast arrives in the ascending aorta). A separate test bolus acquisition goes along with a number of advantages. They include easier integration of a slow and long breathhold command as described above, a further opportunity to perform and observe the

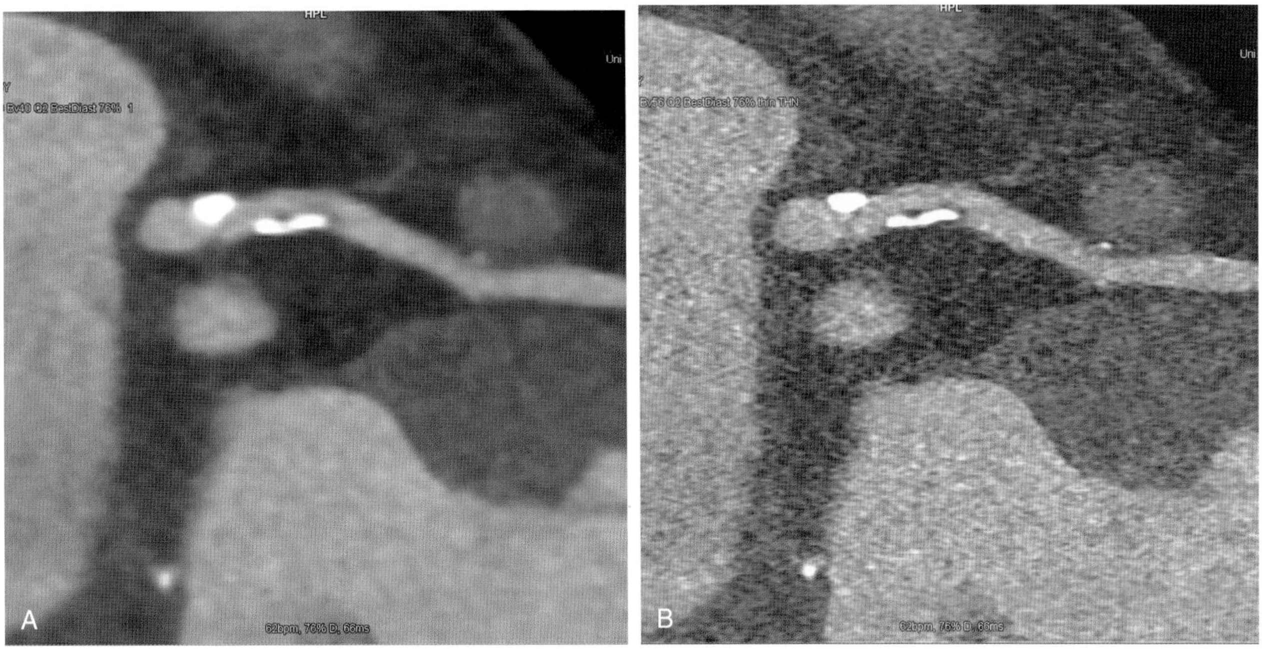

FIG. 6.14 Relationship between spatial resolution and image noise. The same coronary CT angiography dataset (here, ostial left anterior descending coronary artery) reconstructed with lower resolution (0.6-mm slice thickness and low-resolution kernel, A) and higher resolution (0.2-mm slice thickness and high-resolution kernel, B). Panel B shows a substantially better ability to separate calcified plaque and coronary lumen, at the cost of higher image noise.

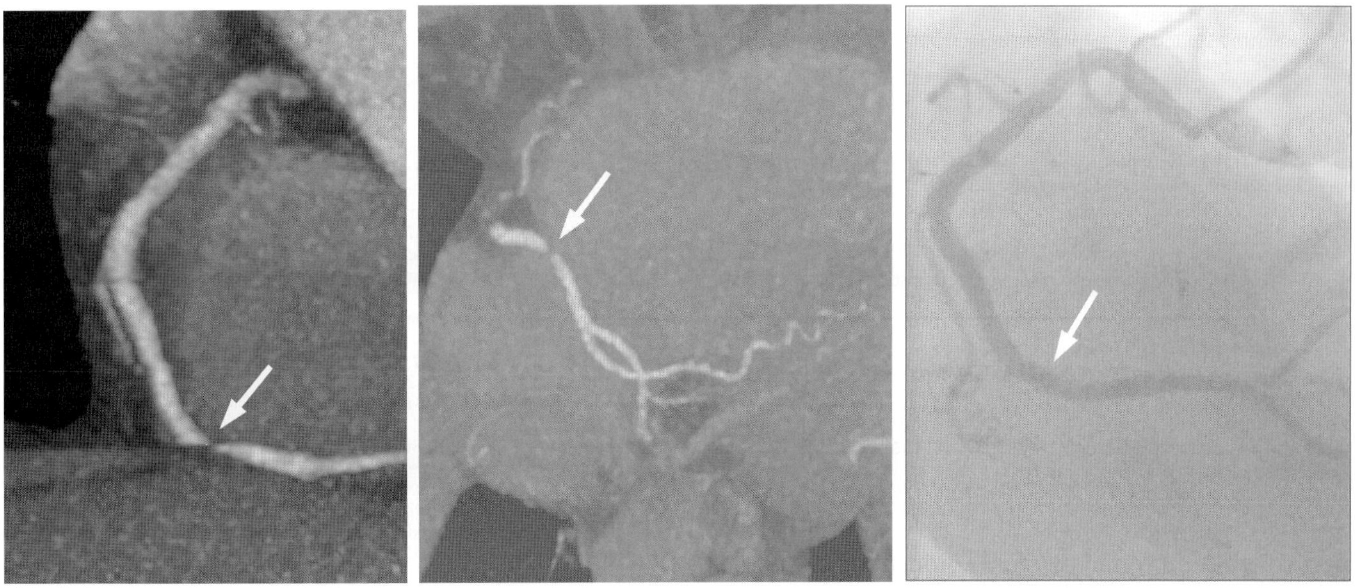

FIG. 6.15 An important concept for image interpretation in coronary CT angiography (CCTA) is to separately assess coronary atherosclerotic plaque on one hand and luminal stenosis on the other. A cursory interpretation of CCTA (*left and middle panel*) may suggest substantial stenosis of the very proximal left anterior descending coronary artery, particularly in cross-section (*arrow*). However, there is substantial positive remodeling, and the lumen of the left anterior descending coronary artery is not substantially smaller than that of the left main coronary artery. This is confirmed in invasive coronary angiography (*right panel*).

required breathhold, and the identification of problems with contrast injection.

IMAGE RECONSTRUCTION, PROCESSING, AND INTERPRETATION

In order to facilitate image interpretation, a set of cross-sectional images reconstructed with the thinnest possible slice thickness should be used for interpretation. Reconstructed slice thickness, reconstruction kernels, and the use of iterative reconstruction substantially influence the balance between spatial resolution and image noise (see Fig. 6.14). Optimal settings are scanner specific and must be individually determined for each CT system. Original, transaxial cross-sectional image data sets must be carefully screened for artifacts, in particular those caused by motion or discontinuity of the coronary arteries in order to avoid misinterpretation of reformatted reconstructions (see Fig. 6.15). If artifacts are present, it may be required to reconstruct further image datasets at different time points in the cardiac cycle in order to minimize artifact, in

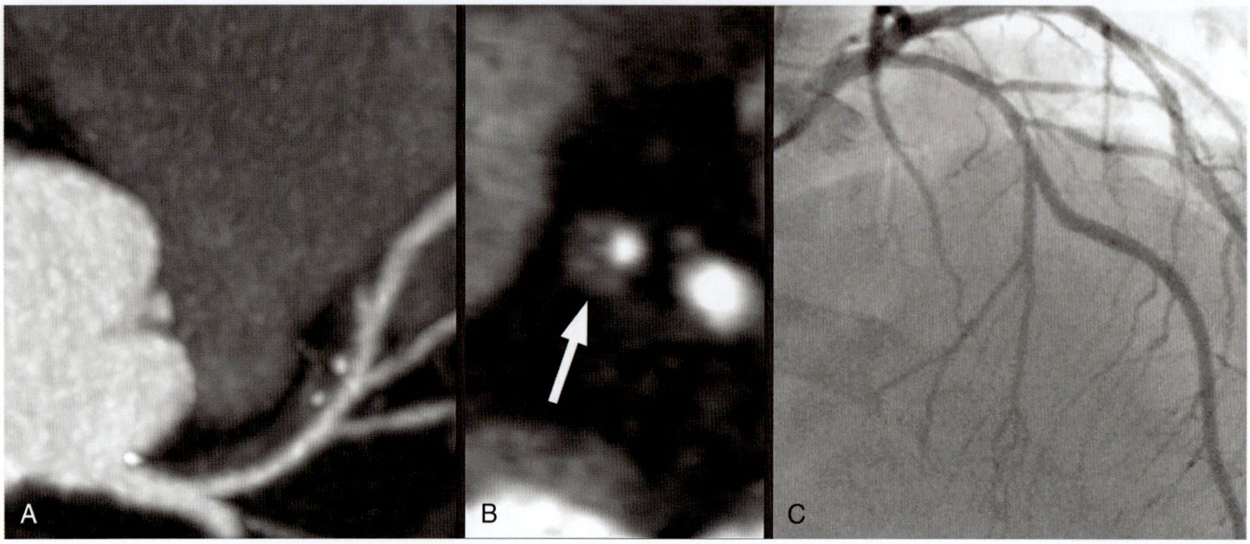

FIG. 6.16 Coronary CT angiography dataset affected by misalignment artifacts (A, B). The misalignment artifact of the right coronary artery is easily detected in a lateral view of the original dataset (A). In a multiplanar reformatted maximum intensity projection, however, it is indiscernible from a coronary artery stenosis (B). Invasive coronary angiography confirms absence of stenosis (C).

TABLE 6.3 Important Factors to Consider in Order to Achieve High-Quality Coronary CT Angiography

Heart rate should be regular and low, ideally <60 beats/min. This will typically require the use of medication such as short-acting beta blockers 1 hour prior to acquisition
Patient must reliably follow breathhold instructions, which is facilitated by thorough practice prior to scanning
Coronary artery dilatation should be achieved by administration of sublingual nitrates, unless contraindicated
Image acquisition protocols, tube potential, and tube current must be adapted to patient factors such as heart rate and body weight. In patients with high or irregular heart rates, end-systole should be included in the data acquisition window
High image noise should be avoided by selecting sufficiently high tube potential and tube current
Contrast should be injected at a high flow rate (5–7 mL/s) and followed by a saline flush of sufficient volume
Image datasets for evaluation should be reconstructed at the smallest available slice thickness
Image datasets must be carefully inspected for the presence of artifacts; readers should not rely solely on postprocessed reconstructions

particular when caused by rapid coronary motion. If necessary, different reconstructions must be used for different segments of the coronary artery tree.

Basic rules for coronary artery interpretation include separately assessing and reporting the presence of luminal stenoses and the presence or absence of coronary plaque (see Fig. 6.16). Importantly, coronary segments must be reported as "unevaluable" unless fully diagnostic image quality is ascertained. Table 6.3 lists advice on how to achieve high-quality CCTA imaging in condensed form.

REFERENCES

1. Gulati M, Levy PD, Mukherjee D, et al. 2021 AHA/ACC/ASE/CHEST/SAEM/SCCT/SCMR guideline for the evaluation and diagnosis of chest pain: a report of the American college of cardiology/American Heart Association Joint Committee on clinical practice guidelines. *J Am Coll Cardiol.* 2021;78(22):e187–e285.
2. Kontos MC, de Lemos JA, Deitelzweig SB, et al. 2022 ACC expert consensus decision pathway on the evaluation and disposition of acute chest pain in the emergency department: a report of the American College of Cardiology Solution Set Oversight Committee. *J Am Coll Cardiol.* 2022;80(20):1925–1960.
3. Winchester DE, Maron DJ, Blankstein R, et al. ACC/AHA/ASE/ASNC/ASPC/HFSA/HRS/SCAI/SCCT/SCMR/STS 2023 multimodality appropriate use criteria for the detection and risk assessment of chronic coronary disease. *J Am Coll Cardiol.* 2023;81(25):2445–2467.
4. Knuuti J, Wijns W, Saraste A, et al. 2019 ESC guidelines for the diagnosis and management of chronic coronary syndromes. *Eur Heart J.* 2020;41(3):407–477.
5. Byrne RA, Rossello X, Coughlan JJ, et al. 2023 ESC guidelines for the management of acute coronary syndromes. *Eur Heart J.* 2023;44(38):3720–3826.
6. Achenbach S, Ropers D, Holle J, Muschiol G, Daniel WG, Moshage W. In-plane coronary arterial motion velocity: measurement with electron-beam CT. *Radiology.* 2000;216(2):457–463.
7. Shechter G, Resar JR, McVeigh ER. Displacement and velocity of the coronary arteries: cardiac and respiratory motion. *IEEE Trans Med Imaging.* 2006;25(3):369–375.
8. Husmann L, Leschka S, Desbiolles L, et al. Coronary artery motion and cardiac phases: dependency on heart rate—implications for CT image reconstruction. *Radiology.* 2007;245(2):567–576.
9. Sun G, Li M, Li L, Li GY, Zhang H, Peng ZH. Optimal systolic and diastolic reconstruction windows for coronary CT angiography using 320-detector rows dynamic volume CT. *Clin Radiol.* 2011;66(7):614–620.
10. Mander GTW, Dobeli K, Steffensen C, Munn Z. Diagnostic accuracy of prospectively gated, 128-slice or greater CTCA at high heart rates: a systematic review and meta-analysis. *J Med Radiat Sci.* 2021;68(4):435–445.
11. Ghekiere O, Nchimi A, Djekic J, et al. Coronary computed tomography angiography: patient-related factors determining image quality using a second-generation 320-slice CT scanner. *Int J Cardiol.* 2016;221:970–976.
12. Li M, Zhang GM, Zhao JS, et al. Diagnostic performance of dual-source CT coronary angiography with and without heart rate control: systematic review and meta-analysis. *Clin Radiol.* 2014;69(2):163–171.
13. Menke J, Kowalski J. Diagnostic accuracy and utility of coronary CT angiography with consideration of unevaluable results: a systematic review and multivariate Bayesian random-effects meta-analysis with intention to diagnose. *Eur Radiol.* 2016;26(2):451–458.
14. Moser LJ, Mergen V, Allmendinger T, Manka R, Eberhard M, Alkadhi H. A novel reconstruction technique to reduce stair-step artifacts in sequential mode coronary CT angiography. *Invest Radiol.* 2024;59(9):622–628. http://doi.org/10.1097/RLI.0000000000001066 Epub ahead of print.
15. Qian W, Liu W, Zhu Y, et al. Influence of heart rate and coronary artery calcification on image quality and diagnostic performance of coronary CT angiography: comparison between 96-row detector dual source CT and 256-row multidetector CT. *J Xray Sci Technol.* 2021;29(3):529–539.
16. Stocker TJ, Deseive S, Leipsic J, et al. Reduction in radiation exposure in cardiovascular computed tomography imaging: results from the PROspective multicenter registry on radiaTion dose Estimates of cardiac CT anglOgraphy iN daily practice in 2017 (PROTECTION VI). *Eur Heart J.* 2018;39(41):3715–3723.
17. Araki S, Kitagawa K, Kokawa T, et al. Radiation exposure in cardiac computed tomography imaging in Mie prefecture in 2021. *Jpn J Radiol.* 2023;41(6):596–604.
18. Abbara S, Blanke P, Maroules CD, et al. SCCT guidelines for the performance and acquisition of coronary computed tomographic angiography: a report of the society of Cardiovascular Computed Tomography Guidelines Committee:

Endorsed by the North American Society for Cardiovascular Imaging (NASCI). *J Cardiovasc Comput Tomogr*. 2016;10(6):435–449.
19. Schuhbaeck A, Schaefer M, Marwan M, et al. Patient-specific predictors of image noise in coronary CT angiography. *J Cardiovasc Comput Tomogr*. 2013;7(1):39–45.
20. Kim H, Park CH, Han KH, Kim TH. Predicting the image noise level of prospective ECG-triggered coronary computed tomography angiography: quantitative measurement of thoracic component versus body mass index. *Int J Cardiovasc Imaging*. 2015;31(Suppl 2):213–221.
21. Kusk MW, Bromark CS, Hestbek-Møller M, Davidsen LØ, Precht H, Brage K. Pill or pump? Nitroglycerin 0.5 mg tablet vs 0.8 mg spray: effect on proximal vessel diameters at Coronary CT Angiography (CCTA). *Radiography (Lond)*. 2023;29(5):918–925.
22. Rengo M, Dharampal A, Lubbers M, et al. Impact of iodine concentration and iodine delivery rate on contrast enhancement in coronary CT angiography: a randomized multicenter trial (CT-CON). *Eur Radiol*. 2019;29(11): 6109–6118.

7 Diagnostic Accuracy of Coronary CT Angiography

RONEN RUBINSHTEIN AND TODD C. VILLINES

KEY POINTS

- Coronary CT angiography is the most sensitive noninvasive method to diagnose anatomically obstructive coronary artery disease, using invasive coronary angiography as the reference standard.
- High negative predictive value allows rapid exclusion of coronary stenosis in patients with chest pain of possible ischemic origin.
- Diagnostic accuracy of coronary CT angiography depends heavily on image quality, which may be improved with both technical solutions and with cardiac pharmacology.
- The rate of nondiagnostic scans is very low with new-generation CT scanners.

BACKGROUND ON NEW-GENERATION SCANNERS AND IMAGE QUALITY

Contrast-enhanced multidetector computed tomography (MDCT), which provides high-quality noninvasive images of the heart, great vessels, and coronary vasculature, has been shown to be useful and reliable in the triage of patients with chest pain of possible ischemic origin[1–3] and specifically in the diagnosis of acute coronary syndrome.[4,5] Current-generation CT scanners (64-slice and higher) require minimal patient cooperation (short breathhold) and deliver excellent image quality and high diagnostic accuracy.[6,7] MDCT can visualize coronary plaques[8] and even calculate coronary hemodynamics.[9]

Cardiac CT angiography is also gaining a role in the evaluation of coronary stents and bypass grafts (see Chapter 10, Evaluation of Coronary Stents and Bypass Grafts) and is frequently performed for evaluation of patients undergoing structural or electrophysiological cardiac interventions[10] (see Chapter 20, Use of Cardiac CT in Structural Heart Disease Interventions [other than transcatheter aortic valve replacement]).

Although the usefulness of MDCT in various clinical scenarios and the technical consideration required in achieving high-quality images are discussed elsewhere in this textbook (see Chapter 2, Advances in Hardware and Reconstruction Techniques for Cardiac CT; see Chapter 6, How to Obtain a High-Quality Coronary CT Angiography), the current chapter aims to describe the diagnostic accuracy of coronary CT angiography (CCTA) with a focus on native coronary arteries and the factors that may impact diagnostic accuracy.

TECHNICAL CONSIDERATION

Although specific protocols and optimal use of MDCT are discussed earlier in this book, it is understandable that diagnostic accuracy depends heavily on image quality. Common artifacts such as motion artifacts or "blooming" artifacts in heavily calcified vessels may significantly decrease diagnostic accuracy and result in nondiagnostic coronary segments.

Despite the fact that clinically important coronary atherosclerotic plaques usually appear in the proximal coronary segments that are often of sufficient sizes to make a diagnosis, the aim of any CCTA analysis is to describe most if not all available coronary segments (e.g., by describing all available segments of at least 1.5 mm in diameter from an 18-segment Society of Cardiovascular CT [SCCT] model and presenting a graded approach for the severity of coronary artery disease [CAD] such as recommended by the CAD-RADS 2 [coronary artery disease reporting and data system]).[11]

New-generation CT scanners allow rapid scanning of the heart by a high gantry rotation speed (>0.25 sec/rotation) and wider coverage of the field of view than older-generation scanners. More rapid acquisition CCTA allows for "freezing" of cardiac motion (improved temporal resolution) and overcomes many previously observed breathing and patient motion artifacts. Some scanners allow a single beat acquisition and very rapid reconstruction of scanned data to be presented to the reader. Preliminary results show that high-resolution scanners (spatial resolution as low as 0.20 mm) have better diagnostic accuracy than standard-resolution CT scanners (spatial resolution of approximately 0.625 mm).[12,13] Therefore diagnostic accuracy of CCTA cannot be evaluated as "one size fits all." The improved spatial resolution of contemporary scanners (see Chapter 2, Advances in Hardware and Reconstruction Techniques for Cardiac CT) may be especially helpful for mitigating calcium blooming artifacts, evaluating coronary stents, and visualizing smaller vessels.

CARDIAC PHARMACOLOGY AND IMAGE QUALITY

Despite the aforementioned technical advances, it is still recommended to lower the patient heart rate to <65 beats per minute to optimize image quality.[2] Moreover, in the absence of contraindications (e.g., severe aortic stenosis, concomitant use of phosphodiesterase inhibitors, or hypotension), it is also recommended to administer sublingual nitroglycerine approximately 3 to 5 minutes prior to scanning to allow coronary vasodilatation and improve coronary visualization. Nitroglycerine, which is an endothelium-independent vasodilator, may not only cause enlargement of the relatively small coronary arteries—hence gaining another "pixel or two" for visual assessment—but may improve coronary opacification by contrast media during diastole.[14] The effect of cardiac pharmacology with beta blockade (or ivabradine or verapamil) plus nitroglycerine is important for improving image quality, and therefore diagnostic accuracy, with previous-generation CT scanners, but its importance with newer systems that provide better spatial and temporal resolution may be less prominent. However, as per SCCT acquisition guidelines recommendations,[2] and as practiced by many experienced readers, these medications should be routinely used to allow for the highest diagnostic accuracy possible.

Of note, an additional beneficial consequence of beta blockade and heart rate lowering may be a decrease in radiation exposure in some scanning protocols.

OPTIMAL SCANNING TO ALLOW HIGH-QUALITY IMAGES

As previously described, the scan itself is performed using ECG gating or ECG triggering to image and reconstruct the heart and the coronary vessels during specific phases in the cardiac cycle, usually a mid-diastolic or end-systolic phase to coincide with cardiac cycle sections that are associated with reduced motion (e.g., ventricular diastasis or isovolumic relaxation). In cases of higher heart rates (>70 bpm), an end-systolic phase (targeting isovolumic relaxation) may be optimal for providing diagnostic images.

After scanning, the reconstructed data can be viewed and manipulated on a dedicated workstation that utilizes software to optimize image display, assist in analysis, and mitigate artifacts. Most software is semiautomatic and allows a variety of analysis modes (e.g., double oblique cross-sectioning using multiplanar reformations) that are then utilized by the experienced reader to achieve maximal diagnostic accuracy.

OVERCOMING IMAGE ARTIFACTS AND IMPROVING ACCURACY

Diagnostic accuracy is heavily dependent on image quality. Poor image quality results in reduced diagnostic accuracy, lower reader certainty, and more subjective findings. Although reader interpretation of the image is the most important step in diagnosis, other factors may affect the interpretation: motion artifacts, heavy calcifications that can lead to beam-hardening or calcium-blooming artifacts, or small vessel size. Regardless of the type of artifacts, image manipulation while utilizing images acquired from several phases of the cardiac cycle (when available) is usually the first step utilized by an experienced CT reader.

However, there are additional techniques that may allow readers to overcome some artifacts: ECG editing tools to overcome motion artifacts, spectral imaging to overcome heavy calcifications, and use of sharp kernels and display-setting optimization to reduce calcium blooming. In some cases, utilizing fractional flow reserve with CT (FFR-CT) or other AI-based assessment of plaque or stenosis may further improve diagnostic accuracy for lesions with intermediate stenosis.[15,16]

OBJECTIVE MEASURES OF IMAGE QUALITY

While relating image quality to diagnostic accuracy, poor vessel opacification or insufficient separation between the coronary vessel and surrounding tissue may be measured objectively with dedicated software, thus allowing an objective assessment of image quality. Several parameters have been used to objectively evaluate image quality: image noise, signal-to-noise ratio (SNR), and contrast-to-noise ratio (CNR). Calculation of SNR and CNR is most commonly performed as the following: 10 mm^2 circular regions of interest (ROI) is placed in the lumen of the left main coronary artery (LM) and the proximal right coronary artery (RCA), and mean attenuation in Hounsfield units (HU) is calculated for each vessel. To assess contrast, another 2 ROIs of 10 mm^2 are placed in the perivascular area near LM and near RCA or in soft tissue at the same axial plane. Contrast is calculated as [signal in HU within the vessel] − [signal in HU in the corresponding perivascular area] and the average from the two vessels calculated. Image noise is defined as the standard deviation (SD) of the attenuation in an ROI of 1 cm^2 placed in the ascending aorta. CNR is then calculated as: [mean (LM and RCA) contrast] / [Image noise]. SNR is calculated as: [mean (LM and RCA) signal] / [Image noise].[17] The higher the SNR and CNR and lower the noise, image quality is considered better and may translate to improved diagnostic accuracy of CCTA.

DIAGNOSTIC PERFORMANCE OF CCTA

Coronary CT angiography is the noninvasive test with the highest sensitivity to diagnose coronary plaque and stenosis when compared to invasive coronary angiography as the reference standard. This test has a very high negative predictive value (97–100%), making it a useful tool to rule out coronary stenosis when compared with invasive coronary angiography. On the other hand, due to the qualitative assessment of stenosis, which may at times be affected by motion artifacts and coronary calcifications, the positive predictive value is somewhat lower but still very good (85–92%)[18] (Fig. 7.1).

Beyond evaluation of the native coronary vessels, coronary CT angiography can evaluate the patency of coronary stents, especially stents that are ≥3 mm wide, albeit with reduced diagnostic accuracy related to metallic artifacts. Diagnostic accuracy is very high in coronary artery bypass grafts but can be negatively affected by the presence of metallic clips in distal anastomosis regions, and the accuracy of CCTA is also lower in native coronary segments due to the diffuse nature of calcified coronary atherosclerosis in patients who have undergone coronary artery bypass graft surgery. Although the specific aspects of CCTA in patients post revascularization is discussed elsewhere in this book (see Chapter 10, Evaluation of Coronary Stents and Bypass Grafts), it is important to mention that the rate of unassessable coronary segments on CCTA is higher in

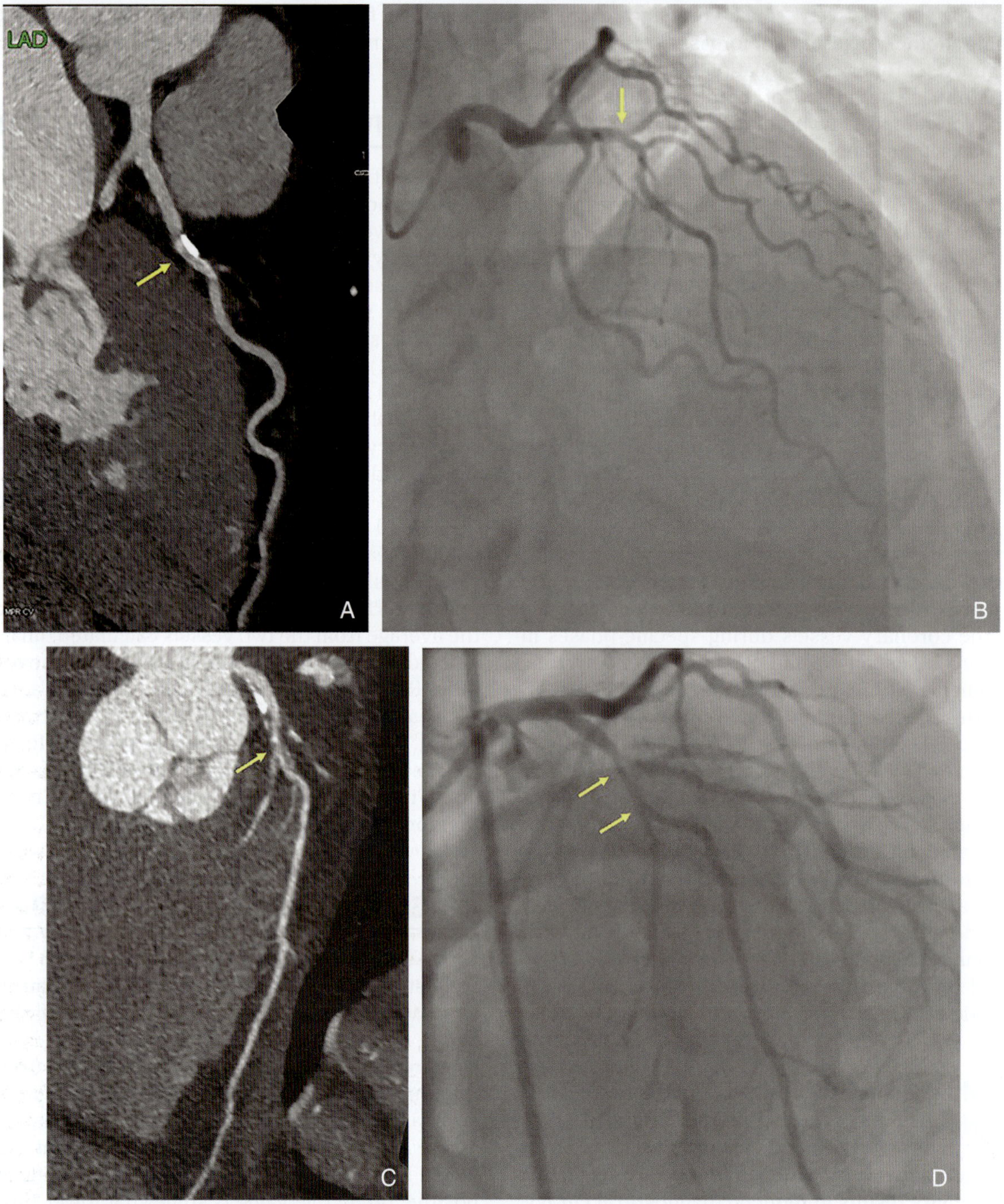

FIG. 7.1 False-positive and true-positive coronary CT angiography findings. (A) Curved multiplanar reformatted image of the left anterior descending artery (LAD) demonstrating a calcified plaque (*yellow arrow*) reported as 50% to 69% (moderate) stenosis. (B) Corresponding right anterior oblique image of the LAD on invasive coronary angiography (Panel B) showing no significant angiographic stenosis (*yellow arrow*). The presence of calcium "blooming" resulted in overcalling the degree of luminal stenosis. (C) Curved multiplanar image of a heavily diseased left main and left anterior descending coronary artery with severe (>70%) stenosis in the proximal vessel (*yellow arrow*). (D) Corresponding invasive coronary angiogram showing severe bifurcation stenosis in the proximal and mid LAD (*yellow arrows*). Invasive fractional flow reserve of the LAD was abnormal (0.70).

this group of patients, thus reducing the diagnostic performance of CCTA and therefore its clinical usefulness.

However, with advances in technology (improved spatial and temporal resolution), the rate of unassessable segments has decreased significantly, and advances in CT detector technology, such as with ultra-high-resolution photon-counting CT, may allow for significantly improved accuracy for stenosis and plaque detection and quantification (Figs. 7.2 and 7.3).[13]

While during the early phase of CCTA using 16 to 40 row MDCT scanners the rate of nondiagnostic scans was as high as 20%, the rate of nondiagnostic scans was reported in 2% to 7% when using ≥64-slice scanners.[19] It is now accepted that with new-generation scanners (>64 slice) the rate of nondiagnostic scans has significantly decreased, allowing a clinically useful diagnostic scan in majority of cases (>98%). Previous studies have presented some variability in diagnostic accuracy among different vessels,

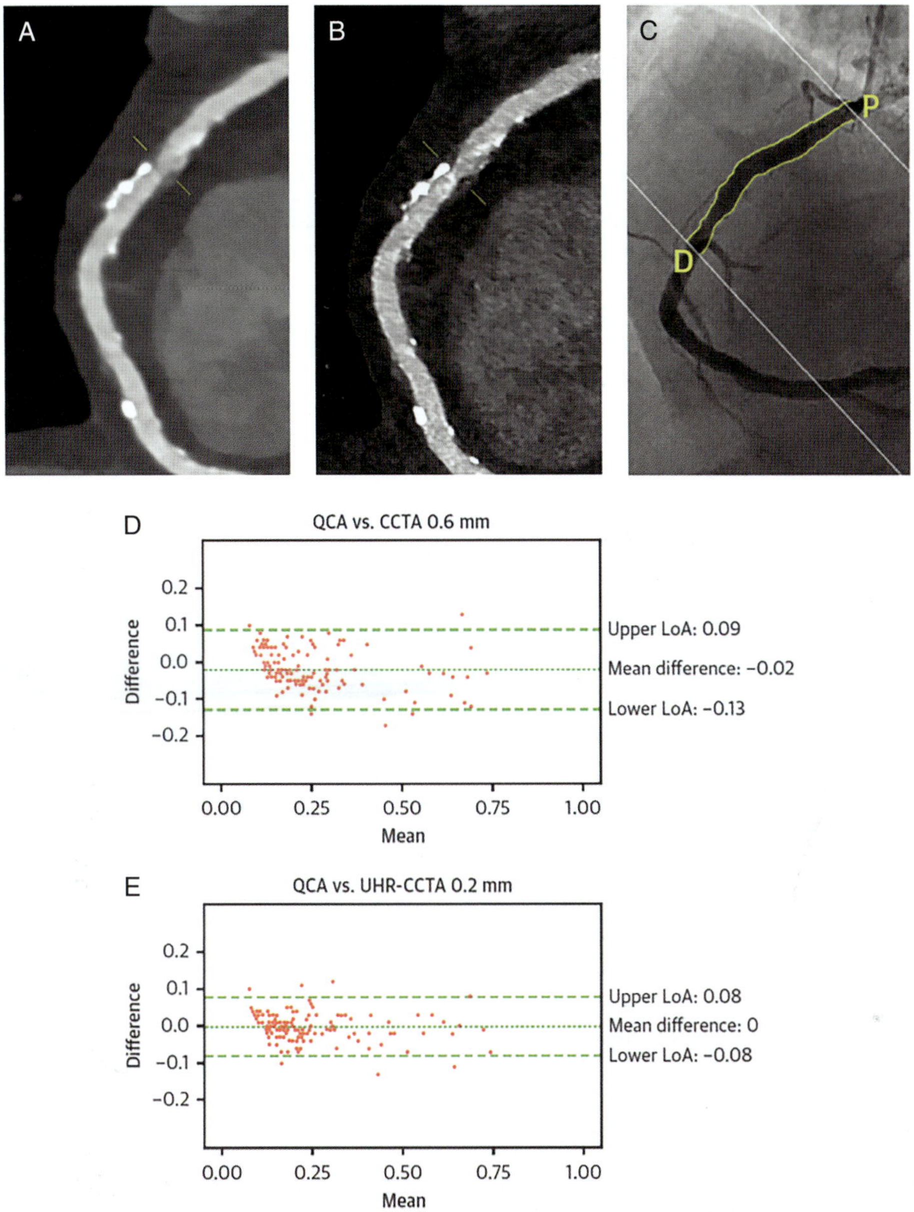

FIG. 7.2 **Coronary CTA and invasive catheter angiography of a 72-year-old female patient with severe aortic stenosis.** Curved reformations at (A) 0.6-mm slice thickness (Bv40 kernel) and (B) 0.2-mm slice thickness (Bv64-kernel) as well as (C) invasive catheter angiography showing a stenosis caused by calcific plaque in the proximal right coronary artery. (D, E) Bland-Altman analyses for quantitative stenosis measurements on standard and UHR coronary CTA. *CCTA*, coronary computed tomography angiography; *LoA*, limits of agreement; *QCA*, quantitative coronary angiography; *UHR*, ultra-high-resolution. (From Eberhard M, Candreva A, Rajagopal R, et al. Coronary stenosis quantification with ultra-high-resolution photon-counting detector CT angiography: comparison with 3D quantitative coronary angiography. *JACC Cardiovasc Imaging*. 2024;17[3]:342–344).

where the left circumflex coronary artery was associated with somewhat lower diagnostic accuracy. However, with improvements in technology, postprocessing software, and training of readers, the performance characteristics of CCTA is now comparable in all three major coronary arteries. As expected, larger, more proximal coronary segments are easier to interpret than smaller, more distal vessels, but because the majority of acute coronary syndromes occur in more proximal segments, the clinical usefulness of CCTA remains high in the majority of case scenarios.

In a metaanalysis of >30 studies evaluating diagnostic accuracy of CCTA in symptomatic patients, performance characteristics of CCTA was high in the majority of studies evaluating ≥64-slice MDCT scanners when compared with >50% or >70% stenosis on invasive coronary angiography: sensitivity was 96%, specificity was 82%, positive predictive value was 89%, and negative predictive value was 98%.[19]

More importantly, studies evaluating diagnostic accuracy of newer-generation MDCT (>64 slices) reported negative predictive value of 99% to 100% on a patient-based analysis.[20]

The high accuracy of CCTA to diagnose anatomically significant CAD when compared to invasive coronary angiography is recognized by both European and U.S. guidelines on chest pain and acute coronary syndromes.[18,21,22]

However, despite the fact that the accuracy of CCTA is very high when compared to an anatomic test (invasive

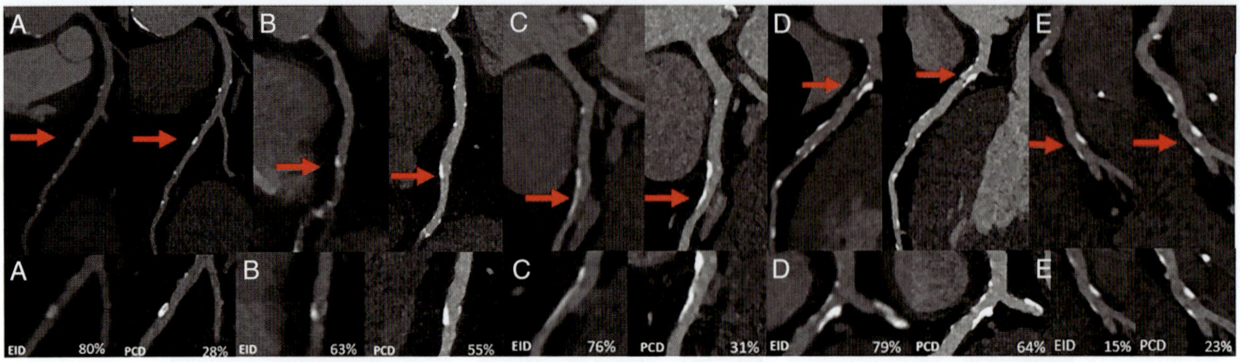

FIG. 7.3 Comparison of coronary CTA images on traditional energy-integrating detector versus photon-counting detector CTA Representative multiplanar reformat patient images (EID (Energy-Integrating Detector), left; PCD (Photon-Counting Detector), right) of the left anterior descending (LAD) (A), right coronary artery (B), LAD (C–E) with calcified plaques that were used for stenosis analysis (*top*). View enlarged at *red arrow* with percent diameter stenosis listed in bottom right for each panel (*bottom*). (Reproduced from Koons EK, Rajiah PS, Thorne JE, et al. Coronary artery stenosis quantification in patients with dense calcifications using ultra-high-resolution photon-counting-detector computed tomography. *J Cardiovasc Comput Tomogr*. 2024;18[1]:56–61).

TABLE 7.1 Performance Characteristics of Different Tests for Anatomically and Functionally Significant Coronary Artery Disease

ANATOMICALLY SIGNIFICANT CAD			FUNCTIONALLY (FFR) SIGNIFICANT CAD (FFR ≤0.80)		
TEST	*SENSITIVITY (%) (95% CI)*	*SPECIFICITY (%) (95% CI)*	*TEST*	*SENSITIVITY (%) (95% CI)*	*SPECIFICITY (%) (95% CI)*
			ICA	68 (60–75)	73 (55–86)
Stress ECG	58 (46–69)	62 (54–69)			
Stress Echo	85 (80–89)	82 (72–89)			
CCTA	97 (93–99)	78 (67–86)	CCTA	93 (89–96)	53 (37–68)
SPECT	87 (83–90)	70 (63–76)	SPECT	73 (62–82)	83 (71–90)
PET	90 (78–96)	85 (78–90)	PET	89 (82–93)	85 (81–88)
Stress CMR	90 (83–94)	80 (69–88)	Stress CMR	89 (85–92)	87 (83–91)

CAD, Coronary artery disease; *CCTA*, coronary computed tomography angiography; *CMR*, cardiac magnetic resonance; *FFR*, fractional flow reserve; *ICA*, invasive coronary angiography; *PET*, positron emission tomography; *SPECT*, single-photon emission computed tomography.
Adapted from Knuuti J, Ballo H, Juarez-Orozco LE, et al. The performance of non-invasive tests to rule-in and rule-out significant coronary artery stenosis in patients with stable angina: a meta-analysis focused on post-test disease probability. *Eur Heart J*. 2018;39:3322–3330.

angiography), it may be lower to diagnose functionally significant CAD (abnormal FFR). In a similar way, invasive coronary angiography is also limited in diagnosing functionally significant CAD, and FFR is recommended for evaluation of stable patients with less than 90% coronary diameter stenosis.[18] Notably, CCTA has higher sensitivity but lower specificity than invasive coronary angiography for diagnosing functionally significant CAD.[23]

Table 7.1 summarizes the performance of different tests including CCTA for anatomically significant coronary artery disease.[23]

SUMMARY

CCTA can identify the presence, extent, and severity of nonobstructive and obstructive CAD, as well as atherosclerotic plaque composition and high-risk features (e.g., positive remodeling, low-attenuation plaque). Furthermore, calculation of FFR-CT can provide an estimation of lesion-specific ischemia.[21] Regardless of the additional information available from CCTA, the sensitivity of CCTA to diagnose obstructive CAD in symptomatic patients is excellent with good specificity. Recent improvements in MDCT technology have significantly reduced the rate of nondiagnostic scans and improved diagnostic accuracy. Consequently, the newest generation of scanners can rule out anatomically obstructive CAD in the majority of cases with very high negative predictive value, thereby further reinforcing the use of CCTA as a first-line test in evaluating patients with both stable CAD and acute coronary syndromes.[18,21,22]

REFERENCES

1. Halon DA, Rubinshtein R, Gaspar T, Peled N, Lewis BS. Current status and clinical applications of cardiac multidetector computed tomography. *Cardiology*. 2008;109:73–84.
2. Abbara S, Blanke P, Maroules CD, et al. SCCT guidelines for the performance and acquisition of coronary computed tomographic angiography: a report of the Society of Cardiovascular Computed Tomography Guidelines Committee: endorsed by the North American Society for Cardiovascular Imaging (NASCI). *J Cardiovasc Comput Tomogr*. 2016;10:435–449.
3. Hecht HS, Cronin P, Blaha MJ, et al. 2016 SCCT/STR guidelines for coronary artery calcium scoring of noncontrast noncardiac chest CT scans: a report of the Society of Cardiovascular Computed Tomography and Society of Thoracic Radiology. *J Cardiovasc Comput Tomogr*. 2017;11:74–82.
4. Rubinshtein R, Halon DA, Gaspar T, et al. Impact of 64-slice cardiac computed tomographic angiography on clinical decision-making in emergency department patients with chest pain of possible myocardial ischemic origin. *Am J Cardiol*. 2007;100:1522–1526.
5. Litt HI, Gatsonis C, Snyder B, et al. CT angiography for safe discharge of patients with possible acute coronary syndromes. *N Engl J Med*. 2012;366:1393–1403.
6. Taylor AJ, Cerqueira M, Hodgson JM, et al. ACCF/SCCT/ACR/AHA/ASE/ASNC/NASCI/SCAI/SCMR 2010 appropriate use criteria for cardiac computed tomography. A report of the American college of cardiology foundation appropriate use criteria task force, the society of cardiovascular computed tomography, the American college of Radiology, the American

Heart Association, the American Society of Echocardiography, the American Society of Nuclear Cardiology, the North American Society for Cardiovascular Imaging, the Society for Cardiovascular Angiography and Interventions, and the Society for Cardiovascular Magnetic Resonance. *J Cardiovasc Comput Tomogr*. 2010;4 407.e1–433.e3.

7. Cheruvu C, Precious B, Naoum C, et al. Long term prognostic utility of coronary CT angiography in patients with no modifiable coronary artery disease risk factors: results from the 5 year follow-up of the CONFIRM International Multicenter Registry. *J Cardiovasc Comput Tomogr*. 2016;10:22–27.
8. Motoyama S, Ito H, Sarai M, et al. Plaque characterization by coronary computed tomography angiography and the likelihood of acute coronary events in mid-term follow-up. *J Am Coll Cardiol*. 2015;66:337–346.
9. Min JK, Taylor CA, Achenbach S, et al. Noninvasive fractional flow reserve derived from coronary CT angiography: clinical data and scientific principles. *JACC Cardiovasc Imaging*. 2015;8:1209–1222.
10. Achenbach S, Delgado V, Hausleiter J, Schoenhagen P, Min JK, Leipsic JA. SCCT expert consensus document on computed tomography imaging before transcatheter aortic valve implantation (TAVI)/transcatheter aortic valve replacement (TAVR). *J Cardiovasc Comput Tomogr*. 2012;6:366–380.
11. Cury RC, Leipsic J, Abbara S, et al. CAD-RADS™ 2.0 –2022 coronary artery disease-reporting and data system: an expert consensus document of the Society of Cardiovascular Computed Tomography (SCCT), the American college of cardiology (ACC), the American College of Radiology (ACR), and the North America Society of Cardiovascular Imaging (NASCI). *JACC Cardiovasc Imaging*. 2022;16(6):536–557.
12. Pontone G, Bertella E, Mushtaq S, et al. Coronary artery disease: diagnostic accuracy of CT coronary angiography—a comparison of high and standard spatial resolution scanning. *Radiology*. 2014;271:688–694.
13. Taha Hagar M, Soschynski M, Saffar R, et al. Accuracy of ultrahigh-resolution photon-counting CT for detecting coronary artery disease in a high-risk population. *Radiology*. 2023;307:e223305.
14. Takx RAP, Sucha D, Park J, et al. Sublingual nitroglycerin administration in coronary computed tomography angiography: a systematic review. *Eur Radiol*. 2015;25:3536–3542.
15. Nurmohamed NS, Bom MJ, Jukema RA, et al. AI-Guided Quantitative Plaque Staging Predicts Long-Term Cardiovascular Outcomes in Patients at Risk for Atherosclerotic CVD. *JACC Cardiovasc Imaging*. 2024;17:269–280.
16. Choi AD, Marques H, Kumar V, et al. *J Cardiovasc Comput Tomogr*. 2021;15:470–476.
17. Segev OL, Gaspar T, Halon DA, et al. Image quality in obese patients undergoing 256-row computed tomography coronary angiography. *Int J Cardiovasc Imaging*. 2012;28:633–639.
18. Knuuti J, Wijns W, Saraste A, et al. 2019 ESC guidelines for the diagnosis and management of chronic coronary syndromes. *Eur Heart J*. 2020;41:407–477.
19. Menke J, Kowalski J. Diagnostic accuracy and utility of coronary CT angiography with consideration of unevaluable results: a systematic review and multivariate Bayesian random-effects meta-analysis with intention to diagnose. *Eur Radiol*. 2016;26:451–458.
20. Petcherski O, Gaspar T, Halon DA, et al. Diagnostic accuracy of 256-row computed tomographic angiography for detection of obstructive coronary artery disease using invasive quantitative coronary angiography as reference standard. *Am J Cardiol*. 2013;111:510–515.
21. Gulati M, Levy PD, Mukherjee D, et al. 2021 AHA/ACC/ASE/CHEST/SAEM/SCCT/SCMR guideline for the evaluation and diagnosis of chest pain: a report of the American college of Cardiology/American Heart Association Joint Committee on clinical practice guidelines. *J Cardiovasc Comput Tomogr*. 2022;16:54–122.
22. Collet JP, Thiele H, Barbato E, et al. 2020 ESC guidelines for the management of acute coronary syndromes in patients presenting without persistent ST-segment elevation. *Eur Heart J*. 2021;42:1289–1367.
23. Knuuti J, Ballo H, Juarez-Orozco LE, et al. The performance of non-invasive tests to rule-in and rule-out significant coronary artery stenosis in patients with stable angina: a meta-analysis focused on post-test disease probability. *Eur Heart J*. 2018;39:3322–3330.

8 Coronary CT Angiography for Acute Chest Pain: Clinical Indications, Protocols, and Patient Management

CHRISTOPHER D. MAROULES, ANDREW D. CHOI, AND RICARDO C. CURY

KEY POINTS

- Coronary CT angiography (CCTA) is supported by guidelines for evaluating patients with acute chest pain who have a low-to-intermediate pretest likelihood for acute coronary syndrome, particularly in patients with normal or inconclusive ECG and negative or borderline troponins.
- Evidence-based benefits of CCTA in acute chest pain include emergency department decompression, lower healthcare costs, and a reduction in nonfatal myocardial infarctions.
- CCTA protocols can evaluate more than one life-threatening etiology of acute chest pain.
- Published expert consensus document (CAD-RADS) and guidelines provide terminology for CCTA reporting as well as suggestions for patient management recommendations based on CCTA findings.

INTRODUCTION

Acute chest pain is one of the most common chief complaints in the emergency department, accounting for more than 9 million visits each year in the United States. The challenge for emergency department physicians is to efficiently identify the small number of patients with acute coronary syndrome (ACS) and other life-threatening etiologies in the setting of large chest pain volumes and increasingly overcrowded emergency departments. Missed ACS can have disastrous consequences, leading to unnecessary patient morbidity and mortality and potential malpractice litigation.[1,2]

The role of coronary CT angiography (CCTA) for acute chest pain triage has widely expanded over the past decade and is now recognized as an accurate and efficient tool for select patients presenting to the emergency department. In appropriately selected patients, data from randomized-controlled trials[3–8] demonstrate the role of CCTA to improve efficiency of acute chest pain triage and lower healthcare costs. CCTA allows for rapid evaluation of coronary anatomy, ensuring patients without coronary artery disease (CAD) or those with low-risk anatomy can be safely discharged home in a timely manner, whereas patients with obstructive disease and high-risk anatomy can be routed to the cardiac catheterization lab expeditiously (Table 8.1). As a result of the mounting evidence supporting its clinical utility, CCTA was designated a Class I (Level of Evidence A) indication for acute chest pain evaluation among patients with low-to-intermediate risk for ACS in the 2021 ACC/AHA/Multisociety Chest Pain Guideline.[9] Nevertheless, selecting between CCTA and stress testing requires careful assessment of various clinical parameters, including the likelihood of obtaining good image quality.

CCTA For Acute Chest Pain Triage

An acute chest pain triage strategy that incorporates early use of CCTA, termed *CT First*, has been shown to expedite time to diagnose and reduce emergency department length of stay. Because a large portion of the thorax is commonly imaged during CCTA, other life-threatening etiologies for chest pain can also be evaluated simultaneously, when appropriately protocoled, including pulmonary embolism, aortic dissection, and pneumothorax. Further, CCTA can identify high-risk, nonobstructive coronary plaque that confers a higher risk for future adverse cardiovascular events and warrants medical management. The use of CCTA for patients with suspected ACS was also employed

TABLE 8.1 Value Proposition for Use of Coronary CT Angiography for Evaluating Acute Chest Pain in the Emergency Department

• High accuracy and negative predictive value for diagnosing ACS
• Expedited time to diagnosis
• Expedited time to discharge
• Documented safety
• Warranty period of 5–7 years, or greater, with a normal CCTA exam
• Potentially lower costs
• Reduction in long-term adverse cardiovascular outcomes (e.g., myocardial infarction)
• Exclude other common thoracic etiologies for chest pain

ACS, Acute coronary syndrome; *CCTA*, coronary computed tomographic angiography.

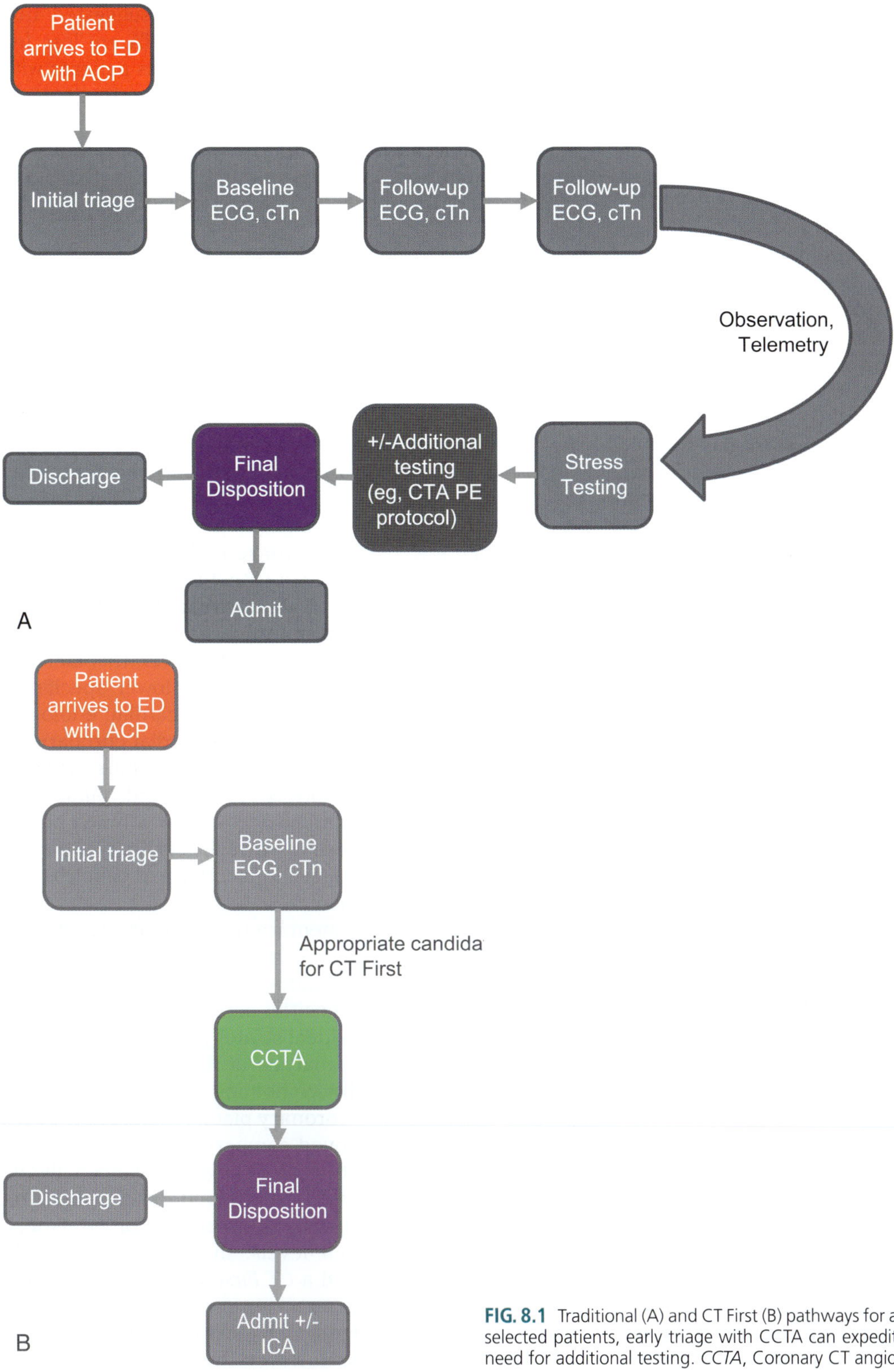

FIG. 8.1 Traditional (A) and CT First (B) pathways for acute chest pain triage. In appropriately selected patients, early triage with CCTA can expedite time-to-diagnosis and eliminate the need for additional testing. *CCTA*, Coronary CT angiography; *ED*, emergency department.

in the COVID era in order to limit unnecessary diagnostic cardiac catheterization procedures while lowering the risk of viral transmission to patients and medical staff during the emergency department encounter.[10]

Traditional acute chest pain triage in the emergency department can be time consuming and less efficient without early incorporation of CCTA (Fig. 8.1). The traditional pathway for acute chest pain triage involves an initial patient assessment with history and physical exam, baseline 12-lead ECG, and cardiac biomarkers. Patients are commonly observed in a chest pain or telemetry unit for several hours and often undergo functional testing once ACS has been excluded by serial troponin draws. Quite often, the etiology for patients' chest pain is never diagnosed during the index visit, and patients are frequently discharged home without an explanation for their symptoms or a tailored treatment plan to prevent further chest pain episodes.

For patients at low-to-intermediate pretest risk for ACS with normal or inconclusive ECG and normal or borderline troponins, the use of CCTA as the initial test of choice has emerged as a safe and efficient strategy for acute chest pain triage, with excellent sensitivity and high accuracy for excluding ACS.[11,12] A reduction in emergency department length of stay with *CT First* has been demonstrated in several trials.[3,4,6,7,13–16] For example, in ROMICAT II,[4] patients with acute chest pain and low-to-intermediate pretest risk for ACS with normal baseline troponins were randomized 1:1 to early CCTA or standard care. Emergency department length of stay was 25% shorter among patients who underwent CCTA. In addition, there was a fourfold increase in the number of direct emergency department discharges within the CCTA arm, with comparable safety to standard care. In CT-STAT,[14] acute chest pain patients at low-to-intermediate pretest risk for ACS were randomized to either early CCTA or stress myocardial perfusion imaging, and time to diagnosis was significantly lower in the CCTA arm (2.9 hr vs. 6.2 hr, $P < .0001$). Nevertheless, one multicenter trial showed that with the introduction of high-sensitivity troponin, the reduction in length of stay associated by use of CCTA was no longer apparent (see below section).[3]

CT First for acute chest pain triage is extremely safe and is associated with a very low rate of missed ACS. In a 2013 metaanalysis by Hulten et al.[17] that reviewed outcomes data from four randomized-controlled trials, there were no deaths among patients who triaged early with CCTA and no differences in incident myocardial infarctions (MI), postdischarge ED visits, or rehospitalizations compared to standard care. In ACRIN PA,[7] the largest of multicenter randomized controlled studies in this area (n = 1392), designed to compare the safety and efficiency of *CT First* to standard care within the emergency department setting, there was 0% risk of death or MI among patients with a normal CCTA exam, compared with a 1.1% risk in the standard care arm. Further, the 28-day risk of major adverse cardiovascular events (MACE) in the ROMICAT II trial[4] was 0.4% in the CCTA arm compared with 1.2% in the standard care arm ($P = .18$). Patients in the CCTA arm had a higher rate of discharge from the ED and shorter length of stay.

Evidence also suggests early triage with CCTA may improve long-term health outcomes. In the CATCH trial,[6] which compared the long-term clinical value of CCTA to functional testing among patients presenting with acute chest pain, 600 patients were randomized 1:1 to either early CCTA or standard care and then followed for 19 months. In the CCTA group, 30 patients (11%) experienced the primary endpoint (a composite of cardiac death, myocardial infarction, hospitalization for unstable angina, late symptom-driven revascularization, and readmission for chest pain), versus 47 patients (16%) in the standard care group ($P = .04$). Further, results from the Scottish Computed Tomography of the HEART Trial (SCOT-HEART) trial 5-year outcomes data[18] demonstrated a 41% decrease in nonfatal myocardial infarction and cardiovascular death for symptomatic patients who underwent CCTA in addition to standard care. However, it should be noted SCOT-HEART only evaluated patients with stable chest pain, not acute chest pain. Additionally, several studies have suggested that changes in medical therapy following CCTA are less frequent in the acute chest pain setting versus patients with stable chest pain who are evaluated in the outpatient setting.[19] Thus, for CCTA to have the greatest impact on long-term outcomes, it is important to ensure that test results are communicated and incorporated in future preventive care beyond the emergency department setting.

The Role OF CCTA With High-sensitivity Troponins

The introduction of high-sensitivity troponin assays has greatly improved the detection of myocardial injury in the setting of ACS. High-sensitivity troponins are now preferred over conventional troponin assays in the emergency department because they enable more rapid detection and exclusion of myocardial injury and improve diagnostic accuracy.[20,21] The time interval from onset of chest pain to a detectable level of troponin using a high-sensitivity assay is much lower, allowing for rapid exclusion or rule-in of ACS.

As their name implies, high-sensitivity assays can measure a 10-fold lower concentration of cardiac troponins compared to conventional assays. However, this increase in sensitivity comes at the expense of lower specificity. There are many other cardiac and noncardiac etiologies for elevated troponins other than epicardial coronary artery disease, including myocarditis, heart failure, arrhythmias, sepsis, rhabdomyolysis, stroke, and pulmonary embolism.[22] These conditions account for a much higher incidence of positive results on high-sensitivity troponin assays when they are utilized for acute chest pain triage in the emergency department.

CCTA can be complementary to high-sensitivity troponin assays by (1) improving specificity for ACS detection and (2) identifying at-risk patients without ACS. Thus pairing CCTA with a highly sensitive serologic test for myocardial injury may offer an ideal strategy for early chest pain triage. In a secondary analysis of ROMICAT II, Ferencik et al.[23] showed that by combining high-sensitivity troponins with advanced coronary plaque features on CCTA, accuracy for ACS improved compared with conventional troponin assays. This study also showed advanced plaque features on CCTA allowed for improved risk stratification among patients with low-to-intermediate, or equivocal, high-sensitivity troponin levels. In the BEACON trial,[3] which directly compared a *CT First* strategy to high-sensitivity troponins for acute chest pain triage, early CCTA was associated with significantly less downstream testing and lower direct costs. However, the use of CCTA in this trial was not associated with a reduction in length of stay, likely reflecting the higher efficiency of care that exists in systems that use high-sensitivity troponins.

Patients with normal high-sensitivity troponin labs may still have vulnerable coronary anatomy, including significant coronary stenosis or the presence of high-risk plaque. Although these patients may not be suffering ACS at the time of their presentation to the emergency department, they will remain at high risk for future cardiovascular events following discharge. Early CCTA allows these at-risk

TABLE 8.2 Recommended Acute Chest Pain Pathways for Patients With No Known Coronary Artery Disease

RISK CATEGORY	APPROPRIATENESS OF CCTA	GOAL OF EVALUATION/ MANAGEMENT
High Risk for ACS • STEMI • ST-changes suggestive of ischemia (no ST-elevation), leading diagnosis NSTE-ACS • Elevated cTn or hs-cTn (>99th percentile)	Usually not appropriate	Invasive coronary angiography CCTA is rarely indicated to determine if an invasive evaluation is appropriate in the setting of (Non-ST-elevation myocardial infarction) NSTE-ACS[a]
Low to Intermediate Risk for ACS[b] • Normal, nonischemic, or nonspecific ECG changes • Normal or equivocal baseline cTn, *or* hs-cTn <99th percentile	CCTA usually appropriate	Detection of coronary plaque and stenosis; detection of high-risk anatomy
Very Low Risk for ACS • Normal or nonischemic ECG • Normal hs-cTn, or • Normal cTn, and leading diagnosis is noncardiac chest pain	Usually not appropriate	No testing required Discharge, +/− outpatient follow-up CCTA is rarely considered to exclude CAD and provide additional risk stratification[a]

[a]Triple rule-out CTA can substitute for coronary CTA if there is reasonable risk for both ACS and either PE or AAS. The CT scanner used must be cardiac capable with a minimum of 64 multidetector units and offer reasonable likelihood for diagnostic quality.
[b]Using a pretest clinical decision assessment tool.
AAS, Acute aortic syndrome; *ACS*, acute coronary syndrome; *CAD*, coronary artery disease; *CCTA*, coronary computed tomographic angiography; *cTn*, cardiac troponin; *hs-cTn*, high-sensitivity cardiac troponin; *PE*, pulmonary embolism; *STEMI*, ST-elevation myocardial infarction.

patients to be identified early, so appropriate medical therapy can be initiated in a timely manner and their future risk for myocardial infarction can be mitigated.

CLINICAL INDICATIONS

Appropriate patient selection is critical to ensuring that the use of CCTA for acute chest pain triage improves health outcomes and optimizes resource utilization in a responsible manner. Not all patients are appropriate candidates for early CCTA, and there are certainly circumstances when CCTA triage is inappropriate. Generally, CCTA offers the greatest value for acute chest pain triage in patients with low-to-intermediate risk for ACS. It is in this population CCTA has been extensively validated and endorsed by Societal guidelines.[9,24–27]

CCTA is the only noninvasive test to be issued a "Class I" endorsement by the 2021 American College of Cardiology (ACC) and American Heart Association (AHA) Chest Pain Guidelines for patients with acute chest pain,[9] supported by "Level A" level of evidence. Although other diagnostic tests also received a Class I endorsement, such as stress myocardial perfusion imaging, their recommendations were only supported by "Level B" quality of evidence. The 2021 ACC/AHA guidelines specifically endorse CCTA as a frontline test for patients considered low-to-intermediate risk for ACS based on initial risk stratification, 12-lead electrocardiography, and cardiac troponins.

In the 2020 European Society of Cardiology (ESC) guidelines for the management of ACS in patients presenting without ST-segment elevation,[24] CCTA was also endorsed as a Class I indication ("Level A" quality of evidence) for patients at low-to-intermediate risk for ACS with normal ECG and negative troponins, as well as for patients with inconclusive or equivocal baseline troponins. The Asian Society of Cardiovascular Imaging also supports CCTA for acutely symptomatic patients suspected of ACS who have high pretest probability for coronary artery disease with normal or equivocal biomarkers.[26]

Assessing pretest risk for ACS is best accomplished in the context of an institutional chest pain algorithm, to ensure timely triage and selection of patients for CCTA or to other alternative modalities based on risk. A three-level algorithm is one such example, which assigns patients to one of three diagnostic pathways (high risk, low-to-intermediate risk, or very low risk for ACS) based on clinical examination, 12-lead ECG, and cardiac biomarkers (Table 8.2).

Patients in the "high-risk" category include those presenting with ST-elevation myocardial infarction (STEMI) and patients in whom the leading diagnosis is non-ST-elevation acute coronary syndrome (NSTE-ACS). In patients presenting with STEMI, urgent cardiac catheterization is proven to be beneficial,[28] and CT imaging should not delay door-to-balloon time. CCTA is rarely indicated as a first-line strategy in the setting of NSTE-ACS to determine whether an invasive approach is appropriate, or when a noninvasive strategy is preferred (e.g., during the COVID-19 pandemic, bleeding risk, vascular access issues, patient preference).[10,29–32] Potential benefits of CCTA within this higher-risk population include (1) rapid and accurate exclusion of obstructive CAD, (2) identification of high-risk plaque and atherosclerosis burden to improve risk prediction, and (3) potential reduction in costs and resource utilization for cases where invasive coronary angiography can be safely avoided.

When considering the use of CCTA in "high-risk" patients, it is important to recognize that early trials on the use of CT for acute chest pain included low-risk patients, and there is a paucity of data on how CCTA might perform within a higher risk cohort. An observational component of the randomized-controlled VERDICT trial[30] examined the accuracy of CCTA among 1023 patients with documented non-ST elevation ACS and determined 33% of patients with non-ST elevation ACS had no clinically significant coronary artery disease, suggesting an opportunity for CCTA to safely defer invasive coronary angiography in nearly one-third of high-risk patients. Similar results were observed in the CARMENTA trial,[32] a prospective, randomized-controlled trial designed to investigate whether cardiac magnetic resonance imaging (CMR) or CCTA could serve as an effective gatekeeper for invasive coronary angiography in patients presenting to the ED with non-ST elevation ACS. Early CCTA safely reduced referrals for invasive coronary angiography by 34% compared with routine clinical care, with no increase in MACE after 1 year.

The Rapid Assessment of Potential Ischaemic Heart Disease with CTCA (RAPID-CTCA) trial randomized 1748 patients to CCTA with standard of care versus standard of care alone with 1 year follow-up in intermediate-to-high risk patients.[33] The inclusion criteria included a prior history of coronary heart disease, troponin >99th percentile, or abnormal electrocardiogram. Fifty-three percent had normal or nonobstructive CAD, whereas 47% had obstructive CAD. This was representative of an intermediate-to-high pretest probability cohort with 34% of patients with prior coronary heart disease. There was no significant difference in the primary outcome of death or MI, although patients in the CCTA group had a lower rate of invasive angiography with HR of 0.81 (0.72–0.92; $P = .001$). Although the study did not meet its primary outcome, this cohort consisted of intermediate-to-high pretest probability of patients, and one-third had known coronary heart disease. This supports the notion that the routine use of CCTA may not benefit patients with established CAD—especially those with prior myocardial infarction, coronary artery bypass grafting (CABG), or percutaneous coronary intervention (PCI).

Low-to-intermediate risk patients include those with no definite evidence of ACS by ECG and troponins. It also includes patients with inadequate or mildly abnormal functional testing during the index ED visit or within the previous 1 year. The majority of trial evidence supporting CCTA includes patients within this low-to-intermediate risk category.[4,6,7,14–16] CCTA is often an appropriate front-line test for these patients, particularly at centers with local expertise and established high-quality CCTA programs. It is in this population that CCTA can be most efficient; approximately 5% to 15% of patients will have obstructive CAD warranting further evaluation with invasive coronary angiography, whereas the majority of patients can be safely discharged from the emergency department with normal or nonobstructive disease. CCTA can safely defer invasive coronary angiography in patients with normal or nonobstructive CAD, which can represent up to 50% of the low-to-intermediate risk chest pain population.[34,35] Among patients found to have nonobstructive disease, early recognition with CCTA offers an opportunity to optimize medical management prior to discharge from the emergency department.[36]

Patients at very low risk for ACS include those for whom a noncardiac etiology of chest pain is the leading diagnosis, with normal or nonischemic ECG and normal baseline high-sensitivity troponin. The 30-day risk of major adverse cardiovascular events in this population is less than 1%.[37] For the majority of very-low-risk patients, further testing for CAD is usually not necessary. However, CCTA may be reasonable in some scenarios to confidently exclude CAD and provide additional risk stratification, for example, patients with recurrent ED visits for chest pain who desire further testing to confidently exclude CAD. Shared decision-making cannot be overemphasized in this patient population, so patients are well informed of the potential risks and benefits of additional testing.

Pretest Risk Stratification

Risk stratification tools—performed as part of a clinical decision pathway (CDP)—can aid in categorizing patients into very-low-risk, low-to-intermediate risk, and high-risk for ACS, providing second-order risk stratification beyond cardiac troponins and ECG. A few of the commonly used CDP tools in the emergency department setting include the HEART (History-ECG-Age-Risk Factors-Troponin) score,[38] Emergency Department Assessment of Chest Pain Score (EDACS),[39] and ADAPT[40] (2-Hour Accelerated Diagnostic Protocol to Assess Patients With Chest Pain Symptoms Using Contemporary Troponins as the Only Biomarker) (based on the Thrombolysis in Myocardial Infarction Risk Score (TIMI) risk score). The HEART score is a validated tool endorsed by recent guidelines that is currently incorporated in many U.S. emergency departments (Table 8.3). Scoring is based on five elements (History, ECG, Age, Risk factors, and Troponins), with a 0, +1, or +2 score for each element, and a total score ranging from 0 to 10, analogous to the Apgar score. As the HEART score increases, there is an incrementally increased risk of 30-day major adverse cardiovascular events. A score between 0 and 3 is considered *low risk* (0.9–1.7% MACE), between 4 and 6 is *moderate risk* (12–16.6% MACE), and between 7 and 10 is *high risk* (50–65% MACE).[38]

Risk stratification should be performed in parallel with serial troponin measurements, preferably high-sensitivity troponin, to exclude myocardial injury or infarction. For high-sensitivity troponin assays, baseline sample collection should be obtained followed by a repeat measurement in 1 to 3 hours. For conventional assays, repeat sample collections are generally advised between 3 and 6 hours.

Safety and Diagnostic Quality Considerations

The principal safety considerations for CCTA include radiation exposure, allergic reactions to iodinated contrast, and contrast-induced nephropathy. The risk of contrast-induced nephropathy is very low, and recent guidelines from the American College of Radiology (ACR) recommend limiting eGFR screening prior to iodinated contrast administration to patients who are older than 60 years, history of renal disease, history of hypertension and taking antihypertensive medication, and diabetes mellitus.[41]

Exposure to radiation should always be weighed against the potential risk of cancer, according to the "as low as reasonably achievable" (ALARA) principle. For example, increased radiation sensitivity in premenopausal women or younger patients may favor stress testing (e.g., stress echocardiography or stress MRI) for early chest pain triage. Similarly, patient characteristics known to impair image quality (i.e., inability to take beta blockers, lack of cooperation, or high body mass index) may favor alternative

TABLE 8.3 HEART Score[38] Risk Stratification for ACS in the Emergency Department

Scoring	• History
	  • Highly suspicious (2 pts)
	  • Moderately suspicious (1 pt)
	  • Slightly or nonsuspicious (0 pts)
	• ECG
	  • Significant ST depression (2 pts)
	  • Nonspecific repolarization (1 pt)
	  • Normal (0 pts)
	• Age
	  • ≥65 yrs (2 pts)
	  • >45–<65 yrs (1 pt)
	  • ≤ 45 yrs (0 pts)
	• Risk factors (DM, current or recent (<1 month) smoker, HTN, HLP, family history of CAD, & obesity)
	  • ≥3 risk factors or history of CAD (2 pts)
	  • 1 or 2 risk factors (1 pt)
	  • No risk factors (0 pts)
	• Troponin (0, 3 hrs)
	  • ≥3x normal limit (2 pts)
	  • >1–<3 normal limit (1 pt)
	  • ≤ normal limit (0 pts)

Troponin	cTn or hs-cTn
Risk Thresholds	
Low risk	• HEART score <3 • Negative 0, 3-hr cTn • Negative 0, 2-hr hs-cTn
Intermediate risk	• HEART score 4–6
High risk	• HEART score 7–10

ACS, Acute coronary syndrome; *CAD*, coronary artery disease; *cTn*, cardiac troponin; *DM*, diabetes mellitus; *hs-cTn*, high-sensitivity cardiac troponin; *HLD*, hyperlipidemia; *HTN*, hypertension.

TABLE 8.4 Contraindications to CCTA

Absolute Contraindications
• Severe allergy to iodinated contrast (anaphylaxis)
• Inability to lay flat
• Inability to perform breath-hold
Relative Contraindications[a]
• Pregnancy or breastfeeding
• Renal insufficiency
• Contraindication to beta blockers, if heart rate elevated
• Contraindication to nitrates (severe aortic stenosis, recent use of erectile dysfunction medications)
• Cardiac arrhythmia, including refractory tachycardia
• Extensive coronary artery calcification

[a]Relative contraindications are scanner dependent and may not be problematic when using modern CT scanner platforms.
CCTA, Coronary computed tomographic angiography.

testing, and clinical judgment by the referring clinician is required for optimal test selection.

Contraindications

There are several scenarios when alternative testing should be considered for acute chest pain triage. For example, the history of severe allergic reaction to iodinated contrast (anaphylaxis) after adequate steroid/antihistamine preparation should be considered an absolute contraindication (Table 8.4). Patients unable to lay flat, unable perform a short breath-hold, and unable to follow technologist commands are not appropriate candidates for CCTA. Relative contraindications leading to potentially nondiagnostic scans include heart rate above the site maximum for reliably diagnostic CCTA, markedly irregular rhythm, high coronary calcium burden, and large body size. Renal insufficiency is another relative contraindication, although patients with estimated glomerular filtration rates above 30, and patients on chronic dialysis, may safely undergo CCTA. Pregnancy or uncertain pregnancy status in premenopausal women is another relative contraindication. However, CTA may be useful in this setting as a noninvasive approach to exclude spontaneous coronary artery dissection (SCAD), which predominantly occurs in young women considered low risk for coronary artery disease.[42]

PROTOCOLS AND WORKFLOW

The essential steps in preparing patients with acute chest pain for CCTA include: evaluation, education, medication and reevaluation after premedication.[43] Clinical judgment, scanner technology, and institutional experience should help guide and tailor patient preparation. The goal is to achieve high diagnostic accuracy with the lowest possible radiation dose. CCTA is sensitive to motion, requiring slow, steady heart rates and patient cooperation. Higher heart rates require scan protocols that are less sensitive to movement, such as retrospective ECG-gated scan protocols, but these may result in higher radiation doses.

Patient Evaluation and Education

Patients should be evaluated by medical staff to ensure no absolute contraindications exist. It should be clear the patient understands the nature of the examination and can cooperate with breath-holding instructions. Baseline vital signs should be used to design a prescan medication protocol to achieve heart rate targets based on the scanner model to be used. Staff should ascertain the patient's previous medications. If the baseline heart rate is within target range, a mild stress, for example, 30 seconds of hard hand-grip on a towel, may be considered to ensure heart rate does not rise unduly.[44]

Patients should be informed about the nature of the CCTA exam, its objectives, possible risks including radiation dose, their required cooperation, and potential sensations they are likely to feel. Patients should be given a chance to request an alternative diagnostic test if they feel unable or unwilling to proceed. This process should be repeated after premedication and before scanning, to ensure patients remember breath-hold instructions and are prepared for the sensations likely to occur from nitroglycerin and contrast administration.

Premedication

Premedication should be considered prior to CCTA to improve image quality, including (1) heart rate–lowering medication to minimize coronary motion, generally beta blockers, and (2) nitroglycerin to dilate the coronary arteries (Table 8.5). Generally, a target heart rate of 65 beats per minute or less is preferred for most CCTA studies.[45] However, institutional protocols will vary depending on target heart rates required by the scanner model being utilized, with some tolerance for higher heart rates with modern scanners.

Beta blockers are most commonly used to establish heart rate control and reduce heart rate variability prior to CCTA. Oral short-acting metoprolol administration is the usual practice, with 50 to 100 mg by mouth 45 to 60 minutes prior to imaging.[45] Alternatively, IV metoprolol can be used to achieve target heart rate (5 mg IV, followed by repeated 5 mg doses as necessary, typically up to 20–25 mg total). However, IV metoprolol must be administered while the patient is on the scanner table, which may slow CT throughput in the emergency department.

Ivabradine, a direct I(f) current inhibitor, can be used in lieu of beta blockers for heart rate control prior to CCTA. Ivabradine can effectively lower heart rate with a lesser impact on myocardial contractility and blood pressure as metoprolol.[46] This makes ivabradine an attractive alternative for patients with low blood pressure. A sample protocol is 15 mg orally 60 to 75 minutes prior to scanning.[47] Although ivabradine may be more effective than metoprolol in patients treated with chronic beta blockers, it is ineffective in patients who are not in sinus rhythm, as it acts through direct inhibition of the sinoatrial node.

Scan Protocols for Acute Chest Pain

In some patients presenting with acute chest pain, there may be more than one life-threatening condition being considered in the differential. For example, a patient with multiple cardiovascular risk factors may also have a positive D-dimer test and symptoms suggesting pulmonary embolism. In these scenarios, the CCTA protocol can be modified to include the entire thorax and simultaneously opacify the pulmonary arteries, coronary arteries, and aorta. This so-called "triple rule-out" (TRO) protocol can be used to exclude significant disease in all three vascular territories.[48]

Compared to conventional CCTA, TRO is associated with a higher diagnostic yield for pulmonary embolism and aortic dissection and may detect a significant noncoronary diagnosis in 8% to 14% of patients that can explain the patient's chest pain, including findings that may not be detectable on CCTA due to its limited scan coverage.[49] TRO is also accurate for excluding significant coronary artery disease, with comparable accuracy and diagnostic yield to conventional CCTA.[48–50] In some studies, TRO was able to safely eliminate the need for further noninvasive testing.[51]

Depending on the CT scanner, TRO may be performed with an extended contrast infusion to maintain pulmonary artery contrast using a similar contrast infusion rate as CCTA (e.g., 5–7 mL/sec) followed by a reduced rate (3 ml/sec). Alternatively, a two-pass protocol can be implemented in which the first contrast bolus is timed to optimally opacify the pulmonary arteries. Then, a second bolus of contrast is administered with scanning timed to opacify the coronary arteries and aorta.[50]

TRO comes with the downside of increased radiation and contrast dose, and potentially higher incidence of nondiagnostic coronary evaluation, which varies based on the type of CT scanner used.[25,50,52] However, with modern scanners and scan protocols, the additional radiation and contrast associated with TRO are less substantial than previously described.[51] Nevertheless, judicious use of TRO is recommended, and its potential risks and benefits should be considered. If the primary clinical diagnosis under consideration is pulmonary embolism or acute aortic syndrome, strong consideration should be given to dedicated CTA of the pulmonary arteries or aorta, respectively.

The 2021 ACC/AHA/Multisociety Chest Pain Guideline supports tailoring chest pain protocols to the most likely diagnosis with TRO protocols to be applied judiciously.[53] Similarly, the 2015 Multisociety appropriate use guideline for cardiovascular imaging in the emergency department[25]

TABLE 8.5 Sample Premedication Protocols for CCTA in the Emergency Department

HEART RATE CONTROL	ORAL METOPROLOL	IV METOPROLOL	IVABRADINE	DILTIAZEM
Sample premedication protocol	Give 45–60 min prior to imaging, then reassess Baseline HR 55–60, give 25 mg Baseline HR 61–65, give 50 mg Baseline HR >65, give 100 mg	While patient is on the scanner table, give 5 mg slow push every 5 min, up to 20–25 mg total	Give 75 min prior to imaging, then reassess Oral ivabradine 15 mg or 7.5 mg (chronic beta blockade)	While patient is on the scanner table, give 5 mg IV slow push, redoes every 10 min up to 30 mg total
Contraindications	• Conduction abnormalities (e.g., sinoatrial block, sick sinus syndrome) unless functional pacemaker is present • Systolic blood pressure (SBP) <90 mmHg • Known allergy • Severe bronchospasm	• Conduction abnormalities (e.g., sinoatrial block, sick sinus syndrome) unless functional pacemaker is present • SBP <90 mmHg • Known allergy • Severe bronchospasm	• Conduction abnormalities (e.g., sinoatrial block, sick sinus syndrome) unless functional pacemaker is present • Severe liver impairment • Decompensated heart failure • Known allergy	• Do not combine with beta blockers • SBP <90 mmHg • Conduction abnormalities (e.g., sinoatrial block, sick sinus syndrome) • Known allergy
Advantages	Simple oral titration Minimal patient/nurse time in CT scanner suite Well-tolerated Low cost	Simple titration Shorter wait time for full effect Low cost	Simple oral titration Generally well-tolerated in patients with lower BP Minimal hypotensive effect	Shorter wait time for full effect
Disadvantages	Longer wait time for full effect Larger doses may have a hypotensive effect	Longer patient/nurse time in the CT scanner suite Multiple doses (5 mg) may be necessary to achieve target HR Larger doses may have a hypotensive effect	Longest wait time for full effect Expensive	Potential hazardous interaction with beta blockers Hypotensive effect is more common than with beta blockers
VASODILATION	**SUBLINGUAL NITROGLYCERIN**	**TOPICAL NITROPASTE**		
Sample premedication protocol	Give 0.4–0.8 mg (tabs or spray) 3–5 min prior to IV contrast	Apply ½ inch to chest 60 min prior to imaging; remove after CT imaging		
Contraindications	SBP <90 mmHg Known allergy Recent use of erectile dysfunction meds[a] Severe aortic stenosis	SBP <90 mmHg Known allergy Recent use of erectile dysfunction meds[a] Severe aortic stenosis		
Advantages	Simple dosing Rapid onset	No need for nurse or provider to administer in the CT suite		
Disadvantages	Nurse or provider must administer in the CT suite	Longer wait time for full effect		

[a]Omit nitroglycerin in patients with recent intake of phosphodiesterase inhibitors (24 hours for sildenafil, 72 hours for tadalafil).
CCTA, Coronary computed tomographic angiography; *HR*, heart rate; *IV*, intravenous.

designates TRO as "appropriate" in patients with acute chest pain for whom a leading diagnosis is problematic or not possible, and in whom the overall likelihood of ACS, pulmonary embolism, or acute aortic syndrome is not low. This may include patients with history of deep vein thrombosis, malignancy, or immobility and positive D-dimer on laboratory testing (Fig. 8.2). If there is concern for both ACS and aortic dissection but not pulmonary embolism, an extended CCTA scan protocol can be utilized that is timed to image the aorta and coronary arteries, but with an extended craniocaudal field-of-view that includes the aortic arch (termed CCTA with extended scan length [CCTA-XL] protocol) (Fig. 8.3). Sample scan protocols for CCTA, CCTA-XL, and TRO are included in Table 8.6.

Coronary artery calcium (CAC) testing with noncontrast CT is generally not used as a standalone test for the evaluation of patients with acute chest pain but may have a selective role in low-risk patients with acute chest pain (Class 2a by 2021 Chest Pain Guideline). When CAC = 0, the rate of obstructive CAD is low (less than 1%), and long-term prognosis is favorable.[54] However, CAC = 0 cannot definitely exclude ACS, which can occurs in 1% to 3% of patients who have noncalcified plaque.[55,56] Thus, when there is concern for ACS, CCTA may allow for more definitive rule-out of coronary plaque or stenosis.

CT Gating Strategies and Patient-tailored Scanning

All cardiac CT acquisitions are synchronized to the cardiac cycle using ECG leads to minimize coronary motion. Gating strategies include prospective triggering, retrospective gating, and high-pitch helical prospective triggering, which are reviewed in Chapter 1 Image Acquisition Protocols

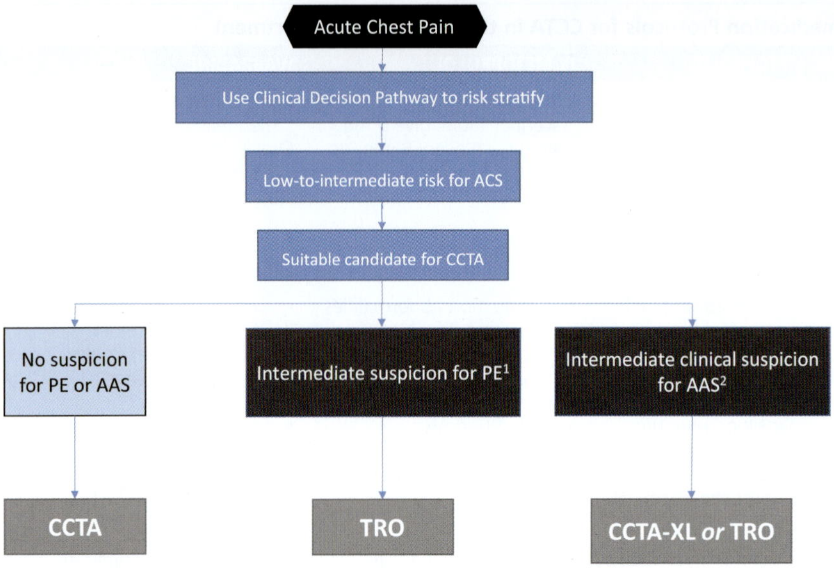

FIG. 8.2A Algorithm for deciding between conventional CCTA, CCTA with an extended field-of-view (CCTA-XL) or triple rule-out (TRO).
1. Intermediate suspicion for PE includes:
   - History of deep vein thrombosis, *or*
   - History of malignancy, *or*
   - Immobility, *or*
   - Age >65 years and tachycardia
2. Intermediate suspicion for AAS includes:
   - History of connective tissue disease (Marfan syndrome, Ehlers Danlos), bicuspid aortic valve, aortic aneurysm, or recent aortic surgery, *or*
   - Clinical symptoms of abrupt onset ripping/stabbing/tearing pain, *or*
   - Physical exam findings of pulse or blood pressure deficit, or new murmur of aortic regurgitation

ACS, Acute coronary syndrome; *AAS*, acute aortic syndrome; *CAD*, coronary artery disease; *CCTA*, coronary computed tomographic angiography; *PE*, pulmonary embolism.

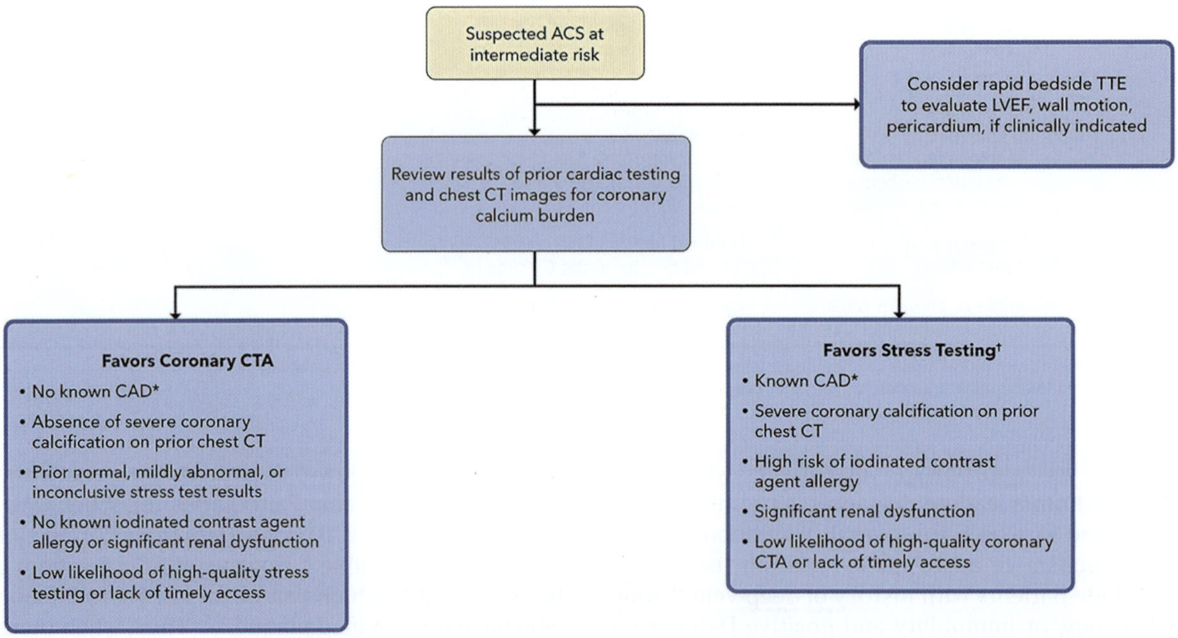

FIG. 8.2B Guideline-Directed Approach to Subsequent Diagnostic Testing in Patients With Suspected ACS at Intermediate Clinical Risk
Prior myocardial infarction, coronary revascularization, or stenosis >50% or extensive nonobstructive CAD on prior ICA/CTA. †Exercise ECG, stress CMR,stress echocardiography, stress perfusion imaging. *ACS,* Acute coronary syndrome; *CAD,* ¼ coronary artery disease; *CT,* computed tomography; *CTA,* computed tomography angiography; *ICA,* internal carotid artery; *LVEF,* left ventricle ejection fraction; *TTE,* transthoracic echocardiogram. (Source: Kontos et al., 2022 ECDP on Evaluation and Disposition of Acute Chest Pain in ED, JACC 2022.)

for Different Types of Cardiac CT. Generally, prospectively triggering should be considered the default scan mode of choice in patients with sufficient heart rate control, including patients with regular rhythms and heart rates less than 65 beats per minute.[45] At higher heart rates (i.e., 66–72 beats per minute), the acquisition window can be widened ("padded") to increase the likelihood of imaging during coronary diastasis. If retrospectively gated scanning is necessary due to high or irregular heart rate, ECG-gated tube current modulation should generally be applied to mitigate

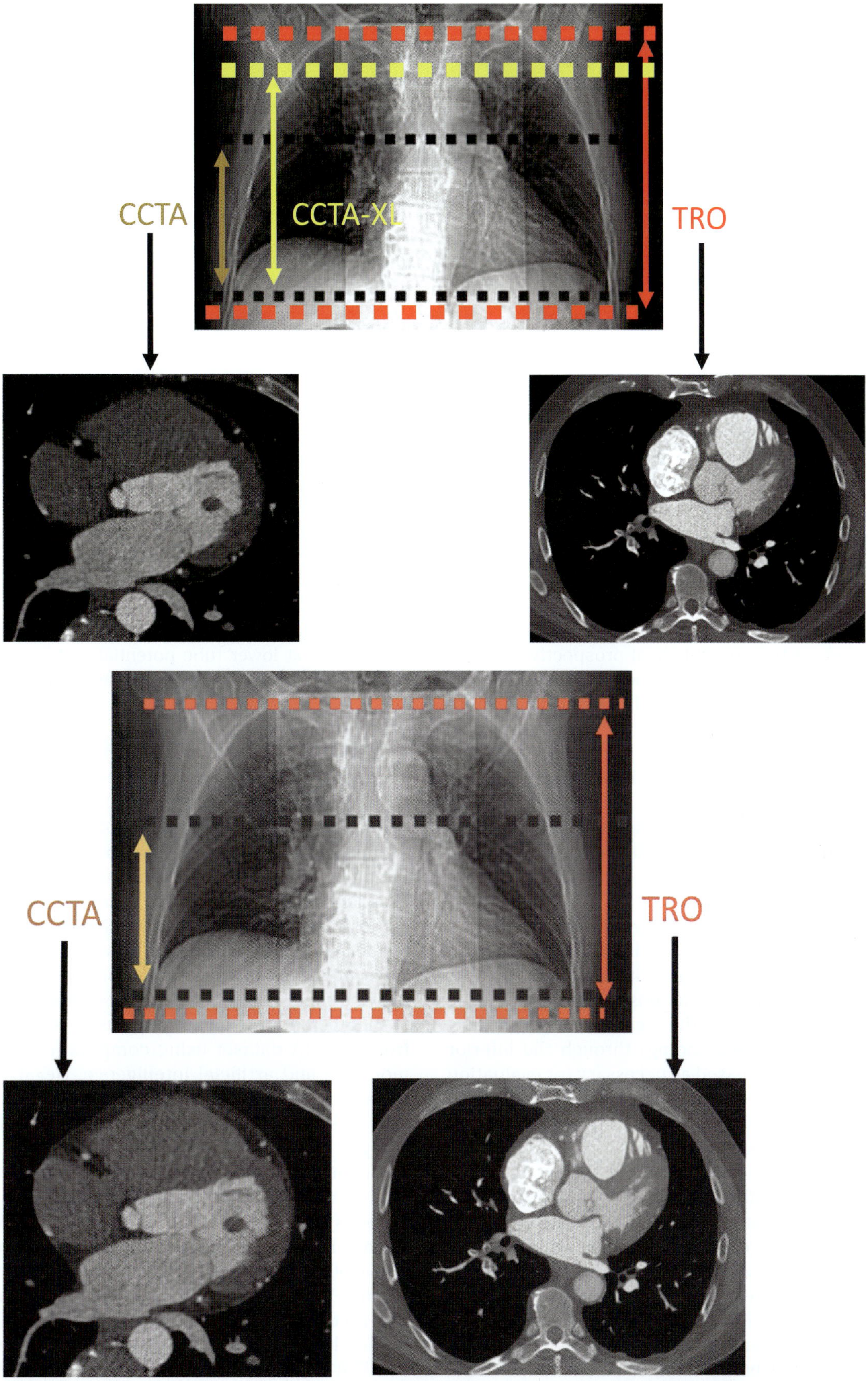

FIG. 8.3 Protocol differences between conventional CCTA, CCTA-XL, and TRO. For TRO, the entire lungs are included within the scan field, from apices through the lung bases. For conventional CCTA, the carina is often used as an anatomic marker on the frontal scout view to indicate the cranial scan limit, whereas for CCTA-XL, the superior scan margin is selected just above the aortic arch. If a single-pass TRO protocol is utilized, approximately 30% more contrast is administered to ensure adequate back-filling of the pulmonary arteries. For CCTA, the right heart and pulmonary arteries are poorly opacified with contrast. Pulmonary artery filling defects are noted within the TRO image (*right*), consistent with acute pulmonary emboli. *CCTA*, Coronary computed tomographic angiography; *CCTA-XL*, coronary computed tomographic angiography with extended scan length; *TRO*, triple rule-out.

TABLE 8.6 Sample Scan Protocols for CCTA, CCTA With Expanded Scan Length and Triple Rule-out

	CCTA	CCTA-XL	TRO (SINGLE INJECTION)	TRO (DUAL INJECTION)
Scan range	Just below carina through inferior border of the heart	Above aortic arch through the inferior heart	Lung apices through the costophrenic angles	1. Lung apices through the costophrenic angles (PE) 2. Above aortic arch through the inferior heart (AD, CAD)
Scan direction	Craniocaudal	Craniocaudal	Caudocranial	1. Craniocaudal (PE) 2. Caudocranial (AD, CAD)
Scan mode	High-pitch helical, prospective triggering, or retrospective gating with ECG triggering	High-pitch helical, prospective triggering, or retrospective gating with ECG triggering	High-pitch helical, prospective triggering, or retrospective gating with ECG triggering	1. Helical (high-pitch preferred) (PE) 2. High-pitch helical, prospective triggering, or retrospective gating with ECG triggering (AD, CAD)
Field of view	150–200 mm	150–200 mm	150–200 mm	1. 150–200 mm (covering both lungs) (PE) 2. 150–200 mm (AD, CAD)
Contrast	Generally, 60–90 ml at 5–7 ml/sec, followed by 50 ml saline flush	Generally 60–100 ml at 5–7 ml/sec, followed by 50 ml saline flush	Generally, 80–120 ml at 5–7 ml/sec, followed by 50 ml saline flush	1. 50–75 mL at 5–7 mL, followed by 50 mL saline flush (PE) 2. 50–75 mL at 5–7 mL, followed by 50 mL saline flush (AD, CAD)
Procedure	Bolus tracking or test bolus	Bolus tracking or test bolus	Bolus tracking or test bolus	Bolus tracking (at main pulmonary artery for PE evaluation, ascending aorta for AD/CAD evaluation) or test bolus

AD, Aortic dissection; *CAD*, coronary artery disease; *CCTA*, coronary computed tomographic angiography; *CCTA-XL*, coronary computed tomographic angiography with expanded scan length; *PE*, pulmonary embolism; *TRO*, triple rule-out.

radiation exposure. With modern scanners, low-dose scan techniques such as high-pitch helical prospective triggering and wide-detector single heart beat scanning may be options for patients meeting standards for target heart rate and body habitus, allowing diagnostic CT angiograms to be acquired at doses as low as <1 mSv.[57–59]

Patient-specific modifications to the scan protocol are recommended to minimize radiation while maintaining diagnostic image quality. This includes modification of scan length, timing and infusion rate of the contrast bolus, and alteration of tube potential and tube current based on patient characteristics.

Scan length can be determined by the initial topogram or by the noncontrast calcium scoring CT scan. As scan length has a linear relationship with radiation dose it should be decreased as much as possible, to include the heart from above the level of the highest coronary artery (often the left anterior descending) through the inferior heart. Scan length is increased as necessary for evaluation of bypass grafts (to include the origin of the left internal mammary artery) or the aorta and pulmonary arteries (in TRO and CCTA-XL protocols).[60]

As radiation dose varies approximately as the square of the change in tube potential, as opposed to linearly with tube current or scan length, small incremental decreases in tube potential may lead to large reductions in radiation dose. Routine use of 100 kV tube potential is generally possible when the patient's weight is below 100 kg and the body mass index ≤30 kg/m sq.[45] In addition to weight-based and body mass index–based tube voltage selection, automated methods for tube voltage selection based on attenuation values in the scout images are available on modern scanners. In smaller adults and pediatric patients, reducing tube potential to 80 kVp can lower radiation exposure and maintain diagnostic image quality, while substantially lowering radiation exposure by as much as 30% to 50%.[45] Iterative and model-based reconstruction techniques reduce image noise, allowing for CT imaging at lower tube potential and lower tube current with preservation of diagnostic image quality.

Sequential Testing With FFR-CT or Stress CTP

The addition of CT-based fractional flow reserve (FFR-CT)[61–64] or stress myocardial CT perfusion (CTP)[8,65,66] to CCTA may (see Chapter 13, FFR-CT, and Chapter 15, CT Perfusion) be appropriate in situations where the determination of ischemia would be helpful to guide management. This includes in cases where there is intermediate-severe stenosis (40–90%) and flow-limiting lesions are clinically suspected.[9] Both techniques have the potential to eliminate unnecessary invasive coronary angiograms by improving specificity for obstructive coronary artery disease.

FFR-CT offers evaluation of lesion-specific physiology from a CCTA dataset using computational flow dynamic modeling and artificial intelligence. Negative FFR-CT results are associated with good prognosis and may serve as a gatekeeper for cardiac catheterization. In a post hoc analysis of ROMICAT II,[67] FFR-CT in the ED setting was able to downgrade severely stenotic lesions (>70% stenosis) on CCTA by more than half. In addition, over one-third of patients with mild coronary stenosis (25–49%) were found to have hemodynamically significant flow limitation (FFR-CT <0.80). In another single-center observational study, when FFR-CT was added to CCTA in the ED setting, there was no difference in MACE compared to CCTA alone, and no deaths or myocardial infarctions occurred with negative FFR-CT when revascularization was deferred.[64]

Stress myocardial CTP following vasodilator stress has also been validated to identify functionally significant coronary artery disease, and emerging data highlight its potential role for acute chest pain evaluation.[8,66,68–70] In a prospective trial of 145 ED patients who underwent combined stress myocardial CTP and CCTA or single-photon emission computed tomography (SPECT) myocardial perfusion imaging,[65] mean length of stay was 28% shorter and mean direct costs were 44% lower with stress CTP/CCTA compared to SPECT. In the CATCH-2 trial,[8] 300 patients hospitalized for acute chest pain were randomized to combined stress myocardial CTP and CCTA or CCTA alone, and the primary endpoint was frequency of coronary revascularization among patients referred for invasive coronary angiography. Although there was no observed difference in the primary endpoint, combined stress CTP/CCTA resulted in significantly fewer referrals for invasive coronary angiography compared to CCTA alone (14% vs. 30%, $P < .0001$), with similar outcomes after a median follow-up of 1.5 years, highlighting a potential gatekeeping role for stress myocardial CTP.

REPORTING AND PATIENT MANAGEMENT

Interpretation of CCTA exams for the evaluation of acute chest pain should make use of the Coronary Artery Disease Data and Reporting System 2.0 (CAD-RADS).[71,72] Each coronary vessel should be consciously and algorithmically evaluated, with a statement on plaque morphology (i.e., calcified, noncalcified, mixed, or high-risk plaque) and a quantitative or semiquantitative estimate of stenosis expressed as maximal percent diameter narrowing (i.e., no stenosis, minimal <25%, mild 25–49%, moderate 50–69%, severe ≥70%, or total occlusion). For the left main coronary artery, ≥50% diameter narrowing represents severe stenosis. Reports should include final impression statements on (1) the presence or absence of obstructive CAD, (2) the presence or absence of high-risk plaque, and (3) a semiquantitative or quantitative measure of total plaque burden. Any potentially life-threatening findings should be communicated urgently and directly to emergency department staff. This includes coronary findings, as well as emergent noncardiac findings such as aortic dissection and acute pulmonary emboli.

A final CAD-RADS assessment should be included at the end of the report, which summarizes the key findings and directs patient management[72] (Table 8.7). CAD-RADS is the standardized reporting system for patients undergoing CCTA that links imaging findings with specific management recommendations.[71] The primary goal of CAD-RADS is to improve patient care by facilitating communication of CCTA results to referring physicians. It also provides a framework that may benefit education, research, peer review, and quality assurance. The classification is applied on a per-patient basis for the clinically most relevant coronary stenosis. Assessment categories range from CAD-RADS 0 (denoting complete absence of coronary plaque and stenosis) to CAD-RADS 5 (denoting the presence of at least one totally occluded coronary artery). In addition to the numeric assessment category, the most recent CAD-RADS guidelines also incorporate a quantitative summary of coronary plaque burden when plaque is detected on CCTA, ranging from P1 (mild burden) to P4 (extensive burden).[72] Patients with normal coronary arteries (CAD-RADS 0) have an excellent long-term prognosis with a warranty period of at least 2 years for developing clinically significant coronary artery disease.[73,74]

Modifiers incorporated into the CAD-RADS lexicon include the presence or absence of high-risk plaque (modifier "HRP"), the presence or absence of ischemia when CT fractional flow reserve or myocardial CT perfusion are performed (modifier "I"), prior coronary stent (modifier "S"), prior coronary artery bypass grafting (modifier "G"), and one or more nondiagnostic coronary segments (modifier "N"). Abnormal ischemia evaluation, designated "I+", includes an abnormal FFR-CT ≤0.75 or the presence of a stress myocardial perfusion inducible defect on stress CTP that resolves on rest perfusion images. Ischemia testing with FFR-CT or stress myocardial CTP should be considered when coronary stenoses between 50% and 90% are detected, to better define if the lesion is hemodynamically significant.

Management

The CAD-RADS recommendations include management considerations based on the results of the CCTA exam. Although the extent of coronary plaque on CCTA will influence preventive management recommendations, including the titration of preventive pharmacotherapy, acute management in the emergency department is influenced primarily by the severity and extent of coronary stenosis, depicted by the CAD-RADS assessment category, as well as the presence of high-risk plaque. The clinical suggestions provided by CAD-RADS are meant to complement existing clinical guidelines and should not replace clinical judgment, as there are many patient-specific factors that may influence further management. Further, CAD-RADS is not a substitute for the impression section of the report provided by the reading physician. CAD-RADS is complementary in nature and should always be interpreted in conjunction with the more detailed and patient-specific information found in the report and the impression.

CASE VIGNETTES

The following cases illustrate key concepts regarding appropriate patient selection, preparation, image interpretation and management for CCTA in the setting of acute chest pain.

CASE 1

A 44-year-old active male presented to the emergency department with angina that developed while running a half marathon. He had no known cardiovascular risk factors. On initial triage, his 12-lead ECG was normal. Baseline hs-cTn was detectable but below the 99th percentile upper limit. HEART score was 2 and the patient was considered "Low-to-Intermediate Risk."

The patient was selected for early CCTA after excluding contraindications. On evaluation of the noncontrast CT, the patient's total coronary calcium score was zero. On evaluation of the CCTA (Fig. 8.4), there was noncalcified plaque in the mid right coronary artery (RCA) resulting in focal occlusion (100% stenosis). The left anterior descending (LAD)and left circumflex (LCx) were unremarkable without evidence of plaque or stenosis. The study was reported as CAD-RADS 5/P3 and was interpreted as "ACS very likely." Urgent cardiology consultation was initiated, and the patient's CCTA findings were confirmed by invasive coronary angiography. The RCA lesion was successfully treated with a drug-eluting stent, and the patient had a short hospital course with successful discharge with goal directed medical therapy.

TABLE 8.7 CAD-RADS 2.0 Reporting and Data System for Patients Presenting With Acute Chest Pain

CATEGORY	DEGREE OF MAXIMAL CORONARY STENOSIS	INTERPRETATION	CARDIAC INVESTIGATION	MANAGEMENT CONSIDERATIONS
CAD-RADS 0	0%	ACS highly unlikely	• No further evaluation of ACS is required • If Tn (+), consider other sources of increased troponin (See Table 9)	• Reassurance
CAD-RADS 1	1–24%[a]	ACS unlikely	• No further evaluation of ACS is required • If Tn(+), consider other sources of increased troponin (See Table 9)	• P1 or P2: Referral for outpatient follow-up for risk factor modification and preventive pharmacotherapy • P3 or P4: Referral for outpatient follow-up for aggressive risk factor modification and preventive pharmacotherapy
CAD-RADS 2	25–49%	ACS less likely	• No further evaluation of ACS is required • If clinical suspicion of ACS is high, Tn (+) or HRP features, consider hospital admission with cardiology consultation.	• P1 or P2: Referral for outpatient follow-up for risk factor modification and preventive pharmacotherapy • P3 or P4: Referral for outpatient follow-up for aggressive risk factor modification and preventive pharmacotherapy
CAD-RADS 3	50–69%	ACS possible	• Consider hospital admission with cardiology consultation. • Consider FFR-CT, CTP, or stress testing	• P1, P2, P3, or P4: Preventive management, including aggressive preventive pharmacotherapy. Other treatments, including antianginal therapies, should be considered per guideline directed care.[b] • When modifier I+, consider ICA.
CAD-RADS 4	A - 70%–99% or B - Left main ≥50% or 3- VD	ACS likely	• Hospital admission with cardiology consultation. • A: Consider ICA or functional assessment • B: ICA is recommended	• P1, P2, P3, or P4: Preventive management, including aggressive preventive pharmacotherapy • Other treatments, including antianginal therapies and options of revascularization, should be considered per guideline directed care[b]
CAD-RADS 5	100% (Total occlusion)	ACS very likely	• Hospital admission with cardiology consultation. Expedited ICA and revascularization if suspected acute occlusion	• P1, P2, P3, or P4: Preventive management, including aggressive preventive pharmacotherapy. • Other treatments (including antianginal therapies and options of revascularization) should be considered per guideline-directed care[b]
CAD-RADS N	Nondiagnostic study	ACS cannot be excluded	Additional or alternative evaluation for ACS is needed	
	OVERALL AMOUNT OF CORONARY PLAQUE	**CAC**	**SIS[a]**	**VISUAL[a]**
P1	Mild	1–100	≤2	1–2 vessels with mild amount of plaque
P2	Moderate	101–300	3–4	1–2 vessels with moderate amount; 3 vessels with mild amount of plaque
P3	Severe	301–999	5–7	3 vessels with moderate amount; 1 vessel with severe amount of plaque
P4	Extensive	>1000	≥8	2–3 vessels with severe amount of plaque

[a]CAD-RADS 0 denotes absence of stenosis or plaque, therefore P0 is not required as a classification.
[b]As there is currently no one single method that should be used to identify the overall amount of plaque, CAD-RADS recommends that imagers select the technique which is considered most appropriate at a given institution.
ACS, Acute coronary syndrome; *CAC*, coronary artery calcium score; *CTP*, CT perfusion; *HRP*, high-risk plaque; *ICA*, invasive coronary angiography; *SIS*, segment involvement score; *Tn*, cardiac troponin.
Adopted from Cury RC, Blankstein R, Leipsic J, et al. CAD-RADS™ 2.0 – 2022 Coronary artery disease—reporting and data system an expert consensus document of the Society of Cardiovascular Computed Tomography (SCCT), the American College of Cardiology (ACC), the American College of Radiology (ACR) and the North America society of cardiovascular imaging (NASCI). *J Cardiovasc Comput Tomogr*. 2022;16(6):536–557.

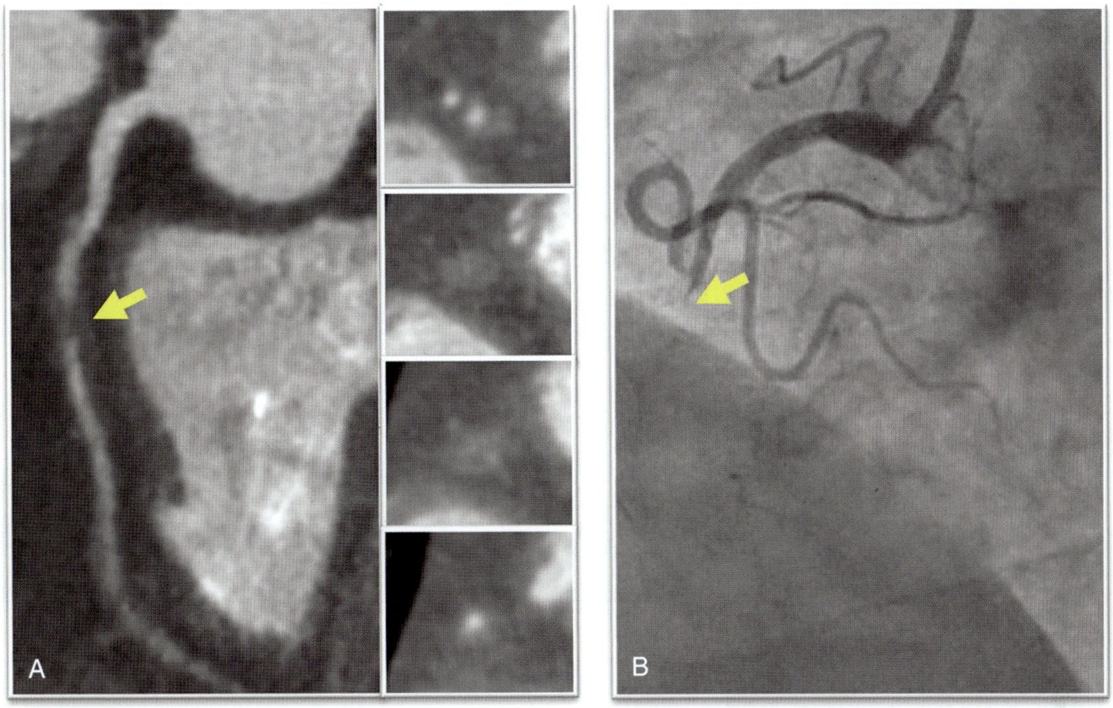

FIG. 8.4 Case 1 CCTA images. Curved multi-planar reformats (MPR) image of the RCA demonstrated focal noncalcified plaque resulting in complete occlusion (100% stenosis) within the mid-segment (A). A diminutive contrast stream distal to the stenosis likely represents collateral flow. Invasive coronary angiography confirmed coronary occlusion in the mid-RCA (B). *CCTA*, Coronary computed tomographic angiography; *RCA*, right coronary artery.

CASE 2

A 48-year-old female presented to the emergency department with shortness of breath and dyspnea. Her cardiovascular risk factors included hypertension, hyperlipidemia, and obesity. The patient also recently completed a round of chemotherapy for non-Hodgkin lymphoma. On initial triage, the patient was mildly diaphoretic with nonspecific T-wave inversions on 12-lead ECG. Baseline hs-cTn was detectable but below the 99th percentile upper limit. HEART score was 4, and the patient's chest pain was considered "Low-to-Intermediate Risk."

Early TRO is selected for further evaluation after excluding contraindications. Based on the patient's heart rate of 82 beats per minute, 100 mg of oral metoprolol was administered. After 45 minutes, the patient's heart rate dropped to 62 beats per minute during a practice breath-hold, and the patient was transferred to the CT scanner for imaging.

On evaluation of TRO images, there was focal calcified plaque in the proximal LAD associated with minimal stenosis. Extensive filling defects were identified throughout her pulmonary arteries consistent with acute pulmonary embolism (Fig. 8.5) as well as significant right ventricular enlargement and RV/LV ratio of ≥1. Although the study was graded CAD-RADS 1/P1, the ED physician was promptly notified of the critical findings. The patient was admitted with submassive pulmonary embolism and was treated promptly with thrombolytics and anticoagulation.

CASE 3

A 55-year-old male patient without any traditional risk factors for coronary artery disease arrived at the emergency department with acute chest pain that began while playing soccer with his children. Baseline 12-lead ECG demonstrated nonspecific repolarization, and baseline hs-cTn was detectable but below the 99th percentile upper limit. HEART score was 4, and the patient's chest pain was considered "Low-to-Intermediate Risk," prompting further investigation with CCTA.

The patient's baseline heart rate was 88 beats per minute, and blood pressure 115/83. On screening, the patient endorsed a history of poorly controlled asthma resulting in multiple prior admissions to the emergency department. Due to the potential risk of exacerbating bronchospasm with metoprolol, oral ivabradine (15 mg) was administered prior to CCTA to lower his heart rate. After waiting 70 minutes for the medication to reach peak effect, the patient's heart rate decreased to 62 beats per minute, and he was transferred to the scanner table.

A noncontrast CT scan demonstrated mild burden of coronary plaque with a total coronary calcium score of 15. Review of the CCTA demonstrated focal severe stenosis of the proximal LAD, greater than 90% due to predominantly noncalcified plaque. Focal mixed plaque at the site of stenosis demonstrated positive remodeling and spotty calcification, consistent with HRP (Fig. 8.6). No plaque or stenosis was identified elsewhere in the coronary tree. The study was graded CAD-RADS 4A/P1/HRP, and the patient was admitted to the hospital. Invasive coronary angiography confirmed focal severe stenosis of the proximal LAD, and the patient was treated with a drug-eluting stent.

CASE 4

A 62-year-old female arrived at the emergency department with exertional chest pain that radiated to her back. Her cardiovascular risk factors included hypertension and hyperlipidemia. Baseline 12-lead ECG and cardiac troponins were unremarkable. HEART score was 3 and the patient's chest pain was considered "Low-to-Intermediate Risk." The patient was selected for CCTA-XL to exclude both coronary artery disease and acute aortic syndrome. Evaluation of the coronary arteries was unremarkable, with no plaque or stenosis throughout the coronary tree (CAD-RADS 0). However, a Stanford Type B aortic dissection was identified along the descending thoracic aorta that extends into the abdominal aorta (Fig. 8.7). The ED physician was promptly notified, and the patient was admitted for management of acute aortic syndrome. She was treated with medical management and endovascular aortic repair.

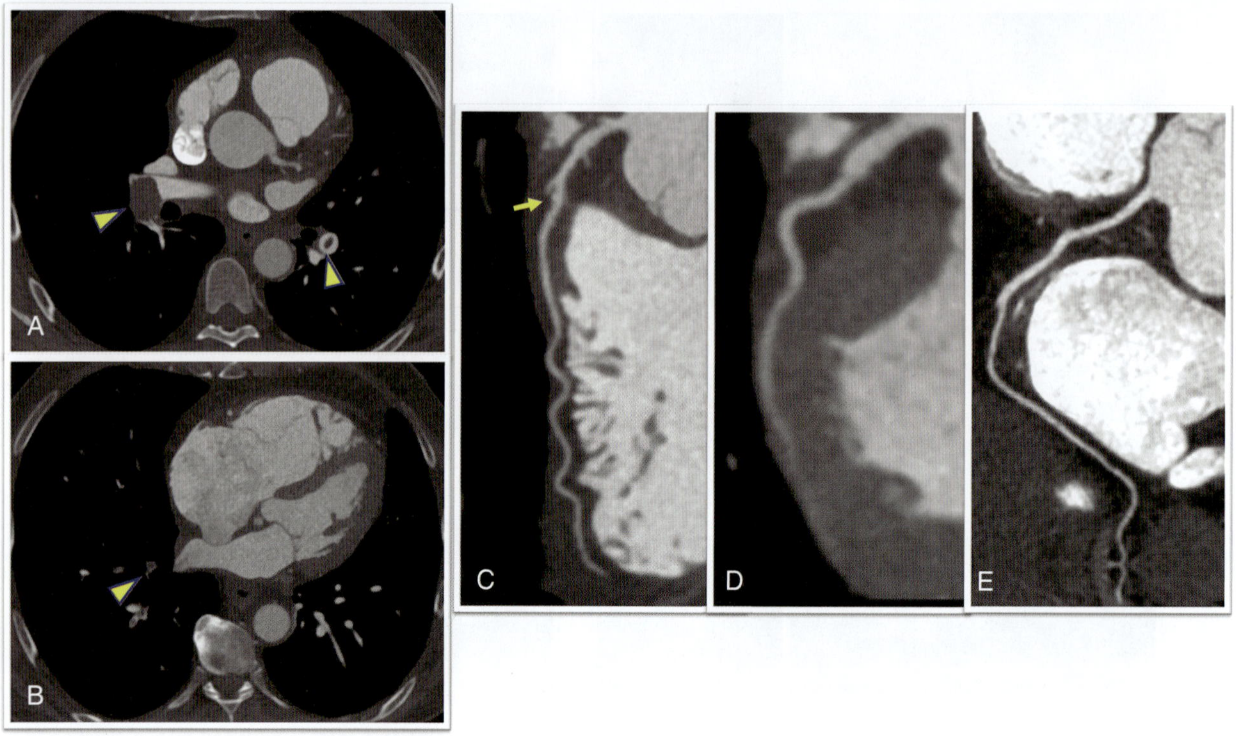

FIG. 8.5 Case 2 TRO images. (A, B) Axial triple rule-out (TRO) images through the chest. Acute pulmonary emboli were present throughout multiple bilateral pulmonary arteries (*arrowheads*), and there was evidence of right atrial and right ventricular chamber enlargement, with bowing of the interatrial septum into the left atrium, and bowing of the interventricular septum into the left ventricle. (C– E) Curved MPR images of the LAD (C), LCx (D), and RCA (E) demonstrate minimal stenosis of the proximal LAD (*arrow*). *LAD*, Left anterior descending; *LCx*, left circumflex; *RCA*, right coronary artery; *TRO*, triple rule-out.

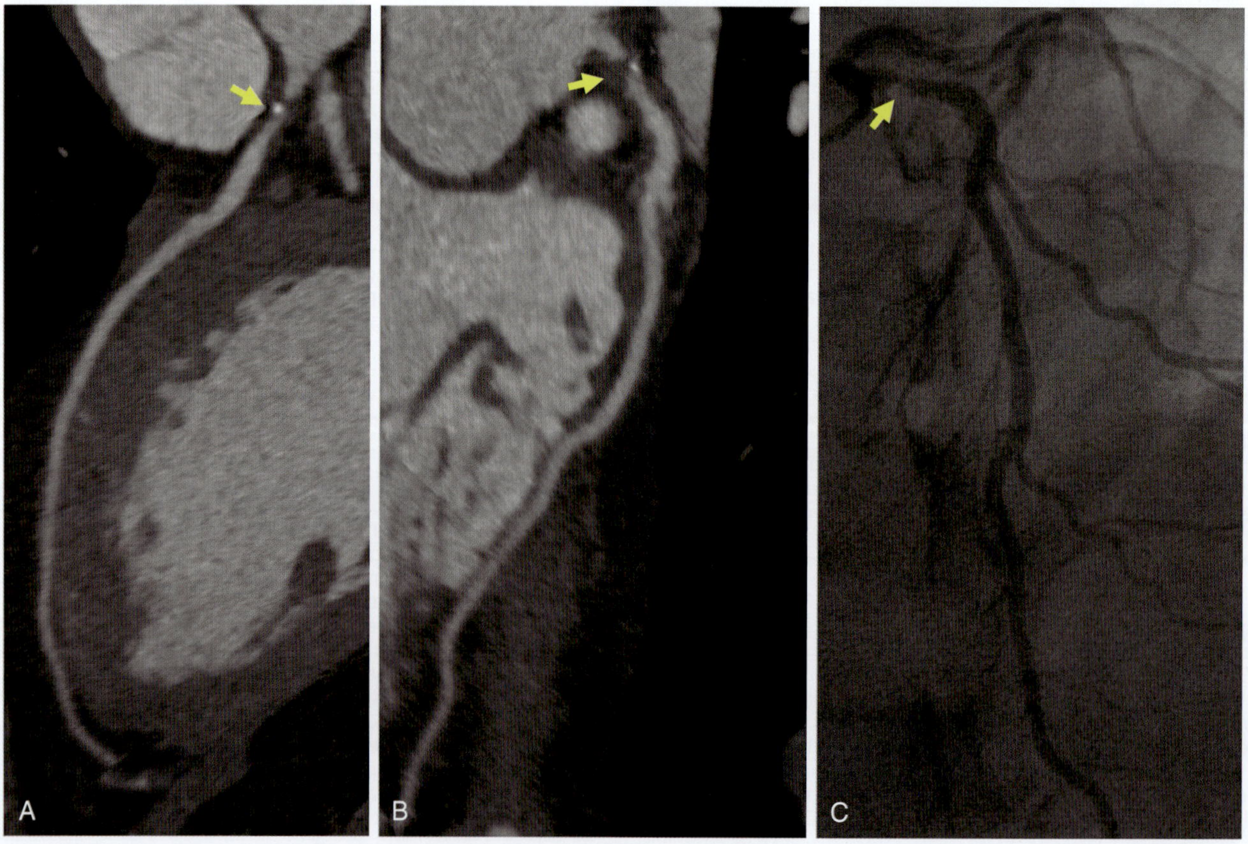

FIG. 8.6 Case 3 CCTA images. Curved multi-planar reformat (MPR) images of the LAD (A, B) demonstrated focal severe stenosis of the proximal LAD with high-risk plaque (*arrow*). Invasive coronary angiography (C) confirms severe stenosis of the proximal LAD, estimated 90% narrowing. The lesion was subsequently treated with percutaneous coronary intervention (*not shown*). *CCTA*, Coronary computed tomographic angiography; *LAD*, left anterior descending.

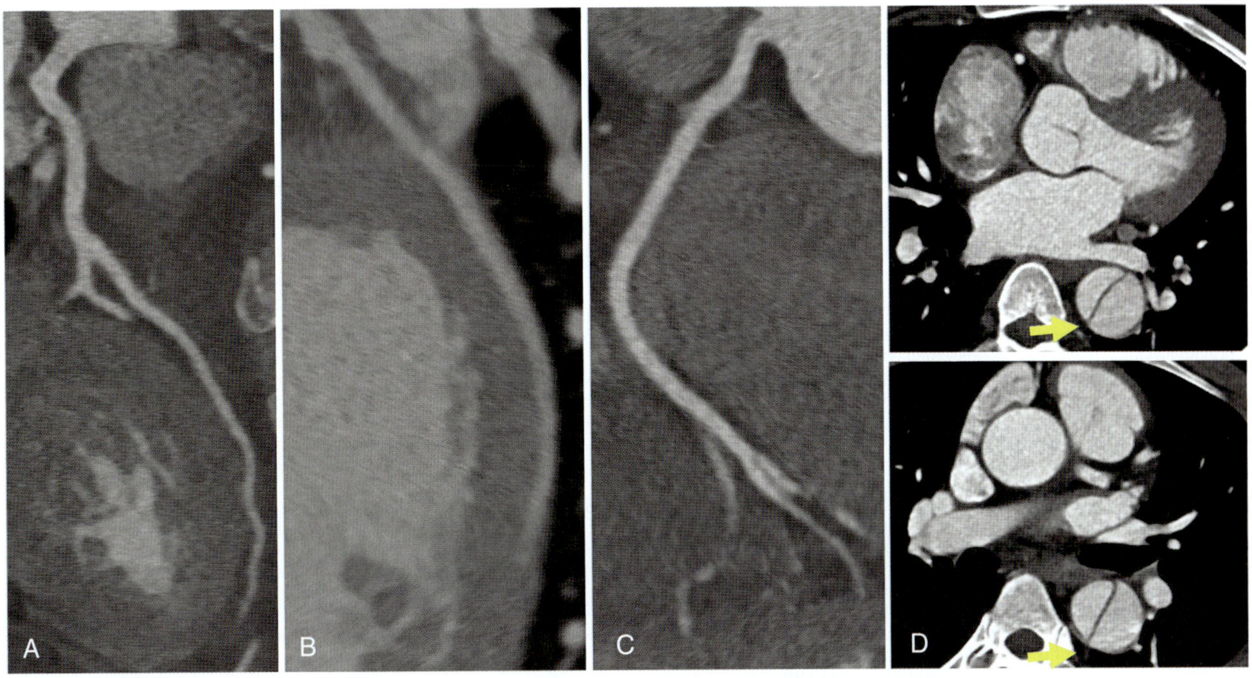

FIG. 8.7 Case 4 CCTA-XL images. Curved multi-planar reformat (MPR) images of the LAD (A), LCx (B), and RCA (C) showed no evidence of coronary plaque or stenosis. Axial images of through the chest (D) demonstrated a Stanford Type B aortic dissection (*arrows*). *CCTA-XL*, Coronary computed tomographic angiography with extended scan length; *LAD*, left anterior descending; *LCx*, left circumflex; *RCA*, right coronary artery.

SUMMARY

CCTA is now a front-line test for acute chest pain triage in selected patients, with the potential to improve patient outcomes, lower healthcare costs, and decompress busy emergency departments. Multidisciplinary collaboration is essential for establishing a successful CCTA program in the emergency department, with stakeholders engaged from cardiology, radiology, and emergency medicine. Algorithmic chest pain pathways with institutional premedication and screening protocols ensure high-quality CCTA studies are safely performed in the right patients. Structured reporting using CAD-RADS ensures results from CCTA exams are clearly and consistently communicated to ordering clinicians, with tailored management recommendations. As technology rapidly expands in the era of artificial intelligence, promising new strategies are likely to further impact diagnosis and clinical management using the use of CCTA for acute chest pain triage.

REFERENCES

1. National Hospital Ambulatory Medical Care Survey: 2010 Emergency Department Summary Tables; 2010. https://archive.cdc.gov/www_cdc_gov/nchs/data/ahcd/nhamcs_emergency/2010_ed_web_tables.pdf.
2. Bhuiya FA, Pitts SR, McCaig LF. Emergency department visits for chest pain and abdominal pain: United States, 1999–2008. *NCHS Data Brief.* 2010; (43):1–8.
3. Dedic A, Lubbers MM, Schaap J, et al. Coronary CT angiography for suspected ACS in the era of high-sensitivity troponins: randomized multicenter study. *J Am Coll Cardiol.* 2016;67:16–26. http://doi.org/10.1016/j.jacc.2015.10.045.
4. Hoffmann U, Truong QA, Schoenfeld DA, et al. Coronary CT angiography versus standard evaluation in acute chest pain. *N Engl J Med.* 2012;367:299–308. http://doi.org/10.1056/NEJMoa1201161.
5. Levsky JM, Spevack DM, Travin MI, et al. Coronary computed tomography angiography versus radionuclide myocardial perfusion imaging in patients with chest pain admitted to telemetry: a randomized trial. *Ann Intern Med.* 2015;163:174–183. http://doi.org/10.7326/M14-2948.
6. Linde JJ, Hove JD, Sorgaard M, et al. Long-term clinical impact of coronary CT angiography in patients with recent acute-onset chest pain: the randomized controlled CATCH trial. *JACC Cardiovasc Imaging.* 2015;8:1404–1413. http://doi.org/10.1016/j.jcmg.2015.07.015.
7. Litt HI, Gatsonis C, Snyder B, et al. CT angiography for safe discharge of patients with possible acute coronary syndromes. *N Engl J Med.* 2012;366:1393–1403. http://doi.org/10.1056/NEJMoa1201163.
8. Søgaard MH, Linde JJ, Kühl JT, et al. Value of myocardial perfusion assessment with coronary computed tomography angiography in patients with recent acute-onset chest pain. *JACC Cardiovasc Imaging.* 2018;11:1611–1621. https://doi.org/10.1016/j.jcmg.2017.09.022.
9. Gulati M, Levy PD, Mukherjee D, et al. 2021 AHA/ACC/ASE/CHEST/SAEM/SCCT/SCMR guideline for the evaluation and diagnosis of chest pain: a report of the American College of Cardiology/American Heart Association Joint Committee on clinical practice guidelines. *J Cardiovasc Comput Tomogr.* 2022;16:54–122. http://doi.org/10.1016/j.jcct.2021.11.009.
10. Choi AD, Abbara S, Branch KR, et al. Society of Cardiovascular Computed Tomography guidance for use of cardiac computed tomography amidst the COVID-19 pandemic Endorsed by the American College of Cardiology. *J Cardiovasc Comput Tomogr.* 2020;14:101–104. http://doi.org/10.1016/j.jcct.2020.03.002.
11. Arbab-Zadeh A, Di Carli MF, Cerci R, et al. Accuracy of computed tomographic angiography and single-photon emission computed tomography-acquired myocardial perfusion imaging for the diagnosis of coronary artery disease. *Circ Cardiovasc Imaging.* 2015;8:e003533. http://doi.org/10.1161/circimaging.115.003533.
12. Neglia D, Rovai D, Caselli C, et al. Detection of significant coronary artery disease by noninvasive anatomical and functional imaging. *Circ Cardiovasc Imaging.* 2015;8:e002179. http://doi.org/10.1161/CIRCIMAGING.114.002179.
13. Chang SA, Choi SI, Choi EK, et al. Usefulness of 64-slice multidetector computed tomography as an initial diagnostic approach in patients with acute chest pain. *Am Heart J.* 2008;156:375–383. http://doi.org/10.1016/j.ahj.2008.03.016.
14. Goldstein JA, Chinnaiyan KM, Abidov A, et al. The CT-STAT (Coronary computed tomographic angiography for systematic triage of acute chest pain patients to treatment) trial. *J Am Coll Cardiol.* 2011;58:1414–1422. http://doi.org/10.1016/j.jacc.2011.03.068.
15. Goldstein JA, Gallagher MJ, O'Neill WW, Ross MA, O'Neil BJ, Raff GL. A randomized controlled trial of multi-slice coronary computed tomography for evaluation of acute chest pain. *J Am Coll Cardiol.* 2007;49:863–871. doi:10.1016/j.jacc.2006.08.064 https://doi.org/S0735-1097(06)03007-5 [pii].
16. Hamilton-Craig C, Fifoot A, Hansen M, et al. Diagnostic performance and cost of CT angiography versus stress ECG—a randomized prospective study of suspected acute coronary syndrome chest pain in the emergency department (CT-COMPARE). *Int J Cardiol.* 2014;177:867–873. https://doi.org/10.1016/j.ijcard.2014.10.090.
17. Hulten E, Pickett C, Bittencourt MS, et al. Outcomes after coronary computed tomography angiography in the emergency department: a systematic review and meta-analysis of randomized, controlled trials. *J Am Coll Cardiol.* 2013;61:880–892. https://doi.org/10.1016/j.jacc.2012.11.061.

18. Newby DE, Adamson PD, Berry C, et al. Coronary CT angiography and 5-year risk of myocardial infarction. *N Engl J Med.* 2018;379:924–933. https://doi.org/10.1056/NEJMoa1805971.
19. Pursnani A, Celeng C, Schlett CL, et al. Use of coronary computed tomographic angiography findings to modify statin and aspirin prescription in patients with acute chest pain. *Am J Cardiol.* 2016;117:319–324. https://doi.org/10.1016/j.amjcard.2015.10.052.
20. Cullen L, Mueller C, Parsonage WA, et al. Validation of high-sensitivity troponin I in a 2-hour diagnostic strategy to assess 30-day outcomes in emergency department patients with possible acute coronary syndrome. *J Am Coll Cardiol.* 2013;62:1242–1249. https://doi.org/10.1016/j.jacc.2013.02.078.
21. Twerenbold R, Boeddinghaus J, Nestelberger T, et al. Clinical use of high-sensitivity cardiac troponin in patients with suspected myocardial infarction. *J Am Coll Cardiol.* 2017;70:996–1012. https://doi.org/10.1016/j.jacc.2017.07.718.
22. Long B, Long DA, Tannenbaum L, Koyfman A. An emergency medicine approach to troponin elevation due to causes other than occlusion myocardial infarction. *Am J Emerg Med.* 2020;38:998–1006. https://doi.org/10.1016/j.ajem.2019.12.007.
23. Ferencik M, Liu T, Mayrhofer T, et al. hs-Troponin I followed by CT angiography improves acute coronary syndrome risk stratification accuracy and work-up in acute chest pain patients: results from ROMICAT II trial. *JACC Cardiovasc Imaging.* 2015;8:1272–1281. https://doi.org/10.1016/j.jcmg.2015.06.016.
24. Collet JP, Thiele H, Barbato E, et al. 2020 ESC guidelines for the management of acute coronary syndromes in patients presenting without persistent ST-segment elevation. *Eur Heart J.* 2021;42(14):1289–1367. https://doi.org/10.1093/eurheartj/ehaa575.
25. Rybicki FJ, Udelson JE, Peacock WF, et al. 2015 ACR/ACC/AHA/AATS/ACEP/ASNC/NASCI/SAEM/SCCT/SCMR/SCPC/SNMMI/STR/STS appropriate utilization of cardiovascular imaging in emergency department patients with chest pain. A Joint Document of the American College of Radiology Appropriateness Criteria Committee and the American College of Cardiology Appropriate Use Criteria Task Force. *J Am Coll Cardiol.* 2016;67:853–879. https://doi.org/10.1016/j.jacc.2015.09.011.
26. Beck KS, Kim JA, Choe YH, et al. 2017 multimodality appropriate use criteria for noninvasive cardiac imaging: expert consensus of the Asian Society of Cardiovascular Imaging. *Korean J Radiol.* 2017;18:871–880. https://doi.org/10.3348/kjr.2017.18.6.871.
27. Maroules CD, Rybicki FJ, Ghoshhajra BB, et al. 2022 use of coronary computed tomographic angiography for patients presenting with acute chest pain to the emergency department: an expert consensus document of the Society of Cardiovascular Computed Tomography (SCCT): endorsed by the American College of Radiology (ACR) and North American Society for Cardiovascular Imaging (NASCI). *J Cardiovasc Comput Tomogr.* 2023;17(2):P146–P163. https://doi.org/10.1016/j.jcct.2022.09.003.
28. O'Gara PT, Kushner FG, Ascheim DD, et al. 2013 ACCF/AHA guideline for the management of ST-elevation myocardial infarction. A report of the American College of Cardiology Foundation/American Heart Association Task Force on Practice Guidelines. *Circulation.* 2013;61:e78–e140. https://doi.org/10.1016/j.jacc.2012.11.019.
29. Kühl JT, Hove JD, Kristensen TS, et al. Coronary CT angiography in clinical triage of patients at high risk of coronary artery disease. *Scand Cardiovasc J.* 2017;51:28–34. https://doi.org/10.1080/14017431.2016.1207799.
30. Linde JJ, Kelbæk H, Hansen TF, et al. Coronary CT angiography in patients with non-ST-segment elevation acute coronary syndrome. *J Am Coll Cardiol.* 2020;75:453–463. https://doi.org/10.1016/j.jacc.2019.12.012.
31. MacLachlan H, Thomas R, Langtree J, Hare C, Mitchell AR. Is there a role for a local inpatient CT coronary angiography service in selected patients with acute coronary syndrome? A cohort analysis of inpatient tertiary centre referrals for invasive coronary angiography. *Open Heart.* 2016;3:e000389. https://doi.org/10.1136/openhrt-2015-000389.
32. Smulders MW, Kietselaer B, Wildberger JE, et al. Initial imaging-guided strategy versus routine care in patients with non-ST-segment elevation myocardial infarction. *J Am Coll Cardiol.* 2019;74:2466–2477. https://doi.org/10.1016/j.jacc.2019.09.027.
33. Gray AJ, Roobottom C, Smith JE, et al. Early computed tomography coronary angiography in patients with suspected acute coronary syndrome: randomised controlled trial. *BMJ (Clinical Research ed).* 2021;374:n2106. https://doi.org/10.1136/bmj.n2106.
34. Gray AJ. Early coronary CT angiography in patients with suspected or provisionally diagnosed acute coronary syndrome—RAPID CTCA. In: *American Heart Association Virtual Scientific Sessions 2020*; 2020. https://pubmed.ncbi.nlm.nih.gov/36062819/.
35. Gray AJ, Roobottom C, Smith JE, et al. The RAPID-CTCA trial (Rapid Assessment of Potential Ischaemic Heart Disease with CTCA)—a multicentre parallel-group randomised trial to compare early computerised tomography coronary angiography versus standard care in patients presenting with suspected or confirmed acute coronary syndrome: study protocol for a randomised controlled trial. *Trials.* 2016;17:579. https://doi.org/10.1186/s13063-016-1717-2.
36. Williams MC, Dweck MR, Newby DE. Coronary computed tomography angiography to triage patients with non-ST-segment elevation acute coronary syndrome. *J Am Coll Cardiol.* 2021;77:1053–1056. https://doi.org/10.1016/j.jacc.2020.12.050.
37. Allen BR, Christenson RH, Cohen SA, et al. Diagnostic performance of high-sensitivity cardiac troponin T strategies and clinical variables in a multisite US cohort. *Circulation.* 2021;143:1659–1672. https://doi.org/10.1161/CIRCULATIONAHA.120.049298.
38. Mahler SA, Riley RF, Hiestand BC, et al. The HEART pathway randomized trial. *Circ Cardiovasc Qual Outcomes.* 2015;8:195–203. https://doi.org/10.1161/CIRCOUTCOMES.114.001384.
39. Than MP, Pickering JW, Aldous SJ, et al. Effectiveness of EDACS versus ADAPT accelerated diagnostic pathways for chest pain: a pragmatic randomized controlled trial embedded within practice. *Ann Emerg Med.* 2016;68:93–102.e101. https://doi.org/10.1016/j.annemergmed.2016.01.001.
40. Than M, Aldous S, Lord SJ, et al. A 2-hour diagnostic protocol for possible cardiac chest pain in the emergency department: a randomized clinical trial. *JAMA Intern Med.* 2014;174:51–58. https://doi.org/10.1001/jamainternmed.2013.11362.
41. Media ACoDaC. *ACR Manual on Contrast Media 2021.* ACR; 2021.
42. Gupta S, Meyersohn NM, Wood MJ, et al. Role of coronary CT angiography in spontaneous coronary artery dissection. *Radiol Cardiothorac Imaging.* 2020;2:e200364. https://doi.org/10.1148/ryct.2020200364.
43. Halliburton SS, Abbara S. Practical tips and tricks in cardiovascular computed tomography: patient preparation for optimization of cardiovascular CT data acquisition. *J Cardiovasc Comput Tomogr.* 2007;1:62–65. doi:10.1016/j.jcct.2007.04.004 https://doi.org/S1934-5925(07)00005-6 [pii].
44. Cauwenberghs N, Cornelissen V, Christle JW, et al. Impact of age, sex and heart rate variability on the acute cardiovascular response to isometric handgrip exercise. *J Hum Hypertens.* 2021;35:55–64. https://doi.org/10.1038/s41371-020-0311-y.
45. Abbara S, Blanke P, Maroules CD, et al. SCCT guidelines for the performance and acquisition of coronary computed tomographic angiography: a report of the Society of Cardiovascular Computed Tomography Guidelines Committee: Endorsed by the North American Society for Cardiovascular Imaging (NASCI). *J Cardiovasc Comput Tomogr.* 2016;10:435–449. https://doi.org/10.1016/j.jcct.2016.10.002.
46. Celik O, Atasoy MM, Erturk M, et al. Comparison of different strategies of ivabradine premedication for heart rate reduction before coronary computed tomography angiography. *J Cardiovasc Comput Tomogr.* 2014;8:77–82. https://doi.org/10.1016/j.jcct.2013.12.005.
47. Guler EC, Yam Y, Jia K, et al. Effectiveness of point-of-care oral ivabradine for cardiac computed tomography. *J Cardiovasc Comput Tomogr.* 2021;15:226–231. https://doi.org/10.1016/j.jcct.2020.09.006.
48. Ayaram D, Bellolio MF, Murad MH, et al. Triple rule-out computed tomographic angiography for chest pain: a diagnostic systematic review and meta-analysis. *Acad Emerg Med.* 2013;20:861–871. https://doi.org/10.1111/acem.12210.
49. Wnorowski AM, Halpern EJ. Diagnostic yield of triple-rule-out CT in an emergency setting. *AJR Am J Roentgenol.* 2016;207:295–301. https://doi.org/10.2214/AJR.15.15717.
50. Burris AC, Boura JA, Raff GL, Chinnaiyan KM. Triple rule out versus coronary CT angiography in patients with acute chest pain: results from the ACIC consortium. *JACC Cardiovasc Imaging.* 2015;8:817–825. https://doi.org/10.1016/j.jcmg.2015.02.023.
51. Halpern EJ. Triple-rule-out CT angiography for evaluation of acute chest pain and possible acute coronary syndrome. *Radiology.* 2009;252:332–345. https://doi.org/10.1148/radiol.2522082335.
52. Gruettner J, Fink C, Walter T, et al. Coronary computed tomography and triple rule out CT in patients with acute chest pain and an intermediate cardiac risk profile. Part 1: impact on patient management. *Eur J Radiol.* 2013;82:100–105. https://doi.org/10.1016/j.ejrad.2012.06.001.
53. Gulati M, Levy PD, Mukherjee D, et al. 2021 AHA/ACC/ASE/CHEST/SAEM/SCCT/SCMR guideline for the evaluation and diagnosis of chest pain. *J Am Coll Cardiol.* 2021;144(22):e368–e454. https://doi.org/10.1016/j.jacc.2021.07.053.
54. Chaikriangkrai K, Palamaner Subash Shantha G, Jhun HY, et al. Prognostic value of coronary artery calcium score in acute chest pain patients without known coronary artery disease: systematic review and meta-analysis. *Ann Emerg Med.* 2016;68:659–670. https://doi.org/10.1016/j.annemergmed.2016.07.020.
55. Pursnani A, Chou ET, Zakroysky P, et al. Use of coronary artery calcium scanning beyond coronary computed tomographic angiography in the emergency department evaluation for acute chest pain: the ROMICAT II trial. *Circ Cardiovasc Imaging.* 2015;8(3):e002225. https://doi.org/10.1161/circimaging.114.002225.
56. Bittner DO, Mayrhofer T, Bamberg F, et al. Impact of coronary calcification on clinical management in patients with acute chest pain. *Circ Cardiovasc Imaging.* 2017;10(5):e005893. https://doi.org/10.1161/circimaging.116.005893.
57. Achenbach S, Marwan M, Ropers D, et al. Coronary computed tomography angiography with a consistent dose below 1 mSv using prospectively electrocardiogram-triggered high-pitch spiral acquisition. *Eur Heart J.* 2010;31:340–346. https://doi.org/10.1093/eurheartj/ehp470.
58. Kang EJ, Lee KN, Kim DW, et al. Triple rule-out acute chest pain evaluation using a 320-row-detector volume CT: a comparison of the wide-volume and helical modes. *Int J Cardiovasc Imaging.* 2012;28(Suppl 1):7–13. https://doi.org/10.1007/s10554-012-0072-y.
59. Cecco CND, Meinel FG, Chiaramida SA, Costello P, Bamberg F, Schoepf UJ. Coronary artery computed tomography scanning. *Circulation.* 2014;129:1341–1345. https://doi.org/10.1161/CIRCULATIONAHA.113.002835.
60. Takakuwa KM, Halpern EJ. Evaluation of a "triple rule-out" coronary CT angiography protocol: use of 64-Section CT in low-to-moderate risk emergency department patients suspected of having acute coronary syndrome. *Radiology.* 2008;248:438–446. https://doi.org/10.1148/radiol.2482072169.

61. Graby J, Metters R, Kandan SR, et al. Real-world clinical and cost analysis of CT coronary angiography and CT coronary angiography-derived fractional flow reserve (FFR(CT))-guided care in the National Health Service. *Clin Radiol.* 2021;76(11):862.e19–862.e28. https://doi.org/10.1016/j.crad.2021.06.009.
62. Curzen N, Nicholas Z, Stuart B, et al. Fractional flow reserve derived from computed tomography coronary angiography in the assessment and management of stable chest pain: the FORECAST randomized trial. *Eur Heart J.* 2021;42(37):3844–3852. https://doi.org/10.1093/eurheartj/ehab444.
63. Patel MR, Nørgaard BL, Fairbairn TA, et al. 1-year impact on medical practice and clinical outcomes of FFR(CT): the ADVANCE registry. *JACC Cardiovasc Imaging.* 2020;13:97–105. https://doi.org/10.1016/j.jcmg.2019.03.003.
64. Chinnaiyan KM, Safian RD, Gallagher ML, et al. Clinical use of CT-derived fractional flow reserve in the emergency department. *JACC Cardiovasc Imaging.* 2020;13:452–461. https://doi.org/10.1016/j.jcmg.2019.05.025.
65. Grandhi GR, Batlle JC, Maroules CD, et al. Combined stress myocardial CT perfusion and coronary CT angiography as a feasible strategy among patients presenting with acute chest pain to the emergency department. *J Cardiovasc Comput Tomogr.* 2021;15:129–136. https://doi.org/10.1016/j.jcct.2020.06.195.
66. Patel AR, Bamberg F, Branch K, et al. Society of cardiovascular computed tomography expert consensus document on myocardial computed tomography perfusion imaging. *J Cardiovasc Comput Tomogr.* 2020;14:87–100. https://doi.org/10.1016/j.jcct.2019.10.003.
67. Ferencik M, Lu MT, Mayrhofer T, et al. Non-invasive fractional flow reserve derived from coronary computed tomography angiography in patients with acute chest pain: subgroup analysis of the ROMICAT II trial. *J Cardiovasc Comput Tomogr.* 2019;13:196–202. https://doi.org/10.1016/j.jcct.2019.05.009.
68. Feuchtner GM, Plank F, Pena C, et al. Evaluation of myocardial CT perfusion in patients presenting with acute chest pain to the emergency department: comparison with SPECT-myocardial perfusion imaging. *Heart.* 2012;98:1510–1517. https://doi.org/10.1136/heartjnl-2012-302531.
69. Ko SM, Choi JW, Song MG, et al. Myocardial perfusion imaging using adenosine-induced stress dual-energy computed tomography of the heart: comparison with cardiac magnetic resonance imaging and conventional coronary angiography. *Eur Radiol.* 2011;21:26–35. https://doi.org/10.1007/s00330-010-1897-1.
70. Parikh R, Patel A, Lu B, Senapati A, Mahmarian J, Chang SM. Cardiac computed tomography for comprehensive coronary assessment: beyond diagnosis of anatomic stenosis. *Methodist Debakey Cardiovasc J.* 2020;16:77–85. https://doi.org/10.14797/mdcj-16-2-77.
71. Cury RC, Abbara S, Achenbach S, et al. CAD-RADS(TM) coronary artery disease—reporting and data system. An expert consensus document of the Society of Cardiovascular Computed Tomography (SCCT), the American College of Radiology (ACR) and the North American Society for Cardiovascular Imaging (NASCI). Endorsed by the American College of Cardiology. *J Cardiovasc Comput Tomogr.* 2016;10:269–281. https://doi.org/10.1016/j.jcct.2016.04.005.
72. Cury RC, Blankstein R, Leipsic J, et al. CAD-RADS™ 2.0 – 2022 coronary artery disease—reporting and data system an expert consensus document of the Society of Cardiovascular Computed Tomography (SCCT), the American College of Cardiology (ACC), the American College of Radiology (ACR) and the North America society of cardiovascular imaging (NASCI). *J Cardiovasc Comput Tomogr.* 2022;16(6):536–557. https://doi.org/10.1016/j.jcct.2022.07.002.
73. Nasis A, Meredith IT, Sud PS, Cameron JD, Troupis JM, Seneviratne SK. Long-term outcome after CT angiography in patients with possible acute coronary syndrome. *Radiology.* 2014;272:674–682. https://doi.org/10.1148/radiol.14132680.
74. Schlett CL, Banerji D, Siegel E, et al. Prognostic value of CT angiography for major adverse cardiac events in patients with acute chest pain from the emergency department: 2-year outcomes of the ROMICAT trial. *JACC Cardiovasc Imaging.* 2011;4:481–491. https://doi.org/10.1016/j.jcmg.2010.12.008.

9 The Role of Coronary Computed Tomography Angiography in Patients With Stable Chest Pain

ARTHUR SHIYOVICH, RON BLANKSTEIN, AND DANIEL S. BERMAN

KEY POINTS

- Coronary CT angiography (CCTA) has emerged as a frontline noninvasive modality for the evaluation of intermediate- to high- risk patients with suspected stable coronary artery disease (CAD).
- Among patients with stable CAD, CCTA can be used for diagnosis of both nonobstructive and obstructive CAD, for risk stratification, and to help decide on the role of preventive therapies and coronary revascularization.
- The use of CCTA is safe and is associated with favorable patient outcomes compared with stress imaging or direct invasive coronary angiography (ICA).
- Fractional flow reserve computed tomography (FFR_{CT}) provides lesion-specific, functional evaluation to support decision-making in patients with intermediate or inconclusive lesions at CCTA.
- The long-term costs of a CCTA strategy for the outpatient evaluation of patients with suspected CAD are overall similar to those associated with stress imaging.
- Quantitative coronary plaque assessment using AI tools may prove helpful in guiding intensity of medical management and assessing effects of therapy.

INTRODUCTION

Coronary artery disease (CAD) is characterized by accumulation of atherosclerotic plaque in the coronary vasculature. In some cases this can lead to anatomic obstruction or limitations in blood flow, whereas in other cases, nonobstructive lesions may lead to plaque rupture and myocardial infarction.[1] It is a chronic progressive disease of dynamic nature and variability in clinical presentation that is often classified as either acute coronary syndrome (ACS) or stable CAD, a term that has recently been replaced with "chronic coronary syndrome" or "chronic coronary disease."[1] Stable CAD often refers to chronic, relatively constant symptoms with consistent precipitants (e.g., exertion). More than 8.7 million Americans are evaluated annually for symptoms suspected of stable CAD, usually stable chest pain or a chest pain equivalent, most commonly dyspnea on exertion, resulting in substantial healthcare burden and economic expenditure.[2,3] The differential diagnosis of chest pain or chest pain equivalents is wide, and only a minority of patients are found to have obstructive CAD.[4] An initial noninvasive test can substantially lower the number of patients who require invasive coronary angiography (ICA).[4–6] Accordingly, accurate diagnosis and detailed characterization of CAD, preferably in a noninvasive manner, plays a pivotal role in the evaluation and management of patients with suspected CAD.[1–3,7] With recent technological advances, improving quality of image acquisition and postprocessing, coronary CT angiography (CCTA) offers a broad spectrum of applications in patients with stable chest pain[8] (Fig. 9.1), including determining the presence, severity, and extent of CAD, characterizing plaque, and evaluating for lesion-specific physiological significance. Due to its demonstrated ability to improve patient outcomes, CCTA has the highest class of recommendation ([COR] 1 level of evidence [(LOE] A) by the AHA/ACC Chest Pain guidelines[4] and has emerged as the frontline strategy for evaluation of patients with stable chest pain.[1,4,6] However, appropriate patient selection, accurate interpretation of CCTA findings, and ensuring appropriate patient management after testing are crucial for optimizing patient outcomes.

DIAGNOSTIC ACCURACY AND PROGNOSTIC IMPLICATIONS

The diagnostic accuracy of CCTA is well established. When used in the appropriate patient population, a sensitivity of 97% with a specificity of 78% for detecting >50% stenosis was previously reported by a metaanalysis.[9] Furthermore, among all current noninvasive modalities, CCTA has the highest sensitivity to detect stenosis, making it highly effective in ruling out obstructive CAD (see Chapter 7, Diagnostic Accuracy of CCTA). However, the diagnostic accuracy to detect hemodynamically significant ("obstructive") CAD, as defined by an invasive fractional flow reserve (FFR) ≤0.80, is lower with a sensitivity 93% (89–96) and specificity of 53% (37–68).[9] The specificity can be significantly improved by the addition of indirect CT assessments of fractional flow reserve (CT-FFR) or CT perfusion (see section below on advanced uses of CCTA and Chapters 13, Cardiac Computed Tomography Fractional Flow Reserve (CT-FFR) Current Clinical Evidence and Limitations and 15, Myocardial Perfusion Imaging).[8,10]

One of the major advantages of CCTA for patients with stable CAD is the robust prognostic information.[8] A normal CCTA (no plaque or stenosis) is associated with a very low risk for subsequent adverse coronary events with a "warranty period" of at least 2 years.[4,11] When CAD is present, its severity and extent are important predictors of subsequent events both in patients with nonobstructive and obstructive disease.[8,12] For patients with obstructive disease, the number of involved vessels and severity of obstruction are associated with adverse patient outcomes.[11,12] Similarly, for patients with nonobstructive disease, a continuum of

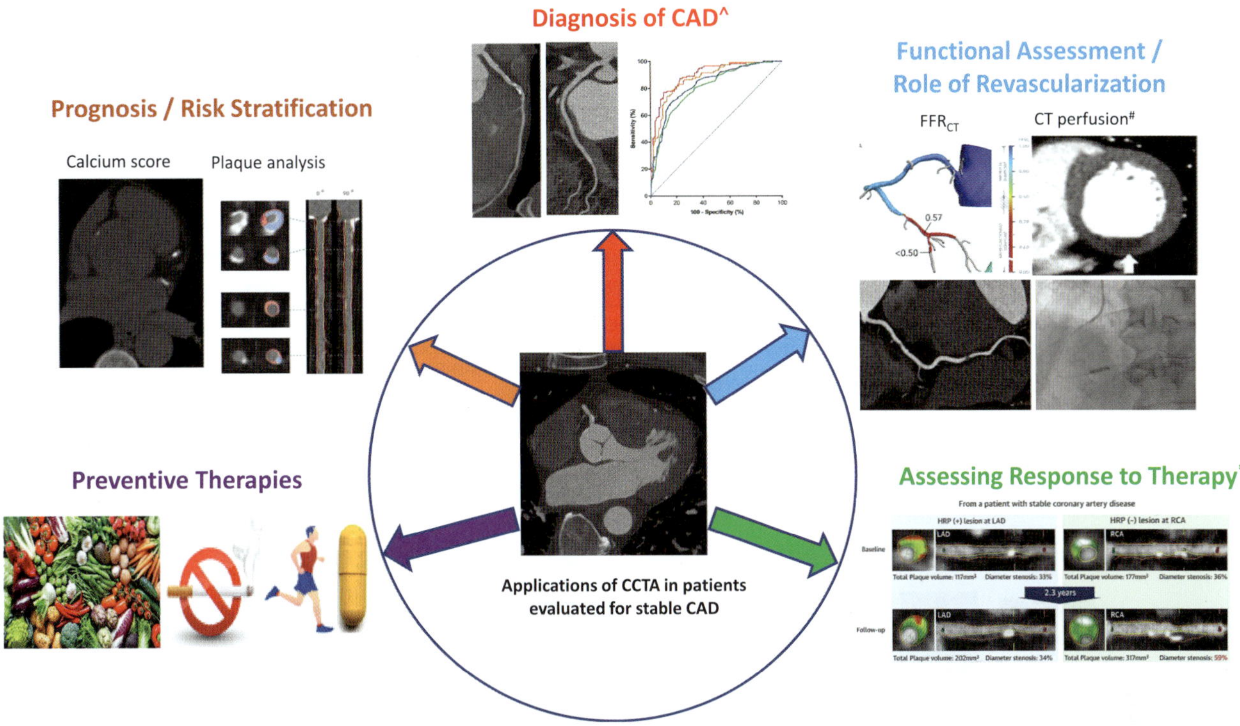

FIG. 9.1 The Applications of CCTA in Stable Patients Evaluated for CAD. Displayed are the main applications of CCTA in patients evaluated for stable CAD. In these patients CCTA can be used for diagnosis of CAD, prognosis/risk stratification, functional assessment (i.e., fractional flow reserve computed tomography), decisions regarding preventive and interventional therapies, and assessing response to therapy. *CAD*, Coronary artery disease; *CCTA*, coronary computed tomography angiography; FFR_{CT}, fractional flow reserve calculated from computed tomography.
^Adapted from Bom MJ, Driessen RS, Kurata A, et al. Diagnostic value of comprehensive on-site and off-site coronary CT angiography for identifying hemodynamically obstructive coronary artery disease. *J Cardiovasc Comput Tomogr*. 2021;15[1]:37–45.
#Adapted from Serruys PW, Hara H, Garg S, et al. Coronary computed tomographic angiography for complete assessment of coronary artery disease: JACC state-of-the-art review. *J Am Coll Cardiol*. 2021;78[7]:713–736.
*Adapted from Lee S-E, Sung JM, Andreini D, et al. Differences in progression to obstructive lesions per high-risk plaque features and plaque volumes with CCTA. *JACC Cardiovasc Imaging*. 2020;13[6]:1409–1417.

risk has been found with the extent and severity of CAD.[13] Notably, patients with extensive nonobstructive CAD have been found to have a similar risk as those with 1-vessel obstructive CAD.[14,15]

A comprehensive evaluation of disease extent and severity can be achieved either by semiquantitative methods or advanced quantitative methods (see section below on advanced uses of CCTA). Both approaches provide incremental prognostic data beyond standard methods that rely on the presence of CAD or the degree of stenosis.[16–18] Semiquantitatively, plaque burden can be measured by summed involvement score, indicating the extent of plaque in the coronary tree and severity by the number of stenosed vessels. High-risk plaque (formerly vulnerable plaque) is associated with adverse outcomes, independent of stenosis. It is usually defined as having two or more of the following four features: positive remodeling of the coronary wall, low attenuation plaque, "spotty" plaque calcification, and the napkin ring sign (i.e., eccentric structure with low attenuation representing a necrotic core surrounded by a thin ring-like hyperattenuating rim) is also associated higher risk of adverse events (see Chapter 11 for further detail).[19]

Coronary Artery Calcium (CAC)

The calcium score (CAC) is assessed from a noncontrast gated scan, integrating the total area and the attenuation values of coronary calcifications (Fig. 9.1)[20] and in many centers routinely performed at the time of CCTA. Accordingly, the CAD-RADS 2.0 document provides an option for use of the CAC score for grading the overall plaque burden when assessing coronary CTA studies (see Table 9.1).

The degree of CAC provides substantial information over that provided by global risk scores in assessing the pretest probability (PTP) of obstructive CAD.[21,22] In most reported studies, a large proportion of patients presenting for evaluation of possible CAD with stable chest pain have no coronary calcium (CAC score), almost 50% in a recent series,[23] and a very low reported prevalence of obstructive CAD (~3%) as well as a very low subsequent event rate (0.1%). Accordingly, the concept of the "power of zero," which refers to the excellent negative predictive value of CAC = 0, has been extended to patients with stable chest pain.[24,25] In this context, CAC testing may be used as a gatekeeper to identify patients who may or may not require further testing, including CCTA.[26] The 2021 Chest Pain Guideline[4] recommends that patients with stable chest pain and no known CAD be categorized as low risk, and CAC testing is reasonable as a first-line test for excluding calcified plaque and identifying patients with a low likelihood of obstructive CAD (COR 2a LOE B-R).

Patients with CAC >0 are at higher risk for major adverse cardiovascular events (MACE), and the risk increases with every increasing category of CAC.[23] Importantly, by defining the presence of atherosclerosis, the presence and amount of CAC has been shown to affect preventive treatment

TABLE 9.1 Different Methods to Categorize the Overall Amount of Coronary Plaque

	OVERALL AMOUNT OF CORONARY PLAQUE	CAC	SIS*	VISUAL†
P1	Mild	1–100	≤2	1–2 vessels with mild amount of plaque
P2	Moderate	101–300	3-4	1–2 vessels with moderate amount; 3 vessels with mild amount of plaque
P3	Severe	301–999	5–7	3 vessels with moderate amount; 1 vessel with severe amount of plaque
P4	Extensive	>1000	≥8	2–3 vessels with severe amount of plaque

Note: Categories may not always correspond across different scores; if discrepant, use coronary artery calcium (CAC) or total plaque burden quantification, if available.
*Please note that CAD-RADS 0 denotes absence of stenosis or plaque, therefore P0 is not required as a classification.
†As there is currently no one single method that should be used to identify the overall amount of plaque, CAD-RADS recommends that imagers select the technique that is considered most appropriate at a given institution.
SIS, Segment involvement score.
Adapted from Cury RC, Leipsic J, Abbara S, et al. CAD-RADS™ 2.0 - 2022 coronary artery disease-reporting and data system: an expert consensus document of the Society of Cardiovascular Computed Tomography (SCCT), the American College of Cardiology (ACC), the American College of Radiology (ACR), and the North America Society of Cardiovascular Imaging (NASCI). *JACC Cardiovasc Imaging*. 2022;15(11):1974–2001.

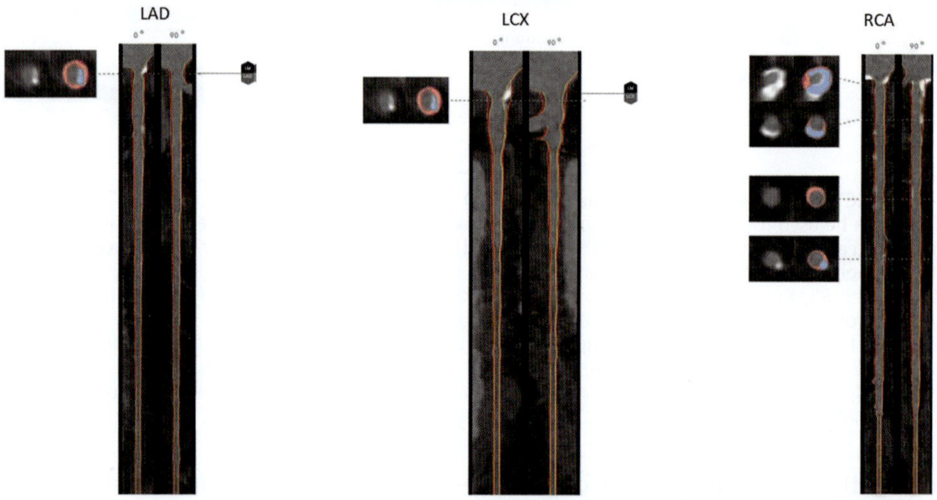

CORONARY SYSTEM (including branches)	TOTAL PLAQUE MM³	CALCIFIED PLAQUE	NON-CALCIFIED PLAQUE	LOW ATTENUATION PLAQUE
Left Main	20	12	8	0
Left Anterior Descending	85	17	68	3
Left Circumflex	42	10	32	2
Right Coronary	448	139	309	9
Total	595	178	417	14

PLAQUE CHARACTERISTICS: calcified plaque; non-calcified plaque; low attenuation plaque
VESSEL BOUNDARY: lumen boundary; outer wall boundary

FIG. 9.2 Plaque Analysis and Quantification. Quantitative and qualitative plaque analysis (Heartflow INC, Los Angeles, CA, USA) from a 74-year-old male with a positive stress test showing an overall large amount of calcified, noncalcified, and low-attenuation plaque in the major epicardial arteries, mainly in the right coronary artery. *LAD*, Left anterior descending; *LCx*, left circumflex.

recommendations and patient compliance as well as to inform the need for further testing.[27] In addition, CAC can complement noninvasive functional testing by identification of nonobstructive coronary atherosclerosis that would otherwise be missed in patients with normal stress tests. A trial that included 4897 symptomatic patients, of whom 91% were of intermediate PTP for CAD, found that 69% of patients with normal myocardial perfusion imaging test had CAC >0 and 15% had CAC >400.[28] Indeed, there are now several studies showing that the addition of CAC testing can improve both the diagnostic and prognostic value of myocardial perfusion imaging.[29,30] Accordingly, the 2021 AHA/ACC Chest Pain Guideline provides a class 2a recommendation that "For intermediate to high-risk patients with stable chest pain and no known CAD undergoing stress testing, the addition of CAC testing can be useful."

CCTA ASSESSMENTS BEYOND STENOSIS

Plaque Analysis

CCTA is the only widely available noninvasive diagnostic modality that accurately detects nonobstructive coronary plaque and enables robust plaque evaluation throughout the entire epicardial coronary tree[4,16,19] (see Chapter 11, Approaches to Plaque Imaging by CCTA).[8,19] Quantification of plaque burden and subtypes (Figs. 9.2 and 9.3) among stable patients evaluated for CAD can enhance cardiovascular risk assessment beyond disease detection alone, luminal stenosis, and risk scores.[8,16,18,31] Moreover, the quantitative methods provide an evaluation of plaque progression by serial CCTA scans that may become used as a surrogate marker for treatment response (Fig. 9.1),[32] although additional studies

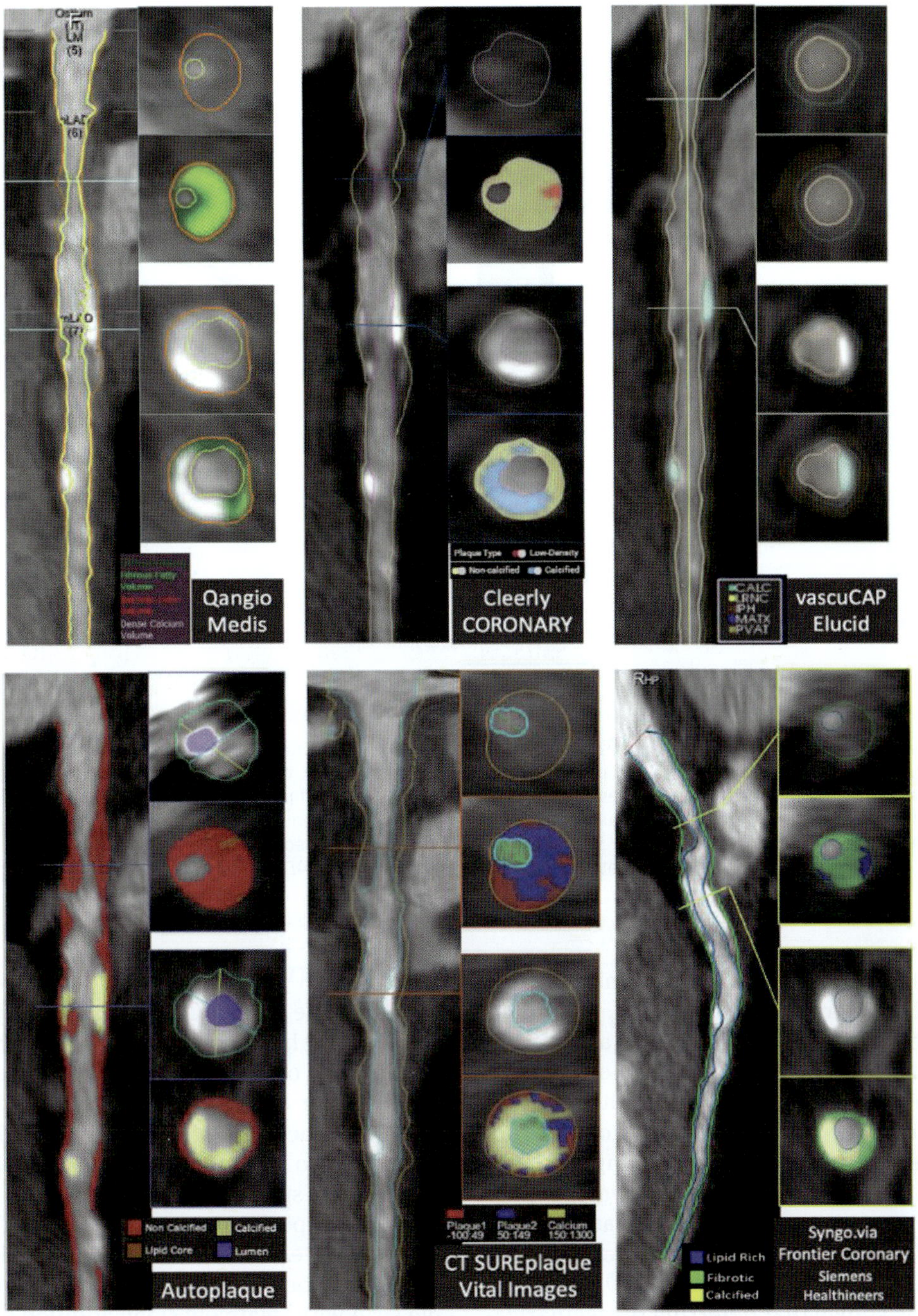

FIG. 9.3 Plaque Analysis and Quantifications by Various Software. An example case assessed using six of the most commonly used software. Curved planar reformations and cross-sectional images from the left anterior descending coronary artery of a 43-year-old male who presented to the emergency department with acute chest pain. Software from left to right: QAngio, Medis Medical Imaging Systems; Cleerly CORONARY, Cleerly Healthcare; vascuCAP, Elucid Bioimaging; Autoplaque, Cedars-Sinai Medical Center; CT SUREplaque, Vital Images; Syngo.via Frontier Coronary, Siemens Healthineers. With thanks to Dr Basel Yacoub, MD, from The Medical University of South Carolina for Elucid Bioimaging and Siemens Healthineers images. (Courtesy of Siemens Medical Solutions USA, Inc.)

are needed in this area. Currently, several vendors are providing artificial intelligence–based semiautomatic software for assessment of total plaque burden and plaque subtypes.

CT Assessment of Fractional Flow Reserve Computed Tomography

FFR, measured invasively during ICA, is considered the gold standard for functional assessment of CAD and can inform decision-making, particularly regarding revascularization.[33] The most commonly used method for CT-FFR is FFR_{CT} (Heartflow INC, Los Angeles, CA, USA), which is based on an integration of computational fluid dynamics and the anatomical data from CCTA to enable the calculation of a three-dimensional pressure map. FFR_{CT} provides an accurate lesion-specific tool for noninvasive FFR estimation, improving the diagnostic yield and reducing the need for invasive testing (Fig. 9.4)[34,35] (see Chapter 13, CT-FFR: Current Clinical Evidence and Limitations). FFR_{CT} has been shown to improve diagnostic performance of standard CCTA and to outperform single-photon emission computerized tomography (SPECT) and positron emission

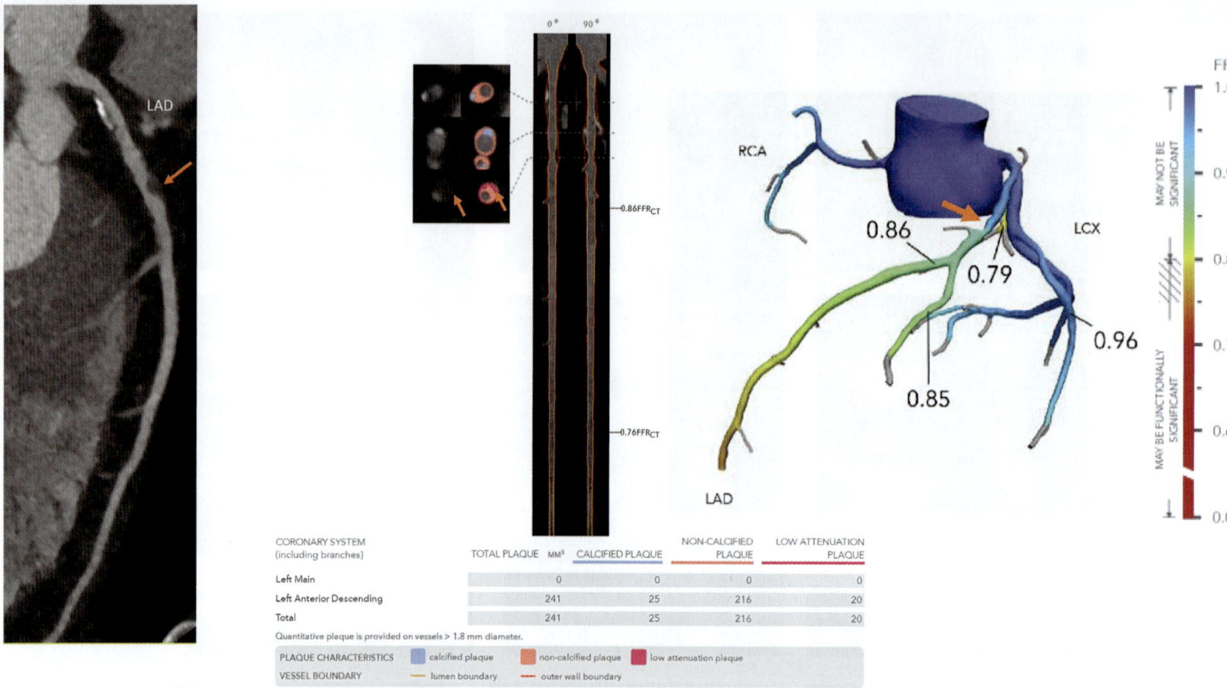

FIG. 9.4 Plaque Analysis and FFR$_{CT}$. Curved multiplanar reconstruction of the LAD (A), qualitative and quantitative plaque analysis (Heartflow INC, Los Angeles, CA, USA) (B), and FFR$_{CT}$ (C) from a 59-year-old male with multiple cardiovascular risk factors presenting with stable chest pain. Images show a medium-large amount of calcified and noncalcified plaque resulting in mild stenosis (25–49%) of proximal LAD and moderate stenosis (50–69%) of the mid LAD (*arrows*). The mid-LAD plaque (*arrows*) is a high-risk plaque (positive remodeling and low-attenuation plaque) as can be appreciated visually and by plaque analysis. Despite the high-risk plaque features, the moderate stenosis in the mid LAD was assessed by FFR$_{CT}$ as not being hemodynamically significant (FFR$_{CT}$ distal to the lesion 0.86). *FFR$_{CT}$*, Fractional flow reserve calculated from computed tomography; *LAD*, left anterior descending; *LCx*, left circumflex.

tomography (PET) for vessel-specific ischemia.[36] In patients from the PROMISE trial, abnormal FFR$_{CT}$ was found to be a strong predictor of revascularization and MACE, beyond significant stenosis (>50%).[37] Furthermore, in the PLATFORM study, the use of FFR$_{CT}$ resulted in less referrals to ICA and lower rates of ICA with nonobstructive CAD compared with CCTA alone among patients who planned to undergo ICA; however, in symptomatic patients in whom a noninvasive strategy was planned (stress testing or CCTA), there was no difference in the rates of ICA or of ICA without obstructive CAD.[38] The ADVANCE registry[39] has shown that deferring revascularization based on a normal FFR$_{CT}$ result (FFR$_{CT}$ >0.8) is safe and associated with no MACE within 90 days, whereas the risk following positive FFR$_{CT}$ was significantly higher (hazard ratio [HR] 19.75, $P = .0008$). However, the limitations of using FFR$_{CT}$ are that it requires very good image quality, and results in substantial additional costs. Importantly, FFR$_{CT}$, much like invasive FFR, has a continuous relationship with the hemodynamic significance of a coronary lesion rather than being dichotomous as used in most trials.[40] Practically, this means that borderline FFR$_{CT}$ values (i.e., 0.76–0.80 or slightly lower) may require additional information for optimal decision-making. CT-based assessment of the presence of flow-limiting coronary lesions as surrogates of catheter-based FFR that are based on AI plaque quantitation have been described and validated as predictors of vessel-specific ischemia.[41,42]

CT Myocardial Perfusion

It is possible to use CT to evaluate myocardial enhancement during hyperemia in order to establish the functional significance of CAD, similar to other perfusion modalities (see Chapter 15, Myocardial Perfusion Imaging Using Stress CT). Pharmacologic stress CT myocardial perfusion (CTP) was found to be incremental over CTA alone for detecting functionally significant CAD with similar diagnostic accuracy to other perfusion modalities.[43,44] CT myocardial perfusion has several advantages, which include: (1) the ability to evaluate both physiologic and anatomic data from a single scan with relatively small addition of radiation, and (2) that it is less dependent on image quality and not limited by coronary calcifications or stents. However, clinical data on this modality are limited and it is not widely adopted. Therefore its use in stable patients would probably be limited to centers with the required experience and expertise and in a setting where FFR$_{CT}$ is not available or technically not possible.[8] Unlike FFR$_{CT}$, CTP requires a separate CCTA acquisition that adds to the length of a study for both the patient and the laboratory and requires extra time on the CT scanner that may be difficult in busy laboratories.

INDICATIONS AND SELECTION OF APPROPRIATE CANDIDATES FOR CCTA

Evaluation of symptomatic patients with suspected stable CAD relies on pretest probability (PTP) of obstructive CAD.[1,4]

TABLE 9.2 Indications for CCTA in Stable Patients as Provided by 2019 ESC and 2021 AHA/ACC Guidelines

CLINICAL SETTING	2019 EUROPEAN SOCIETY OF CARDIOLOGY GUIDELINE[1]	COR	LOE
Initial diagnostic management of symptomatic patients with suspected coronary artery disease	Noninvasive functional imaging for myocardial ischemic or coronary CTA is recommended as the initial test to diagnose CAD in symptomatic patients in whom obstructive CAD cannot be excluded by clinical assessment alone.	I	B
	CCTA should be considered as an alternative to invasive angiography if another noninvasive test is equivocal or nondiagnostic.	IIa	C
	Risk stratification, preferably using stress imaging or coronary CTA (if permitted by local expertise and availability), or alternatively exercise stress ECG (if significant exercise can be performed and the ECG is amenable to the identification of ischaemic changes) is recommended in patients with suspected or newly diagnosed CAD.	I	B
Investigations of patients with suspected vasospastic angina	Invasive angiography or coronary CTA is recommended in patients with characteristic episodic resting angina and ST-segment changes, which resolve with nitrates and/or calcium antagonists, to determine the extent of underlying coronary disease.	I	C
	2021 AMERICAN HEART ASSOCIATION/AMERICAN COLLEGE OF CARDIOLOGY GUIDELINE[4]		
Patients with stable chest pain and no known CAD	For intermediate- to high-risk patients with stable chest pain and no known CAD, CCTA is effective for diagnosis of CAD, for risk stratification, and for guiding treatment decisions.	1	A
	For intermediate- to high-risk patients with stable chest pain after an inconclusive or abnormal exercise ECG or stress imaging study, CCTA is reasonable.	2a	B-NR
	For intermediate- to high-risk patients with stable chest pain and no known CAD undergoing stress testing, the addition of CAC testing can be useful.	2a	B-NR
	For intermediate- to high-risk patients with stable chest pain after a negative stress test but with high clinical suspicion of CAD, CCTA or ICA may be reasonable.	2b	C-EO
	For patients with known coronary stenosis from 40% to 90% on CCTA, FFR_{CT} can be useful for diagnosis of vessel-specific ischemia and to guide decision-making regarding the use of ICA.	2a	B-NR
Patients with stable chest pain and prior revascularization	For patients who have stable chest pain with previous coronary revascularization, CCTA is reasonable to evaluate bypass graft or stent patency (for stents ≥3 mm).	2a	B-NR
	In patients who have had prior CABG surgery presenting with stable chest pain who are suspected to have myocardial ischemia, it is reasonable to perform stress imaging or CCTA to evaluate for myocardial ischemia or graft stenosis or occlusion.	2a	C-LD
Patients with stable chest pain and prior nonobstructive plaque	For symptomatic patients with known nonobstructive CAD who have stable chest pain, CCTA is reasonable for determining atherosclerotic plaque burden and progression to obstructive CAD and guiding therapeutic decision-making.	2a	B-NR

CABG, Coronary artery bypass graft; *CAD*, coronary artery disease; *CCTA*, coronary computed tomography angiography; *COR*, class of recommendation, *ETT*, electrocardiogram exercise tolerance test; FFR_{CT}, fractional flow reserve computed tomography; *ICA*, invasive coronary angiography; *LOE*, level of evidence.

Many global risk scores, particularly the ones based on older equations, have been shown to overestimate the PTP of having obstructive CAD.[1,45–48] More contemporary data derived from 15,815 symptomatic patients were used to create the PTP tool used by the 2019 European Society of Cardiology (ESC) Chronic Coronary Syndrome guideline and the 2021 AHA/ACC chest pain guideline.[4,47] Notably, the PTP predicted by this tool is approximately one-third of that predicted by older models.[1,48] Another contemporary risk score, the PROMISE Minimal Risk Score (PMRS), may further down-classify more than one-third of patients in the 5% to 15% PTP group by identifying a group with very low prevalence of obstructive CAD and adverse events.[49] As noted above, estimates of the PTP can be significantly augmented by the use of CAC, whether obtained from a dedicated CAC exam or if estimated from available noncardiac chest CT exams.[23] Specifically, the absence of CAC can identify a patient with a low PTP, whereas the presence of extensive CAC can identify patients who have intermediate-high PTP and who may therefore be referred for further diagnostic testing.[4]

Guidelines-based Recommendations for CCTA

The 2019 ESC guideline (Table 9.2) for the diagnosis and management of chronic coronary syndromes state that patients with PTP ≤5% can be assumed to have such a low probability of disease that diagnostic testing should be performed only for compelling reasons. For patients with PTP, 5% to 15% testing may be considered, particularly if symptoms are limiting. These guidelines provide a class I LOE B recommendation for CCTA or other noninvasive functional imaging as the initial test for diagnosing CAD in symptomatic patients in whom obstructive CAD cannot be excluded by clinical assessment alone. The selection of the initial test by these guidelines should be based on the clinical likelihood of CAD, with CCTA being preferred over stress imaging in patients with lower clinical likelihood of CAD. These guidelines also recommend using CCTA, or functional testing for risk stratification of patients with suspected or newly diagnosed CAD (class I LOE B). A class IIa LOE C recommendation was also given to CCTA as an alternative to ICA among symptomatic patients in whom another test is equivocal or nondiagnostic.

The adoption of the ESC chronic coronary syndrome guideline recommendations regarding CCTA was evaluated among 5156 patients in 73 centers from 24 ESC member countries throughout 2019 to 2020.[50] The authors found that the diagnostic pathway used in real-world practice did not adhere with these guidelines in 44% of the study participants. In the group in whom the guidelines were not adhered to, referral to stress imaging (21% vs. 58%; $P < .001$) or CCTA (Coronary computed tomography angiography) (17% vs. 30%; $P < .001$) was less frequent, whereas exercise ECG (43% vs. 22%; $P < .001$) and ICA (48% vs. 15%; $P < .001$) were more frequently performed. The adoption of guidelines was associated with fewer ICAs, higher proportion of diagnosis of obstructive CAD (60% vs. 39%, $P < .001$) and revascularization (54% vs. 37%, $P < .001$), higher quality of life, and less additional testing.

The 2021 AHA/ACC chest pain guideline (Table 9.2) indicates that diagnostic testing can be deferred in patients with stable chest pain and no known CAD who have a low PTP (i.e., <15%) of obstructive CAD (COR 1 LOE B-NR). It is noteworthy that a COR 2a LOE B-R is provided for CAC or exercise treadmill testing in these patients. For patients with intermediate-high PTP with stable chest pain and no known CAD, a COR 1 LOE A recommendation is provided for CCTA for the diagnosis of CAD, risk stratification, and for guiding treatment decisions.

The guidelines also indicate that CCTA is reasonable (1) after an inconclusive or abnormal exercise ECG or stress imaging study in intermediate- to high-risk patients with stable chest pain (COR 2a LOE B-NR); (2) after a negative stress test but with high clinical suspicion of CAD (COR 2b LOE C-EO); (3) for patients with previous coronary revascularization, to evaluate bypass graft or stent patency (for stents ≥3 mm) (COR 2a, LOE B-NR); and (4) for patients with known prior nonobstructive CAD, for determining atherosclerotic plaque burden and progression to obstructive CAD, and guiding therapeutic decision-making (COR 2a LOE B-NR). A more extensive discussion of indications and recommendations based on expert opinion can be found in an SCCT 2021 Expert Consensus Document on Coronary Computed Tomographic Angiography and in Table 9.3, adapted from that document.[8]

The contraindications to CCTA[4] include severe contrast allergy, severe renal dysfunction (glomerular filtration rate <30 mL/min/1.73 m^2), or uncontrolled tachycardia. Relative contraindications include clinical instability, the presence of irregular heart rate, inability to cooperate with acquisition protocol (e.g., breath-holding commands), significant obesity, extensive coronary calcifications, or any other condition that makes obtaining good image quality unlikely.

CORONARY CTA STRATEGIES AND PATIENT OUTCOMES

Multiple randomized controlled trials (RCT) among patients with suspected stable CAD have evaluated the use of CCTA as an initial strategy compared with functional testing or versus ICA (Table 9.4).

TABLE 9.3 Summary of SCCT CCTA Expert Consensus Recommendations for Patients With Stable CAD

Evaluation of Stable Coronary Artery Disease: CCTA in Native Vessels
• It is appropriate to perform CTA as the first-line test for evaluating patients with no known CAD who present with stable typical or atypical chest pain, or other symptoms which are thought to represent a possible anginal equivalent (e.g., dyspnea on exertion, jaw pain).
• It is appropriate to perform CTA as a first-line test for evaluating patients with known CAD who present with stable typical or atypical chest pain, or other symptoms that are thought to represent a possible anginal equivalent (e.g., dyspnea on exertion, jaw pain).
• It is appropriate to perform coronary CTA following a nonconclusive functional test, in order to obtain more precision regarding diagnosis and prognosis, if such information will influence subsequent patient management.
• It is recommended to perform CTA as the first-line test when considering evaluation for revascularization strategies using the ISCHEMIA Trial.
• It may be appropriate to perform CTA in selected asymptomatic high-risk individuals, especially in those who have a higher likelihood of having a large amount of noncalcified plaque.
• It is rarely appropriate to perform coronary CTA in very-low-risk symptomatic patients, for example, <40 years of age with noncardiac symptoms (chest wall pain, pleuritic chest pain).
• It is rarely appropriate to perform CTA in low- and intermediate-risk asymptomatic patients.
Evaluation of Stable Coronary Artery Disease: Coronary CTA Post Revascularization
• It is appropriate to perform coronary CTA in symptomatic patients with intracoronary stent diameter ≥3.0 mm. Measures to improve accuracy of stent imaging should be utilized, to include strict heart rate control (goal <60 bpm), iterative reconstruction, sharp kernel reconstruction, and monoenergetic reconstructions (when available). Protocols to optimize stent imaging should be developed and followed.
• It may be appropriate to perform coronary CTA in symptomatic patients with stents <3.0 mm, especially those known to have thin stent struts (<100 μm) in proximal, nonbifurcation locations.
• It is appropriate to perform CTA for evaluation of patients with prior CABG, particularly if graft patency is the primary objective.
• It is appropriate to perform CTA to visualize grafts and other structures prior to redo cardiac surgery.
Evaluation of Stable Coronary Artery Disease: Coronary CTA with FFR or CT Perfusion (CTP)
• It may be appropriate to perform CT-derived FFR and CT myocardial perfusion imaging to evaluate the functional significance of intermediate stenoses on CTA (30–90% diameter stenosis) particularly in the setting of multivessel disease to help guide ICA referral and revascularization treatment planning. LM (Left main) stenosis ≥50% and severe triple vessel disease should undergo invasive coronary angiography.

TABLE 9.3 Summary of SCCT CCTA Expert Consensus Recommendations for Patients With Stable CAD–cont'd

- Adding FFRCT and stress-CTP to CTA increases specificity, positive predictive value, and diagnostic accuracy over regular CTA.
- FFRCT and stress-CTP may be largely comparable in diagnostic utility. CTP is a potentially valuable alternative particularly when CT-FFR is technically difficult (e.g., suboptimal CTA quality, prior revascularization).

Evaluation of Stable Coronary Artery Disease: Coronary CTA in Other Conditions

- It is appropriate to perform CTA for coronary artery evaluation prior to noncoronary cardiac surgery as an equivalent alternative to invasive angiography in selected patients, for example, low-intermediate probability of CAD, younger patients with primarily nondegenerative valvular conditions.
- CTA may be considered an appropriate alternative to other noninvasive tests for evaluation of selected patients prior to noncardiac surgery.
- It is appropriate to perform CTA to exclude coronary artery disease in patients with suspected nonischemic cardiomyopathy.
- It may be appropriate to perform late enhancement CT imaging to detect infiltrative heart disease or scar in selected patients who have nonischemic or ischemic cardiomyopathy and who cannot undergo cardiac MRI. Such imaging may be performed if it has the potential to impact the diagnosis and/or treatment (e.g., planning for ablation therapy)
- It may be appropriate to perform CTA as an alternative to invasive coronary angiography for the screening of patients for coronary allograft vasculopathy in selected clinical practice settings.
- It is appropriate to perform CTA for the evaluation of coronary anomalies.
- It is appropriate to EKG gate aortic dissection and aneurysm CTA, as well as pulmonary embolus studies in men >45 years and women >55 years, and analyze and report the coronary arteries.
- CTA with a limited delayed image (60–90 sec) is an appropriate alternative to trans-esophageal echocardiogram (TEE) when the primary aim is to exclude left atrial/left atrial appendage thrombus and in patients where the risks associated with TEE outweigh the benefits. In all situations, CTA and TEE should be discussed with the patient in the setting of shared decision-making.
- It may be appropriate to perform late enhancement CT imaging for the evaluation of myocardial viability in selected patients who cannot undergo cardiac MRI. Such imaging may be performed if it has the potential to impact the diagnosis and/or treatment (e.g., planning for revascularization).

Reporting on CTA: Coronary and Noncoronary Information

- The CAD-RAD reporting is recommended.
- It is appropriate to report prior myocardial infarction when its features are evident on CTA.
- It is appropriate to report remote myocardial infarction when fatty metaplasia or calcification within an area of infarction are present.

CABG, Coronary artery bypass graft; *CAD*, coronary artery disease; *CCTA*, coronary computed tomography angiography; *CTA*, computed tomography angiography; *FFR*, fractional flow reserve; FFR_{CT}, fractional flow reserve calculated from computed tomography; *ICA*, invasive coronary angiography; *SSCT*, Society of Cardiovascular Computed Tomography.
Adapted from Narula J, Chandrashekhar Y, Ahmadi A, et al. SCCT 2021 expert consensus document on coronary computed tomographic angiography: a report of the Society of Cardiovascular Computed Tomography. *J Cardiovasc Comput Tomogr*. 2021;15(3):192–217.

TABLE 9.4 Randomized Controlled Trials of Coronary Computed Tomography in Patients With Stable Chest Pain

STUDY NAME	AUTHOR, YEAR	N	FOLLOW-UP	AIM	MAIN FINDINGS
Coronary Computed Tomography Angiography Versus Stress Imaging Testing					
Min et al.[10]	Min et al. 2012	180	55 ± 34 days	To compare CCTA vs. MPI	CCTA vs. MPI: • Comparable improvements in angina-specific health status • Increased initiation of preventive therapies with aspirin (22% vs. 8%, *P* = .04) and statin (7% vs. −3.5%, *P* = .03) • Similar rates of CAD-related hospitalization and ICA • Increased revascularization (8% vs. 1%, *P* = .03) • Lower costs ($781 vs. $1214, *P* < .001) • Lower effective radiation (7.4 mSv vs. 13.3 mSv, *P* < .0001).
CAPP[51]	McKavanagh et al. 2015	500	1-year	To compare CCTA vs. ETT	CCTA vs. ETT: • Improved angina stability (mean difference −6.8, *P* = .03) and quality of life (mean difference −4.9, *P* = .04) assessed using the Seattle Angina Questionnaires • More revascularizations • No significant differences in MACE, but fewer visits to the emergency department and re-admissions
PROMISE[53]	Douglas et al. 2015	10,003	25 months	CCTA vs. functional testing (ETT, MPI or stress echocardiography)	CCTA vs. functional • No difference in the composite primary endpoint of death, MI, hospitalization for unstable angina or major procedural complication (3.3% vs. 3.0%; HR, *P* = .75) • Higher rate of ICA within 90 days after randomization (12.2% vs. 8.1%) • Fewer ICA showing no obstructive CAD compared to functional testing (3.4% vs. 4.3%, *P* = .02) • lower median cumulative radiation (10 mSv vs. 11.3 mSv)

Continued

TABLE 9.4 Randomized Controlled Trials of Coronary Computed Tomography in Patients With Stable Chest Pain–cont'd

STUDY NAME	AUTHOR, YEAR	N	FOLLOW-UP	AIM	MAIN FINDINGS
CRESCENT[26]	Lubbers et al. 2016	350	1.2-year	CAC/CCTA vs. functional tests	CCTA vs. functional • Less anginal complaints (*P* = .012) • Higher event free survival (96.7% vs. 89.8%, *P* = .011). • Higher cumulative radiation dose (6.6+8.7 vs. 6.1+9.3 mSv; *P* < .0001). • More rapid diagnosis, less frequent downstream testing (25% vs. 53%), and lower cumulative costs (*P* < .0001 for all).
SCOT-HEART 5 years[54]	Newby et al. 2018	4146	4.8 years	Standard care +CCTA vs. standard care	Standard care +CCTA vs. standard care • Lower rate of the primary endpoint (death from coronary heart disease or nonfatal MI) compared to standard of care (2.3% vs. 3.9%; HR 0.59, 95% CI 0.41–0.84, *P* = .004) • No significant differences in the rates of cardiovascular or noncardiovascular deaths or deaths from any cause • More initiation of preventive (odds ratio [OR], 1.40, 95% CI 1.19–1.65) and anti- anginal (OR 1.27, 95% CI 1.05–1.54) therapies • Rates of ICA (HR 1.00, 95% CI 0.88–1.13) and coronary revascularization (HR 1.07, 95% CI 0.91–1.27) were similar at 5 years between the two groups
CRESCENT II[52]	Lubbers et al. 2019	268	6 months	Tiered CAC/CCTA/ MPI vs. functional tests	Tiered CAC/CCTA/MPI vs. functional tests • The rate of invasive coronary angiograms without a European Society of Cardiology class I indication for revascularization, was (2 of 130 [1.5%] vs. 10 of 138 [7.2%]; *P* = .035) • Proportion of invasive angiograms with revascularization indication was higher (88% vs. 50%; *P* = .017). • Lower rate required further testing (13 vs. 37%, *P* < .001). • The adverse event rate was similar (3% vs. 3%; *P* = 1) • The median cumulative radiation dose was higher for the CT group (3.1 mSv • [interquartile range: 1.6 to 7.8] vs. 0 mSv [interquartile range: 0.0 to 7.1]; *P* < .001).
Coronary Computed Tomography Angiography Versus Invasive Coronary Angiography					
CAD-MAN[58]	Dewey et al. 2016	340	3.3 years	To compare CCTA vs. ICA in intermediate-risk patients.	CCTA vs. ICA • Reduced the need for coronary angiography from 100% to 14% (95% CI: 9–20%, *P* < .001) • Greater diagnostic yield from coronary angiography: 75% (53–90%) vs. 15% (10–22%), *P* < .001 • Major procedural complications were uncommon (0.3%) and similar across groups • Less common minor complications: 3.6% (1–8%) vs. 10.5% (6–16%), *P* = .014 • Similar rate of MACE between groups (4.2% vs. 3.7%, *P* = .86) • Similar radiation exposure: 5.0 mSv vs. 6.4 mSv *P* = .45.
CONSERVE[59]	Chang et al. 2018	1631	1 year	To compare CCTA vs. ICA among patients referred for ICA	CCTA vs. ICA • Similar MACE rate between the arms of the trial (4.6% vs. 4.6%; hazard ratio: 0.99; 95% CI l: 0.66–1.47). • Following CCTA, only 23% went on to ICA • Coronary revascularization occurred less often (13% vs. 18%; *P* < .001) • Lower rate of normal ICA (24.6% vs. 61.1% in the, *P* < .001)
CAT-CAD[61]	Rudzinski et al. 2022	120	3 years	To compare CCTA vs. ICA among high-risk patients and indication for ICA	CCTA vs. ICA • Similar rate of MACE (15.5% vs. 16.7%, log-rank *P* = .89) • Similar cumulative number of serious adverse events (36 vs. 38, *P* = .79)
DISCHARGE[60]	Maurovich-Horvat et al. 2022	3561	3.5 years	To compare CCTA vs. ICA in intermediate-risk patients.	CCTA vs. ICA • Similar rate of MACE (2.1% vs. 3.0% *P* = .1) • Lower rate of procedure-related complications (0.5% vs. 1.9%, hazard ratio, 0.26; 95% CI, 0.13–0.55) • Similar rate of angina during the final 4 weeks of follow-up (8.8% vs. in 7.5%, odds ratio, 1.17; 95% CI, 0.92–1.48)

TABLE 9.4 Randomized Controlled Trials of Coronary Computed Tomography in Patients With Stable Chest Pain–cont'd

STUDY NAME	AUTHOR, YEAR	N	FOLLOW-UP	AIM	MAIN FINDINGS
Coronary Computed Tomography Angiography With Selective FFRCT Versus Standard Clinical Pathway					
FORCAST[63]	Curzen et al. 2021	1400	9 months	To compare CCTA with selective FFR_{CT} versus standard clinical pathway among patients with stable chest pain	• CCTA with selective FFRCT versus standard clinical pathway • Initial CCTA 96% vs. 63% • FFR_{CT} was used in 38% of the experimental group • Mean total cardiac costs: £1605 vs. £1491 (P = .10). • MACCE: 10.2 vs. 10.6 (P = .8) • Angina and quality of life improved to a similar degree • ICA: 19% vs. 25% (P = .01)
PRECISE[64]	Douglas et al. 2022 (presented)	2103	11.8 months	To compare precision strategy (guideline-based recommendations) with usual care in patients with nonacute chest pain or equivalent requiring testing for suspected CAD	Precision strategy vs. usual care • Initial test CCTA+ FFR_{CT}: 31% vs. 0.4% • Primary endpoint (death, MI, or ICA without obstructive CAD): 4.2% vs. 11.3% (P < .001) • Death or MI: 1.7% vs. 1.1% • All cause death: 0.5% vs. 0.7% • Nonfatal MI: 1.2% vs. 0.5% • ICA without obstructive CAD: 2.6% vs. 10.2%

CAC, Coronary artery calcium score; *CAD*, coronary artery disease; *CCTA*, coronary computed tomography angiography; *CI*, confidence interval; *ETT*, electrocardiogram exercise tolerance test; *FFR_{CT}*, fractional flow reserve computed tomography; *ICA*, invasive coronary angiography; *MACE*, major adverse cardiovascular events; *MACCE*, major adverse cardiac and cerebrovascular events; *MI*, myocardial infarction; *MPI*, myocardial perfusion imaging.

Coronary CTA Versus Functional Testing

A study by Min et al.,[10] the CAPP study,[51] CRESCENT,[26] and CRESCENT II[52] studies (Table 9.3) were relatively small RCTs (n = 180–500) comparing CCTA versus functional testing that generally showed more rapid diagnosis, reduced rate of downstream testing and costs, improved patient symptoms, and increased use of prevention therapies following CCTA compared with functional tests (Figs. 9.5 and 9.6). The largest RCTs comparing CCTA and functional testing

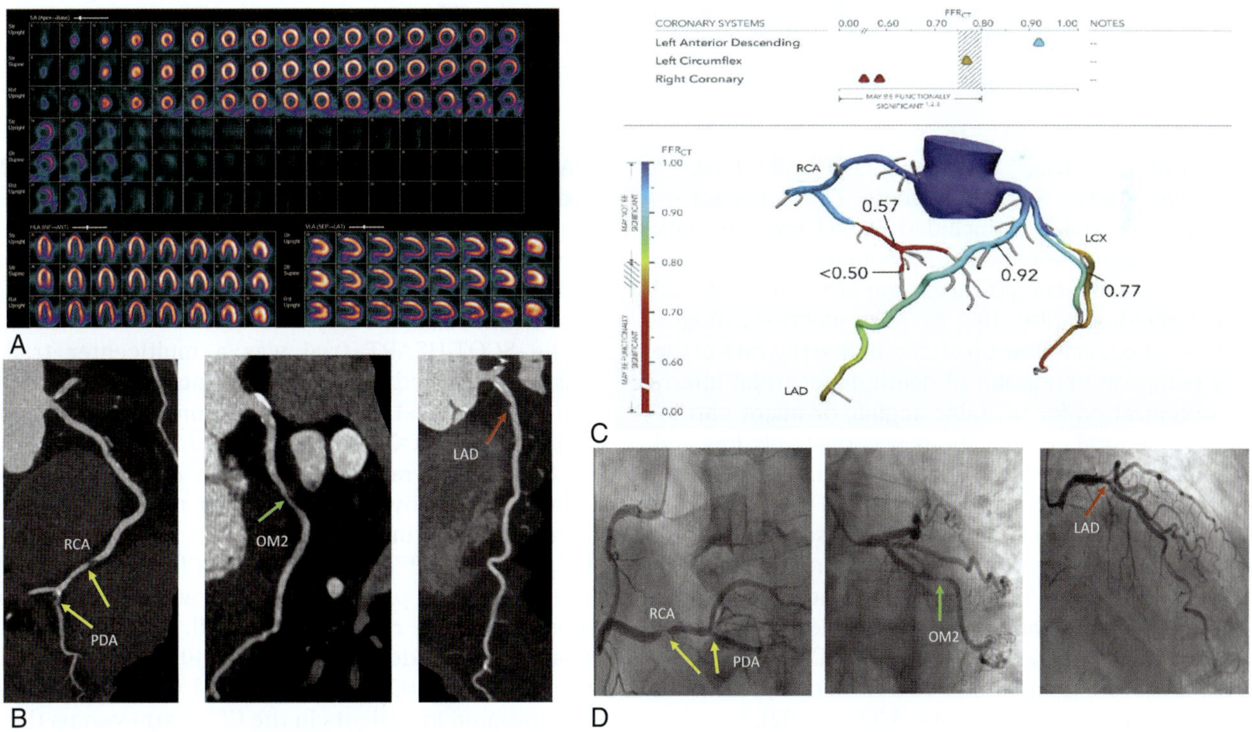

FIG. 9.5 Discordant Findings of Stress Imaging and CCTA. Myocardial perfusion single-photon emission computerized tomography (SPECT) (A), curved multiplanar reconstruction from a CCTA (B), FFR_{CT} (C), and invasive coronary angiography (D) of a 72-year-old male evaluated for stable chest pain. The findings show discordance between stress imaging (SPECT) and CCTA. The SPECT shows no definite perfusion defects on the stress or rest images. The CCTA shows a medium amount of calcified and noncalcified plaque in the proximal LAD resulting in mild (25–49%) stenosis (*orange arrow*), a large amount of noncalcified plaque in the OM2 (Second Obtuse Marginal branch) resulting in severe (70–99%) stenosis (*green arrow*), a medium amount of mostly calcified plaque resulting in minimal (1–24%) stenosis of the proximal right coronary artery RCA (Right coronary artery), a large amount of mostly noncalcified plaque resulting in severe (70–99%) stenosis of the distal RCA, and a moderate (50–69%) stenosis of the ostial PDA (Posterior Descending Artery) (*yellow arrows*). FFR_{CT} showed a hemodynamically significant lesion in the proximal OM2 branch with an abnormal FFR_{CT} value of 0.77 and a hemodynamically significant lesion in the distal RCA with an abnormal FFR_{CT} value of 0.57. ICA showed findings highly consistent with those of CCTA. Patient underwent revascularization of distal RCA and OM2. *CCTA*, Coronary computed tomography angiography; *FFR_{CT}*, fractional flow reserve calculated from computed tomography; *LAD*, left anterior descending.

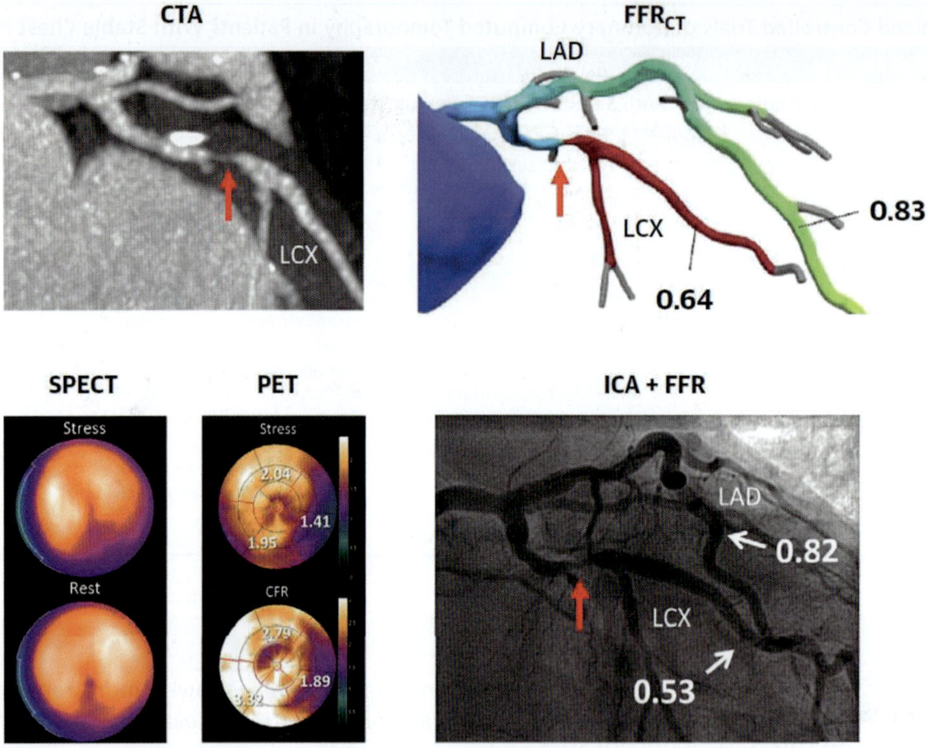

FIG. 9.6 Concordant Findings of Stress Imaging and CCTA. Representative imaging results of a 57-year-old male with typical angina and a history of smoking. Multiplanar reformat of a coronary CTA demonstrating obstructive stenosis of the proximal LCX artery and a corresponding reduced FFR$_{CT}$ value of 0.64, next to a FFR$_{CT}$ value of 0.83 for the LAD artery. Myocardial perfusion imaging with SPECT and PET show, respectively, a reversible defect and a diminished stress MBF and CFR in the inferolateral territory. ICA with FFR measurements confirm the obstructive lesion and detrimental FFR value of 0.53 in the LCX. *CFR*, Coronary flow reserve; *CTA*, computed tomography angiography; *FFR*, fractional flow reserve; *FFR$_{CT}$*, fractional flow reserve calculated from computed tomography; *ICA*, invasive coronary angiography; *LAD*, left anterior descending; *LCx*, left circumflex; *MBF*, myocardial blood flow; *PET*, positron emission tomography; *SPECT*, single-photon emission computed tomography. (Adapted from Driessen RS, Danad I, Stuijfzand WJ, et al. Comparison of coronary computed tomography angiography, fractional flow reserve, and perfusion imaging for ischemia diagnosis. *J Am Coll Cardiol*. 2019;73[2]:161–173.)

were the PROMISE trial[53] and the SCOT-HEART trial.[54–56] The PROMISE study[53] was a multicenter (193 sites across North America) trial that included 10,003 patients with symptoms suggestive of stable CAD who were assigned to CCTA or functional testing (67% nuclear stress testing, 27% stress echocardiography, 10% exercise electrocardiography). Over a median follow-up of 25 months, the rate of the primary composite endpoint of death, myocardial infarction, hospitalization for unstable angina, or major cardiovascular procedural complications was relatively low and did not differ between the two study arms (3.3% and 3%, respectively; HR 1.04, 95% confidence interval [CI]: 0.83–1.29, P = .75). However, the use of CCTA was associated with a lower rate of death or myocardial infarction at 12 months (HR 0.66, P = .049). It is noteworthy that more patients in the CCTA group underwent ICA 90 days following randomization (12.2% vs. 8.1%). However, fewer ICA without obstructive CAD were found in the CCTA arm compared with the functional testing arm (3.4% vs. 4.3%, P = .02).

The PROMISE trial failed to show superiority of a CCTA strategy in patients with stable chest pain symptoms over stress testing modalities. However, PROMISE ended up not being sufficiently powered to show significant differences in the primary outcome between the two arms, due to the relatively short follow-up period and the low event rate, only 3% instead of anticipated 8%. It is noteworthy that although the estimated PTP of patients enrolled in the CCTA arm of PROMISE was 53.3%, only 10.7% had ≥50% stenosis on CCTA.

A prespecified post-hoc analysis from the PROMISE study evaluated outcomes among 2144 patients with diabetes. The risk for cardiovascular death or MI was lower among patients with diabetes in the CCTA arm compared with the function stress testing arm (CCTA: 1.1% vs. 2.6%; hazard ratio: 0.39; P = .01).[57]

The SCOT-HEART trial was a multicenter trial (12 sites in the United Kingdom) that included 4146 patients with suspected stable CAD randomized to standard of care (SOC) or SOC and CCTA. After a median follow-up of 4.8 years, the rate of the primary composite endpoint defined as cardiovascular death or nonfatal MI was significantly lower in the CCTA group compared with the SOC (2.3% vs. 3.9%; HR = 0.59, 95% CI:0.41–0.84, P = .004). This decrease in primary endpoint was mainly driven by a decrease in the rate of nonfatal MI. Of note, higher rate of preventive (odds ratio [OR], 1.40, 95% CI: 1.19–1.65) and antianginal (OR 1.27, 95% CI: 1.05–1.54) treatments were initiated in patients in the CCTA arm versus the SOC arm. Although being higher in the CCTA group at 2 years, the rates of ICA and coronary revascularization of both groups were similar at 4.8 years. These findings were further reinforced by recent reports demonstrating sustained benefits at 10-year follow-up.[56] A prominent limitation of the SCOT-HEART trial is the high rate of patients evaluated by an exercise treadmill test (90%), which is not currently considered the standard of care, and the relatively low rate of stress imaging.

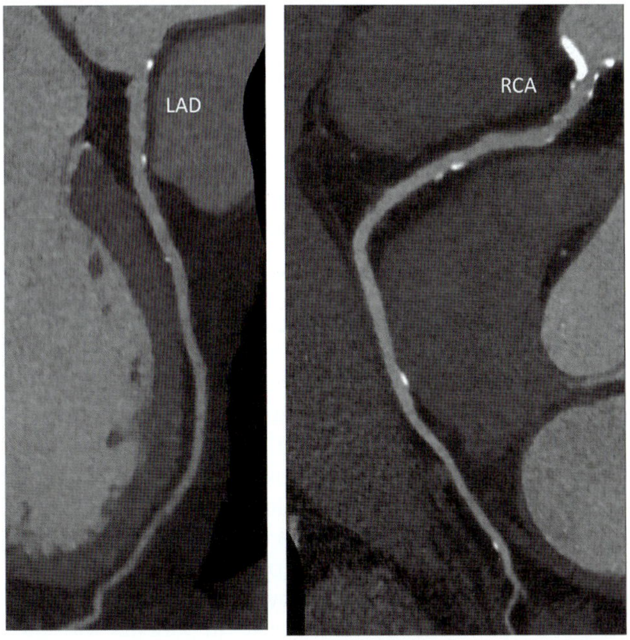

FIG. 9.7 Nonobstructive Coronary Artery Disease. Curved multiplanar reconstructions from a CCTA of a 74-year-old male with multiple risk factors and nonanginal chest pain showing moderate-large amount of calcified and noncalcified plaque in the RCA and a small amount of mostly calcified plaque in the LAD without significant stenosis. CAD-RADS classification: CAD-RADS 1 (minimal stenosis), P3 (large amount of plaque). *CCTA*, Coronary computed tomography angiography; *LAD*, left anterior descending.

CCTA Versus ICA

Two relatively small randomized controlled trials (CAD-MAN[58] and CONSERVE[59]) of CCTA versus ICA among intermediate-risk stable patients have shown an increased rate of ICA with obstructive CAD, reduction in revascularization procedures, and similar clinical outcomes in CCTA first strategy compared with ICA (Table 9.4). The DISCHARGE trial[60] was a pragmatic trial comparing CCTA with ICA, as the initial diagnostic imaging strategy for guiding the treatment of intermediate-PTP patients with stable chest pain who were referred for ICA at one of 26 European centers. Over 3.5 years, the primary composite outcome, which included cardiovascular death, nonfatal myocardial infarction, or nonfatal stroke, occurred in 2.1% in the CCTA arm and 3% in the ICA arm (HR 0.7; 95% CI: 0.46–1.07, $P = .1$). The frequency of major procedure-related complications was lower with an initial CT strategy versus ICA (0.5% vs. 1.9%, HR = 0.26; 95% CI: 0.13–0.55). The frequency of angina during the final 4 weeks of follow up did not differ between the two groups (odds ratio, 1.17; 95% CI: 0.92–1.48). This finding of no difference in cardiovascular outcomes between the two strategies probably results from the limited effect of revascularization on cardiovascular events among most patients with stable CAD.[7] Notably, even though all patients assigned to the CCTA were, by design, referred for invasive angiography, following CCTA, only 22% underwent CCTA. Similarly, in the CONSERVE study, only 23% of patients who were referred for CCTA ultimately underwent invasive angiography.

The CAT-CAD[61] trial was a small study (n = 120) that enrolled patients with high PTP for CAD and an indication for ICA. Patients were randomized with an allocation ratio of 1:1 to CCTA and ICA. Over 3 years, there were no significant differences between both diagnostic strategies in terms of neither the long-term efficacy nor the long-term safety.

A metaanalysis[62] of these four studies showed there were no statistically significant differences between groups with regard to MACE (OR: 0.84, 95% CI: 0.63–1.13, $P = .25$), MI (OR: 1.12, 95% CI: 0.65–1.94, $P = .68$), stroke (OR: 0.51, 95% CI: 0.26–1.03, $P = .06$), or cardiovascular death (OR: 0.53, 95% CI: 0.23–1.24, $P = .14$). However, coronary CTA was associated with lower major procedure-related complications compared with ICA (0.4% vs. 1.3%; OR: 0.30, 95% CI: 0.12–0.75, $P < .05$). A metaanalysis by Machado et al.[5] further showed that the use of CCTA versus invasive angiography was also associated with a lower rate of stroke.

CCTA With Selective CT-FFR

In the FORECAST trial[63] (Table 9.4), overall 1400 patients with stable chest pain in 11 centers were randomized to initial testing with CCTA with selective CT-FFR (experimental group) or standard clinical care pathways (standard group). The primary endpoint was total cardiac costs at 9 months. Secondary endpoints were angina status, quality of life, major adverse cardiac and cerebrovascular events, and use of invasive coronary angiography. Most patients had an initial CTCA: 439 (63%) in the standard group versus 674 (96%) in the experimental group, of whom 254 (38%) underwent FFR_{CT}. There was no statistically significant difference in the mean total cardiac costs between both groups. There was also no significant difference in the rate of major adverse cardiac and cerebrovascular events between the groups and angina, and quality of life improved to a similar degree over follow-up in both randomized groups. Invasive angiography was reduced significantly in the experimental group (19% vs. 25%, $P = .01$).

The PRECISE trial[64] (Table 9.4) randomized 2103 symptomatic patients who required testing for suspected CAD into an arm of usual testing as determined by treating clinicians or to the Precision strategy, which comprised of an initial risk assessment (using the aforementioned PMRS) to identify low-risk individuals[65] in whom testing can be deferred. All other patients in the precision strategy arm were sent to CCTA with subsequent selective use of FFR_{CT} for lesions that had 30% to 90% stenosis. As expected, the rate of deferred testing was higher in the Precision arm (16.5% vs. 6.5%), although only 64% of patients who advised to defer testing had no testing performed. Over a median follow-up of 11.8 months the primary composite endpoint of all-cause death, nonfatal MI, or ICA without obstructive CAD occurred in 4.2% of the Precision group and 11.3% of the usual testing group (HR = 0.35, 95% CI: 0.25–0.5, $P < .001$). However, this was driven mainly by a ~76% reduction of ICA without obstructive CAD. Patients with very low likelihood of disease were excluded from the CCTA arm but not from the stress testing arm, potentially biasing the study toward a superior result in the CCTA arm.

Mechanisms of Improved Outcomes Following CCTA

The major improvement in patient outcomes observed with CCTA in the aforementioned studies has prompted questions about the underlying mechanisms behind this improvement. Because there is little evidence that revascularization improves patient outcomes with respect to subsequent cardiac events, the mechanism most likely responsible for the improved outcomes is an increase in preventive therapies. There are numerous observational studies and clinical trials indicating that identification of CAD, whether obstructive or nonobstructive (Figure 7), by CCTA leads to higher use of preventive therapies known to improve outcomes.[66]

Support of this concept was observed in a post-hoc analysis of the SCOT-HEART trial that showed that patients who were randomized to undergo CCTA had higher rates of preventive therapies throughout the trial.[67] In terms of appropriateness of therapy in the CCTA group, the rates of antiplatelet and statin therapy use were almost threefold higher in those with CAD versus without CAD (despite identical risk scores). Thus more targeted use of therapies to patients who actually had CAD and were at high risk may explain the improved outcomes following CCTA.[67]

In SCOT-HEART, coronary revascularization was more frequent in the CCTA arm during the first year after randomization, driven by early detection of obstructive CAD including left main and triple-vessel CAD. It is possible that earlier identification by CCTA and therapy of these higher-risk patients might have contributed to the improved outcomes observed in the CCTA group.[67]

MANAGEMENT FOLLOWING CCTA

The goals of CCTA in the evaluation of patients with chest pain and suspected CAD can be summarized as follows: to diagnose the cause of symptoms, identify patients who may benefit from coronary revascularization, identify patients who may benefit from initiation or intensification of preventive measures, and to determine the need for medical treatment to reduce ischemia. All of these goals can be achieved with the use of CCTA, although subsequent testing following CCTA is needed when the CCTA results are inconclusive, as discussed below. A comprehensive format for CCTA-based classification and decision-making is provided by the Coronary Artery Disease Reporting & Data System (CAD-RADS 2.0) and is presented in Table 9.5.[19] Fig. 9.8 summarizes patient management recommendations following CCTA consistent with contemporary guidelines. Patients with chest pain due to microvascular disease are one group for whom CCTA may not be helpful in identifying. Such patients are more accurately assessed by stress PET or CMR myocardial perfusion imaging.

Medical Therapy and Preventive Measures Guided by CCTA

Current guidelines emphasize the importance of guideline-directed medical therapy (GDMT) among stable patients who are found to have either nonobstructive or obstructive CAD on CCTA. The importance of classifying and treating patients with nonobstructive CAD as having stable CAD is a relatively newer concept in contemporary cardiology guidelines. The 2021 AHA/ACC Chest Pain guideline provides a class 1 recommendation based on expert opinion that "for patients with known nonobstructive CAD and stable chest pain, it is recommended to optimize preventive therapies."[4] The 2023 AHA/ACC Guideline for the Management of Patients with Chronic Coronary Diseases (CCD)[68] also supports this concept and states that CCD should include patients diagnosed with CAD based on imaging tests (CCTA and stress testing).

Although there are currently no guidelines that specifically address the management of nonobstructive CAD, adherence to the 2019 atherosclerotic cardiovascular prevention guidelines and the 2023 Chronic Coronary Disease Guideline is recommended.[68–70]

In general, preventive therapies should include both lifestyle modifications and pharmacological interventions to halt the progression of CAD and mitigate its impact, as illustrated in Fig. 9.9. Indeed, the detection and guiding management of both nonobstructive and obstructive CAD is considered one of the major advantages of CCTA over stress imaging studies, as well as one of the mechanisms for the improved outcomes observed with CCTA versus stress testing.

The importance of aggressive preventive therapies in patients with stable CAD defined by noninvasive testing was well illustrated in the ISCHEMIA trial.[7] In patients with moderate to severe ischemia and at least a 50% stenosis on CCTA, the trial showed that an initial invasive strategy was not associated with a reduction in the primary composite outcome of cardiovascular death, myocardial infarction, hospitalization for unstable angina, hospitalization for heart failure, or resuscitated cardiac arrest over a median follow-up of 3.3 years compared with an initial conservative strategy. Although the ISCHEMIA trial did not specifically evaluate the yield of a CCTA strategy for patients with stable CAD, these findings strongly support the use of aggressive medical therapy in most stable patients after CCTA prior to considering interventional options. However, the ISCHEMIA trial results, the 2021 chest pain guidelines, as well as the CAD-RADS 2.0 document all support that high-risk CAD patients (left main stenosis ≥50%, or anatomically significant three-vessel disease [≥70% stenosis]), or those with frequent angina, should be referred to ICA, for further evaluation and decision-making.[4]

Guideline-directed medical therapy in secondary prevention is associated with a >50% reduction in cardiovascular events in stable CAD[71]; however, adherence to medical therapy in secondary prevention populations is known to be low.[72] In ISCHEMIA, application of secondary preventive care medications was protocolized and monitored throughout the duration of the trial. Behavioral interventions focused on smoking cessation, nutrition, physical activity, weight control, and medication adherence, which was monitored at every visit. The aggressive prevention measures in the trial may have affected the prognostic relationship between ischemia and outcomes compared with that observed in observational registries.[73–75] It has been suggested that the impact of a patient being told or seeing in images that they have CAD (as opposed to possibly having disease) is motivational to patients to adhere to preventive medications and adopt healthier lifestyles.

Subsequent Noninvasive Testing

Among symptomatic patients with intermediate stenosis (e.g., 40–70% or at times even greater) or inconclusive CCTA (e.g., due significant coronary calcification; Figs. 9.4

TABLE 9.5 CAD-RADS 2.0 Reporting and Data System for Patients Presenting With Stable Chest Pain

CATEGORY	DEGREE OF MAXIMAL CORONARY STENOSIS	INTERPRETATION	FURTHER CARDIAC INVESTIGATION	MANAGEMENT CONSIDERATIONS
CAD-RADS 0	0% (No plaque or stenosis)	Absence of CAD[a]	None	Reassurance. Consider nonatherosclerotic causes of symptoms
CAD-RADS 1	1–24% (Minimal stenosis or plaque with no stenosis)[b]	Minimal nonobstructive CAD[b]	None	• Consider nonatherosclerotic causes of symptoms • P1: Consider risk factor modification and preventive pharmacotherapy • P2: Risk factor modification and preventive pharmacotherapy • P3 or P4: Aggressive risk factor modification and preventive pharmacotherapy
CAD-RADS 2	25–49% (Mild stenosis)	Mild nonobstructive CAD	None	• Consider nonatherosclerotic causes of symptoms • P1 or P2: Risk factor modification and preventive pharmacotherapy • P3 or P4: Aggressive risk factor modification and preventive pharmacotherapy
CAD-RADS 3	50–69% (Moderate stenosis)	Moderate stenosis	Consider functional assessment[c]	• P1, P2, P3, or P4: Aggressive risk factor modification and preventive pharmacotherapy • Other treatments (including antianginal therapy) should be considered per guideline directed cared • When modifier I+, consider ICA, especially if frequent symptoms persist after guideline-directed medical therapy
CAD-RADS 4	A – 70–99% stenosis or B - Left main ≥50% or 3-vessel obstructive (≥70%) disease	Severe stenosis	A: Consider ICA[e] or functional assessment B: ICA is recommended	• P1, P2, P3, or P4: Aggressive risk factor modification and preventive pharmacotherapy • Other treatments (including antianginal therapy and options of revascularization) should be considered per guideline-directed carec
CAD-RADS 5	100% (total occlusion)	Total coronary occlusion or subtotal occlusion	Consider ICA, functional, and/or viability assessment	
CAD-RADS N	Nondiagnostic study	Obstructive CAD cannot be excluded	Additional/alternative evaluation may be needed	

The CAD-RADS classification should be applied on a per-patient basis for the clinically most relevant (usually highest-grade) stenosis.
All vessels greater than 1.5 mm in diameter should be graded for stenosis severity. CAD-RADS will not apply for smaller vessels (1.5 mm in diameter).
[a]CAD, Coronary artery disease.
[b]CAD-RADS 1 - This category should also include the presence of plaque with positive remodeling and no evidence of stenosis.
[c]Functional Assessment includes CT-FFR, CTP, stress testing (ETT, stress echocardiogram, SPECT, PET, cardiac MRI), or invasive FFR.
[d]Guideline-directed care per 2021 AHA/ACC Chest Pain Guideline 2012 ACC/AHA Guideline for the diagnosis and management of patients with stable ischemic heart disease and 2019 ACC/AHA Prevention Guidelines. Further evaluation of CAD-RADS 3 and 4A with functional imaging or invasive coronary angiography should be considered to identify a target lesion (if unknown) and if the patient has persistent symptoms despite adequate medical therapy.
[e]ICA – invasive coronary angiography may be favored if high-grade stenosis (>90%), high-risk plaque features or I+ (presence of lesion-specific ischemia on CT FFR or perfusion defects by CTP) or concordant ischemia by other stress tests and a candidate for revascularization. It should be clarified that benefit of revascularization should be confined to patients with persistent symptoms despite optimal medical therapy.
Adapted from Cury RC, Leipsic J, Abbara S, et al. CAD-RADS™ 2.0 - 2022 coronary artery disease-reporting and data system: an expert consensus document of the Society of Cardiovascular Computed Tomography (SCCT), the American College of Cardiology (ACC), the American College of Radiology (ACR), and the North America Society of Cardiovascular Imaging (NASCI). *JACC Cardiovasc Imaging*. 2022;15(11):1974–2001.

and 9.5),[4,8] additional stress testing, FFR_{CT} or plaque-based ischemia measures can be performed.[4,8,19,76] However, such testing is not always indicated, especially when patients do not have frequent angina, have good exercise capacity, or the lesions with potential obstruction are in small vessels or in a distal location (i.e., less likely to result in significant angina and/or to benefit from coronary revascularization). The guidelines state that among patients with 40% to 90% stenosis in proximal or middle coronary segment on CCTA and ongoing symptoms, FFR_{CT} can be useful for diagnosis of vessel-specific ischemia and to guide decision-making regarding the use of coronary revascularization (COR 2a LOE B-NR)[4] when the functional implications of the stenoses is uncertain. However, FFR_{CT} might not always be available, and imaging quality might not always enable its performance. Of note, the measurement of functional significance of stenoses on CCTA is not limited to FFR_{CT}. Methods for diagnosis of ischemia on CCTA based on coronary plaque have been developed using artificial intelligence algorithms.[42,76] Stress imaging is also a reasonable option for patients with stable chest pain after inconclusive CCTA receiving the same COR as FFR_{CT} (COR 2a LOE B-NR).[4] Data regarding the performance of various tests as second-line options is scarce. In addition, there are limited data comparing between FFR_{CT} and stress imaging modalities in this setting, although the aforementioned PRECISE trial suggests that the use of CCTA with FFR_{CT} may be associated with lower use of invasive angiography when compared with usual stress testing. When comparing FFR_{CT} and stress testing, FFR_{CT} may have some advantages when evaluating the hemodynamic consequences of single lesions that are located in the proximal to mid-segments of a vessel. However,

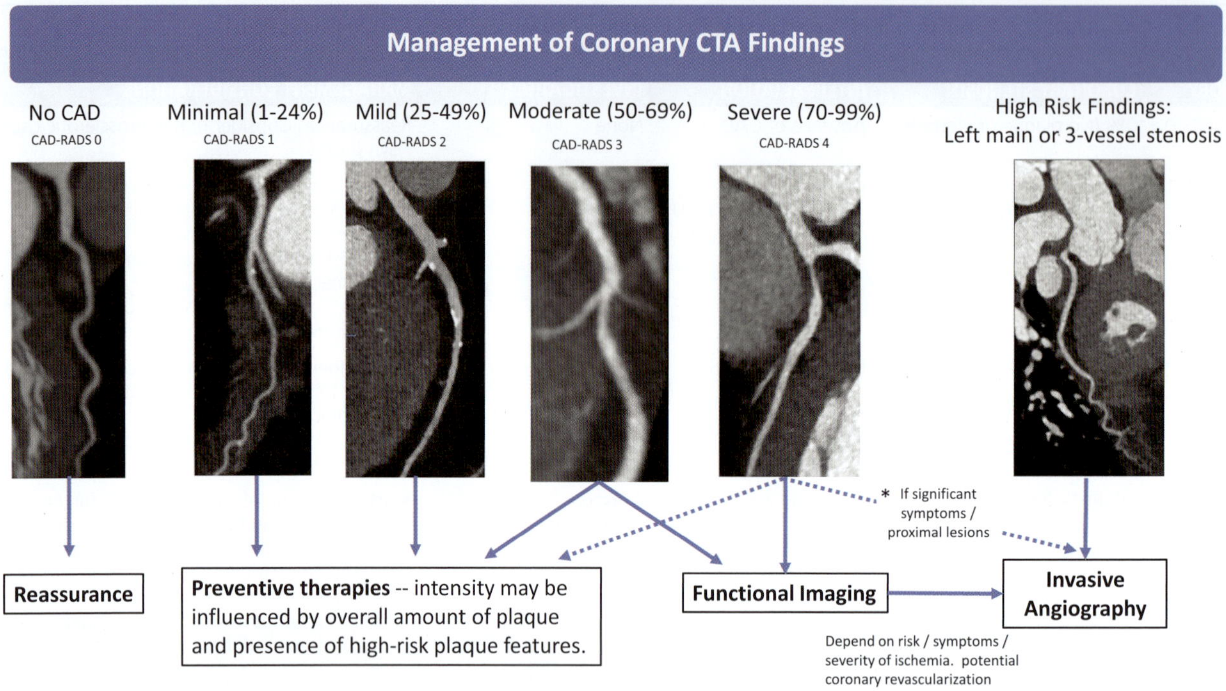

FIG. 9.8 Patient Management Recommendations Following CCTA in Stable Chest Pain. *CTA*, Computed tomography angiography. (Reprinted with permission from *Braunwald's Heart Disease*, 12th ed. Elsevier; 2022.)

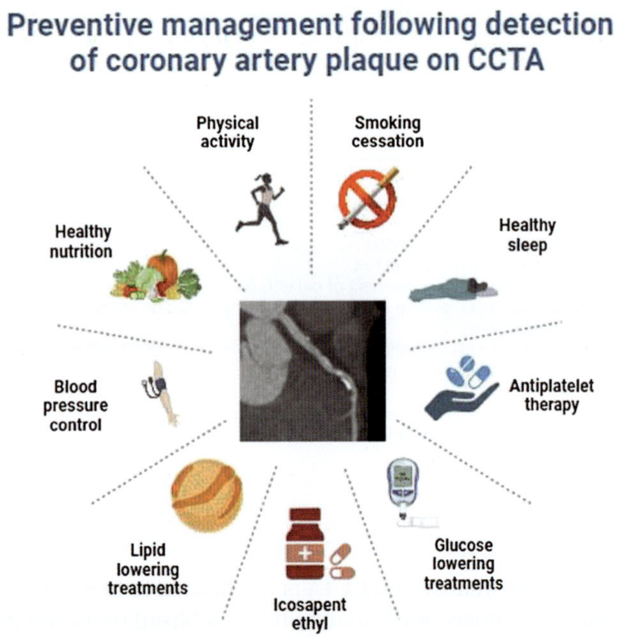

FIG. 9.9 Preventive Management to Consider Following Detection of Coronary Artery Plaque on CCTA. *CCTA*, Coronary computed tomography angiography.

stress testing may be useful when there is diffuse disease and multiple lesions or when microvascular disease is considered as a possibility for a patient's symptoms. In these cases, stress imaging may help evaluate the significance of these lesions as well as detect microvascular disease if myocardial blood flow quantification is performed.

Regarding stress imaging modalities, the Danish study of Non-Invasive Testing in Coronary Artery Disease (Dan-NICAD) 1[77] was an RCT that evaluated the accuracy of single-photon emission computed tomography (SPECT) and CMR (1.5Tesla) in low/intermediate-risk patients with suspected CAD based on CCTA findings. Patients underwent ICA with invasive FFR that served as reference standard (FFR ≤0.80 or >90% diameter stenosis by visual assessment). The study found similar low-moderate sensitivities (36% [95% CI: 24–50] and 41% [95% CI: 28–54]) but high specificities (94% [95% CI: 87–98] and 84% [95% CI: 75–91]) for SPECT and CMR, respectively.

The Dan-NICAD 2 trial[78] was a similarly designed trial evaluating 3Tesla-CMR and adenosine ^{82}Rubidium PET, following a CCTA with suspected CAD. The sensitivities for CMR and PET were 59% (95% CI: 51–67) and 64% (95% CI: 56–71), $P = .21$, respectively, and specificities 84% (95% CI: 78–89) and 89% (95% CI: 84–93), $P = .08$, respectively. The overall accuracy was slightly higher for PET compared to CMR (73% vs. 78%, $P = .03$). These two trials, designed in a way that is consistent with the guideline recommendation of CCTA as a frontline test, show an attenuated accuracy for well-established imaging modalities following CCTA, compared with previously published accuracy measures for these tests.[4,79] However, previous studies evaluated these modalities primarily as initial tests rather than second-line tests as applied in the Dan-NICAD trials. This reduced diagnostic accuracy can result from a variety of reasons such as broad definition for categorizing a test as positive, testing of patients after an abnormal CCTA that resulted in higher prevalence of CAD, selection bias derived from different rates of performance of both tests, and imperfect reference standard. Additional studies comparing how different tests perform following initial use of CCTA are needed. In addition to the available literature supporting the use of FFR_{CT} and more advanced stress testing options (PET or stress CMR), considerations of test selection should account for local availability and expertise in addition to patient suitability and preference.

Invasive Evaluation and Management Guided by CCTA

The purpose of revascularization in patients with stable CAD is improving symptoms of angina, and possibly improvement in outcomes, by increasing exercise capacity and quality of life as well as reducing the risk of MACE.[1] Accordingly, in most patients with stable CAD (unless high-risk anatomy is present) revascularization would be indicated for symptoms that are frequent or refractory to optimal GDMT. Considering that ICA should ideally only be offered to patients who may benefit from revascularization, the rate of normal or nonobstructive ICAs remains high (up to ~50%), even in modern practice.[8,62] Although stenosis severity is the primary parameter for therapeutic decisions, the addition of physiologic data to determine hemodynamic significance (e.g., FFR_{CT}) can significantly improve decision-making. Thus physiologic information from FFR_{CT} or CTP in addition to CCTA can serve as a robust gatekeeper optimizing downstream ICA referral. A post-hoc subanalysis of the PROMISE trial has shown that FFR_{CT} ≤0.8 was a better predictor of MACE or revascularization than stenosis alone on CCTA.[37] Reserving ICA for patients with FFR_{CT} ≤0.8 could decrease ICA without ≥50% stenosis by 44% and increase the proportion of ICA leading to revascularization by 24%.[37] The PLATFORM study has shown a 61% reduction in ICA referral and a reduction in nonobstructive disease from 73% to 12% with the use of FFR_{CT} in patients for whom invasive angiography was planned before CCTA. However, there was no difference in the frequency of nonobstructive disease in the patients for whom a noninvasive strategy was planned.[34,38] As previously noted in the PRECISE trial,[64] there was a reduction of composite endpoint driven mainly by reduction of ICA without obstructive CAD by the Precision strategy (CCTA ± FFR_{CT}) versus usual care (mostly functional tests) arm; as noted above, however, patients with a very low likelihood of obstructive CAD were eliminated from further testing only in the Precision strategy. Similarly, the aforementioned FORECAST trial[63] reported a reduction in ICA without significant change in other outcomes or costs with the selective use of FFR_{CT} versus standard clinical care pathway. Similar findings regarding the rate of ICA after CCTA were also shown by the CRESCENT II trial,[52] in which the addition of CTP when >50% stenosis was shown by CCTA, resulted in a decrease in the rate of ICA without a class I indication for revascularization.

One advantage to combining anatomic and physiologic data from CCTA +FFR_{CT} is that it can help procedural planning and decision-making prior to the cath lab. This can be aided by calculating a comprehensive CT-based SYNTAX score that is highly consistent with the ICA-based SYNTAX score.[80,81] Collectively, the evaluation of the various parameters that CCTA offers by the heart team before ICA may help with planning of potential revascularization procedures by assessing lesion-specific ischemia, estimating stent sizing and choosing the landing zones of stents. Further, CCTA can be used to identify patients in whom ICA is likely to be complex (e.g., bifurcation lesions or lesions requiring plaque modification prior to stent insertion) and evaluating the likelihood of functional impact of PCI (Percutaneous Coronary Intervention).[82,83]

COST-VALUE CONSIDERATIONS

The costs of CCTA strategy for the outpatient evaluation of patients suspected with CAD are overall similar to those of stress imaging strategy when compared over a long-term period (2–3 years).[84,85] As shown by the PROMISE trial, the higher costs of increased ICA following CCTA are matched by increased downstream testing in the functional group.[4,85] Findings from the SCOT-HEART trial showed a mildly higher cost of $462 in the CCTA group.[75] However, the increased costs did not result from increased additional services or the use of medications.[75]

A tiered strategy, as applied in the CRESCENT trial that comprised of a CAC test followed by CCTA only for patients with CAC >0 or high PTP, resulted in higher rate of diagnostic testing (approximately twofold) following electrocardiogram exercise tolerance test (ETT) compared to CAC/CCTA and 16% higher cost of the ETT strategy.[26] Notably approximately 40% of the CAC/CCTA group were found to have CAC = 0 and did not undergo a subsequent CCTA, which contributed to the cost savings in the CCTA group.

A selective referral to ICA using CCTA strategy has been shown to save approximately 57% in costs when compared with direct use of ICA as shown in the CONSERVE trial.[59]

FUTURE AREAS OF RESEARCH

Subsequent Diagnostic and Therapeutic Strategies Based on CCTA Findings

Following the adoption of CCTA as a leading frontline strategy for the evaluation of stable patients for CAD, there is a growing need in prospective randomized trials evaluating the optimal application of CCTA in these patients, as well as subsequent diagnostic and therapeutic strategies based on CCTA findings.

IDENTIFICATION AND MANAGEMENT OF LOW-RISK PATIENTS

Low-risk patients represent more than 50% of all patients with stable chest pain.[86] Guidelines generally recommend against additional testing in this group and offer the option to pursue exercise testing or CAC.[4] However, there is controversy as to how to best identify low-risk patients, and significant limitations of current risk scores, despite improvements with some recent novel scores such as PMRS.[49,86,87] Despite guidelines and appropriate use criteria, in clinical practice, CCTA and other imaging modalities are often used in low-risk patients. Thus additional studies are needed to determine the best way to identify low-risk stable patients and to establish safe and acceptable evidence-based diagnostic pathways for this large group of patients. These is also a need to examine whether CCTA can improve outcomes in selected asymptomatic group. The SCOT-HEART 2 study is currently examining this question, with expected results by 2027.

THRESHOLDS QUANTIFICATION OF CORONARY PLAQUE FOR MANAGEMENT AND FOLLOW-UP IN PATIENTS WITH NONOBSTRUCTIVE CAD

The risk associated with nonobstructive CAD, especially when extensive, is significantly higher compared with having no coronary atherosclerosis.[14,88] Moreover, the identification of nonobstructive CAD is considered a unique advantage of CCTA and often drives the initiation or intensification of preventive therapies. However, standardization with regard to the quantitative and qualitative plaque analysis in these scenarios is insufficient. The commercial availability of quantitative assessments of coronary plaque (Fig. 9.3) is leading to broad interest in their clinical use; however, to date, there is a paucity of indicating how these methods will influence patient management or change outcomes. Additional studies are needed to determine optimal thresholds relating the amount or type of plaque with the potential benefit of various preventive therapies, as well as to evaluate the therapeutic effects of various preventive and therapeutic interventions by serial CCTA scans.

APPLICATIONS OF CCTA+CT-FFR IN HIGH-RISK PATIENTS

A significant number of patients at high-risk for stable CAD are referred to ICA, without an attempt to optimize GDMT or a prior noninvasive test. An initial evaluation with CCTA is safe and is not associated with worse outcomes.[62] Furthermore, even in these high-risk patients there is a substantial rate of ICAs without subsequent revascularization. However, even when such patients are evaluated with a CCTA and found to have obstructive CAD, therapeutic decisions or even discussions (e.g., heart teams) are often performed only after ICA. An integration of high-quality anatomic and functional assessment by the combination of CCTA and CT-FFR (or in some cases CCTA and stress testing) could assist in better selection of high-risk patients who may benefit from ICA.

However, it is important to recognize that most CCTA outcomes studies have been in lower risk cohorts. Thus additional studies are needed to evaluate the use of CCTA (with or without CT-FFR) versus stress testing in high-risk patients. In addition, studies are needed to examine the benefit of routine CCTA prior to planned coronary intervention. One such trial using CT-FFR is currently in progress (Precise Procedural and PCI Plan (P4); Clinicaltrials.gov)

Use of CCTA Among Older Patients

The 2021 AHA/ACC chest pain guideline favors CCTA for patients <65 years of age, whereas stress imaging is preferred in patients ≥65 years.[4] The use of CCTA in older individuals is often hindered by increased risk for contrast-induced nephropathy, higher likelihood of dense calcifications of the coronary arteries, and difficulties complying with breath-holding protocols. On the other hand, stress imaging modalities are often not feasible in this population due to deconditioning or contraindications to pharmacological stress. A metaanalysis of 5332 patients, which included 1434 patients aged 65 to 75 years and 462 patients aged >75 years, reported relatively high accuracy of CCTA for the diagnosis of obstructive CAD among the elderly (aged 65–75 years: sensitivity 94.8%, specificity 80.5%, >75 years: sensitivity 93.6%, specificity 77.4%), particularly considering that older studies were included the analysis.[89] Studies evaluating CCTA versus other modalities in terms of cardiovascular outcomes among older patients are scarce, and additional studies are necessary to establish whether technological advancements would improve diagnostic accuracy in this population and to determine the parameters for choosing the optimal strategy in this age group across various clinical scenarios.

Diagnostic Yield Among Patients With Significant Calcification

The diagnostic accuracy of CCTA can significantly decrease when there are focal areas of dense coronary calcifications or coronary stents. For instance, in the CORE 64 study, the specificity to detect significant CAD decreased to 56% and 57% with a calcium score of ≥600 or the presence of stents, respectively, versus 91% in patients without stents or severe calcification.[90] The use of CT-FFR for detecting hemodynamically significant lesions by FFR has been shown to be lower in patients with high CAC scores. The FACC study evaluated 260 stable patients with CAC score >399 showed concordant CT-FFR accuracy, sensitivity, and specificity of 71%, 87%, and 54%, respectively. Due to the low specificity, myocardial perfusion imaging methods with PET, SPECT, or MRI might be preferred methods for assessing ischemia in the territory of high CAC. Of note, the FACC study examined patients with a high overall CAC score.[91] Further studies examining the various levels of high CAC scores in individual lesions (rather than overall scores) are needed. The recently introduced photon-counting CTs (see Chapter 2, Advances in Hardware and Reconstruction Techniques for Cardiac CT for details) have the potential to improve the aforementioned limitations of CCTA, particularly with respect to decreased calcium blooming, and improved accuracy to detect stenosis in the presence of coronary calcifications.[8,92,93]

Application in Patients With Known Obstructive CAD

CCTA is becoming increasingly used in patients with known CAD, particularly patients with coronary stents (see Chapter 10, Coronary Stents and Bypass Grafts). Decreased diagnostic accuracy for assessing in-stent restenosis compared to vessels without stents has been well described and is most pronounced in patients with stents <3 mm in diameter. Further study is needed to assess how CCTA affects the management and outcomes of these patients. As with densely calcified lesions, photon-counting CT has shown promising results for detecting in-stent stenosis.

CONCLUSIONS

Coronary computed tomography angiography has emerged as a first-line strategy for the evaluation of patients with suspected stable CAD. CCTA has broad applications in this clinical setting, and several studies have shown CCTA to be associated with favorable patient outcomes compared with stress imaging or direct invasive coronary angiography. Furthermore, CCTA is considered to be cost effective and has not been found to be associated with increased costs compared with stress imaging. With recent technological advancements, CCTA enables accurate, highly detailed, characterization and quantification of plaque in patients with obstructive and nonobstructive disease, providing robust diagnostic and prognostic data to augment decision-making and future follow-up. Moreover, it can also provide lesion-specific accurate functional information in the form of CT-FFR that could be of value among patients with intermediate or inconclusive coronary lesions. Additional studies using contemporary technologies are needed to accurately evaluate the applications of CCTA in various subgroups of patients (e.g., low- and high-risk, older individuals, significant coronary calcifications, coronary stents). In addition, future studies and clinical trials should focus on the use of quantitative plaque measurements in patient management following CCTA and determine appropriate thresholds for management decision. Such studies would further support CCTA as a leading strategy for individualized evaluation and management of patients with stable CAD.

REFERENCES

1. Knuuti J, Wijns W, Saraste A, et al. 2019 ESC guidelines for the diagnosis and management of chronic coronary syndromes. *Eur Heart J*. 2020; 41(3):407–477.
2. Tsao CW, Aday AW, Almarzooq ZI, et al. Heart disease and stroke statistics-2022 update: a report from the American Heart Association. *Circulation*. 2022;145(8):e153–e639.
3. Benjamin EJ, Virani SS, Callaway CW, et al. Heart disease and stroke statistics-2018 update: a report from the American Heart Association. *Circulation*. 2018;137(12):e67–e492.
4. Gulati M, Levy PD, Mukherjee D, et al. 2021 AHA/ACC/ASE/CHEST/SAEM/SCCT/SCMR guideline for the evaluation and diagnosis of chest pain: a report of the American College of Cardiology/American Heart Association Joint Committee on clinical practice guidelines. *J Am Coll Cardiol*. 2021;78(22):e187–e285.
5. Machado MF, Felix N, Melo PHC, et al. Coronary computed tomography angiography versus invasive coronary angiography in stable chest pain: a meta-analysis of randomized controlled trials. *Circ Cardiovasc Imaging*. 2023;16(11):e015800.
6. Vrints C, Andreotti F, Koskinas KC, et al. 2024 ESC Guidelines for the management of chronic coronary syndromes. *Eur Heart J*. 2024;45(36):3415–3537.
7. Maron DJ, Hochman JS, Reynolds HR, et al. Initial invasive or conservative strategy for stable coronary disease. *N Engl J Med*. 2020;382(15):1395–1407.
8. Narula J, Chandrashekhar Y, Ahmadi A, et al. SCCT 2021 expert consensus document on coronary computed tomographic angiography: a report of the society of cardiovascular computed tomography. *J Cardiovasc Comput Tomogr*. 2021;15(3):192–217.
9. Knuuti J, Ballo H, Juarez-Orozco LE, et al. The performance of non-invasive tests to rule-in and rule-out significant coronary artery stenosis in patients with stable angina: a meta-analysis focused on post-test disease probability. *Eur Heart J*. 2018;39(35):3322–3330.
10. Min JK, Koduru S, Dunning AM, et al. Coronary CT angiography versus myocardial perfusion imaging for near-term quality of life, cost and radiation exposure: a prospective multicenter randomized pilot trial. *J Cardiovasc Comput Tomogr*. 2012;6(4):274–283.
11. Andreini D, Pontone G, Mushtaq S, et al. A long-term prognostic value of coronary CT angiography in suspected coronary artery disease. *JACC Cardiovasc Imaging*. 2012;5(7):690–701.
12. Min JK, Dunning A, Lin FY, et al. Age- and sex-related differences in all-cause mortality risk based on coronary computed tomography angiography findings results from the International Multicenter CONFIRM (Coronary CT Angiography Evaluation for Clinical Outcomes: an International Multicenter Registry) of 23,854 patients without known coronary artery disease. *J Am Coll Cardiol*. 2011;58(8):849–860.
13. Mortensen MB, Steffensen FH, Bøtker HE, et al. Heterogenous distribution of risk for cardiovascular disease events in patients with stable ischemic heart disease. *JACC Cardiovasc Imaging*. 2021;14(2):442–450.
14. Jespersen L, Hvelplund A, Abildstrøm SZ, et al. Stable angina pectoris with no obstructive coronary artery disease is associated with increased risks of major adverse cardiovascular events. *Eur Heart J*. 2012;33(6):734–744.
15. Bittencourt MS, Hulten E, Ghoshhajra B, et al. Prognostic value of nonobstructive and obstructive coronary artery disease detected by coronary computed tomography angiography to identify cardiovascular events. *Circ Cardiovasc Imaging*. 2014;7(2):282–291.
16. Williams MC, Kwiecinski J, Doris M, et al. Low-attenuation noncalcified plaque on coronary computed tomography angiography predicts myocardial infarction: results from the multicenter SCOT-HEART trial (Scottish Computed Tomography of the HEART). *Circulation*. 2020;141(18):1452–1462.
17. Cho I, Al'Aref SJ, Berger A, et al. Prognostic value of coronary computed tomographic angiography findings in asymptomatic individuals: a 6-year follow-up from the prospective multicentre international CONFIRM study. *Eur Heart J*. 2018;39(11):934–941.
18. Nurmohamed NS, Bom MJ, Jukema RA, et al. AI-guided quantitative plaque staging predicts long-term cardiovascular outcomes in patients at risk for atherosclerotic CVD. *JACC Cardiovasc Imaging*. 2024;17(3):269–280.
19. Cury RC, Leipsic J, Abbara S, et al. CAD-RADS™ 2.0 – 2022 coronary artery disease-reporting and data system: an expert consensus document of the Society of Cardiovascular Computed Tomography (SCCT), the American College of Cardiology (ACC), the American College of Radiology (ACR), and the North America Society of Cardiovascular Imaging (NASCI). *JACC Cardiovasc Imaging*. 2022;15(11):1974–2001.
20. Agatston AS, Janowitz WR, Hildner FJ, Zusmer NR, Viamonte Jr M, Detrano R. Quantification of coronary artery calcium using ultrafast computed tomography. *J Am Coll Cardiol*. 1990;15(4):827–832.
21. Winther S, Schmidt SE, Foldyna B, et al. Coronary calcium scoring improves risk prediction in patients with suspected obstructive coronary artery disease. *J Am Coll Cardiol*. 2022;80(21):1965–1977.
22. Miller RJH, Gransar H, Rozanski A, et al. Simplified approach to predicting obstructive coronary disease with integration of coronary calcium: development and external validation. *J Am Heart Assoc*. 2023;12(24):e031601.
23. Koopman MY, Reijnders JJW, Willemsen RTA, et al. Coronary calcium scoring as first-line test to detect and exclude coronary artery disease in patients presenting to the general practitioner with stable chest pain: protocol of the cluster-randomised CONCRETE trial. *BMJ Open*. 2022;12(4): e055123.
24. Agha AM, Pacor J, Grandhi GR, et al. The prognostic value of CAC zero among individuals presenting with chest pain: a meta-analysis. *JACC Cardiovasc Imaging*. 2022;15(10):1745–1757.
25. Hulten E, Bittencourt MS, Ghoshhajra B, et al. Incremental prognostic value of coronary artery calcium score versus CT angiography among symptomatic patients without known coronary artery disease. *Atherosclerosis*. 2014;233(1):190–195.
26. Lubbers M, Dedic A, Coenen A, et al. Calcium imaging and selective computed tomography angiography in comparison to functional testing for suspected coronary artery disease: the multicentre, randomized CRESCENT trial. *Eur Heart J*. 2016;37(15):1232–1243.
27. Winther S, Schmidt SE, Mayrhofer T, et al. Incorporating coronary calcification into pre-test assessment of the likelihood of coronary artery disease. *J Am Coll Cardiol*. 2020;76(21):2421–2432.
28. Engbers EM, Timmer JR, Ottervanger JP, Mouden M, Knollema S, Jager PL. Prognostic value of coronary artery calcium scoring in addition to single-photon emission computed tomographic myocardial perfusion imaging in symptomatic patients. *Circ Cardiovasc Imaging*. 2016;9(5):e003966.
29. Chang SM, Nabi F, Xu J, et al. The coronary artery calcium score and stress myocardial perfusion imaging provide independent and complementary prediction of cardiac risk. *J Am Coll Cardiol*. 2009;54(20):1872–1882.
30. Bavishi C, Argulian E, Chatterjee S, Rozanski A. CACS and the frequency of stress-induced myocardial ischemia during MPI: a meta-analysis. *JACC Cardiovasc Imaging*. 2016;9(5):580–589.
31. Tzimas G, Gulsin GS, Everett RJ, et al. Age- and sex-specific nomographic CT quantitative plaque data from a Large International Cohort. *JACC Cardiovasc Imaging*. 2024;17(2):165–175.
32. Gu H, Gao Y, Hou Z, et al. Prognostic value of coronary atherosclerosis progression evaluated by coronary CT angiography in patients with stable angina. *Eur Radiol*. 2018;28(3):1066–1076.
33. De Bruyne B, Pijls NH, Kalesan B, et al. Fractional flow reserve-guided PCI versus medical therapy in stable coronary disease. *N Engl J Med*. 2012;367(11):991–1001.
34. Douglas PS, De Bruyne B, Pontone G, et al. 1-year outcomes of FFRCT-guided care in patients with suspected coronary disease: the PLATFORM study. *J Am Coll Cardiol*. 2016;68(5):435–445.
35. Patel MR, Nørgaard BL, Fairbairn TA, et al. 1-year impact on medical practice and clinical outcomes of FFR(CT): the ADVANCE registry. *JACC Cardiovasc Imaging*. 2020;13(1 Pt 1):97–105.
36. Driessen RS, Danad I, Stuijfzand WJ, et al. Comparison of coronary computed tomography angiography, fractional flow reserve, and perfusion imaging for ischemia diagnosis. *J Am Coll Cardiol*. 2019;73(2):161–173.
37. Lu MT, Ferencik M, Roberts RS, et al. Noninvasive FFR derived from coronary CT angiography: management and outcomes in the PROMISE trial. *JACC Cardiovasc Imaging*. 2017;10(11):1350–1358.
38. Douglas PS, Pontone G, Hlatky MA, et al. Clinical outcomes of fractional flow reserve by computed tomographic angiography-guided diagnostic strategies vs. usual care in patients with suspected coronary artery disease: the prospective longitudinal trial of FFR(CT): outcome and resource impacts study. *Eur Heart J*. 2015;36(47):3359–3367.
39. Fairbairn TA, Nieman K, Akasaka T, et al. Real-world clinical utility and impact on clinical decision-making of coronary computed tomography angiography-derived fractional flow reserve: lessons from the ADVANCE registry. *Eur Heart J*. 2018;39(41):3701–3711.
40. Nørgaard BL, Fairbairn TA, Safian RD, et al. Coronary CT Angiography-derived fractional flow reserve testing in patients with stable coronary artery disease: recommendations on interpretation and reporting. *Radiol Cardiothorac Imaging*. 2019;1(5):e190050.
41. Varga-Szemes A, Schoepf UJ, Maurovich-Horvat P, et al. Coronary plaque assessment of Vasodilative capacity by CT angiography effectively estimates fractional flow reserve. *Int J Cardiol*. 2021;331:307–315.

42. Nurmohamed NS, Danad I, Jukema RA, et al. Development and validation of a quantitative coronary CT angiography model for diagnosis of vessel-specific coronary ischemia. *JACC Cardiovasc Imaging*. 2024;17(8):894–906.
43. Bamberg F, Becker A, Schwarz F, et al. Detection of hemodynamically significant coronary artery stenosis: incremental diagnostic value of dynamic CT-based myocardial perfusion imaging. *Radiology*. 2011;260(3):689–698.
44. Lu M, Wang S, Sirajuddin A, Arai AE, Zhao S. Dynamic stress computed tomography myocardial perfusion for detecting myocardial ischemia: a systematic review and meta-analysis. *Int J Cardiol*. 2018;258:325–331.
45. Juarez-Orozco LE, Saraste A, Capodanno D, et al. Impact of a decreasing pre-test probability on the performance of diagnostic tests for coronary artery disease. *Eur Heart J Cardiovasc Imaging*. 2019;20(11):1198–1207.
46. Bittencourt MS, Hulten E, Polonsky TS, et al. European society of cardiology-recommended coronary artery disease consortium pretest probability scores more accurately predict obstructive coronary disease and cardiovascular events than the diamond and forrester score: the partners registry. *Circulation*. 2016;134(3):201–211.
47. Juarez-Orozco LE, Saraste A, Capodanno D, et al. Impact of a decreasing pre-test probability on the performance of diagnostic tests for coronary artery disease. *Eur Heart J. Cardiovascular Imaging*. 2019;20(11):1198–1207.
48. Foldyna B, Udelson JE, Karády J, et al. Pretest probability for patients with suspected obstructive coronary artery disease: re-evaluating Diamond-Forrester for the contemporary era and clinical implications: insights from the PROMISE trial. *Eur Heart J Cardiovasc Imaging*. 2019;20(5):574–581.
49. Rasmussen LD, Fordyce CB, Nissen L, et al. The PROMISE minimal risk score improves risk classification of symptomatic patients with suspected CAD. *JACC Cardiovasc Imaging*. 2022;15(8):1442–1454.
50. Neglia D, Liga R, Gimelli A, et al. Use of cardiac imaging in chronic coronary syndromes: the EURECA imaging registry. *Eur Heart J*. 2023;44(2):142–158.
51. McKavanagh P, Lusk L, Ball PA, et al. A comparison of cardiac computerized tomography and exercise stress electrocardiogram test for the investigation of stable chest pain: the clinical results of the CAPP randomized prospective trial. *Eur Heart J Cardiovasc Imaging*. 2015;16(4):441–448.
52. Lubbers M, Coenen A, Kofflard M, et al. Comprehensive cardiac CT with myocardial perfusion imaging versus functional testing in suspected coronary artery disease: the multicenter, randomized CRESCENT-II trial. *JACC Cardiovasc Imaging*. 2018;11(11):1625–1636.
53. Douglas PS, Hoffmann U, Patel MR, et al. Outcomes of anatomical versus functional testing for coronary artery disease. *N Engl J Med*. 2015;372(14):1291–1300.
54. Newby DE, Adamson PD, Berry C, et al. Coronary CT angiography and 5-year risk of myocardial infarction. *N Engl J Med*. 2018;379(10):924–933.
55. CT coronary angiography in patients with suspected angina due to coronary heart disease (SCOT-HEART): an open-label, parallel-group, multicentre trial. *Lancet (London, England)*. 2015;385(9985):2383–2391.
56. Williams MC, Wereski R, Tuck C, et al. Coronary CT angiography-guided management of patients with stable chest pain: 10-year outcomes from the SCOT-HEART randomised controlled trial in Scotland. *Lancet (London, England)*. 2025;405(10475):329–337.
57. Sharma A, Coles A, Sekaran NK, et al. Stress testing versus CT angiography in patients with diabetes and suspected coronary artery disease. *J Am Coll Cardiol*. 2019;73(8):893–902.
58. Dewey M, Rief M, Martus P, et al. Evaluation of computed tomography in patients with atypical angina or chest pain clinically referred for invasive coronary angiography: randomised controlled trial. *BMJ (Clinical Research ed.)*. 2016;355:i5441.
59. Chang HJ, Lin FY, Gebow D, et al. Selective referral using CCTA versus direct referral for individuals referred to invasive coronary angiography for suspected CAD: a randomized, controlled, open-label trial. *JACC Cardiovasc Imaging*. 2019;12(7 Pt 2):1303–1312.
60. Maurovich-Horvat P, Bosserdt M, Kofoed KF, et al. CT or invasive coronary angiography in stable chest pain. *N Engl J Med*. 2022;386(17):1591–1602.
61. Rudziński PN, Kruk M, Demkow M, et al. Efficacy and safety of coronary computed tomography angiography in patients with a high clinical likelihood of obstructive coronary artery disease. *Kardiologia Polska*. 2022;80(1):56–63.
62. Kheiri B, Simpson TF, Osman M, German DM, Fuss CS, Ferencik M. Computed tomography vs invasive coronary angiography in patients with suspected coronary artery disease: a meta-analysis. *JACC Cardiovasc Imaging*. 2022;15(12):2147–2149.
63. Curzen N, Nicholas Z, Stuart B, et al. Fractional flow reserve derived from computed tomography coronary angiography in the assessment and management of stable chest pain: the FORECAST randomized trial. *Eur Heart J*. 2021;42(37):3844–3852.
64. Douglas PS, Nanna MG, Kelsey MD, et al. Comparison of an initial risk-based testing strategy vs usual testing in stable symptomatic patients with suspected coronary artery disease: the PRECISE randomized clinical trial. *JAMA Cardiol*. 2023;8(10):904–914.
65. Fordyce CB, Douglas PS, Roberts RS, et al. Identification of patients with stable chest pain deriving minimal value from noninvasive testing: the PROMISE minimal-risk tool, a secondary analysis of a randomized clinical trial. *JAMA Cardiol*. 2017;2(4):400–408.
66. Generoso G, Agarwal V, Shaw LJ, Cardoso R, Blankstein R, Bittencourt MS. Changes in use of preventive medications after assessment of chest pain by coronary computed tomography angiography: a meta-analysis. *J Cardiovasc Comput Tomogr*. 2024;18(3):233–242.
67. Adamson PD, Williams MC, Dweck MR, et al. Guiding therapy by coronary CT angiography improves outcomes in patients with stable chest pain. *J Am Coll Cardiol*. 2019;74(16):2058–2070.
68. Virani SS, Newby LK, Arnold SV, et al. 2023 AHA/ACC/ACCP/ASPC/NLA/PCNA guideline for the management of patients with chronic coronary disease: a report of the American Heart Association/American College of Cardiology Joint Committee on clinical practice guidelines. *J Am Coll Cardiol*. 2023;82(9):833–955.
69. Arnett DK, Blumenthal RS, Albert MA, et al. 2019 ACC/AHA guideline on the primary prevention of cardiovascular disease: a report of the American College of Cardiology/American Heart Association Task Force on clinical practice guidelines. *J Am Coll Cardiol*. 2019;74(10):e177–e232.
70. Grundy SM, Stone NJ, Bailey AL, et al. 2018 AHA/ACC/AACVPR/AAPA/ABC/ACPM/ADA/AGS/APhA/ASPC/NLA/PCNA guideline on the management of blood cholesterol: a report of the American College of Cardiology/American Heart Association Task Force on clinical practice guidelines. *J Am Coll Cardiol*. 2019;73(24):e285–e350.
71. Montalescot G, Sechtem U, Achenbach S, et al. 2013 ESC guidelines on the management of stable coronary artery disease: the Task Force on the management of stable coronary artery disease of the European Society of Cardiology. *Eur Heart J*. 2013;34(38):2949–3003.
72. Bansilal S, Castellano JM, Garrido E, et al. Assessing the impact of medication adherence on long-term cardiovascular outcomes. *J Am Coll Cardiol*. 2016;68(8):789–801.
73. Ladapo JA, Hoffmann U, Lee KL, et al. Changes in medical therapy and lifestyle after anatomical or functional testing for coronary artery disease. *J Am Heart Assoc*. 2016;5(10):e003807.
74. Blankstein R, Bittencourt MS, Bhatt DL. Coronary CTA in the evaluation of stable chest pain: clear benefits, but not for all. *J Am Coll Cardiol*. 2017;69(14):1771–1773.
75. Williams MC, Hunter A, Shah ASV, et al. Use of coronary computed tomographic angiography to guide management of patients with coronary disease. *J Am Coll Cardiol*. 2016;67(15):1759–1768.
76. Lin A, van Diemen PA, Motwani M, et al. Machine learning from quantitative coronary computed tomography angiography predicts fractional flow reserve-defined ischemia and impaired myocardial blood flow. *Circ Cardiovasc Imaging*. 2022;15(10):e014369.
77. Nissen L, Winther S, Westra J, et al. Diagnosing coronary artery disease after a positive coronary computed tomography angiography: the Dan-NICAD open label, parallel, head to head, randomized controlled diagnostic accuracy trial of cardiovascular magnetic resonance and myocardial perfusion scintigraphy. *Eur Heart J Cardiovasc Imaging*. 2018;19(4):369–377.
78. Rasmussen LD, Winther S, Eftekhari A, et al. Second-line myocardial perfusion imaging to detect obstructive stenosis: head-to-head comparison of CMR and PET. *JACC Cardiovasc Imaging*. 2023;16(5):642–655.
79. Yang K, Yu SQ, Lu MJ, Zhao SH. Comparison of diagnostic accuracy of stress myocardial perfusion imaging for detecting hemodynamically significant coronary artery disease between cardiac magnetic resonance and nuclear medical imaging: a meta-analysis. *Int J Cardiol*. 2019;293:278–285.
80. Collet C, Onuma Y, Miyazaki Y, Morel MA, Serruys PW. Integration of non-invasive functional assessments with anatomical risk stratification in complex coronary artery disease: the non-invasive functional SYNTAX score. *Cardiovasc Diagn Ther*. 2017;7(2):151–158.
81. Kerner A, Abadi S, Abergel E, et al. Direct comparison between coronary computed tomography and invasive angiography for calculation of SYNTAX score. *EuroIntervention*. 2013;8(12):1428–1434.
82. Andreini D, Belmonte M, Penicka M, et al. Impact of coronary CT image quality on the accuracy of the FFR(CT) planner. *Eur Radiol*. 2024;34(4):2677–2688.
83. Safian RD. Computed tomography-derived physiology assessment: state-of-the-art review. *Int Cardiol Clin*. 2023;12(1):95–117.
84. Mark DB, Federspiel JJ, Cowper PA, et al. Economic outcomes with anatomical versus functional diagnostic testing for coronary artery disease. *Ann Intern Med*. 2016;165(2):94–102.
85. Xie JX, Shaw LJ. Measuring diagnostic health care costs in stable coronary artery disease: should we follow the money? *Ann Intern Med*. 2016;165(2):147–148.
86. Redberg RF, Guduguntla V. A PROMISE to reduce low-value testing. *JACC Cardiovasc Imaging*. 2022;15(8):1455–1457.
87. Udelson JE, Kelsey MD, Nanna MG, et al. Deferred testing in stable outpatients with suspected coronary artery disease: a prespecified secondary analysis of the PRECISE randomized clinical trial. *JAMA Cardiol*. 2023;8(10):915–924.
88. Shaw LJ, Blankstein R, Bax JJ, et al. Society of cardiovascular computed tomography /North American society of cardiovascular imaging—expert consensus document on coronary CT imaging of atherosclerotic plaque. *J Cardiovasc Comput Tomogr*. 2021;15(2):93–109.
89. Haase R, Schlattmann P, Gueret P, et al. Diagnosis of obstructive coronary artery disease using computed tomography angiography in patients with stable chest pain depending on clinical probability and in clinically important subgroups: meta-analysis of individual patient data. *BMJ (Clinical Research ed.)*. 2019;365:l1945.
90. Arbab-Zadeh A, Miller JM, Rochitte CE, et al. Diagnostic accuracy of computed tomography coronary angiography according to pre-test probability of coronary artery disease and severity of coronary arterial calcification. The CORE-64 (Coronary Artery Evaluation Using 64-Row Multidetector Computed Tomography Angiography) International Multicenter Study. *J Am Coll Cardiol*. 2012;59(4):379–387.
91. Mickley H, Veien KT, Gerke O, et al. Diagnostic and clinical value of FFR(CT) in stable chest pain patients with extensive coronary calcification: the FACC study. *JACC Cardiovasc Imaging*. 2022;15(6):1046–1058.
92. Latina J, Shabani M, Kapoor K, et al. Ultra-high-resolution coronary CT angiography for assessment of patients with severe coronary artery calcification: initial experience. *Radiol Cardiothorac Imaging*. 2021;3(4):e210053.
93. Hagar MT, Soschynski M, Saffar R, et al. Accuracy of ultrahigh-resolution photon-counting CT for detecting coronary artery disease in a high-risk population. *Radiology*. 2023;307(5):e223305.

10 Coronary Stents and Bypass Grafts

KOEN NIEMAN, FILIPPO CADEMARTIRI, AND BRIAN BURNS GHOSHHAJRA

KEY POINTS

- Visualization of coronary stents by coronary CT angiography (CCTA) can be challenging due to calcifications and noise. When CCTA is performed in such cases, it is essential to ensure appropriate patient selection (e.g., larger stents, nonoverlapping stents) and to optimize all scan parameters.
- CCTA accurately detects obstructive disease in bypass grafts.
- Following bypass surgery, assessment of the native coronary arteries by CCTA is often challenging due to diffuse atherosclerotic disease.

BACKGROUND

In the United States every year, 200,000 patients undergo coronary bypass graft surgery (CABG), and nearly 1 million undergo percutaneous coronary interventions (PCI). Although the long-term outcome of CABG as well as PCI by contemporary techniques is good, graft failure, in-stent restenosis, or progression of native coronary disease can occur. Many patients who underwent coronary revascularization in the past will at some point return with symptoms and the need for evaluation of obstructive disease. The diagnostic evaluation and subsequent therapeutic decision-making for patients with prior revascularizations is challenging by any imaging technique, anatomical or functional, invasive or noninvasive.

CARDIAC CT AFTER PERCUTANEOUS CORONARY INTERVENTION

Consideration of coronary CTA (CCTA) after stent placement requires understanding of the nuances of the clinical situation, as well as the limitations of CT physics. Although CCTA for native coronary arteries enjoys very robust supporting data, its performance in stented vessels bears significant limitations. These limitations are evolving along with CT technology and are highly specific to locally available scanner technology.[1]

When clinically questioning the possibility of additional or untreated disease progression in the native, unstented coronary vessels, CCTA is a useful adjunct and will perform similarly to published data, with the caveat that the pretest probability is high due to the presence of prior known disease requiring treatment. Thus CCTA may be reliably called upon to answer these focused questions, when they arise.

However, the evaluation of previously stented coronary segments warrant careful consideration of the likelihood of a useful test result. The limitations of CCTA in stented segments is twofold: first, the presence of prior disease warranting PCI implies a higher likelihood of densely calcified plaque at the site of PCI. Densely calcified plaque alone can cause significant blooming artifacts, rendering a difficult to evaluate or nonevaluable vessel lumen. Second, the stent struts themselves may be dense and cause beam hardening/blooming artifacts, which similarly limit the possibility of successful visualization of the stent lumen. Older stents, particularly bare metal stents, tend to be thicker and cause more artifacts; more modern stents tend to be thinner and cause less artifacts. Stent size also plays a role, with published data using more mature scanner technology verifying a higher likelihood of success in stents of 2.5 to 3.0 mm or higher.[2,3] Indeed, the 2021 Chest Pain guidelines deem the use of CCTA reasonable to evaluate patients with previous coronary revascularization (bypass grafts and stent patency for stents ≥3 mm).[7] Bioresorbable stents without significant metal components are less well studied and are not used widely throughout the world, but thought to present far less challenges.

If undertaking post-PCI imaging, careful pretest selection and discussion of the benefits and risks of the exam are warranted. For instance, if the primary question is to assess for new disease in proximal segments, the decision may favor CCTA. On the other hand, concerns for distal lesions or stented segment evaluation in older, smaller stents will favor alternative means of imaging such as functional (stress) imaging or invasive angiography. If CCTA is deemed appropriate, maximal image quality via optimization of spatial resolution and heart rate lowering—when necessary—is vital. Spatial resolution can be significantly improved with newer platforms including photon-counting CT,[4,5] which is an emerging method that allows much higher x-ray photon detection efficiency (see Chapter 2 for further detail). Sharper reconstruction kernels and iterative reconstruction algorithms are thought to confer advantages when imaging within metallic stents and are highly specific to each scanner platform. Additional practical considerations include particularly challenging situations such as overlapping stents and patients with additional surgical hardware such as adjacent bypass graft clips or extracardiac hardware such as spinal fusion rods that contribute to unavoidable beam hardening and attenuation.

Larger patients and patients with positional limitations, such as the inability to raise an arm, and patients with arrhythmia and tachycardia will present challenges for all CTA, but the detriment to image quality may be significantly higher when imaging stents. Fig. 10.1 shows the potential of photon-counting CT to successfully image-stented segments; Fig. 10.1A offers an example of successful stent imaging, whereasFigs. 10.1B and 10.1C show additional successful examples. They also highlight the challenge of surrounding dense calcium, as well as the utility of CCTA to assess native vessel disease that is either new or untreated (Fig. 10.1B)—the success of older technology may be variable in these settings but still have high yield to evaluate native vessels.

Fig. 10.2 shows three examples of patients who underwent modern photon-counting CT but also underwent less successful previous scans using older, traditional, energy integrating detector CT scanners. The challenges in the setting of dense calcification around the stents (Fig. 10.2A), overlapping stents (Fig. 10.2B), and small vessel size (Fig. 10.2C) are readily apparent when comparing these selected images obtained using older versus newer technology in the same patients. The data that inform current applicable guidelines are based on the accuracy of more traditional CT scanners.[6–8] As these relatively new scanners[9–11] are more widely studied, the expected success rates and diagnostic performance are predicted to improve accordingly.[12]

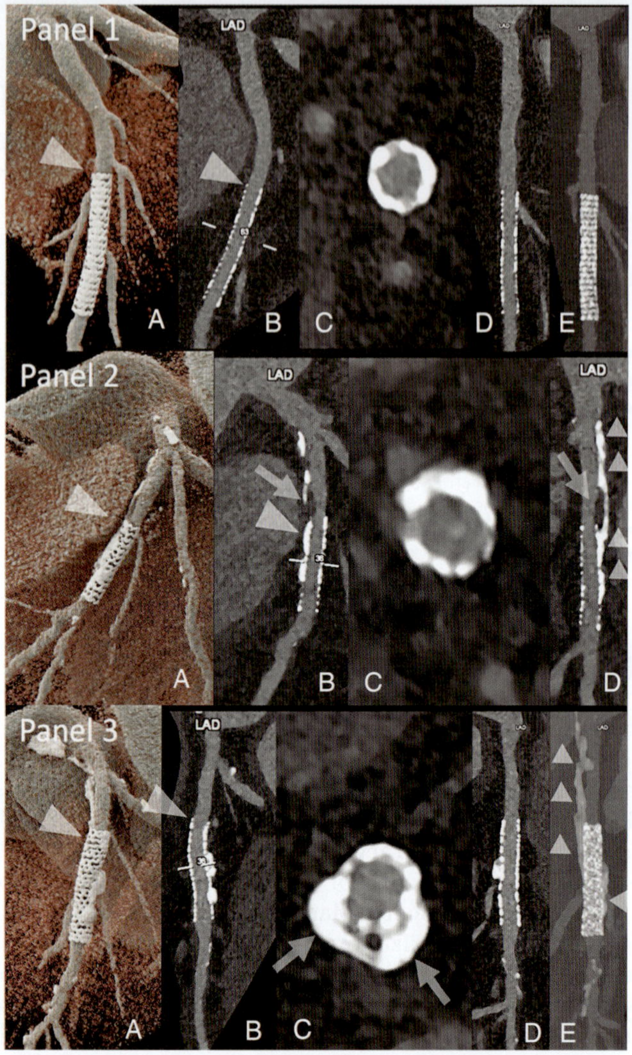

FIG. 10.1 Examples of cardiac/coronary CT angiography performed with a photon counting CT (Naeotom Alpha, Siemens Healthineers).
The scan was performed on a commercial whole-body dual source photon counting CT scanner (Naeotom Alpha, Siemens Healthineers) with 0.2 mm slice thickness (0.1 mm reconstruction increment, FOV 140 mm, Matrix 1024 × 1024, Kernel B60-72v, QIR level 4); the scan was performed with retrospective ECG gating with tube current modulation.

The upper panel (Panel 1) shows a stent in mid LAD (*arrowhead*; A, B) with cinematic rendering (A) and curved MPR reconstruction (B), short-axis lumen MPR (C), stretched longitudinal MPR (D), and thick slab longitudinal MIP (E); there is no evidence of endoluminal neointimal hyperplasia or in-stent restenosis.

The middle panel (Panel 2) shows a long stent in a severely diseased mid LAD (*arrowhead*; A, B) with cinematic rendering (A) and curved MPR reconstruction (B), short-axis lumen MPR (C), stretched longitudinal MPR (D); there is no evidence of endoluminal neointimal hyperplasia or overt in-stent restenosis, however, the large eccentric noncalcified plaque burden in the native proximal vessels extends to the proximal edge of the stent (B, D; *arrow*); a long calcified longitudinal plaque (D; *arrowheads*) extends into the stented segment.

The lower panel (Panel 3) shows a stent in a severely diseased proximal LAD (*arrowhead*; A, B) with cinematic rendering (A) and curved MPR reconstruction (B), short-axis lumen MPR (C), stretched longitudinal MPR (D), and thick slab longitudinal MIP (E); although the stent is completely patent and there is no evidence of endoluminal neointimal hyperplasia or overt in-stent restenosis, it is evident the large eccentric calcified plaque burden around the body of the stent (C; *arrow*), which is part of a much longer calcified longitudinal plaque (E; *arrowheads*) that extends around the stent; no resultant luminal narrowing. These densely calcified plaques, as well as metallic stent struts, can cause beam hardening artifacts that are more pronounced when using older technology and can be mitigated by advanced techniques such as photon-counting CT. *CT*, Computed tomography; *MIP*, maximum intensity projections; *MPR*, multiplanar reconstructions; *PCCT*, photon counting CT; *QIR*, quantum iterative reconstructions.

CARDIAC CT AFTER CORONARY ARTERY BYPASS GRAFT SURGERY

Coronary Artery Bypass Graft Surgery

Coronary artery bypass graft surgery was first performed in the 1970s and became widely available in the 1980s. Until the 1990s, CABG was the primary coronary revascularization technique, after which percutaneous coronary interventions gained momentum. Despite advantages in terms of shorter physical recovery after PCI, long-term outcome of CABG remains superior. CABG remains the preferred method of coronary revascularization in patients with three-vessel disease and reduced left ventricular function, and especially in the presence of diabetes, and is performed 200,000 times per year in the United States. Arterial grafts have excellent survival. Use of the left internal mammary artery is recommended for revascularization of the left anterior descending coronary artery (LAD), with a 10-year patency rate of >90%. Reversed saphenous vein grafts have a higher failure rate. Up to 25% will occlude within 1 year, and after 5 years only half are patent.[13] Although graft failure over time is not uncommon, not all occluded grafts will cause symptoms. As time since surgery increases, recurrence of symptoms can also result from progression of native coronary artery disease.

Conduits and Graft Configurations

Practiced techniques and graft configurations have evolved over time and vary between surgeons, institutions, and regions. Therefore, physicians interpreting CT scans of patients who have undergone CABG need to anticipate a wide range of possible approaches. It is strongly recommended to obtain surgical reports, ideally prior to the performance of the scan. The most common conduits used for coronary

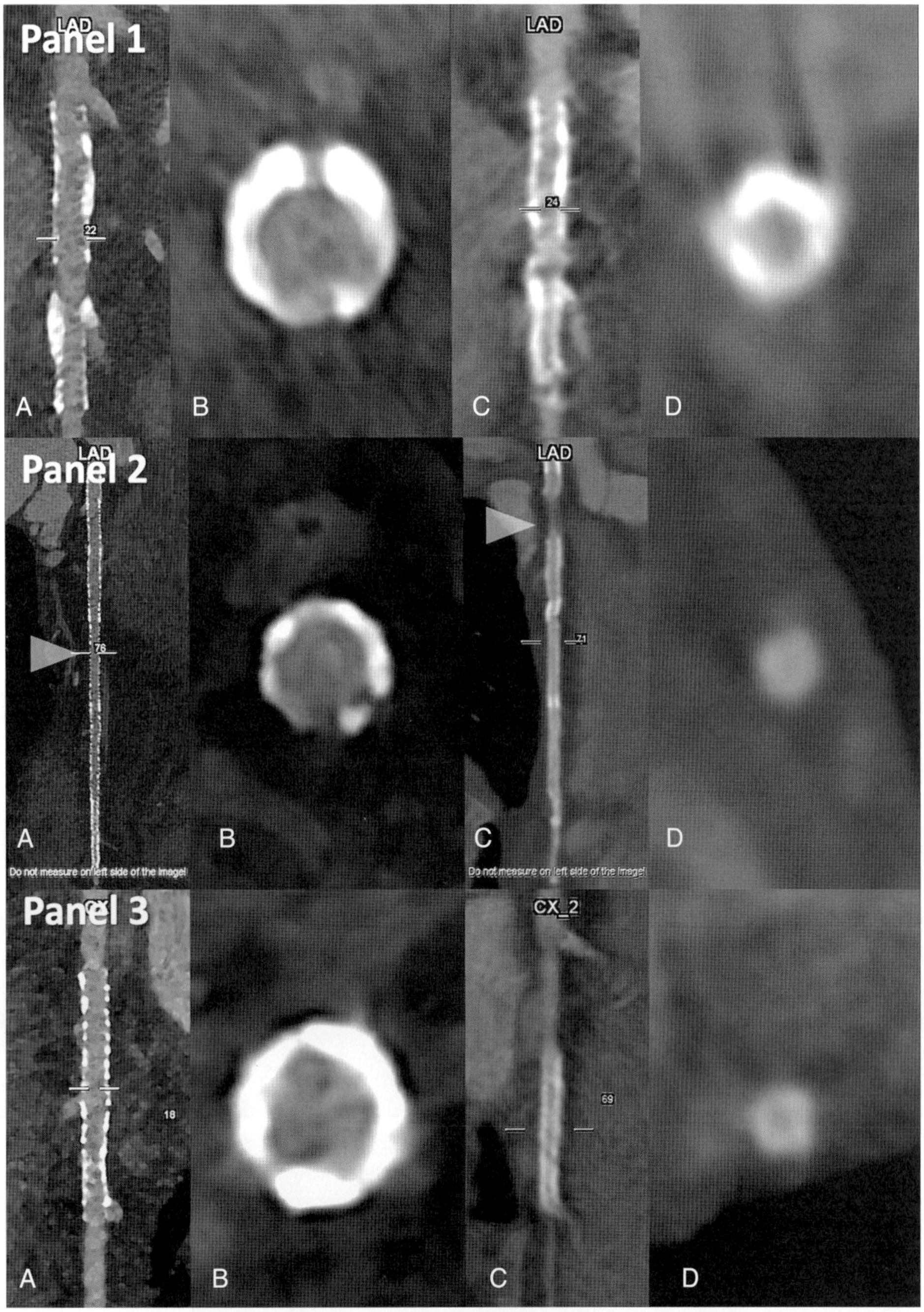

FIG. 10.2 Examples of cardiac/coronary CT angiography performed in the same patients with photon counting CT (Naeotom Alpha, Siemens Healthineers) and traditional energy integrating detector CT. The PCCT scan was performed on a commercial whole-body dual source photon counting CT scanner (Naeotom Alpha, Siemens Healthineers) with 0.2 mm slice thickness (66 ms temporal resolution, 0.1 mm reconstruction increment, FOV 140 mm, Matrix 1024 × 1024, Kernel B60-72v, QIR level 4); the scan was performed with retrospective ECG gating with tube current modulation.

The upper panel (Panel 1) shows two stents (nonoverlapped) in the proximal LAD visualized with PCCT (A – longitudinal stretched MPR, B – orthogonal cross section MPR) and with an older energy integrating detector 256-row multidetector CT scanner (C – longitudinal stretched MPR, D – orthogonal cross section MPR) GEHC; 0.28 s rotation time, 16 cm acquisition, 0.625 mm slice thickness, matrix 512 × 512). PCCT clearly depicts the two separated stents with surrounding calcifications without detriment to the luminal visualization, whereas the older scanner yields a much more difficult luminal assessment.

The middle panel (Panel 2) shows a "full-metal jacket" LAD with multiple overlapping stents. At the site of interest (*arrowhead*; A, B), the LAD well-visualized with PCCT (A – longitudinal stretched MPR, B – orthogonal cross section MPR) and with a traditional energy-integrating detector 320-slice multidetector CT scanner (C – longitudinal stretched MPR, D – orthogonal cross section MPR); 0.35 s rotation time, 16 cm acquisition, 0.625 mm slice thickness, matrix 512 × 512). PCCT allows the assessment of the stent lumen even in the tapering mid LAD, whereas traditional energy-integrating detector CT scanner images depict even the previously unstented more proximal LAD lumen with less detail.

The lower panel (Panel 3) shows a proximal circumflex stent (2.5 mm diameter) LAD visualized with PCCT (A – longitudinal stretched MPR, B – orthogonal cross section MPR) and with the older energy-integrating detector 320-row multidetector CT scanner (C – longitudinal stretched MPR, D – orthogonal cross section MPR); 0.35 s rotation time, 16 cm acquisition, 0.625 mm slice thickness, matrix 512 × 512). PCCT reveals a homogeneous texture of the stent struts and of the intra-stent lumen, whereas the previous generation CT scanner does not result in a confident endoluminal evaluation. *CT*, Computed tomography; *CX*, left circumflex coronary artery; *LAD*, left anterior descending coronary artery; *MIP*, maximum intensity projections; *MPR*, multiplanar reconstructions; *PCCT*, photon counting CT; *QIR*, quantum iterative reconstructions.

bypass surgery are the left and right internal mammary artery, the radial artery, and saphenous vein grafts (Fig. 10.3). Less commonly used grafts are the gastroepiploic and inferior epigastric arteries. The left internal mammary artery (LIMA), which originates from the subclavian artery and runs close to the sternal border along the anterior chest wall, is typically reserved for the LAD. The LIMA is used as an in situ graft; the proximal part is left intact and the distal artery is detached from the chest wall for anastomosis to the coronary artery. The LIMA provides the intercostal arteries, and after ligation of these side branches metal clips are often visible along the course of the LIMA graft (Fig. 10.3). The right internal mammary artery (RIMA) can be similarly harvested as an in situ graft for instance to supply the RCA (Fig. 10.3). The RIMA may also be used as a free graft with a proximal anastomosis to the ascending aorta or anastomosed as a Y-graft to the LIMA. Free radial artery graft can be used in a similar fashion. Venous grafts are harvested from the upper or lower leg and need to be anastomosed in a reversed direction because of the presence of valves. Each graft may supply a single coronary branch, or a single graft can sequentially supply multiple coronary branches using side-to-side anastomoses.

Scan Techniques

The data acquisition protocol after CABG is similar to a standard CCTA scan, except that the scan range needs to be extended cranially to include the proximal grafts. As a result, more contrast medium and a longer breath hold are required. In the past, exams on scanners with limited longitudinal coverage benefited from a caudo-cranial scan direction to avoid motion artifacts at the level of the heart due to an incomplete breath hold. Heart rate modulation and nitroglycerin remain important to optimize image quality, particularly for interpretation of the coronary anastomoses and distal runoffs.

Image Interpretation

Various postprocessing tools can be used for image interpretation after CABG (Fig. 10.3). Axial scrolling will provide a

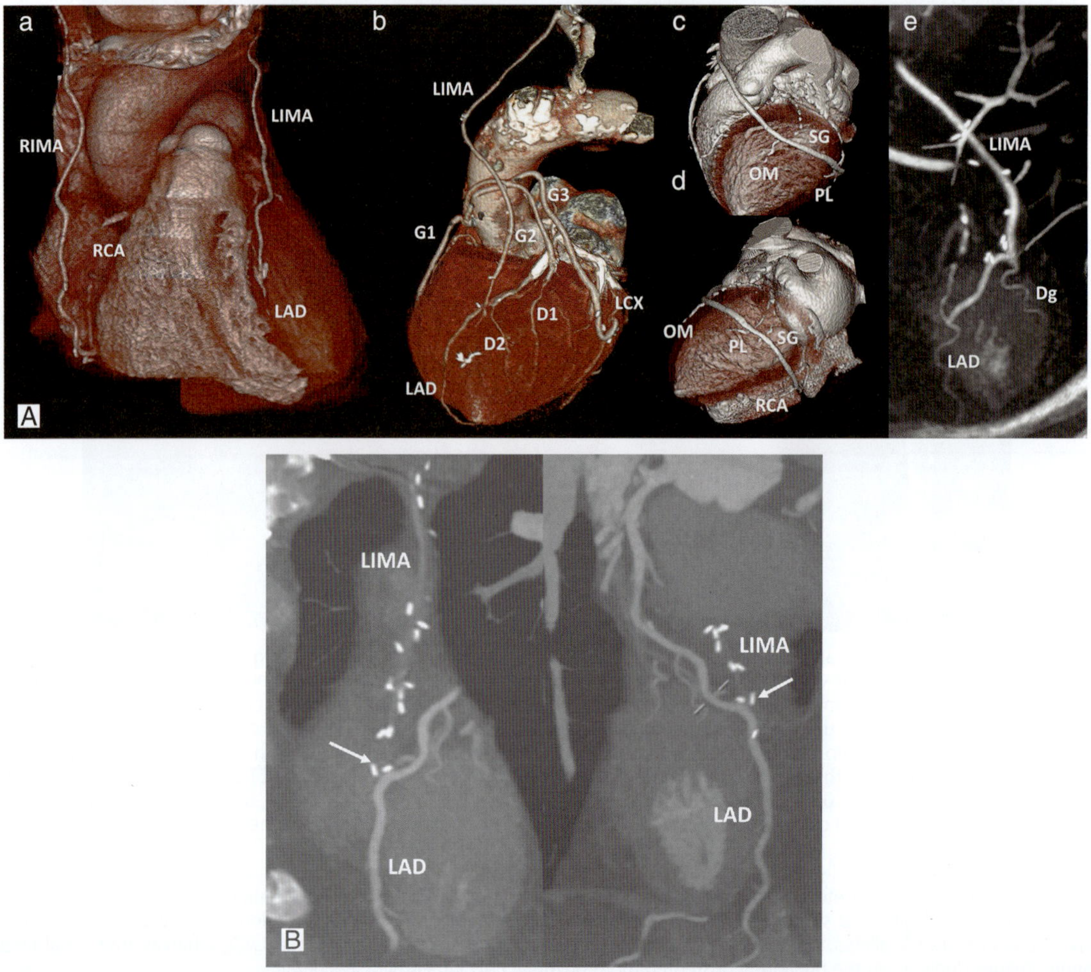

FIG. 10.3 Examples of bypass graft surgery. (A): (a) Arterial revascularization with the right internal mammary artery (RIMA) anastomosed to the right coronary artery (RCA) and the left internal mammary artery (LIMA) anastomosed to the left anterior descending coronary artery (LAD). (b) Single grafts including a LIMA to the second diagonal branch (D2) and three free grafts (G1-3) proximally anastomosed to the aorta and distally to the RCA (out of view), the first diagonal branch (D1), and the marginal branch of the left circumflex branch (LCX), respectively. (c and d) Sequential saphenous vein graft (SG) anastomosed to an obtuse marginal branch (OM), a left posterolateral branch (PL), and finally the posterior descending artery of the RCA. (e) LIMA sequentially anastomosed to a diagonal branch (Dg) and the distal LAD. (B): Occluded LIMA. The left internal mammary artery (LIMA) anastomosed (*arrow*) to the left anterior descending coronary artery (LAD) is functionally occluded, faint contrast enhancement can be seen in the proximal section. This may be the result of competitive flow through the native LAD, which shows only moderately obstructive disease.

first impression of the location and patency of the grafts. Further interrogation using double-oblique multiplanar reformations along the course of the graft and distal run-off provide a better overview of the angiographic integrity. Longer vessels segments can be depicted in a single image using thin-slab maximum-intensity projection. Curved multiplanar reformations provide a complete overview of the graft and distal runoffs. Three-dimensional volume-rendered reconstructions are also helpful to identify grafts and depict their exact course. Application of advanced display methods may require more manual editing because automated algorithms often do not recognize bypass grafts.

After cardiothoracic surgery various sorts of surgical material may be encountered in the chest, some of which may challenge interpretation of the scan. Radiopaque indicators may be present in the ascending aorta near the proximal graft anastomoses. Intended to help locate grafts during invasive angiography, they may result in substantial artifacts on CT scans. Vascular clips can interfere with interpretation of the LIMA, particularly near the anastomosis to the coronary artery. Other metal objects, such as sternal wires, pacemaker, and implantable cardioverter-defibrillator (ICD) electrodes, may also cause artifacts that affect grafts in their proximity.

A comprehensive evaluation systematically includes assessment of graft patency and distal coronary disease. In case of an occluded graft, it is also important to consider alternative blood supply by the native proximal coronary artery (Fig. 10.4), by distal graft segments that have remained patent, or by coronary collaterals.

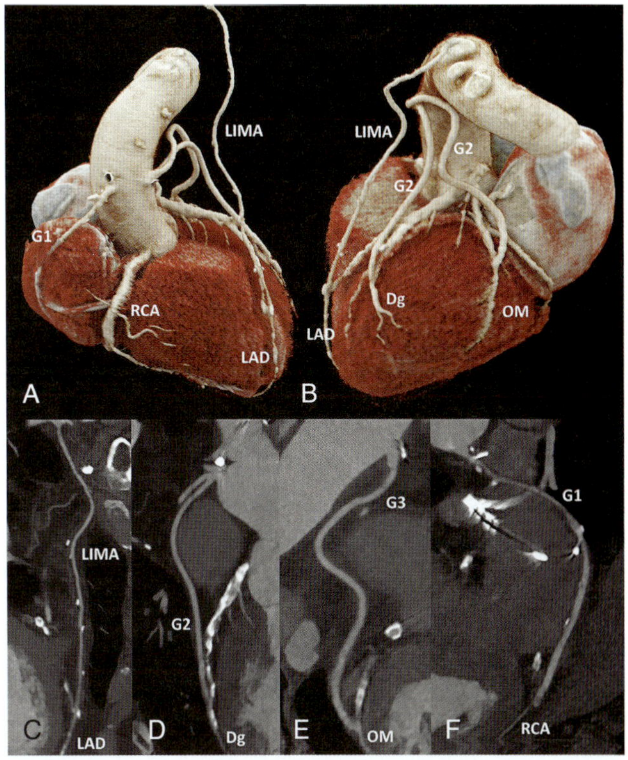

FIG. 10.4 Normal bypass grafts. Three-dimensional volume-rendered reconstructions (A, B) and curved reconstructions (C–F) of a CT angiogram after 4-vessel bypass graft surgery. The left internal mammary artery (LIMA) anastomosed to the left anterior descending coronary artery (LAD). Bright structures along the LIMA are vascular clips to close the (inter-costal) side branches. Two free grafts (G2 and G3) with a joint connection to the aorta are anastomoses to a diagonal branch (Dg) and a marginal branch (OM), respectively. The proximal LAD and diagonal branch show diffuse calcific coronary artery disease (D). A free graft (G1) with mild narrowing of the proximal segment is anastomosed to the distal RCA.

Detection of Bypass Graft Disease

Because of their larger size and limited displacement, CCTA can accurately detect bypass graft disease (Fig. 10.5). For complete graft occlusion, the sensitivity and specificity of CCTA approaches 100% (Table 10.1).[14–21] In case of sequential grafts, only a segment of the graft may be occluded. Graft stenosis can be detected with high accuracy as well; however, for stenosis quantification of saphenous vein grafts, the naturally varying diameter size needs to be taken into account. Assessment of the distal graft anastomoses can be challenging due to cardiac motion and vascular clips.[15] In most technical validation studies, >50% narrowing was considered significant stenosis. Often the diameter of the graft is larger than the target coronary artery, in which case moderate graft narrowing should not cause significant flow obstruction. In a clinical context, angiographic significance may be more appropriately defined as graft narrowing with a residual lumen diameter that is less than 50% of the diameter of the target coronary artery.[22] In addition to thrombotic or atherosclerotic graft disease, obstruction may be mechanical due to compression, kinking, or tethering. Rare aneurysms of bypass grafts can grow to a considerable size. Overall, no difference in CT performance has been reported for imaging of arterial versus venous grafts.[23] Diagnostic performance is decreased in the presence of arrhythmia.[17] Several studies included evaluation of the native coronary artery disease and reported overall lower performance compared to studies performed in patients without prior CABG.[16, 18, 24]

Clinical Indications for Cardiac CT After Bypass Graft Surgery

Early after surgery, cardiac CT can identify general complications from cardiothoracic surgery and specific graft-related issues such as early occlusion or a leaking anastomosis. In a consecutive cohort of 192 patients who underwent CCTA 1 week after CABG, 6% of arterial and 11% of venous graft had silently failed.[25] For symptomatic patients with suspected obstructive disease, cardiac CT can reliably assess graft failure. In patients who have had prior CABG, the 2021 AHA/ACC/ASE/CHEST/SAEM/SCCT/SCMR Guideline for the Evaluation and Diagnosis of Chest Pain consider it reasonable to perform CCTA in patients presenting with stable chest pain and are suspected to have myocardial ischemia (Class 2a), consider CCTA effective in patients presenting with acute chest pain who do not have an acute coronary syndrome (ACS) (Class 1), and evaluate for graft stenosis or occlusion. More challenging is the interpretation of the native coronary arteries. Distal coronary runoffs as well as nongrafted coronary branches may be diffusely diseased with extensive calcific plaque. Identification of the culprit lesion that is responsible for newly developed symptoms is often not straightforward. Failed grafts that are encountered on a CT scan may have occluded subclinically and be in that state for a long time. Moderate stenosis of a large-sized graft may not cause functional obstruction. Stress imaging may be necessary to identify the lesion that causes ischemia and determine further management. At the present time there are no CT-based fractional flow reserve applications suitable for post-CABG patients. There is no extensive experience with CT myocardial perfusion imaging after bypass graft surgery. Assessment of myocardial viability should be considered before revascularization of failed grafts or progressive coronary artery disease (CAD) is considered. Myocardial infarction may be evident by thinning of the myocardium or a perfusion defect on CCTA. Alternatively, although not commonly performed, a late-enhancement scan can better delineate the transmural extent of the scar. In preparation of CABG, valuable information about the availability of arterial graft material or the extent of aortic calcification can be obtained from CT scans. Before redo cardiothoracic surgery, cardiac CT can be valuable to avoid complications by evaluating the distance between the sternal wires and the right ventricle as well as bypass grafts. In case a patent bypass graft runs close to or crosses the sternum, an alternative surgical approach may be elected (Fig. 10.6). Cardiac CT has been used as an end point in a number of clinical trials investigating interventions to prevent graft failure.[26–28]

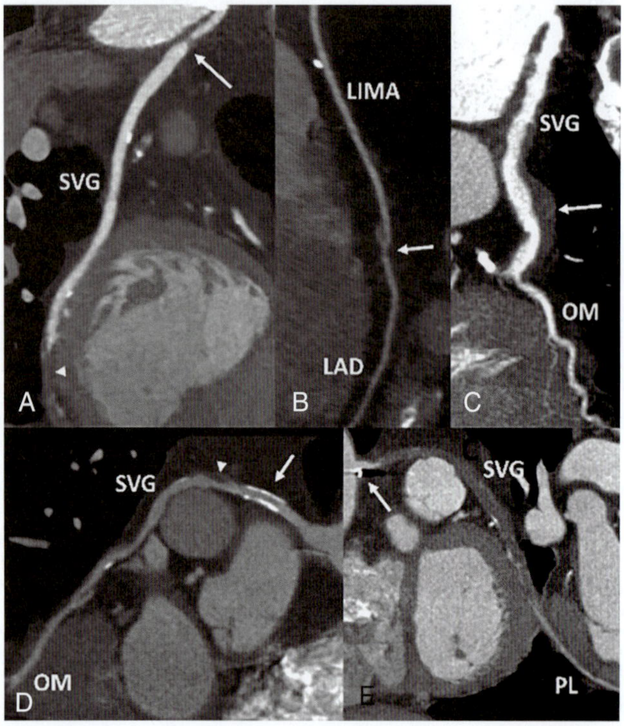

FIG. 10.5 Graft pathology. (A) Saphenous vein graft (SVG) with a proximal stenosis (*arrow*) and acute occlusion of the distal segment (*arrowhead*). (B) Mild stenosis of the left anterior descending coronary artery (LAD) distal to the anastomosis site of the left internal mammary artery (LIMA). (C) Outwardly remodeled SVG with suspected thrombus anastomosed to an obtuse marginal branch (OM). (D) SVG to a marginal branch after stenting with residual, mildly obstructive disease (*arrowhead*). (E) Occluded SVG to a posterolateral branch (PL). The distal vessel is retrogradely filled by collaterals. At the proximal anastomosis site a radiopaque marker causes a high-density artifact (*arrow*).

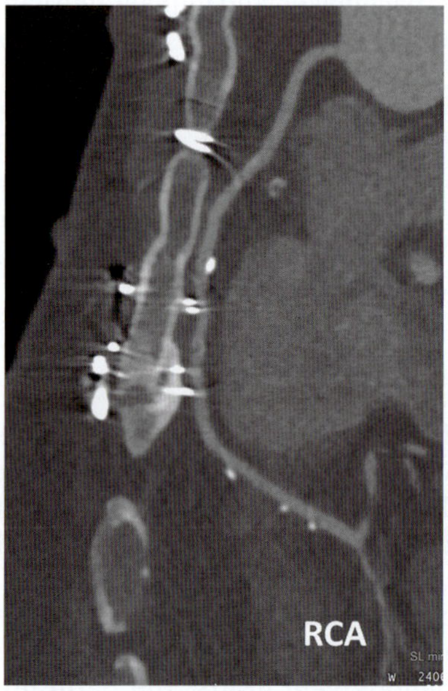

FIG. 10.6 CCTA before redo thoracic surgery. Proximity of the saphenous vein graft (SVG) to the sternum is relevant before redo thoracotomy. *RCA*, Right coronary artery.

TABLE 10.1 CCTA Performance in Bypass Graft Disease

LEAD AUTHOR, YEAR	N	GRAFTS	SCANNER	EXCLUDED	SENSITIVITY	SPECIFICITY
Ropers, 2006	50	139	64 SSCT	–	100%	97%
Jabara, 2007	50	147	64 SSCT	17%	93/100%[a]	100%
Malagutti, 2007	52	109	64 SSCT	–	99%	96%
Meyers, 2007	138	418	64 SSCT	–	97%	97%
Onuma, 2007	54	146	64 SSCT	5%	100%	98%
Weustink, 2009	52	152	64 DSCT	–	100%	96%
Andreini, 2012	119	277	64 SSCT	–	100%	99%

[a]Sensitivity for graft occlusion and graft stenosis, respectively.
Selected studies validating CCTA against invasive angiography. Sensitivity and specificity per graft or graft segment. scanner technology: 64-slice single-source (64-SSCT) and dual-source CT (DSCT).

REFERENCES

1. Abbara S, Blanke P, Maroules CD, et al. SCCT guidelines for the performance and acquisition of coronary computed tomographic angiography: a report of the society of Cardiovascular Computed Tomography Guidelines Committee: endorsed by the North American Society for Cardiovascular Imaging (NASCI). *J Cardiovasc Comput Tomogr.* 2016;10(6):435–449. doi:10.1016/j.jcct.2016.10.002.
2. Hecht HS, Gade C. Current and evolving stent evaluation by coronary computed tomographic angiography. *Catheter Cardiovasc Interv.* 2011;77(6):843–859. doi:10.1002/ccd.22897.
3. Nieman K. Noninvasive stent imaging with MSCT. *EuroIntervention.* 2009;5(Suppl D):D107–D111.
4. Decker JA, O'Doherty J, Schoepf UJ, et al. Stent imaging on a clinical dual-source photon-counting detector CT system-impact of luminal attenuation and sharp kernels on lumen visibility. *Eur Radiol.* 2023;33(4):2469–2477. doi:10.1007/s00330-022-09283-4.
5. Mannil M, Hickethier T, von Spiczak J, et al. Photon-counting CT: high-resolution imaging of coronary stents. *Invest Radiol.* 2018;53(3):143–149. doi:10.1097/RLI.0000000000000420.
6. Park D-W, Kim Y-H, Yun S-C, et al. Complexity of atherosclerotic coronary artery disease and long-term outcomes in patients with unprotected left main disease treated with drug-eluting stents or coronary artery bypass grafting. *J Am Coll Cardiol.* 2011;57(21):2152–2159. ISSN 0735-1097. https://doi.org/10.1016/j.jacc.2011.01.033.7. https://www.sciencedirect.com/science/article/pii/S073510971101179X.
7. Gulati M, Levy PD, Mukherjee D, et al. 2021 AHA/ACC/ASE/CHEST/SAEM/SCCT/SCMR guideline for the evaluation and diagnosis of chest pain: a report of the American College of Cardiology/American Heart Association joint committee on clinical practice guidelines. *Circulation.* 2021;144(22):e368–e454. doi:10.1161/CIR.0000000000001029.
8. Akers SR, Panchal V, Ho VB, et al. ACR appropriateness criteria® chronic chest pain-high probability of coronary artery disease. *J Am Coll Radiol.*. 2017;14(5S):S71–S80. doi:10.1016/j.jacr.2017.01.034.
9. Hagar MT, Soschynski M, Saffar R, et al. Accuracy of ultrahigh-resolution photon-counting CT for detecting coronary artery disease in a high-risk population. *Radiology.* 2023;307(5):e223305. doi:10.1148/radiol.223305.
10. Si-Mohamed SA, Boccalini S, Lacombe H, et al. Coronary CT angiography with photon-counting CT: first-in-human results. *Radiology.* 2022;303(2):303–313. doi:10.1148/radiol.211780.
11. Meloni A, Cademartiri F, Positano V, et al. Cardiovascular applications of photon-counting CT technology: a revolutionary new diagnostic step. *J Cardiovasc Dev Dis.* 2023;10(9):363. doi:10.3390/jcdd10090363.
12. Andreini D, Collet C, Leipsic J, et al. Pre-procedural planning of coronary revascularization by cardiac computed tomography: an expert consensus document of the Society of Cardiovascular computed tomography. *J Cardiovasc Comput Tomogr.* 2022;16(6):558–572. doi:10.1016/j.jcct.2022.08.003.
13. Fitzgibbon GM, Kafka HP, Leach AJ, Keon WJ, Hooper GD, Burton JR. Coronary bypass graft fate and patient outcome: angiographic follow-up of 5,065 grafts related to survival and reoperation in 1,388 patients during 25 years. *J Am Coll Cardiol.* 1996;28(3):616–626. doi:10.1016/0735-1097(96)00206-9.
14. Ropers D, Pohle FK, Kuettner A, et al. Diagnostic accuracy of noninvasive coronary angiography in patients after bypass surgery using 64-slice spiral computed tomography with 330-ms gantry rotation. *Circulation.* 2006;114(22):2334–2341; quiz 2334. doi:10.1161/CIRCULATIONAHA.106.631051.
15. Jabara R, Chronos N, Klein L, et al. Comparison of multidetector 64-slice computed tomographic angiography to coronary angiography to assess the patency of coronary artery bypass grafts. *Am J Cardiol.* 2007;99(11):1529–1534. doi:10.1016/j.amjcard.2007.01.026.
16. Malagutti P, Nieman K, Meijboom WB, et al. Use of 64-slice CT in symptomatic patients after coronary bypass surgery: evaluation of grafts and coronary arteries. *Eur Heart J.* 2007;28(15):1879–1885. doi:10.1093/eurheartj/ehl155.
17. Meyer TS, Martinoff S, Hadamitzky M, et al. Improved noninvasive assessment of coronary artery bypass grafts with 64-slice computed tomographic angiography in an unselected patient population. *J Am Coll Cardiol.* 2007;49(9):946–950. doi:10.1016/j.jacc.2006.10.066.
18. Onuma Y, Tanabe K, Chihara R, et al. Evaluation of coronary artery bypass grafts and native coronary arteries using 64-slice multidetector computed tomography. *Am Heart J.* 2007;154(3):519–526. doi:10.1016/j.ahj.2007.04.054.
19. Opolski MP, Kim WK, Liebetrau C, et al. Diagnostic accuracy of computed tomography angiography for the detection of coronary artery disease in patients referred for transcatheter aortic valve implantation. *Clin Res Cardiol.* 2015;104(6):471–480. doi:10.1007/s00392-014-0806-z.
20. Weustink AC, Nieman K, Pugliese F, et al. Diagnostic accuracy of computed tomography angiography in patients after bypass grafting: comparison with invasive coronary angiography. *JACC Cardiovasc Imaging.* 2009;2(7):816–824. doi:10.1016/j.jcmg.2009.02.010 Erratum in: JACC Cardiovasc Imaging. 2010;3(5):553. Meijboom, Bob W [corrected to Meijboom, W Bob].
21. Andreini D, Pontone G, Mushtaq S, et al. Diagnostic performance of two types of low radiation exposure protocol for prospective ECG-triggering multidetector computed tomography angiography in assessment of coronary artery bypass graft. *Int J Cardiol.* 2012;157(1):63–69. doi:10.1016/j.ijcard.2010.11.015.
22. FitzGibbon GM, Burton JR, Leach AJ. Coronary bypass graft fate: angiographic grading of 1400 consecutive grafts early after operation and of 1132 after one year. *Circulation.* 1978;57(6):1070–1074.
23. Chan M, Ridley L, Dunn DJ, et al. A systematic review and meta-analysis of multidetector computed tomography in the assessment of coronary artery bypass grafts. *Int J Cardiol.* 2016;221:898–905. doi:10.1016/j.ijcard.2016.06.264.
24. Weustink AC, Nieman K, Pugliese F, et al. Diagnostic accuracy of computed tomography angiography in patients after bypass grafting: comparison with invasive coronary angiography. *JACC Cardiovasc Imaging.* 2009;2(7):816–824 doi:10.1016/j.jcmg.2009.02.010. Erratum in: JACC Cardiovasc Imaging. 2010;3(5):553. Meijboom, Bob W [corrected to Meijboom, W Bob].
25. Zientara A, Rings L, Bruijnen H, et al. Early silent graft failure in off-pump coronary artery bypass grafting: a computed tomography analysis†. *Eur J Cardiothorac Surg.* 2019;56(5):919–925. doi:10.1093/ejcts/ezz112.
26. Perrault LP, Carrier M, Voisine P, et al. Sequential multidetector computed tomography assessments after venous graft treatment solution in coronary artery bypass grafting. *J Thorac Cardiovasc Surg.* 2019:S0022-5223(19)32503-6. 10.1016/j.jtcvs.2019.10.115.
27. Willemsen LM, Janssen PWA, Peper J, et al. Effect of adding ticagrelor to standard aspirin on saphenous vein graft patency in patients undergoing coronary artery bypass grafting (POPular CABG): a randomized, double-blind, placebo-controlled trial. *Circulation.* 2020;142(19):1799–1807. doi:10.1161/CIRCULATIONAHA.120.050749 Retracted and republished in: Circulation. 2021;144(2):e36.
28. Zhao Q, Zhu Y, Xu Z, et al. Effect of ticagrelor plus aspirin, ticagrelor alone, or aspirin alone on saphenous vein graft patency 1 year after coronary artery bypass grafting: a randomized clinical trial. *JAMA.* 2018;319(16):1677–1686. doi:10.1001/jama.2018.3197.

11 Approaches to Plaque Imaging by CCTA

ANDREW LIN, ANDREW D. CHOI, AND PÁL MAUROVICH-HORVAT

KEY POINTS

- Coronary computed tomography angiography (CCTA) enables noninvasive assessment of atherosclerotic plaque across the entire coronary tree.
- Visualization of the presence and extent of nonobstructive plaque and identification of high-risk plaque features can be performed during routine clinical reporting.
- Software-based quantitative plaque analysis provides a more robust assessment of plaque burden and morphology than visual evaluation alone.
- Plaque characterization and quantification by CCTA has prognostic value for lesion-specific and patient-level risk of major cardiovascular events.
- Serial quantitative plaque measurements can be used to assess plaque progression or regression and track the effects of medical therapies.

INTRODUCTION

The paradigm for coronary CT angiography (CCTA) imaging has evolved beyond luminal stenosis assessment to the imaging of atherosclerosis within the vessel wall.[1,2] Recent advancements in CT scanner technology now enable whole heart characterization and quantification of atherosclerotic plaque with high accuracy when compared with invasive reference standards. Coronary plaque burden and composition influence cardiovascular risk and outcomes and could potentially be used as surrogate endpoints to guide preventative care and assess response to therapies.[3] In this chapter, we synthesize the burgeoning evidence regarding CCTA imaging of atherosclerosis, discuss clinical implications, highlight advantages and limitations of current plaque assessment techniques, and identify emerging technologies in this progressive field.

TECHNICAL CONSIDERATIONS FOR PLAQUE IMAGING

For image interpretation, an appropriate window level and window width setting is required for accurate grayscale differentiation between the contrast-enhanced lumen and calcified plaque as well as the vessel wall and noncalcified plaque. Guidelines from the Society of Cardiovascular Computed Tomography (SCCT) recommend an initial window width of 800 Hounsfield units (HU) and window level of 300 HU, with subsequent adjustments by the clinician depending on the extent of calcification, contrast intensity, and visual differentiation of stenosis and plaque morphologies.[4] Plaque assessment should be systematically undertaken in epicardial coronary arteries ≥2.0 mm, using the SCCT 16-segment model of the coronary tree for a per segment analysis.[2]

Quantitative plaque analysis has been validated against intravascular ultrasound (IVUS) using both early and latest generation scanners, across a range of heart rates (≥60 beats per minute),[5,6] and using standard tube voltages (100 and 120 kV).[7] Tube voltage, especially lower values (80 kV), has been shown to exert both direct and indirect (via increased luminal contrast attenuation) effects on calcified and noncalcified plaque attenuation,[8] an important consideration when performing plaque assessment on such scans.

HIGH-RISK PLAQUE FEATURES

Definitions

The concept of the "vulnerable plaque" arose in the 1980s from autopsy studies following fatal acute myocardial infarction (MI). Histological features of culprit coronary lesions in these patients included a thin fibrous cap, large lipid-rich necrotic core, positive remodeling, and microcalcification,[9,10] as will be further discussed in Chapter 12 (Plaque on CCTA: Lessons From Histology). Intracoronary imaging modalities such as IVUS and optical coherence tomography (OCT), which focus on depicting a still frame of the plaque structure, can reliably identify some of these features.[11] However, invasive plaque characterization is technically complex, does not allow assessment of the entire coronary tree, and has modest positive predictive value for future acute coronary syndrome (ACS).[11]

CCTA enables noninvasive whole heart evaluation of plaque composition and morphology, including the classification of plaque as calcified or noncalcified[12] and the detection of specific high-risk plaque (HRP) features (Fig. 11.1), including:

- Positive remodeling (PR): present when the outer vessel diameter of the lesion is ≥10% larger than the diameter of a nondiseased proximal reference segment, that is, remodeling index ≥1.1.[13]
- Low-attenuation plaque (LAP): a central focal area within noncalcified plaque that has low CT attenuation. The

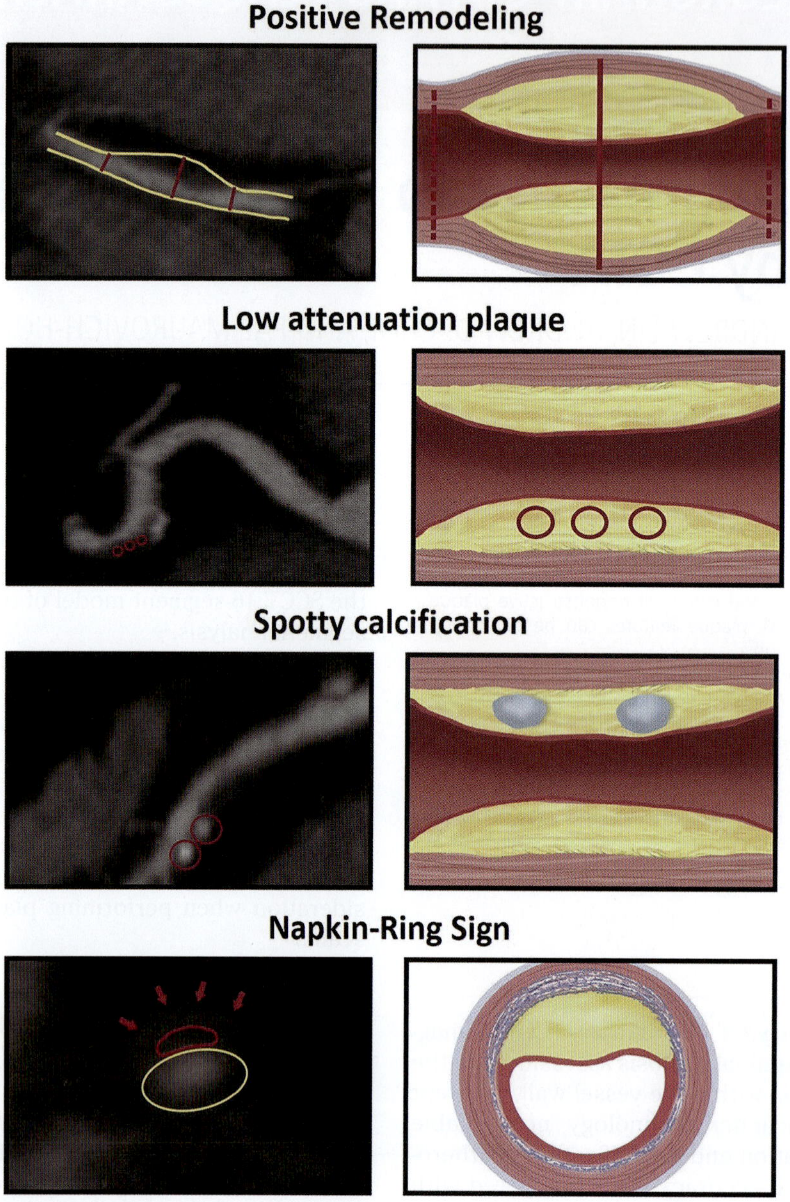

FIG. 11.1 High-risk plaque features. Representative images of positive remodeling, low-attenuation plaque, spotty calcification, and napkin-ring sign. (Modified from Puchner SB, Liu T, Mayrhofer T, et al. High-risk plaque detected on coronary CT angiography predicts acute coronary syndromes independent of significant stenosis in acute chest pain: results from the ROMICAT-II trial. *J Am Coll Cardiol*. 2014;64[7]:684–692.)

most widely used definition of low CT attenuation is a single voxel <30 HU,[14] whereas an alternative method requires three random region-of-interest measurements (0.5–1 mm^2) with a mean CT number of <30 HU.[15]

- Spotty calcification (SC): most commonly defined as any visually detectable calcification ≤3 mm in any direction within a plaque[13]; or alternatively, calcification with length <1.5 times the vessel diameter and width <2/3 the vessel diameter.[16]
- Napkin-ring sign (NRS): a ring-like morphology of noncalcified plaque with a central region of hypoattenuation that abuts the lumen and is surrounded by a rim of higher-attenuation noncalcified plaque tissue.[17]

CCTA-derived HRP features have been shown to associate with advanced atherosclerotic lesions, thin-cap fibroatheroma, and large necrotic cores when referenced by histological and invasive standards.[17–20] HRP features on CCTA are commonly observed in the culprit lesions of patients presenting with ACS[12,13,16,21] and are also associated with lesion-specific ischemia.

Although early CCTA studies included only PR and LAP[13,14] in their definitions of HRP, subsequent criteria have incorporated SC and NRS.[15,22,23] These features can be readily determined using a combination of visual assessment and simple distance and HU measurements on a standard workstation. Interobserver agreement for the presence of HRP has been reported as moderate-to-good (Cohen's kappa = 0.56–0.69).[22,24] Differences exist in interobserver variability for the identification of individual HRP features, with PR yielding the highest overall agreement.[21]

Established Prognostic Value of High-risk Plaque

The predictive value of HRP for future ACS in stable chest pain patients is well established. In a seminal study by

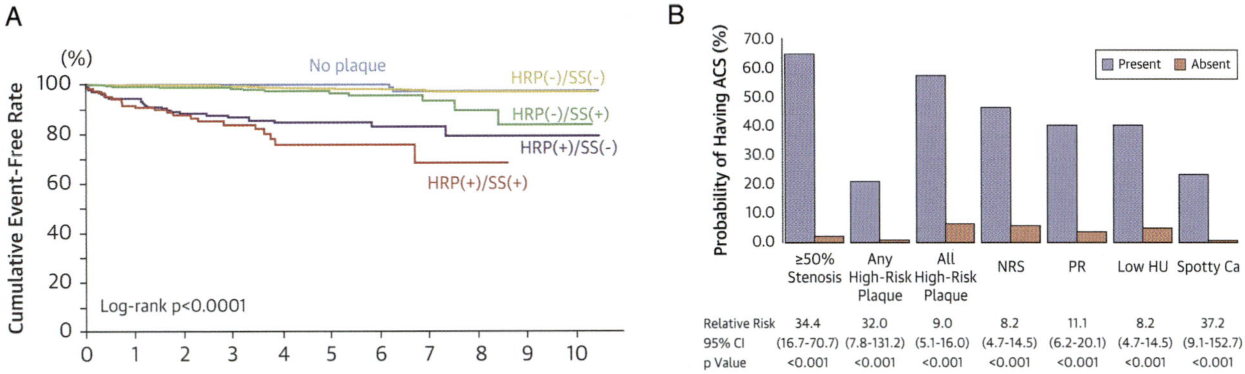

FIG. 11.2 High-risk plaque features and risk of acute coronary syndrome. (A) Kaplan-Meier event-free survival curves stratified by CCTA-verified high-risk plaque (HRP) and significant stenosis (SS) ≥70%. (B) Probability of acute coronary syndrome (ACS) during index hospitalization according to stenosis ≥50% and present of HRP features. *CCTA*, Coronary CT angiography. (Modified from [A] Motoyama S, Ito H, Sarai M, et al. Plaque characterization by coronary computed tomography angiography and the likelihood of acute coronary events in mid-term follow-up. *J Amn Coll Cardiol*. 2015;66[4]:337–346 and [B] Puchner SB, Liu T, Mayrhofer T, et al. High-risk plaque detected on coronary CT angiography predicts acute coronary syndromes independent of significant stenosis in acute chest pain: results from the ROMICAT-II trial. *J Am Coll Cardiol*. 2014;64[7]:684–692.)

Motoyama et al.[14] of 1059 patients undergoing clinically indicated CCTA, the presence of both PR and LAP conferred an ~23-fold higher risk of ACS during a mean follow-up interval of 27 months. The same authors extended these findings to 3158 patients with approximately 4 years of follow-up, in whom the presence of HRP (defined by PR and/or LAP) was associated with an eightfold greater risk of ACS, independent of severe stenosis and clinical risk factors[25] (Fig. 11.2A). The incidence of ACS was significantly higher in patients with two HRP features compared with patients with one HRP feature.

In a post-hoc analysis of 4415 patients from the PROMISE (Prospective Multicenter Imaging Study for Evaluation of Chest Pain) trial who were randomized to CCTA, the presence of HRP (defined by PR, LAP, and/or the NRS) was associated with an ~70% greater risk of major adverse cardiovascular events (MACE; defined as death, MI, or unstable angina).[22] Among patients with nonobstructive coronary artery disease, the presence of HRP increased MACE risk ~4-fold. There was also a stronger association of HRP with MACE in women than in men and in younger (<60 years) versus older (≥60 years) patients.

Investigators in the landmark SCOT-HEART (Scottish Computed Tomography of the HEART) randomized controlled trial showed in a post-hoc analysis that patients with CCTA-verified HRP (defined by PR and/or LAP) had a threefold greater risk of fatal or nonfatal MI over a median of 4.7 years of follow-up.[26] Notably, this association was not independent of the coronary artery calcium (CAC) score, a surrogate measure of overall plaque burden.

The predictive value of CCTA-derived HRP in the emergency department setting was evaluated in a secondary analysis of the ROMICAT-II (Rule Out Myocardial Infarction/Ischemia Using Computer-Assisted Tomography II) trial.[15] Among 472 patients presenting with acute chest pain but without evidence of MI, the presence of HRP was associated with an ~9-fold greater risk of ACS during the index admission, after adjustment for obstructive stenosis and clinical risk factors. All individual HRP features were associated with ACS, and patients with at least one HRP feature were 32 times more likely to have ACS during the index hospitalization (Fig. 11.2B).

A major limitation to the use of HRP for cardiovascular risk prediction is their high prevalence: 15% to 34% in the overall stable chest pain population, increasing to 63% to 75% among patients with severe stenosis.[22,26] Further, HRP has low positive predictive value for subsequent ACS,[22] and in the study by Motoyama et al.[25] the cumulative number of ACS patients without HRP was similar to patients with HRP. There are several possible explanations for these findings. First, plaques undergo continuous remodeling, and HRPs may stabilize with or without subclinical rupture, particularly in response to medical therapies such as statins. Thus identification of plaque characteristics at a single time point by CCTA may not be sufficient to predict long-term event risk. Second, lesion-specific HRP evaluation does not account for the overall coronary atherosclerotic disease burden, which has emerged as a major predictor of outcomes in patients with stable CAD.[27] This is reflected by the limitation of focal HRP to retain independent prognostic value in the SCOT-HEART subanalysis following adjustment for the CAC score.[26]

SEMIQUANTITATIVE PLAQUE ASSESSMENT

Estimating Plaque Burden

The Agatston CAC score derived from noncontrast CT is a surrogate measure of total atherosclerotic plaque burden and a predictor of major cardiovascular outcomes in both asymptomatic patients and patients with stable CAD, as discussed in Chapter 3 (Coronary Artery Calcium Scanning: Indications and Patient Management) However, whereas coronary calcifications are a highly specific feature of atherosclerosis, the Agatston score does not account for noncalcified plaque burden or HRP features, which are associated with greater patient-level risk of future ACS.[1] Further, coronary calcium scoring alone does not provide any information on luminal stenosis severity.

A practical problem in the visual assessment of coronary plaque on CCTA has been how to quantify and report atherosclerotic features for use in clinical reporting and prognosis estimation models. The most common approach is to divide the coronary tree into 16 segments and then score each segment according to certain simple criteria, which has given rise to several semiquantitative composite plaque burden scores. The segment involvement score (SIS) summarizes the total number of segments exhibiting plaque, irrespective of the stenosis severity within each segment (total score ranging from 0 to 16).[28] Meanwhile, the segment stenosis score (SSS) incorporates weighting factors for stenosis severity (scores from 0 to 3), and the stenosis scores of all 16 individual segments are summed to yield a total score ranging from 0 to 48.[28] The CT-adapted Leaman score accounts for coronary dominance, plaque location, degree of stenosis (obstructive versus nonobstructive), and type of plaque (calcified, noncalcified, or mixed).[29] The modified Duke CAD Index, also adopted for CCTA, integrates the number of affected vessels and the location of lesions with ≥50% stenosis.[28]

Prognostic Importance of Nonobstructive CAD

Nonobstructive CAD is uniquely identified by CCTA, the presence and extent of which associates with clinical outcomes. A recent metaanalysis of 17 studies with 49,957 patients showed the annualized rate of events (cardiac or all-cause mortality, ACS, or revascularization) for patients with nonobstructive CAD to be ~1.6%, compared with 0.2% for those with no plaque or stenosis.[2] Another metaanalysis of 11 studies with 7335 patients showed that each additional coronary segment containing plaque is associated with ~20% increase in the risk of future cardiovascular events (~30% increase for each segment containing noncalcified plaque).[30]

The semiquantitative plaque burden scores have also been prognostically validated in cohort studies of patients undergoing CCTA for suspected CAD. Bittencourt et al. showed that among patients with nonobstructive CAD, those with extensive plaque (defined by SIS >4) experienced a higher rate of cardiovascular death or MI than those with nonextensive plaque (SIS ≤4).[31] Notably, the event risk conferred by nonobstructive extensive disease was similar to that observed among patients with obstructive stenosis. Mushtaq et al.[29] showed a high CT-adapted Leaman score (>5) to be associated with a greater than fivefold risk of cardiac death or MI over mean follow-up of 4.3 years, independent of clinical risk factors. Patients with nonobstructive CAD and a high CT-adapted Leaman score had similar event-free survival to those with obstructive CAD. Finally, Min et al. demonstrated that an SSS >5 predicted a 5% higher absolute rate of all-cause mortality among 1127 stable chest pain patients followed up for a mean of 15 months.[28] In the same cohort, an increasing level of plaque as measured by the modified Duke CAD index was associated with a graded reduction in cumulative survival. These findings suggest that regardless of whether obstructive or nonobstructive disease is present, the extent of plaque detected by coronary computed tomography angiography enhances risk assessment.

QUANTITATIVE PLAQUE MEASUREMENT

Semiautomated Plaque Analysis

Quantitative plaque analysis from CCTA provides a more robust assessment of atherosclerotic plaque burden and morphology than composite plaque scores or HRP features. Plaque quantification can be performed using various semiautomated software solutions (Table 11.1 and the CAD-RADS), with measurements of plaque volume and composition demonstrating good agreement with the invasive reference standard of IVUS.[5,32,33] Although plaque quantification evaluation has previously been in the domain of research tools,[2] commercial software services for CCTA analysis are now clinically available.[34]

The workflow for semiautomated plaque assessment across the different platforms involves several common steps. First is coronary artery centerline extraction using

TABLE 11.1 Characteristics of Commonly Used Quantitative Plaque Analysis Software Platforms

SOFTWARE	VENDOR	METHOD	ACCESS	PLAQUE OUTPUT
SurePlaque	Canon Medical Systems, Japan	Computer assisted, semiautomated	Software license	Stenosis, plaque volume, vessel volume, plaque characteristics
QAngio	Medis Medical Systems, Netherlands	Computer assisted, semi-automated	Software license	Stenosis, plaque volume, vessel volume, plaque characteristics, remodeling index
Autoplaque	Cedars-Sinai Medical Center, USA	AI-enabled, automated	Software license	Stenosis, plaque volume, composition and burden, vessel volume, remodeling index, contrast density drop, plaque characteristics
vascuCAP	Elucid Bioimaging, USA	Computer assisted, semiautomated	Software license	Stenosis, plaque volume, vessel volume, remodeling index, plaque characteristics
Cleerly Coronary	Cleerly Healthcare, USA	AI-enabled, fully automated	Software service	Stenosis, plaque volume, vessel volume, remodeling index, plaque characteristics
Artificial Intelligence-Plaque Analysis	HeartFlow, USA	AI-enabled, automated	Software service	Stenosis, plaque volume, vessel volume, remodeling index, plaque characteristics
Syngo.via Frontier	Siemens Healthineers, Germany	Computer assisted, semiautomated	Software license	Stenosis, plaque volume, vessel volume, remodeling index, plaque characteristics

Adapted from Williams MC, Earls JP, Hecht H. Quantitative assessment of atherosclerotic plaque, recent progress and current limitations. *J Cardiovasc Comput Tomogr.* 2022;16(2):124–137.

automated algorithms. This is followed by automated detection of the lumen and outer vessel wall boundaries using mathematical or rule-based approaches; the coronary artery lumen is typically segmented using cross-sectional CCTA images, transforming the entire length of the vessel into a single volume. Next, the detected boundaries are manually adjusted by the reader in multiplanar reconstructed or cross-sectional views, with the extent of adjustment depending on CCTA image quality. Plaque is identified as all voxels between the lumen and vessel wall boundaries, then automatically measured by the software. Examples of several plaque assessment platforms with plaque components are shown in Fig. 11.3.

There is currently no standardized nomenclature for describing plaque volumes or plaque components and thus the terminology varies across different software vendors. Plaque size is typically measured volumetrically in cubic millimeters (mm^3), with analysis performed on a per-lesion,

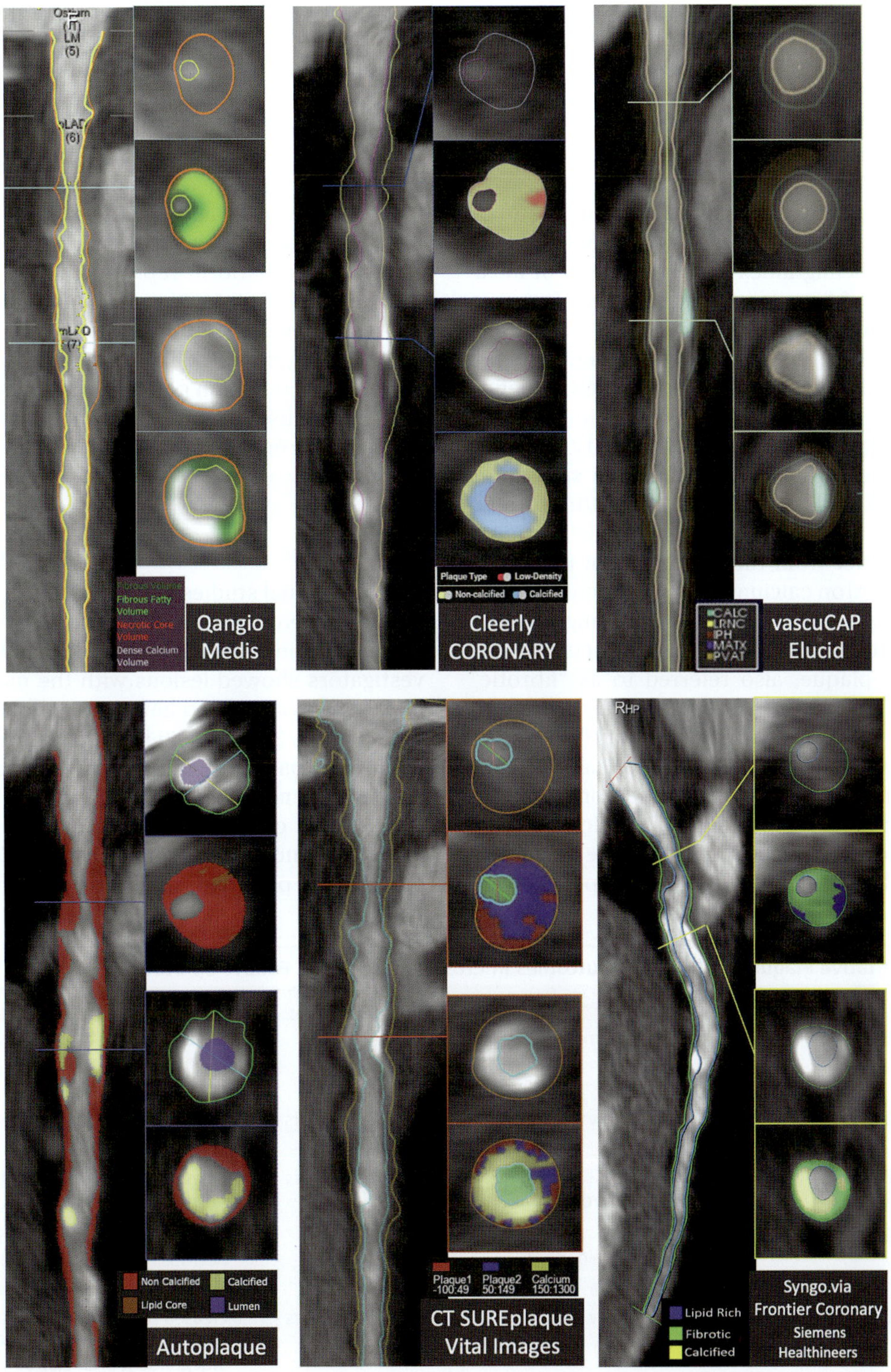

FIG. 11.3 Quantitative plaque analysis using semiautomated software. Curved planar reformations and cross-sectional views showing a case example of the left anterior descending artery analyzed by six of the most commonly used plaque analysis software platforms. (Courtesy of Siemens Medical Solutions USA, Inc.)

per-coronary segment, per-vessel, or per-patient level. In addition, the amount of plaque on a 2D CCTA cross-section can be determined by planimetry as plaque area (mm^2). Similar to IVUS methodology, the percentage of the overall vessel volume occupied by plaque on CCTA can be calculated as total plaque volume/vessel volume × 100%. This is termed "percent atheroma volume," "plaque burden volume ratio," or simply "plaque burden." The vessel volume (mm^3) used for indexation can represent either the analyzed segment of interest or the entire measurable vessel. Normalizing plaque volume to vessel volume reduces variability in this metric by accounting for differences in patient sex and body size and may be a more optimal method of reporting coronary atherosclerotic plaque burden.[35] On 2D cross-sectional plaque analysis, plaque area is indexed to vessel area (mm^2) to calculate the "cross-sectional plaque burden"; most commonly at the site of maximal stenosis.

Additional parameters automatically calculated by plaque analysis software include plaque length, plaque thickness, and remodeling index that is the ratio of maximal vessel dimension (diameter or area) within a lesion to that at a proximal "normal" reference point.

A high degree of heterogeneity exists among software vendors in the terminology and thresholds used to define plaque components. Calcified plaque, sometimes called "dense calcium," is generally defined by density ≥350 HU. Studies have reported additional calcification subgroups of 351–699, 700–1000, and >1000 HU, with the latter termed "1K plaque" and demonstrating very dense calcification.[36] These thresholds differ from the categories of HU densities used for the Agatston calcium score in noncontrast-enhanced CT scans, as contrast use during CT angiography is known to increase the attenuation of all vascular structures. Noncalcified plaque, also referred to as "fibrotic" or "medium density" plaque, is often subcategorized into fibrous (131–350 HU) and fibro-fatty (31–130 HU) components. Low-density noncalcified plaque, typically <30 HU but sometimes <60 HU, has the most varied nomenclature including "necrotic core," "lipid rich," "lipid rich necrotic core," or simply "low-attenuation plaque." The aforementioned HU thresholds for defining plaque components are set as default for most software platforms; however, they can be adjusted by the user. Some of the vendors utilize adaptive scan-specific thresholds that are automatically adjusted based on lumen attenuation[33]; this is particularly useful given that lumen attenuation influences the absolute HU of plaque components.[7]

The accuracy and reproducibility of software-based plaque measurements may be influenced by image quality and reader experience. Puchner et al. showed iterative reconstruction algorithms to improve image quality by reducing image noise, with resultant CCTA-derived cross-sectional plaque burden correlating more strongly with IVUS compared with traditional filtered back projection.[24] Meanwhile, in an ex vivo study, Stolzmann and colleagues showed plaque burden by CCTA to have excellent interreader reproducibility and high correlation with IVUS, irrespective of reconstruction algorithm.[37] Various software vendors have demonstrated close intraobserver and interobserver agreement for total and compositional plaque volumes using their respective platforms.[23,38,39] Data on interplatform reproducibility of plaque measurements, however, is lacking.[40] The interscan repeatability of per-lesion level quantitative plaque analysis has also been shown using serial CCTA scans with both matched[38] and different[41] acquisition parameters. Together, these findings support the use of CCTA for serial quantitative assessment of plaque progression, as will be discussed later in this chapter.

Association With Clinical Outcomes

Cross-sectional studies have demonstrated the association of quantitative plaque measurements with ACS and culprit lesions (Table 11.2). In a post-hoc analysis, ROMICAT II investigators showed lesions with the most severe stenosis in patients with ACS to have higher volumes of low-attenuation plaque (at both <30 HU and <60 HU thresholds) compared with patients without ACS.[42] Culprit lesions also had greater volumes of plaque <30 HU than nonculprit lesions.[21] Further, the cross-sectional plaque burden at the site of maximal stenosis using an optimized CCTA-specific threshold of 55% provided significantly higher discriminatory

TABLE 11.2 Quantitative Plaque Analysis and Outcomes in Cross-sectional and Follow-up Studies

STUDY	YEAR	N	COHORT	OUTCOME	FOLLOW-UP	FINDINGS
ROMICAT II	2015	260	Emergency department	ACS	–	Increased volume of plaque with attenuation <60 HU or <30 HU in the most severe stenosis in ACS patients
Nadjiri et al.	2016	1168	Suspected coronary artery disease	MACE	5.7 years	Increased NCP volume and LAP (<30 HU) volume in patients with MACE
ICONIC	2018	234	234 ACS 234 matched controls	ACS	3.4 years	Increased volume of fibrofatty (30–130 HU) and necrotic core (–30 to 30 HU) in ACS patients
de Knegt et al.	2019	855	274 asymptomatic 254 acute chest pain, no ACS 327 ACS	ACS	–	Increased total, fibrofatty (76–130 HU), and necrotic (–30 to 75 HU) plaque volume across clinical risk groups
SCOT-HEART	2020	1769	Suspected coronary artery disease	MI	4.7 years	Increased plaque burden (total, calcified, NCP, LAP) in patients with MI. LAP burden is an independent predictor of MI.

ACS, Acute coronary syndrome; *MACE*, major adverse cardiovascular events; *MI*, myocardial infarction.
Adapted from Williams MC, Earls JP, Hecht H. Quantitative assessment of atherosclerotic plaque, recent progress and current limitations. *J Cardiovasc Comput Tomogr.* 2022;16(2):124–137.

value for ACS compared with a traditional IVUS based threshold of 70% (area under the receiver operating characteristic curve [AUC] 0.83 versus 0.68).[21] In a mixed cohort study, de Knegt and colleagues[22] performed quantitative plaque analysis in 274 asymptomatic individuals, 254 patients with acute chest pain without ACS, and 327 patients with ACS. They showed a graded increase in total plaque volume across the clinical risk profiles (148 mm^3, 257 mm^3, and 407 mm^3, respectively). Moreover, per-patient proportions of necrotic core (–30 to 75 HU) and fibrofatty plaque (76–130 HU) increased with worsening clinical profile.

Longitudinal observational cohort studies have established the predictive value of plaque quantification for lesion-specific and patient-level risk of future cardiac events. In the recent ICONIC (Incident COroNary Syndromes Identified by Computed Tomography) substudy of the CONFIRM (Coronary CT Angiography Evaluation for Clinical Outcomes: An International Multicenter) registry, 234 patients with incident ACS during mean follow-up of 3.4 years were matched to 234 nonevent controls.[24] Quantitative plaque analysis on baseline CCTA scans showed that although total plaque volume was similar between patients with ACS and controls, the volumes of fibrofatty plaque (31–130 HU; 58.7 versus 41.4 mm^3) and necrotic core (–30 to 30 HU; 6.5 versus 4.2 mm^3) were significantly higher in patients with ACS. Similar findings were observed when plaque volumes were indexed to vessel volume. At a per-lesion level, culprit lesion precursors had greater volumes of fibrofatty plaque and necrotic core when compared with nonculprit lesions in ACS patients and with highest-grade stenosis lesions in controls (Fig. 11.4A). Notably, more than three-quarters of culprit lesion precursors had stenosis <50%, and close to one-third exhibited HRP.

In a post-hoc analysis of the SCOT-HEART trial, investigators performed quantitative plaque assessment on baseline CCTA in 1769 patients.[44] The burden (plaque volume/vessel volume × 100%) of total plaque, calcified plaque, noncalcified plaque, and low-attenuation (<30 HU) plaque

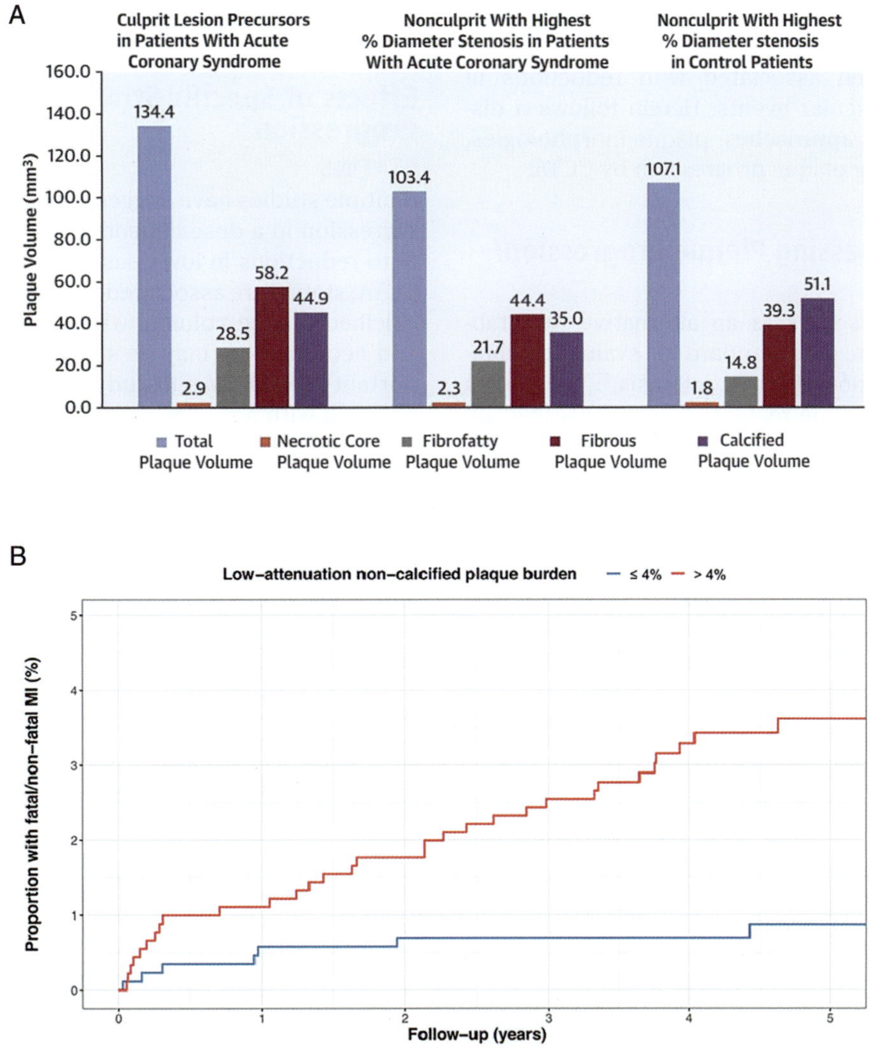

FIG. 11.4 Quantitative plaque parameters and risk of future acute coronary syndrome. (A) Culprit lesion precursors exhibited greater fibrofatty and necrotic core volumes compared with highest baseline percentage diameter stenosis nonculprit lesions in patients with subsequent acute coronary syndrome and with highest percentage diameter stenosis lesions in controls. (B) Kaplan-Meier curves showing cumulative incidence of fatal or nonfatal myocardial infarction in patients with and without low attenuation plaque burden greater than 4%. ([A] Modified from Chang HJ, Lin FY, Lee SE, et al. Coronary atherosclerotic precursors of acute coronary syndromes. *J Am Coll Cardiol*. 2018;71(22):2511–2522 and [B] Williams MC, Kwiecinski J, Doris M, et al. Lowattenuation noncalcified plaque on coronary computed tomography angiography predicts myocardial infarction. *Circulation*. 2020;141[18]:1452–1462.)

was higher in patients with subsequent MI during median follow-up of 4.7 years. Notably, low-attenuation plaque burden conferred the greatest risk for MI, independent of cardiovascular risk score, coronary artery calcium score, and stenosis severity. Patients with a low-attenuation plaque burden greater than 4% had a near fivefold risk of future MI (Fig. 11.4B). Together, the cross-sectional and cohort studies suggest that patients with stable CAD who have a higher overall burden of plaque, in particular low-attenuation plaque, are at greater risk of developing ACS.

ASSESSING PLAQUE PROGRESSION

CCTA offers multiparametric opportunities to track the natural history of atherosclerosis across the entire coronary tree, enabling per-lesion, per-vessel, and per-patient level analysis. The noninvasive nature of CCTA enables evaluation of lower risk patients in whom invasive coronary imaging may not be typically indicated. Treatment with cholesterol-lowering therapies has been associated with morphologic changes that include plaque regression and plaque stabilization. In addition, changes in plaque morphology have been associated with reductions in downstream cardiovascular events. Herein follows a discussion of assessment approaches, plaque morphologies, and evidence regarding plaque progression by CCTA.

Approaches to Assessing Plaque Progression/ Regression

Fundamentally, CCTA serves as an alternative to established IVUS imaging, the gold standard for evaluating clinically relevant progression of atherosclerosis.[45] The effects of statin therapy on plaque regression were assessed by IVUS in several large randomized trials.[46,47] Other invasive techniques with high spatial resolution include the use of OCT to detect thin-cap fibroatheroma, macrophages, and microvessels, and the use of near-infrared spectroscopy (NIRS) to assess and quantify lipid core burden.[48] IVUS has limitations that include resource constraints, high costs, and potential complications of an invasive procedure.[48] The interpretation of IVUS for plaque quantification may be time consuming. IVUS catheters have challenges traversing severely calcified or tortuous lesions as well as smaller side branch vessels.

The largest study to date of CCTA plaque progression is the PARADIGM (Progression of AtheRosclerotic PlAque DetermIned by Computed TomoGraphic Angiography IMaging) study, a prospective, open-label observational registry with 13 participating sites in seven countries.[49,50] The study encompassed 2252 patients with nonobstructive CAD undergoing serial CCTA ≥2 years apart with prospective clinical follow-up. PARADIGM sought to evaluate changes in adverse plaque characteristics through stenosis measures and quantitative plaque assessment. The study primary endpoints included changes in total plaque volume and plaque composition (Table 11.3) with secondary endpoints of major adverse cardiovascular events including cardiac and noncardiac death, myocardial infarction, unstable angina, and revascularization. Plaque quantitation was performed using semiquantitative software (QAngio CT, Research Edition, Medis Imaging, Leiden, the Netherlands) in an independent core laboratory by trained technicians. Each scan typically took several hours to perform plaque analysis.

Effects of Specific Strategies on Plaque Progression

STATINS

Multiple studies have suggested that statins induce plaque regression in a dose-dependent manner and proportionally to reductions in low-density lipoprotein cholesterol. By CCTA, statins are associated with an increase in fibrous and calcified plaque volume, whereas noncalcified, fibrofatty, and necrotic core may be stabilized or reduced. In an important PARADIGM substudy by Lee et al., statins were associated with a slower rate of overall atherosclerosis progression by percent atheroma volume (PAV: 1.76 ± 2.40% per year in statin-naïve versus 2.04 ± 2.37% per year in statin-taking patients, respectively; $P = .002$) but more rapid progression of calcified plaque[51] (Fig. 11.5). Statin therapy was associated with less noncalcified plaque progression and a lower annual incidence of high-risk plaque features but was not associated with a reduction in the rate of lesions becoming obstructive.

TABLE 11.3 Summary of PARADIGM Findings and Plaque Progression Associations

	FACTORS ASSOCIATED WITH PLAQUE PROGRESSION	FACTORS NOT ASSOCIATED WITH PLAQUE PROGRESSION
Quantitative Factors	Baseline percent atheroma volume	
Qualitative Factors		High-risk plaque features
Anatomical factors	Left main coronary artery disease	
Risk Factors	Age Male (noncalcified) Female (calcified) Diabetes mellitus High triglycerides Declining renal function High clinical risk Statin therapy (increased calcified plaque, reduced noncalcified plaque)	Prediabetes Chronic kidney disease Change in BMI >5%

Adapted from Indraratna P, Khasanova E, Gulsin GS, et al. Plaque progression: where, why, and how fast? A review of what we have learned from the analysis of patient data from the PARADIGM registry. *J Cardiovasc Comput Tomogr*. 2022;16(4):294–302.

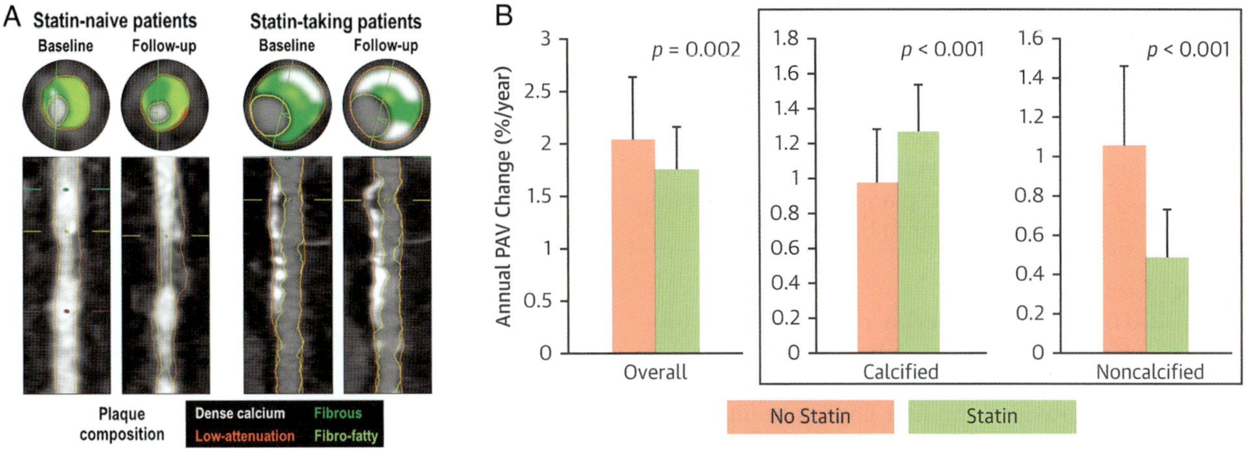

FIG. 11.5 Effects of statins on coronary atherosclerotic plaque. (A) Representative CCTA images of lesions at baseline and follow-up in the PARAGIDM (Progression of AtheRosclerotic PlAque Determined by Computed TomoGraphic Angiography IMaging) study. (B) The annualized change in percent atheroma volume (PAV) per lesion was lower in statin-taking patients (*green bars*) than in statin-naïve patients (*pink bars*). Statin therapy was associated with a 23% increase in calcified plaque volume and 54% decrease in noncalcified plaque volume. *CCTA*, Coronary CT angiography. (Reprinted with permission from Lee SE, Chang HJ, Sung JM, et al. Effects of statins on coronary atherosclerotic plaques: the PARADIGM study. *JACC Cardiovasc Imaging*. 2018;11(10):1475–1484.)

Statin use has been associated with a paradoxical increase in calcified plaque, particularly the coronary artery calcium score. A subgroup of 654 PARADIGM patients (statin naïve [n = 246] and statin taking [n = 408]) with CACS available were analyzed for CACS progression on serial CCTA. The mean CACS increased in both the statin naïve (59 ± 231 to 115 ± 426) and statin-taking groups (146 ± 382 to 252 ± 531).[52] On multivariable analysis, it was found that the change in CACS in the statin-naïve group reflected the progression of both calcified and noncalcified plaque, whereas in the statin-taking group, it reflected only the progression of calcified plaque. A metaanalysis by Andelius et al. of 12 studies found a reduction in noncalcified plaque volume by 8% and an increase in calcified plaque volume by 12% and calcium signal intensity by 22% in patients on statins.[53] It is presumed that measurement of CACS in patients taking statins may overestimate their risk of downstream events.

LIFESTYLE CHANGES AND ATHLETES

Intensive lifestyle interventions have been associated with a favorable change in plaque profile. The Dietary Intervention to Stop Coronary Atherosclerosis in Computed Tomography (DISCO-CT) trial randomized patients to optimal medical therapy + dietician follow-up in comparison to medical therapy alone.[54] At 1.2 years of follow-up, there were significant reductions in noncalcified plaque volume for both interventions (experimental arm ($\Delta = -51.3 \pm 79.5$ mm^3 [-1.7 ± 2.7%]; $P < .001$) and the control arm ($\Delta = -21.3 \pm 57.7$ [-0.7 ± 1.9%]; $P = .018$), but no differences in total percent atheroma volume. Cross-sectional studies assessing plaque composition in athletes have demonstrated higher plaque volume in athletes, whereas sedentary participants have had partially calcified plaque morphologies that are of higher risk for coronary artery events.[55,56] Other prospective trial assessment of diet and plaque progression include aged garlic extract[57] and omega-3 fatty acid[58] in small studies; however, these interventions have not been associated with a reduction in cardiovascular events in large trials.

TESTOSTERONE

Testosterone has been found to have an unfavorable effect on plaque progression by CCTA. In a double-blinded placebo-controlled trial of testosterone gel in older men with low testosterone, Budoff et al. evaluated the progression of noncalcified plaque volume.[59] Among the 138 patients (71 ± 6 years), testosterone was associated with a significantly greater increase in noncalcified plaque volume versus placebo from baseline to 12 months (204 mm^3 to 232 mm^3 versus 317 mm^3 to 325 mm^3, $P = .03$) with an increase in median total plaque volume from 272 mm^3 to 318 mm^3. Although the results were not favorable for testosterone, no major adverse cardiovascular events occurred in either group.

DIRECT ORAL ANTICOAGULANTS

Direct oral anticoagulants (DOACs) have shown favorable associations with plaque inhibition in small observational studies. Lee et al. randomized 97 patients to rivaroxaban versus warfarin and found an increase in total plaque volume at 12 months with vitamin K antagonists (VKA).[60]

Beyer et al. performed a small study of 161 patients with serial CCTA undergoing semiautomated quantification of total plaque volume blinded to patient details with mean scan interval of 3.2 years apart.[61] In comparing 61 control patients versus 50 direct oral anticoagulant patients (31 rivaroxaban, 10 dabigatran, 6 apixaban, and 3 edoxaban) and 50 with warfarin, there was an absolute plaque burden progression of 66.5 ± 136.7 mm^3 in VKA, 27.2 ± 73.6 mm^3 in controls and an inhibition in DOAC users with -7.1 ± 42.1 mm^3 ($P < .001$). Although not directly evaluated, the difference in plaque volume was in line with clinical outcomes with the Cardiovascular Outcomes for People Using Anticoagulation Strategies (COMPASS) trial in which the addition of low-dose anti-Xa inhibition resulted in reduction of cardiac and all-cause mortality.[62]

COLCHICINE

The favorable effect of colchicine plus optimal medical therapy versus optimal medical therapy alone on plaque volume has been prospectively assessed.[63] Vaidya et al.[63] showed 12 months of colchicine led to a significant reduction in low-attenuation plaque volume (15.9 mm^3 versus 6.6 mm^3; $P < .05$) and noncalcified plaque volume, whereas total atheroma volume was similar in both groups.

ICOSAPENT ETHYL (VASCEPA)

The EVAPORATE (Effect of Vascepa on Improving Coronary Atherosclerosis in People with High Triglycerides Taking Statin Therapy) randomized double-blind placebo-controlled trial provided the first important linkage of plaque regression to cardiovascular events.[64,65] It links to the results of 8179 patient REDUCE-IT (Reduction of Cardiovascular Events with EPA–Intervention Trial) that had evaluated icosapent ethyl versus placebo in reducing triglycerides, cardiovascular events, and cardiovascular death in patients at high cardiovascular risk and elevated triglycerides.[65,66] In EVAPORATE, icosapent ethyl was associated with a significant reduction in low-attenuation plaque volume by 17%, whereas in the placebo group low-attenuation plaque volume more than doubled (+109%, $P = .0061$).

HIV AND INFLAMMATORY CONDITIONS

Human immunodeficiency virus (HIV) has been found to be an inflammatory risk enhancer that has renewed interest in evaluating plaque progression in these patients. In a small pilot study, Lo et al.[67] evaluated the effect of atorvastatin in 40 HIV patients versus placebo and found a median change of –8.2 mm^3 versus 6.7 mm^3 ($P = .03$ [–19% versus +20%] $P < .001$) in noncalcified plaque volume. The REPRIEVE trial (Randomized Trial to Prevent Vascular Events in HIV) showed that among persons with human immunodeficiency virus infection, pitavastatin was associated with a lower risk of MACE compared with placebo.[68] The ongoing Mechanistic Substudy of REPRIEVE will examine the effects of pitavastatin on plaque regression by CCTA and the relationship of these changes with serum inflammatory biomarkers.[69]

PCSK-9 INHIBITION

In evaluating plaque progression with proprotein convertase subtilisin/kexin type 9 (PCSK-9), inhibition, there have been many trials by IVUS; however, there are no prospective randomized trials in CCTA to date. The VICTORIAN trial (clinicaltrials.gov: NCT04929249) will assess the role of inclisiran versus usual care in patients with maximally tolerated statin therapy to prospectively track changes in plaque progression. The EPIC-HIV study (Effect of PCSK9 Inhibition on Cardiovascular Risk in Treated HIV Infection) is evaluating alirocumab (PCSK-9 inhibitor) for HIV patients with evidence of vascular inflammation.

STRUCTURED REPORTING OF CORONARY PLAQUE

CAD-RADS 2.0

Standardized reporting of CCTA findings is recommended by multisociety guidelines.[2,48,70] The use of a structured report facilitates communication of important test results to referring physicians. Current guidelines focus on reporting the severity, location, and extent of stenosis and obstructive CAD. Recent guideline level recommendations now expand upon the reporting of nonobstructive CAD and atherosclerotic plaque assessment.

The CAD-RADS™ 2.0 (Coronary Artery Disease-Reporting and Data System) for reporting of CCTA adds modifiers “P1-P4” to denote the extent of plaque beyond stenosis categories as mild (P1), moderate (P2), severe (P3), and extensive (P4) amount of plaque (Table 11.4). To allow flexibility and ensure adoption in clinical practice, there are several options for estimated the overall amount of coronary plaque:

CAC Assessment

When CAC scoring is performed, the summary statement of the report should state total CAC score including risk categories (0: no CAC, 1–99: mild CAC, 100–299: moderate CAC, ≥300: severe CAC). The optional category of minimal CAC (1–9) is also in common use.

Segment Involvement Score

To address the limitations of qualitative visual assessment, the SIS, as previously described, was incorporated into CAD-RADS 2.0 (Table 11.4).

TABLE 11.4 Structured Reporting of Overall Plaque Burden by CAD-RADS 2.0

	OVERALL AMOUNT OF CORONARY PLAQUE	CAC	SIS[a]	VISUAL[a]
P1	Mild amount of plaque	≤100	≤2	1–2 vessels with mild amount of plaque
P2	Moderate amount of plaque	101–300	3–4	1–2 vessel with moderate amount; 3 vessels with mild amount of plaque
P3	Severe amount of plaque	301–999	5–7	3 vessels with moderate amount; 1 vessel with extensive amount of plaque
P4	Extensive amount of plaque	>1000	≥8	2–3 vessels with extensive amount of plaque

[a]As there is currently no one single method that should be used to identify the overall amount of plaque, CAD-RADS (Coronary Artery Disease Reporting and Data System) recommends that imagers select the technique that is considered most appropriate at a given institution.
Risk factor modification and preventive pharmacotherapy, particularly if P2 or greater. Consider more aggressive therapies if P3 or greater.
CAC, Coronary artery calcium; *SIS*, segment involvement score.
Adapted from Cury RC, Leipsic J, Abbara S, et al. CAD-RADS 2.0 - 2022 coronary artery disease-reporting and data system: an expert consensus document of the Society of Cardiovascular Computed Tomography (SCCT), the American College of Cardiology (ACC), the American College of Radiology (ACR), and the North America Society of Cardiovascular Imaging (NASCI). *JACC Cardiovasc Imaging*. 2022;15(11):1974–2001.

Visual Assessment

By CAD-RADS 2.0, a visual assessment of coronary plaque (Table 11.4) includes a description of the coronary location of plaque, the number of vessels involved, and description of the plaque type, including calcified plaque, noncalcified plaque, partially calcified plaque, and features of high-risk plaque (e.g., positive remodeling or low-density noncalcified plaque). Compared with the CAC score, a drawback of visual assessment of coronary plaque on contrast-enhanced CCTA is that it does not easily quantify the overall plaque burden. As visual interpretation is subjective, the reproducibility of this approach—although simple to integrate in routine practice—is likely variable.

High-risk Plaque

The presence of HRP should be included in CCTA reports, as recommended in CAD-RADS, as part of the report summary. When present, HRP should be included in the description of a lesion (using CAD-RADS modifier "HRP"), with the report conclusion noting that the presence of HRP is associated with a higher risk of ACS (when evaluating patients with acute chest pain) or higher risk of future MACE (when evaluating patients with stable chest pain).

Currently, individual HRP features considered in this definition include all features previously described in this chapter (i.e., positive remodeling, low-attenuation plaque, spotty calcification, and napkin-ring sign). The presence of HRP should be reported if at least two features are present in the same plaque to numerical CAD-RADS stenosis category of 1 to 5 and plaque volume category of P1 to P4. The presence of at least two HRP features increases the strength of association with future CAD events. In addition, when significant, the degree of PR may also be described. The presence of individual HRP features at vessel or segment level can be considered for the body of the report.

Structured reporting examples by CAD-RADS 2.0 are shown in Figs. 11.6 and 11.7.

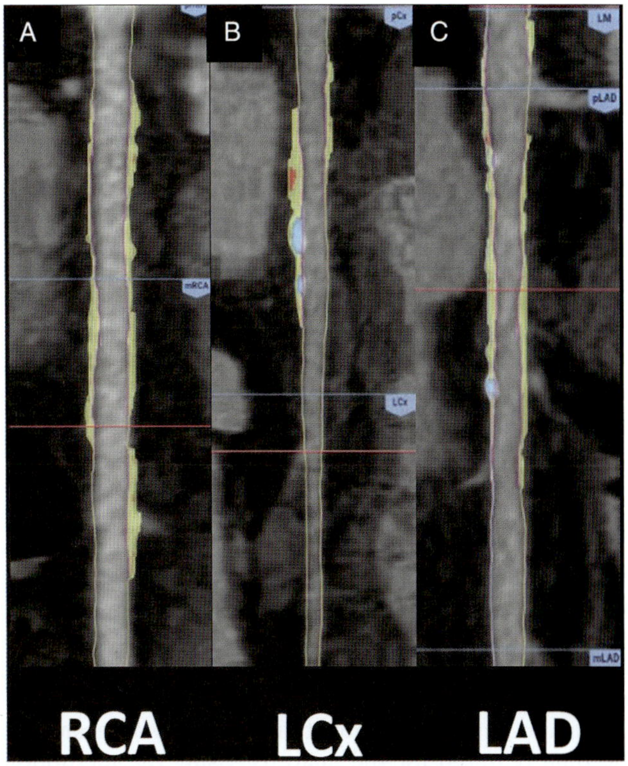

FIG. 11.6 CAD-RADS 2.0 case example. A 58-year-old man presented with acute chest pain and dyspnea. Mild stenosis (25–49%) of right coronary artery (RCA; A), left circumflex (LCx; B) and left anterior descending (LAD; C) with severe amount of plaque. The segment involvement score (SIS) is 6 and severe by visual estimate with three vessels with moderate plaque involvement. There is positive remodeling and low-density plaque consistent with high-risk plaque (HRP). CAD-RADS 2/HRP/P3. Noncalcified plaque is represented in *yellow*, low-density plaque by *red*, and calcified plaque by *blue* (Cleerly, Inc, Denver, CO, USA).

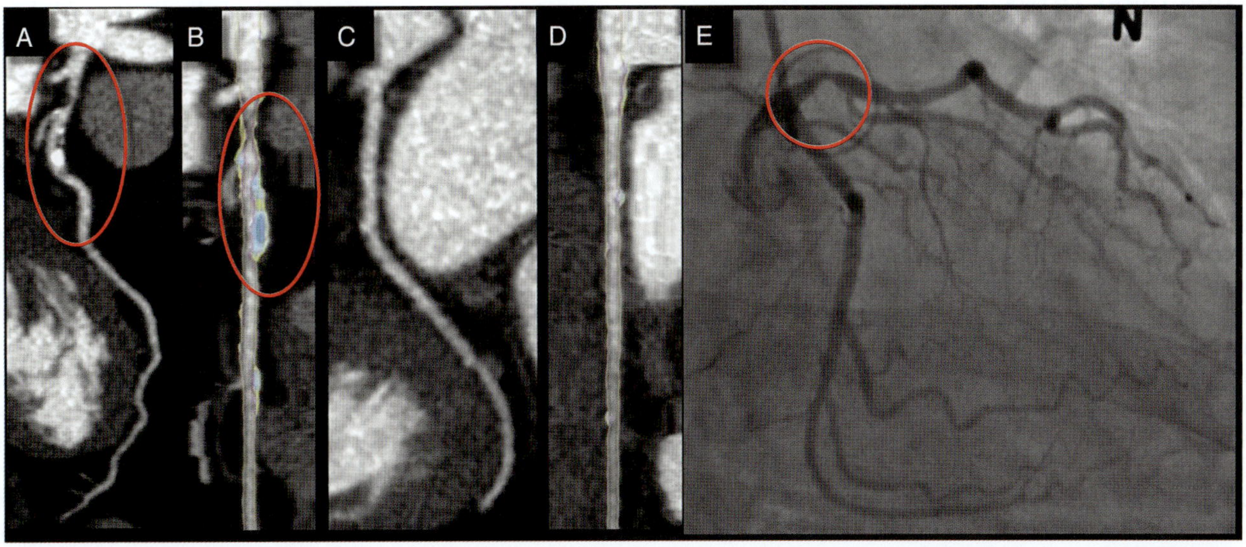

FIG. 11.7 CAD-RADS 2.0 Case example with invasive angiography and FFR correlation. A 72-year-old man presented with acute chest pain. CCTA with severe stenosis (>70%) and high plaque volume by visual estimate including one vessel with a severe amount of plaque with low density and positive remodeling (CAD-RADS 4/HRP/P3) of the proximal LAD (A)/(B). Minimal stenosis (<25%) of the left circumflex (C). Artificial Intelligence Guided Quantitative Computed Tomography (AI-QCT, Cleerly, Denver, CO, USA) shows high plaque volume of both noncalcified (*yellow*) and calcified (*blue*) plaque in (B) and (D). Invasive FFR was hemodynamically significant (0.64). Invasive angiogram (E) is shown with stenosis of the LAD. *CCTA*, Coronary CT angiography; *FFR*, fractional flow reserve; *LAD*, left anterior descending.

LIMITATIONS OF PLAQUE IMAGING

The evaluation of coronary atherosclerosis is limited by the intrinsic spatial resolution of ~0.5 mm that can be achieved with current generation CT scanners.[2] With photon-counting detector CT (PCD-CT; see Chapter 2 (Advances in Hardware and Reconstruction Techniques for Cardiac CT) (for detail) technology, an ~0.2 mm spatial resolution can be achieved, which is expected to improve plaque assessment. Atherosclerotic lesions require a thickness of 0.5 to 1 mm to be detected by CCTA. The detection of noncalcified plaque is limited by low-attenuation differences between plaque tissue and perivascular fat as well as partial volume effects of adjacent calcified plaque.[41,71] Therefore good image quality is important for the detection of coronary plaque, with a lower level of image noise and artifacts required for plaque assessment than for the detection of significant luminal stenosis.

Imaging acquisition parameters and image quality have an impact on plaque quantification and characterization. This is particularly important with the current trend for use of lower peak tube potential imaging in an effort to decrease radiation dose. Recent data have found differences in plaque attenuation with different kV and mA settings.[8] Ideally, a patient undergoing serial imaging should have the scan performed on the same platform with similar scanner settings (especially kV) to reduce this variability.

A major limitation of quantitative plaque assessment is the time required for the analysis. Using the methodology presented in the initial validation studies, the analysis of a single dataset may take several hours in a dedicated core laboratory through software that is not available for clinical use.[48,49] As noted above, further standardization of measurements among software platforms and standardization in reporting of quantitatively defined plaque burden are needed for broad clinical impact.

FUTURE DIRECTIONS

Artificial Intelligence

Artificial intelligence (AI) is a broad term that refers to computing that perform complex tasks to mimic human intelligence.[72] Machine learning (ML) is a subset of AI that encompasses a growing collection of algorithms that allow machines to improve at tasks with experience. At a broad level, ML may be divided into supervised, unsupervised, and reinforcement learning. Deep learning is a subset of machine learning algorithms that permit software to train itself to perform tasks. The application of AI to atherosclerosis imaging aims to enable rapid, accurate automated coronary segmentation, qualitative and quantitative coronary interpretation to enable appropriate and rapid application in clinical practice.[73] Prior plaque semiquantitative methods utilized for much of the evidence described within this book chapter are well-established yet time consuming and require a high level of expertise in a dedicated research core lab. In addition, AI/ML aims to allow for reproducible measurements that may improve upon the variability of clinical reads.

As discussed earlier (Table 11.1 and Fig. 11.3), several quantitative CT software approaches have been developed; the most recent solutions apply AI/ML to perform atherosclerosis analysis.[41] To perform quantitative analysis, it is ideal to use images obtained on a 64-slice or greater CT scanner. Common factors for each software approach includes the automatic depiction the boundary between coronary lumen and vessels, creation of centerlines, and calculation of coronary volumes, stenosis assessment, and adverse plaque characteristics through varied ML and DL algorithms.

Current clinical reporting of CCTA is based on visual assessment of stenosis, but this is subject to significant interreader variability. Kelm et al. developed a random forest ML algorithm to calculate cross-sectional luminal area along centerlines, permitting stenotic segments to be identified and graded as <50% or ≥50% with a per-vessel sensitivity of 98% and average speed of only 1.8 s per case.[74] Hong et al. trained CNNs to automatically quantify minimal luminal area and percentage diameter stenosis; the resultant measurements correlated strongly with manual annotations ($r > 0.95$; $P < .001$), with an average computation speed of 31 s per segment.[75] In the seminal CT EvaLuation by ARtificial Intelligence For Atherosclerosis, Stenosis and Vascular MorphologY (CLARIFY) multicenter study, Choi et al. found that AI-guided quantitative CCTA analysis (AI-QCT) can achieve 98% agreement with expert readers for CAD-RADS category on a per-patient basis and 99% of vessels on a per-vessel basis, with >95% sensitivity for detection of obstructive stenosis.[76]

In order to apply evidence regarding plaque burden and outcomes, new AI/ML approaches have been developed to increase the automation of plaque quantification, identify high-risk features, and provide simplified reporting. Dey et al. combined conventional quantitative plaque and vessel-based metrics in an ML model that provided superior prediction for lesion-specific ischemia compared to stenosis severity alone (AUC 0.84 versus 0.76).[77] The aforementioned CLARIFY study evaluated a broad range of atherosclerosis plaque features using AI analysis.[76] Subsequent initial analysis has further shown that AI detected high-risk features, such as lumen volume and low attenuation, more often than experienced level 3 readers. Griffin et al. demonstrated that AI-QCT allows for rapid direct image analysis, plaque quantification, and characterization with high-accuracy versus core-lab interpreted invasive quantitative coronary angiography and fractional flow reserve (Fig. 11.8) with sensitivity and accuracy of 94% and 84% versus a 50% stenosis threshold, 94% and 86% versus a 70% stenosis threshold.[78] In addition, AI-QCT provided accuracy (AUC 0.9) that is similar to quantitative coronary angiography (QCA) (AUC 0.9) against a standard of FFR <0.8. Lin et al. published data for a multicenter validation of a novel deep learning–based system[79] that assesses coronary stenosis and plaque volumes, with excellent agreement for quantification of plaque subtype and stenosis compared with expert readers with rapid analysis time. There was also excellent agreement between deep learning and IVUS for measurements of total plaque volume (ICC 0.949) and minimal luminal area (ICC 0.904). Prognosis was assessed from patients from the SCOT-HEART trial and identified a total plaque volume threshold of 238.5 mm^3 as associated with increased risk for myocardial infarction

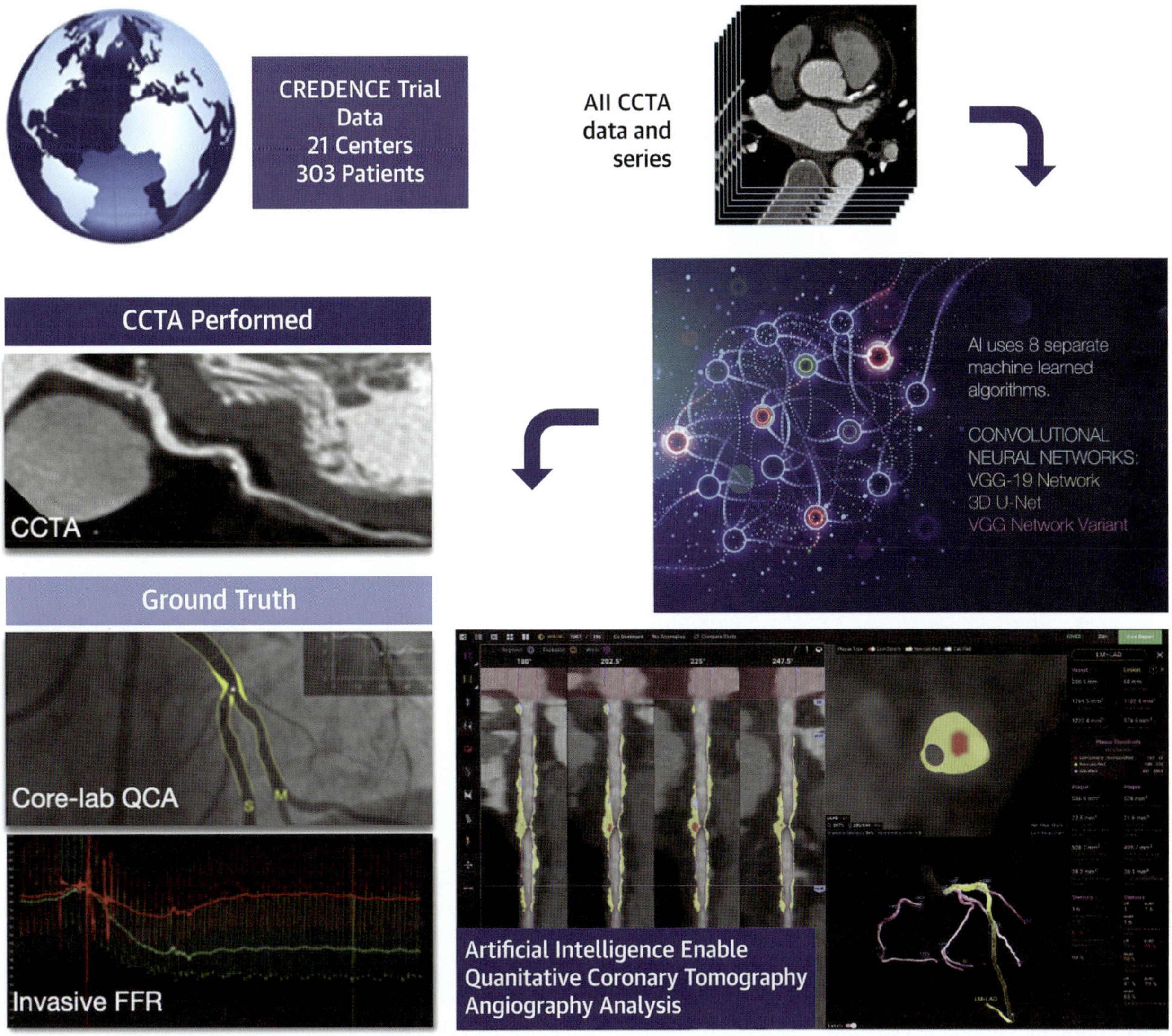

FIG. 11.8 Artificial intelligence–enabled evaluation of coronary artery stenosis. CCTA scans from the CREDENCE (Computed TomogRaphic Evaluation of Atherosclerotic DEtermiNants of Myocardial IsChEmia) trial were analyzed using artificial intelligence–enabled software to determine luminal stenosis. This yielded high performance for detecting stenosis ≥50% and ≥70% referenced by quantitative coronary angiography (QCA) and for predicting invasive fractional flow reserve (FFR) <0.8. (Modified from Griffin WF, Choi AD, Riess JS, et al. AI evaluation of stenosis on coronary CT angiography, comparison with quantitative coronary angiography and fractional flow reserve: a CREDENCE trial substudy. *JACC Cardiovasc Imaging*. 2023;16[2]:193–205.)

(Fig. 11.9). Future clinical integration of quantitative plaque measures would require useful reference values or thresholds to assist with their interpretation and to guide risk stratification and management.[80] Tzimas et al. developed pragmatic age- and sex-specific percentile nomograms for volumes of total plaque and plaque subtypes quantified using an AI-enabled tool.[81] Meanwhile, Min et al. proposed a staging system for coronary atherosclerotic plaque burden (Stages 0–4) based on thresholds of total plaque volume and PAV by AI-QCT, using data on stenosis severity and ischemia from corresponding invasive coronary angiography and FFR assessments.[82] AI-QCT plaque staging was shown to have incremental predictive value for MACE at 10 years, over and above clinical risk factors, CACS, and CAD-RADS 2.0 stenosis grading.[83]

To reframe potential fear and skepticism of AI, it is important to recognize that optimally, these approaches represent advances in computing science with a goal as a clinical support tool to speed up challenging tasks. In the imaging of coronary artery disease, it is important to establish appropriate ground truth standards such as quantitative coronary angiography, fractional flow reserve, invasive ultrasound, and histopathology.[84] In addition, new AI and ML approaches should be validated in randomized controlled trials. It is important that these tools are vetted by the Food and Drug Administration and similar regulatory bodies, through peer-reviewed studies as well as through the professional societies.[85] The field will also need to further develop models for integration into clinical practice, its use as a clinical decision support tool as well as addressing scenarios in which the AI/ML tool disagrees with clinical readers. There is rapid development of new AI applications that include assessment of plaque progression and atherosclerosis-based evaluation of ischemia and coronary flow. Lastly, many of these software have achieved varying levels of regulatory approval resulting

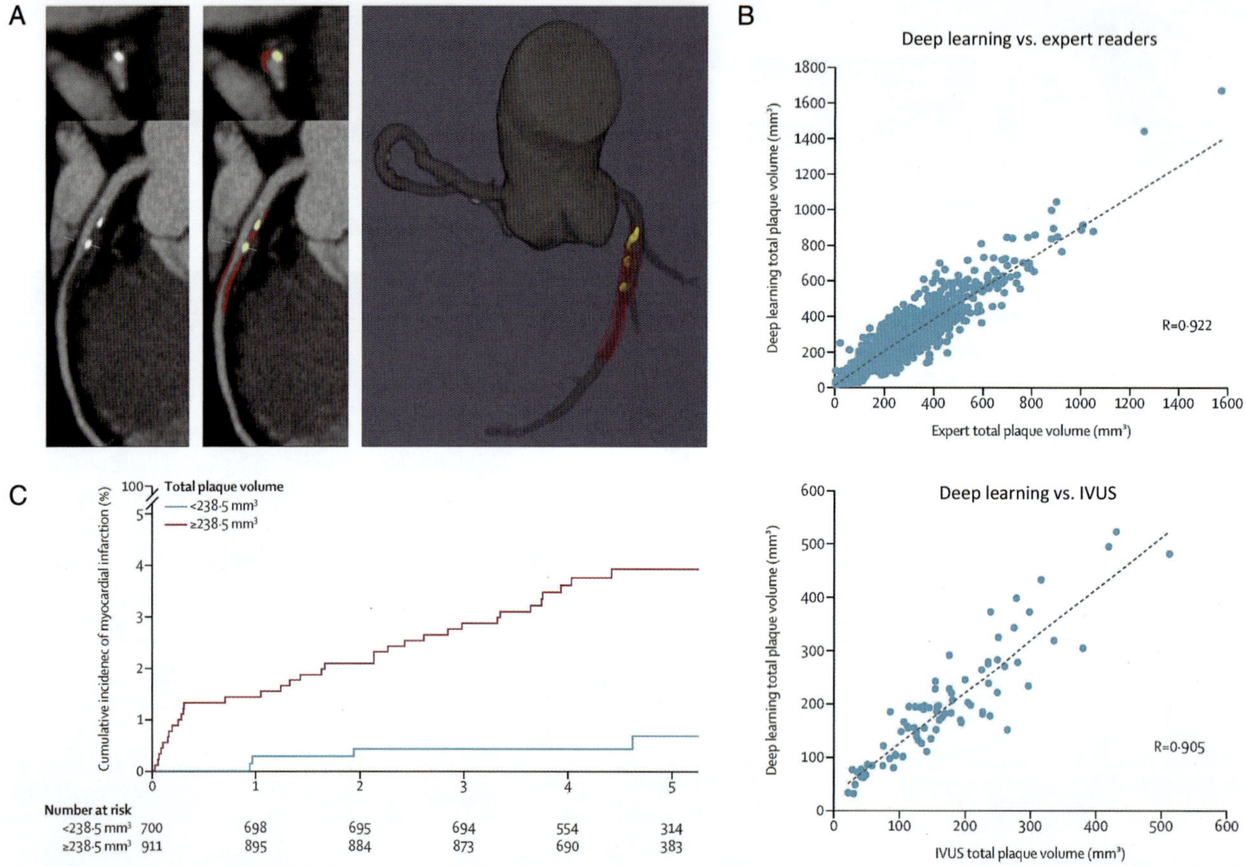

FIG. 11.9 Artificial intelligence–enabled plaque quantification. (A) Case example of automated segmentation of calcified plaque (*yellow*) and noncalcified plaque (*red*) from CCTA using deep learning. (B) Deep learning correlated strongly with expert readers and intravascular ultrasound (IVUS) for measurements of total plaque volume. (C) Kaplan-Meier curves of myocardial infarction in the SCOT-HEART (Scottish Computed Tomography of the HEART) trial stratified by deep learning–based total plaque volume above or below the optimum cutoff value of 238•5 mm³. (Modified from Lin A, Manral N, McElhinney P, et al. Deep learning-enabled coronary CT angiography for plaque and stenosis quantification and cardiac risk prediction: an international multicentre study. *Lancet Digit Health*. 2022;4[4]:e256–e265.)

in rapidly changing clinical access and associated costs in the United States, Europe, Asia, and globally. Future studies are underway to assess the clinical impact of these tools on patient management and outcomes.

Radiomics

The application of radiomics to CCTA for coronary plaque phenotyping is an innovative and exciting field of research. Current quantification of plaque volume and composition is based on absolute voxel attenuation values, without considering the complex spatial relationship between voxels. Radiomics, by extracting thousands of 3D textural and geometric features from CCTA images, can provide an objective mathematical or AI-based description of coronary plaque morphology. This approach has been shown to outperform conventional quantitative CCTA assessment for identifying vulnerable plaques in patients with stable CAD when referenced by intracoronary imaging and histology.[86,87] In a recent prospective study of patients with acute MI undergoing CCTA, radiomics features provided incremental value for discriminating culprit lesions over and above HRP and plaque volumes (AUC 0.86 versus 0.76)[88] (Fig. 11.10). Radiomic phenotyping can also be used to assess temporal changes in plaque morphology beyond volumetric changes on serial CCTA imaging.[89]

CONCLUSION

State-of-the-art CCTA provides a wealth of clinically meaningful information on coronary atherosclerotic plaque. This includes the presence and extent of nonobstructive disease and HRP features, which can be ascertained during routine clinical reads and incorporated in structured reports such as through CAD-RADS 2.0. Software-based quantitative plaque analysis now enables a robust assessment of plaque burden and morphology and has become an important research tool. There is ever-expanding evidence regarding the predictive value of plaque evaluation by CCTA for lesion-specific and patient-level risk of major cardiovascular events. Further, serial quantitative plaque measurements can be used to assess plaque progression or regression and track the effects of conventional or novel medical therapies. The introduction of automated AI systems will improve the speed of plaque quantification and facilitate its clinical adoption. This may be combined with radiomics for the identification of new "high-risk" plaque phenotypes. Finally, integration of plaque analysis with other factors discussed in this book such as stenosis severity, fractional flow reserve with CT, and pericoronary fat attenuation index may further improve the global assessment of cardiovascular risk from CCTA.

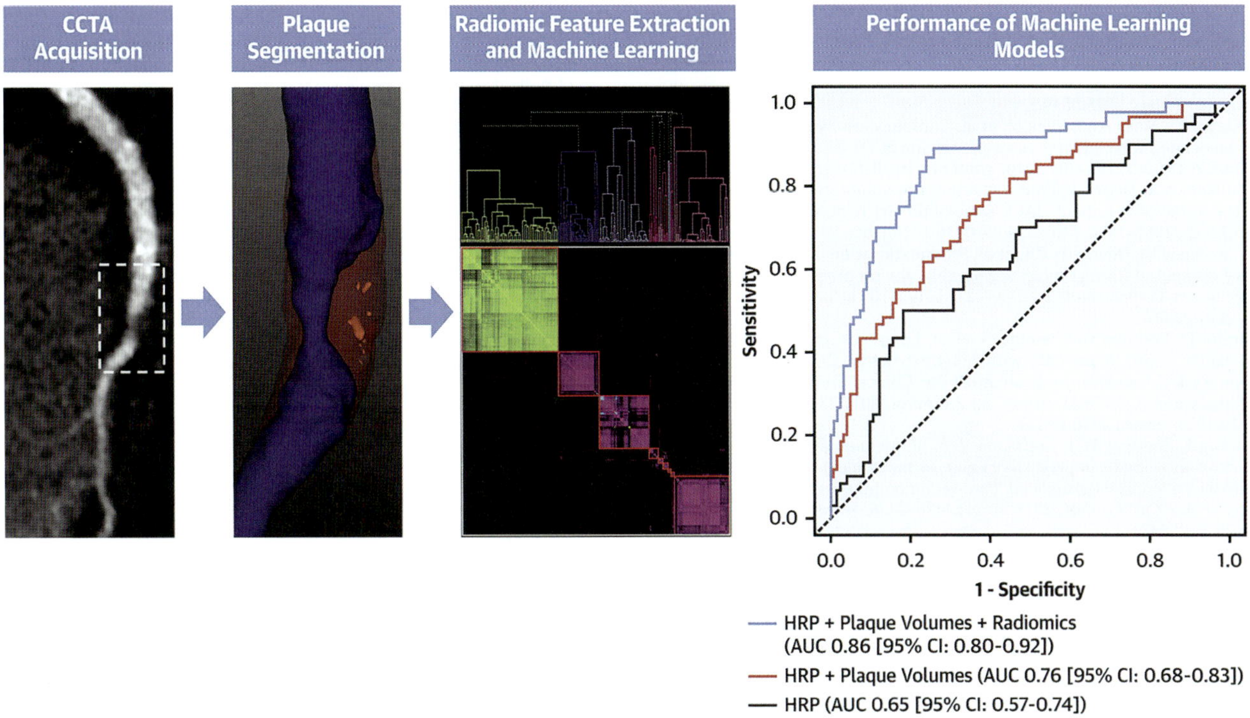

FIG. 11.10 Radiomic analysis in patients with myocardial infarction. Radiomic features were extracted and analyzed from plaque segmentations on CCTA. Machine learning models showed radiomic features to provide incremental value beyond high-risk plaque (HRP) and plaque volumes for discriminating culprit lesions in patients with acute myocardial infarction. *CCTA*, Coronary CT angiography. (Reprinted with permission from Lin A, Kolossváry M, Cadet S, et al. Radiomics-based precision phenotyping identifies unstable coronary plaques from computed tomography angiography. *JACC Cardiovasc Imaging*. 2022;15(5):859–871.)

REFERENCES

1. Maurovich-Horvat P, Ferencik M, Voros S, Merkely B, Hoffmann U. Comprehensive plaque assessment by coronary CT angiography. *Nat Rev Cardiol*. 2014;11(7):390–402. https://doi.org/10.1038/nrcardio.2014.60.
2. Shaw LJ, Blankstein R, Bax JJ, et al. Society of cardiovascular computed tomography /North American society of cardiovascular imaging—expert consensus document on coronary CT imaging of atherosclerotic plaque. *J Cardiovasc Comput Tomogr*. 2021;15(2):93–109. https://doi.org/10.1016/j.jcct.2020.11.002.
3. Kwiecinski J, Tzolos E, Williams Michelle C, et al. Noninvasive coronary atherosclerotic plaque imaging. *JACC Cardiovasc Imaging*. 2023;16(12):1608–1622. https://doi.org/10.1016/j.jcmg.2023.08.021.
4. Leipsic J, Abbara S, Achenbach S, et al. SCCT guidelines for the interpretation and reporting of coronary CT angiography: a report of the Society of Cardiovascular Computed Tomography Guidelines Committee. *J Cardiovasc Comput Tomogr*. 2014;8(5):342–358. https://doi.org/10.1016/j.jcct.2014.07.003.
5. Voros S, Rinehart S, Qian Z. Coronary atherosclerosis imaging by coronary CT angiography: current status, correlation with intravascular interrogation and meta-analysis. *JACC Cardiovasc Imaging*. 2011;4:537.
6. Conte E, Mushtaq S, Pontone G, et al. Plaque quantification by coronary computed tomography angiography using intravascular ultrasound as a reference standard: a comparison between standard and last generation computed tomography scanners. *Eur Heart J Cardiovasc Imaging*. 2020;21(2):191–201. https://doi.org/10.1093/ehjci/jez089.
7. Matsumoto H, Watanabe S, Kyo E, et al. Effect of tube potential and luminal contrast attenuation on atherosclerotic plaque attenuation by coronary CT angiography: in vivo comparison with intravascular ultrasound. *J Cardiovasc Comput Tomogr*. 2019;13(4):219–225. https://doi.org/10.1016/j.jcct.2019.02.004.
8. Takagi H, Leipsic Jonathon A, Indraratna P, et al. Association of tube voltage with plaque composition on coronary CT angiography. *JACC Cardiovasc Imaging*. 2021;14(12):2429–2440. https://doi.org/10.1016/j.jcmg.2021.07.011.
9. Burke AP, Farb A, Malcom GT, Liang YH, Smialek J, Virmani R. Coronary risk factors and plaque morphology in men with coronary disease who died suddenly. *N Engl J Med*. 1997;336(18):1276–1282. https://doi.org/10.1056/nejm199705013361802.
10. Virmani R, Burke AP, Farb A, Kolodgie FD. Pathology of the vulnerable plaque. *J Am Coll Cardiol*. 2006;47(8 Suppl):C13–C18. https://doi.org/10.1016/j.jacc.2005.10.065.
11. Stefanadis C, Antoniou CK, Tsiachris D, Pietri P. Coronary atherosclerotic vulnerable plaque: current perspectives. *J Am Heart Assoc*. 2017;6(3):e005543. https://doi.org/10.1161/JAHA.117.005543.
12. Hoffmann U, Moselewski F, Nieman K, et al. Noninvasive assessment of plaque morphology and composition in culprit and stable lesions in acute coronary syndrome and stable lesions in stable angina by multidetector computed tomography. *J Am Coll Cardiol*. 2006;47(8):1655–1662. https://doi.org/10.1016/j.jacc.2006.01.041.
13. Motoyama S, Kondo T, Sarai M, et al. Multislice computed tomographic characteristics of coronary lesions in acute coronary syndromes. *J Am Coll Cardiol*. 2007;50(4):319–326. https://doi.org/10.1016/j.jacc.2007.03.044.
14. Motoyama S, Sarai M, Harigaya H, et al. Computed tomographic angiography characteristics of atherosclerotic plaques subsequently resulting in acute coronary syndrome. *J Am Coll Cardiol*. 2009;54(1):49–57. https://doi.org/10.1016/j.jacc.2009.02.068.
15. Puchner SB, Liu T, Mayrhofer T, et al. High-risk plaque detected on coronary CT angiography predicts acute coronary syndromes independent of significant stenosis in acute chest pain: results from the ROMICAT-II trial. *J Am Coll Cardiol*. 2014;64(7):684–692. https://doi.org/10.1016/j.jacc.2014.05.039.
16. Kitagawa T, Yamamoto H, Horiguchi J, et al. Characterization of noncalcified coronary plaques and identification of culprit lesions in patients with acute coronary syndrome by 64-slice computed tomography. *JACC Cardiovasc Imaging*. 2009;2(2):153–160. https://doi.org/10.1016/j.jcmg.2008.09.015.
17. Maurovich-Horvat P, Schlett CL, Alkadhi H, et al. The napkin-ring sign indicates advanced atherosclerotic lesions in coronary CT angiography. *JACC Cardiovasc Imaging*. 2012;5(12):1243–1252. https://doi.org/10.1016/j.jcmg.2012.03.019.
18. Kashiwagi M, Tanaka A, Kitabata H, et al. Feasibility of noninvasive assessment of thin-cap fibroatheroma by multidetector computed tomography. *JACC Cardiovasc Imaging*. 2009;2(12):1412–1419. https://doi.org/10.1016/j.jcmg.2009.09.012.
19. Ito T, Terashima M, Kaneda H, et al. Comparison of in vivo assessment of vulnerable plaque by 64-slice multislice computed tomography versus optical coherence tomography. *Am J Cardiol*. 2011;107(9):1270–1277. https://doi.org/10.1016/j.amjcard.2010.12.036.
20. Kröner ES, van Velzen JE, Boogers MJ, et al. Positive remodeling on coronary computed tomography as a marker for plaque vulnerability on virtual histology intravascular ultrasound. *Am J Cardiol*. 2011;107(12):1725–1729. https://doi.org/10.1016/j.amjcard.2011.02.337.
21. Bittner DO, Mayrhofer T, Puchner SB, et al. Coronary computed tomography angiography-specific definitions of high-risk plaque features improve detection of acute coronary syndrome. *Circ Cardiovasc Imaging*. 2018;11(8):e007657. https://doi.org/10.1161/circimaging.118.007657.
22. de Knegt MC, Linde JJ, Fuchs A, et al. Relationship between patient presentation and morphology of coronary atherosclerosis by quantitative multidetector computed tomography. *Eur Heart J Cardiovasc Imaging*. 2019;20(11):1221–1230. doi:10.1093/ehjci/jey146.
23. Ferencik M, Mayrhofer T, Bittner DO, et al. Use of high-risk coronary atherosclerotic plaque detection for risk stratification of patients with stable chest pain: a secondary analysis of the PROMISE randomized clinical trial. *JAMA Cardiol*. 2018;3(2):144–152. https://doi.org/10.1001/jamacardio.2017.4973.
24. Chang HJ, Lin FY, Lee SE, et al. Coronary atherosclerotic precursors of acute coronary syndromes. *J Am Coll Cardiol*. 2018;71(22):2511–2522. https://doi.org/10.1016/j.jacc.2018.02.079.
25. Puchner SB, Ferencik M, Maehara A, et al. Iterative image reconstruction improves the accuracy of automated plaque burden assessment in coronary CT angiography: a comparison with intravascular ultrasound. *Am J Roentgenol*. 2017;208(4):777–784. https://doi.org/10.2214/AJR.16.17187.

26. Motoyama S, Ito H, Sarai M, et al. Plaque characterization by coronary computed tomography angiography and the likelihood of acute coronary events in mid-term follow-up. *J Am Coll Cardiol.* 2015;66(4):337–346. https://doi.org/10.1016/j.jacc.2015.05.069.
27. Williams MC, Moss AJ, Dweck M, et al. Coronary artery plaque characteristics associated with adverse outcomes in the SCOT-HEART study. *J Am Coll Cardiol.* 2019;73(3):291–301. https://doi.org/10.1016/j.jacc.2018.10.066.
28. Arbab-Zadeh A, Fuster V. From detecting the vulnerable plaque to managing the vulnerable patient: JACC state-of-the-art review. *J Am Coll Cardiol.* 2019;74(12):1582–1593. https://doi.org/10.1016/j.jacc.2019.07.062.
29. Min JK, Shaw LJ, Devereux RB, et al. Prognostic value of multidetector coronary computed tomographic angiography for prediction of all-cause mortality. *J Am Coll Cardiol.* 2007;50(12):1161–1170. https://doi.org/10.1016/j.jacc.2007.03.067.
30. Andreini D, Pontone G, Mushtaq S, et al. Long-term prognostic impact of CT-Leaman score in patients with non-obstructive CAD: results from the COronary CT Angiography EvaluatioN For Clinical Outcomes InteRnational Multicenter (CONFIRM) study. *Int J Cardiol.* 2017;231:18–25. https://doi.org/10.1016/j.ijcard.2016.12.137.
31. Bamberg F, Sommer WH, Hoffmann V, et al. Meta-analysis and systematic review of the long-term predictive value of assessment of coronary atherosclerosis by contrast-enhanced coronary computed tomography angiography. *J Am Coll Cardiol.* 2011;57(24):2426–2436. https://doi.org/10.1016/j.jacc.2010.12.043.
32. Bittencourt MS, Hulten E, Ghoshhajra B, et al. Prognostic value of nonobstructive and obstructive coronary artery disease detected by coronary computed tomography angiography to identify cardiovascular events. *Circ Cardiovasc Imaging.* 2014;7(2):282–291. https://doi.org/10.1161/CIRCIMAGING.113.001047.
33. Park HB, Lee BK, Shin S, et al. Clinical feasibility of 3D automated coronary atherosclerotic plaque quantification algorithm on coronary computed tomography angiography: comparison with intravascular ultrasound. *Eur Radiol.* 2015;25(10):3073–3083. https://doi.org/10.1007/s00330-015-3698-z.
34. Matsumoto H, Watanabe S, Kyo E, et al. Standardized volumetric plaque quantification and characterization from coronary CT angiography: a head-to-head comparison with invasive intravascular ultrasound. *Eur Radiol.* 2019;29(11):6129–6139. https://doi.org/10.1007/s00330-019-06219-3.
35. Choi AD, Marques H, Kumar V, et al. CT evaluation by artificial intelligence for atherosclerosis, stenosis and vascular morphology (CLARIFY): a multi-center, international study. *J Cardiovasc Comput Tomogr.* 2021;15(6):470–476. https://doi.org/10.1016/j.jcct.2021.05.004.
36. van Rosendael AR, Lin FY, Ma X, et al. Percent atheroma volume: optimal variable to report whole-heart atherosclerotic plaque burden with coronary CTA, the PARADIGM study. *J Cardiovasc Comput Tomogr.* 2020;14(5):400–406. https://doi.org/10.1016/j.jcct.2020.01.012.
37. van Rosendael AR, Narula J, Lin FY, et al. Association of high-density calcified 1K plaque with risk of acute coronary syndrome. *JAMA Cardiol.* 2020;5(3):282–290. https://doi.org/10.1001/jamacardio.2019.5315.
38. Stolzmann P, Schlett CL, Maurovich-Horvat P, et al. Variability and accuracy of coronary CT angiography including use of iterative reconstruction algorithms for plaque burden assessment as compared with intravascular ultrasound-an ex vivo study. *Eur Radiol.* 2012;22(10):2067–2075. https://doi.org/10.1007/s00330-012-2464-8.
39. Meah MN, Singh T, Williams MC, et al. Reproducibility of quantitative plaque measurement in advanced coronary artery disease. *J Cardiovasc Comput Tomogr.* 2021;15(4):333–338. https://doi.org/10.1016/j.jcct.2020.12.008.
40. Oberoi S, Meinel FG, Schoepf UJ, et al. Reproducibility of noncalcified coronary artery plaque burden quantification from coronary CT angiography across different image analysis platforms. *Am J Roentgenol.* 2013;202(1):W43–W49. https://doi.org/10.2214/AJR.13.11225.
41. Williams MC, Earls JP, Hecht H. Quantitative assessment of atherosclerotic plaque, recent progress and current limitations. *J Cardiovasc Comput Tomogr.* 2022;16(2):124–137. https://doi.org/10.1016/j.jcct.2021.07.001.
42. Lee SE, Park HB, Xuan D, et al. Consistency of quantitative analysis of coronary computed tomography angiography. *J Cardiovasc Comput Tomogr.* 2019;13(1):48–54. https://doi.org/10.1016/j.jcct.2018.09.012.
43. Ferencik M, Mayrhofer T, Puchner SB, et al. Computed tomography-based high-risk coronary plaque score to predict acute coronary syndrome among patients with acute chest pain–Results from the ROMICAT II trial. *J Cardiovasc Comput Tomogr.* 2015;9(6):538–545. https://doi.org/10.1016/j.jcct.2015.07.003.
44. Williams MC, Kwiecinski J, Doris M, et al. Low-attenuation noncalcified plaque on coronary computed tomography angiography predicts myocardial infarction. *Circulation.* 2020;141(18):1452–1462. https://doi.org/10.1161/CIRCULATIONAHA.119.044720.
45. Bose D, von Birgelen C, Erbel R. Intravascular ultrasound for the evaluation of therapies targeting coronary atherosclerosis. *J Am Coll Cardiol.* 2007;49(9):925–932. https://doi.org/10.1016/j.jacc.2006.08.067.
46. Nicholls SJ, Ballantyne CM, Barter PJ, et al. Effect of two intensive statin regimens on progression of coronary disease. *N Engl J Med.* 2011;365(22):2078–2087. https://doi.org/10.1056/NEJMoa1110874.
47. Nissen SE, Nicholls SJ, Sipahi I, et al. Effect of very high-intensity statin therapy on regression of coronary atherosclerosis: the ASTEROID trial. *JAMA.* 2006;295(13):1556–1565. https://doi.org/10.1001/jama.295.13.jpc60002.
48. Dawson LP, Lum M, Nerleker N, Nicholls SJ, Layland J. Coronary atherosclerotic plaque regression: JACC state-of-the-art review. *J Am Coll Cardiol.* 2022;79(1):66–82. https://doi.org/10.1016/j.jacc.2021.10.035.
49. Indraratna P, Khasanova E, Gulsin GS, et al. Plaque progression: where, why, and how fast? A review of what we have learned from the analysis of patient data from the PARADIGM registry. *J Cardiovasc Comput Tomogr.* 2022;16(4):294–302. https://doi.org/10.1016/j.jcct.2021.11.004.
50. Lee SE, Chang HJ, Rizvi A, et al. Rationale and design of the Progression of AtheRosclerotic PlAque DetermIned by Computed TomoGraphic Angiography IMaging (PARADIGM) registry: a comprehensive exploration of plaque progression and its impact on clinical outcomes from a multicenter serial coronary computed tomographic angiography study. *Am Heart J.* 2016;182:72–79. https://doi.org/10.1016/j.ahj.2016.09.003.
51. Lee SE, Chang HJ, Sung JM, et al. Effects of statins on coronary atherosclerotic plaques: the PARADIGM study. *JACC Cardiovasc Imaging.* 2018;11(10):1475–1484. https://doi.org/10.1016/j.jcmg.2018.04.015.
52. Lee SE, Sung JM, Andreini D, et al. Differential association between the progression of coronary artery calcium score and coronary plaque volume progression according to statins: the Progression of AtheRosclerotic PlAque DetermIned by Computed TomoGraphic Angiography Imaging (PARADIGM) study. *Eur Heart J Cardiovasc Imaging.* 2019;20(11):1307–1314. https://doi.org/10.1093/ehjci/jez022.
53. Andelius L, Mortensen MB, Nørgaard BL, Abdulla J. Impact of statin therapy on coronary plaque burden and composition assessed by coronary computed tomographic angiography: a systematic review and meta-analysis. *Eur Heart J Cardiovasc Imaging.* 2018;19(8):850–858. https://doi.org/10.1093/ehjci/jey012.
54. Henzel J, Kepka C, Kruk M, et al. High-risk coronary plaque regression after intensive lifestyle intervention in nonobstructive coronary disease: a randomized study. *JACC Cardiovasc Imaging.* 2021;14(6):1192–1202. https://doi.org/10.1016/j.jcmg.2020.10.019.
55. Aengevaeren VL, Mosterd A, Braber TL, et al. Relationship between lifelong exercise volume and coronary atherosclerosis in athletes. *Circulation.* 2017;136(2):138–148. https://doi.org/10.1161/CIRCULATIONAHA.117.027834.
56. Merghani A, Maestrini V, Rosmini S, et al. Prevalence of subclinical coronary artery disease in masters endurance athletes with a low atherosclerotic risk profile. *Circulation.* 2017;136(2):126–137. https://doi.org/10.1161/CIRCULATIONAHA.116.026964.
57. Matsumoto S, Nakanishi R, Li D, et al. Aged garlic extract reduces low attenuation plaque in coronary arteries of patients with metabolic syndrome in a prospective randomized double-blind study. *J Nutr.* 2016;146(2):427S–432S. https://doi.org/10.3945/jn.114.202424.
58. Alfaddagh A, Elajami TK, Ashfaque H, Saleh M, Bistrian BR, Welty FK. Effect of eicosapentaenoic and docosahexaenoic acids added to statin therapy on coronary artery plaque in patients with coronary artery disease: a randomized clinical trial. *J Am Heart Assoc.* 2017;6(12):e006981. https://doi.org/10.1161/JAHA.117.006981.
59. Budoff MJ, Ellenberg SS, Lewis CE, et al. Testosterone treatment and coronary artery plaque volume in older men with low testosterone. *JAMA.* 2017;317(7):708–716. https://doi.org/10.1001/jama.2016.21043.
60. Lee J, Nakanishi R, Li D, et al. Randomized trial of rivaroxaban versus warfarin in the evaluation of progression of coronary atherosclerosis. *Am Heart J.* 2018;206:127–130. https://doi.org/10.1016/j.ahj.2018.08.007.
61. Beyer C, Wildauer M, Feuchtner G, et al. Relationship of anticoagulant therapies on coronary plaque progression: a longitudinal CTA analysis. *JACC Cardiovasc Imaging.* 2020;13(1 Pt 1):169–170. https://doi.org/10.1016/j.jcmg.2019.07.021.
62. Connolly SJ, Eikelboom JW, Bosch J, et al. Rivaroxaban with or without aspirin in patients with stable coronary artery disease: an international, randomised, double-blind, placebo-controlled trial. *Lancet.* 2018;391(10117):205–218. https://doi.org/10.1016/S0140-6736(17)32458-3.
63. Vaidya K, Arnott C, Martinez GJ, et al. Colchicine therapy and plaque stabilization in patients with acute coronary syndrome: a CT coronary angiography study. *JACC Cardiovasc Imaging.* 2018;11(2 Pt 2):305–316. https://doi.org/10.1016/j.jcmg.2017.08.013.
64. Budoff M, Lakshmanan S, Bhatt DL. The EVAPORATE trial provides important mechanistic data on plaque characteristics that have relevance to the REDUCE-IT results and clinical use of icosapent ethyl. *Eur Heart J.* 2021;42(31):3025–3026. https://doi.org/10.1093/eurheartj/ehab233.
65. Budoff MJ, Bhatt DL, Kinninger A, et al. Effect of icosapent ethyl on progression of coronary atherosclerosis in patients with elevated triglycerides on statin therapy: final results of the EVAPORATE trial. *Eur Heart J.* 2020;41(40):3925–3932. https://doi.org/10.1093/eurheartj/ehaa652.
66. Bhatt DL, Steg PG, Miller M, et al. Cardiovascular risk reduction with icosapent ethyl for hypertriglyceridemia. *N Engl J Med.* 2019;380(1):11–22. https://doi.org/10.1056/NEJMoa1812792.
67. Lo J, Lu MT, Ihenachor EJ, et al. Effects of statin therapy on coronary artery plaque volume and high-risk plaque morphology in HIV-infected patients with subclinical atherosclerosis: a randomised, double-blind, placebo-controlled trial. *Lancet HIV.* 2015;2(2):e52–e63. https://doi.org/10.1016/S2352-3018(14)00032-0.
68. Grinspoon SK, Fitch KV, Zanni MV, et al. Pitavastatin to prevent cardiovascular disease in HIV infection. *N Engl J Med.* 2023;389(8):687–699. https://doi.org/10.1056/NEJMoa2304146.
69. Gilbert JM, Fitch KV, Grinspoon SK. HIV-related cardiovascular disease, statins, and the REPRIEVE trial. *Top Antivir Med.* 2015;23(4):146–149.
70. Cury RC, Leipsic J, Abbara S, et al. CAD-RADS 2.0 –2022 coronary artery disease-reporting and data system: an expert consensus document of the Society of Cardiovascular Computed Tomography (SCCT), the American College of Cardiology (ACC), the American College of Radiology (ACR), and the

North America Society of Cardiovascular Imaging (NASCI). *JACC Cardiovasc Imaging*. 2022;15(11):1974–2001. https://doi.org/10.1016/j.jcmg.2022.07.002.
71. Dalager MG, Bøttcher M, Andersen G, et al. Impact of luminal density on plaque classification by CT coronary angiography. *Int J Cardiovasc Imaging*. 2011;27(4):593–600. https://doi.org/10.1007/s10554-010-9695-z.
72. Dey D, Slomka PJ, Leeson P, et al. Artificial intelligence in cardiovascular imaging: JACC state-of-the-art review. *J Am Coll Cardiol*. 2019;73(11):1317–1335. https://doi.org/10.1016/j.jacc.2018.12.054.
73. Covas P, De Guzman E, Barrows I, et al. Artificial intelligence advancements in the cardiovascular imaging of coronary atherosclerosis. *Front Cardiovasc Med*. 2022;9:839400. https://doi.org/10.3389/fcvm.2022.839400.
74. Kelm BM, Mittal S, Zheng Y, et al. Detection, grading and classification of coronary stenoses in computed tomography angiography. *Med Image Comput Comput Assist Interv*. 2011;14(Pt 3):25–32. https://doi.org/10.1007/978-3-642-23626-6_4.
75. Hong Y, Commandeur F, Cadet S, et al. Deep learning-based stenosis quantification from coronary CT Angiography. *Proc SPIE Int Soc Opt Eng*. 2019;10949. https://doi.org/10.1117/12.2512168.
76. Choi AD, Marques H, Kumar V, et al. CT Evaluation by Artificial Intelligence for Atherosclerosis, Stenosis and Vascular Morphology (CLARIFY): a multi-center, international study. *J Cardiovasc Comput Tomogr*. 2021;15(6):470–476. https://doi.org/10.1016/j.jcct.2021.05.004.
77. Dey D, Gaur S, Ovrehus KA, et al. Integrated prediction of lesion-specific ischaemia from quantitative coronary CT angiography using machine learning: a multicentre study. *Eur Radiol*. 2018;28(6):2655–2664. https://doi.org/10.1007/s00330-017-5223-z.
78. Griffin WF, Choi AD, Riess JS, et al. AI evaluation of stenosis on coronary CT angiography, comparison with quantitative coronary angiography and fractional flow reserve: a CREDENCE trial substudy. *JACC Cardiovasc Imaging*. 2023;16(2):193–205. https://doi.org/10.1016/j.jcmg.2021.10.020.
79. Lin A, Manral N, McElhinney P, et al. Deep learning-enabled coronary CT angiography for plaque and stenosis quantification and cardiac risk prediction: an international multicentre study. *Lancet Digit Health*. 2022;4(4):e256–e265. https://doi.org/10.1016/S2589-7500(22)00022-X.
80. Bienstock S, Lin F, Blankstein R, et al. Advances in coronary computed tomographic angiographic imaging of atherosclerosis for risk stratification and preventive care. *JACC Cardiovasc Imaging*. 2023;16(8):1099–1115. https://doi.org/10.1016/j.jcmg.2023.02.002.
81. Tzimas G, Gulsin GS, Everett RJ, et al. Age- and sex-specific nomographic CT quantitative plaque data from a large international cohort. *JACC Cardiovasc Imaging*. 2023;17(2):165–175. https://doi.org/10.1016/j.jcmg.2023.05.011.
82. Min JK, Chang H-J, Andreini D, et al. Coronary CTA plaque volume severity stages according to invasive coronary angiography and FFR. *J Cardiovasc Comput Tomogr*. 2022;16(5):415–422. https://doi.org/10.1016/j.jcct.2022.03.001.
83. Nurmohamed Nick S, Bom Michiel J, Jukema Ruurt A, et al. AI-guided quantitative plaque staging predicts long-term cardiovascular outcomes in patients at risk for atherosclerotic CVD. *JACC Cardiovasc Imaging*. 2024;17(3):269–280. https://doi.org/10.1016/j.jcmg.2023.05.020.
84. Budoff MJ, Lakshmanan S, Toth PP, et al. Cardiac CT angiography in current practice: an American Society for Preventive Cardiology Clinical Practice Statement*. *Am J Prev Cardiol*. 2022;9:100318. https://doi.org/10.1016/j.ajpc.2022.100318.
85. Dey D, Arnaout R, Antani S, et al. Proceedings of the NHLBI workshop on artificial intelligence in cardiovascular imaging: translation to patient care. *JACC Cardiovasc Imaging*. 2023;16(9):1209–1223. https://doi.org/10.1016/j.jcmg.2023.05.012.
86. Kolossváry M, Park J, Bang J-I, et al. Identification of invasive and radionuclide imaging markers of coronary plaque vulnerability using radiomic analysis of coronary computed tomography angiography. *Eur Heart J Cardiovasc Imaging*. 2019;20(11):1250–1258. https://doi.org/10.1093/ehjci/jez033.
87. Kolossváry M, Karády J, Kikuchi Y, et al. Radiomics versus visual and histogram-based assessment to identify atheromatous lesions at coronary CT angiography: an ex vivo study. *Radiology*. 2019;293(1):89–96. https://doi.org/10.1148/radiol.2019190407.
88. Lin A, Kolossváry M, Cadet S, et al. Radiomics-based precision phenotyping identifies unstable coronary plaques from computed tomography angiography. *JACC Cardiovasc Imaging*. 2022;15(5):859–871. https://doi.org/10.1016/j.jcmg.2021.11.016.
89. Kolossváry M, Gerstenblith G, Bluemke DA, et al. Contribution of risk factors to the development of coronary atherosclerosis as confirmed via coronary CT angiography: a longitudinal radiomics-based study. *Radiology*. 2021;299(1):97–106. https://doi.org/10.1148/radiol.2021203179.

12 Plaque on CCTA: Lessons From Histology

KENJI KAWAI, ALOKE V. FINN, AND RENU VIRMANI

KEY POINTS

- Histologic lesions, divided into nonprogressive nonatherosclerotic lesions (adaptive intimal thickening and intimal xanthoma) and progressive atherosclerotic lesions, consist of pathological intimal thickening, which continues to progress to early and late fibroatheroma, with eventual formation of thin-cap fibroatheroma.
- Thin-cap fibroatheroma is a vulnerable plaque that is prone to rupture.
- High-risk coronary plaques have histologic features of positive remodeling, a large necrotic core, thin-cap fibroatheroma with macrophage infiltration, and fragmented or spotty calcification.
- The most common cause of coronary thrombosis is plaque rupture, followed by plaque erosion and (least frequent) calcified nodules.
- In contrast, stable plaques are rich in collagen and highly calcified with minimal to no necrotic core.

INTRODUCTION

Atherosclerosis is a multifactorial systemic disease that manifests focally, and especially at the site of vascular branches such as abdominal aorta, carotid bifurcation, and left main bifurcation into left anterior descending, left circumflex, and coronary ostia. Atherosclerotic disease is mainly driven by the presence of risk factors including hyperlipidemia, hypertension, smoking, diabetes, renal failure, obesity, family history, advancing age, and sedentary lifestyle. Coronary atherosclerotic disease can manifest as acute coronary syndrome (including acute myocardial infarction and unstable angina pectoris) or sudden death. The burden of atherosclerotic heart disease is worldwide and remains the major cause of morbidity and mortality, despite continued advances in the understanding and treatment of atherosclerosis. Although survival rates have improved, death rates continue to increase globally, reaching 19.05 million in 2020 (accounting for an increase of 18.1% from 2010).[1]

PROGRESSION IN CORONARY PLAQUE

Histologically, the coronary artery wall is made up of three separate layers consisting of intima, media, and adventitia. The intima consists of the endothelial luminal lining and the subendothelial layer, which is composed of a few smooth muscle cells in a proteoglycan-collagen matrix and the internal elastic lamina (IEL). The media consists of a thick muscular layer composed of circumferentially arranged, circularly oriented smooth muscle cells with an outer external elastic lamina (EEL). The outermost layer is the adventitia, which is made up of a few elastic fibers that are surrounded by collagen bundles and fibroblasts. At birth, about 30% of newborns show presence of cell masses consisting of smooth muscle cells in the intima, probably clonal in origin, that may provide a soil for atherosclerosis lesions development.

Atherosclerosis occurs in areas with low shear stress, which slowly progress over time to pathological intima thickening (PIT).[2] The lesions of pathologic intimal thickening show areas of rich in smooth muscle cells (SMC) with interspersed focal areas rich in extracellular matrix (ECM) composed of proteoglycans and collagen type III with a coexisting lipid deposition, that is, lipid pools. The ECM consists primarily of hyaluronan and proteoglycans biglycan, decorin, and versican that are admixed with neutral lipids and free cholesterol. Remnants of apoptotic SMC are generally visualized by a thickened basement membrane on periodic acid–Schiff (PAS) staining and are observed in areas composed of lipid pools. The lipid pool is formed by infiltration and deposition of plasma-derived lipids that on Oil red O staining show microvesicular lipid droplets, whereas areas of macrophages show intracellular globular droplets of lipid.

Lesions of late fibroatheromas show heavy infiltration of globular lipid droplets. Nakagawa and Nakashima have shown presence of apo B and fibrinogen in regions of lipid pools, and such lesions are in the middle and deep intimal layers. The lesions of PIT that show macrophages that are located close to the lumen only stain faintly for apo B or fibrinogen, thus suggesting that extracellular lipids are derived from the plasma, but not from macrophage foam cells.[3] However, our results show that necrotic core lipids are derived both from the macrophages as well as plasma lipids. The plasma lipid may also be the result of hemorrhage within the necrotic core (see "Fibroatheroma").

Macrophage infiltration increases in lesions of fibroatheroma as compared to PIT with macrophages. The number of macrophages is maximum in late fibroatheroma as compared to early fibroatheromas. The lipid pool in a PIT lesion converts into a necrotic core through macrophage infiltration, resulting in the breakdown of the matrix that forms early fibroatheroma lesions. The lesion shows the presence of dying and calcifying macrophages within or at border regions of the necrotic core.[4]

The necrotic core intraplaque hemorrhage occurs from leaking and rupture of intimal microvessels, which are mostly derived from adventitial vasa vasorum, and contribute to the further expansion of the necrotic core. The microvessel density increases with advancing atherosclerotic plaque progression and, commonly, there is incomplete mural cell coverage of the microvessel structural integrity with extensive hemorrhage and macrophage infiltration ensues.[5] We have shown that there is an association between

TABLE 12.1 Morphometric Analysis of 365 Plaques in Coronary Arteries from Patients Who Died Suddenly of Coronary Causes[a]

TYPES OF PLAQUES	NO. OF PLAQUES	GLYCOPHORIN A SCORE[b]	IRON SCORE[b]	SIZE OF NECROTIC CORE, mm²	EXTENT OF MACROPHAGE INFILTRATION
Plaque with pathologic intimal thickening but with no necrotic core	129	0.09 ± 0.04	0.07 ± 0.05	–	0.002 ± 0.001
Fibroatheroma					
Core in early stage of necrosis	79	0.23 ± 0.07	0.17 ± 0.08	0.06 ± 0.02	0.018 ± 0.004
Core in late stage of necrosis	105	0.94 ± 0.11[c]	0.41 ± 0.09[c]	0.84 ± 0.08[c]	0.059 ± 0.007[c]
Thin-cap fibroatheroma	52	1.60 ± 0.20[c]	1.24 ± 0.24[c]	1.95 ± 0.30[c]	0.142 ± 0.016[c]

[a]Plus-minus value are means ± SE.
[b]Scores can range from 0 to 4, with higher scores indicating greater proportions of the analyte.
[c]$P < .001$ for the comparison with fibroatheromas whose cores were in an early stage of necrosis.
Reproduced from Kolodgie FD, Gold HK, Burke AP, et al. Intraplaque hemorrhage and progression of coronary atheroma. *N Eng J Med.* 2003;349:2316–2325.

intraplaque hemorrhage, an increase in the size of the necrotic core, and lesion instability in coronary plaques (Table 12.1).[6] The presence of red cell membranes are responsible for the presence of glycophorin A and are often located around cholesterol clefts. Iron deposition is also observed in the region. The free cholesterol in necrotic cores is likely derived from the red cell membranes.[6]

Histologically, these progressive atherosclerosis stages can be divided into four distinct categories: (1) nonatherosclerotic intimal lesions (intimal thickening, intimal xanthomas), (2) progressive atherosclerotic lesions (pathological intimal thickening, fibroatheroma, and intraplaque hemorrhage or plaque fissure, thin cap fibroatheroma [TCFA]), (3) acute thrombotic lesions, and (4) healing lesions.[2]

The plaque types that are clinically associated with acute thrombosis are plaque rupture (60%), plaque erosion (35%), and calcified nodule (5%).[7] An understanding of the histologic characteristics of these atherosclerotic lesions is important in order to correlate findings on coronary CT imaging. The following section describes the morphologic characteristics of nonatherosclerotic and atherosclerotic lesions (Fig. 12.1), lesions with thrombosis that often present as acute coronary syndromes and sudden death (Fig. 12.2), and other lesions including healed rupture and chronic total occlusion (Fig. 12.3).

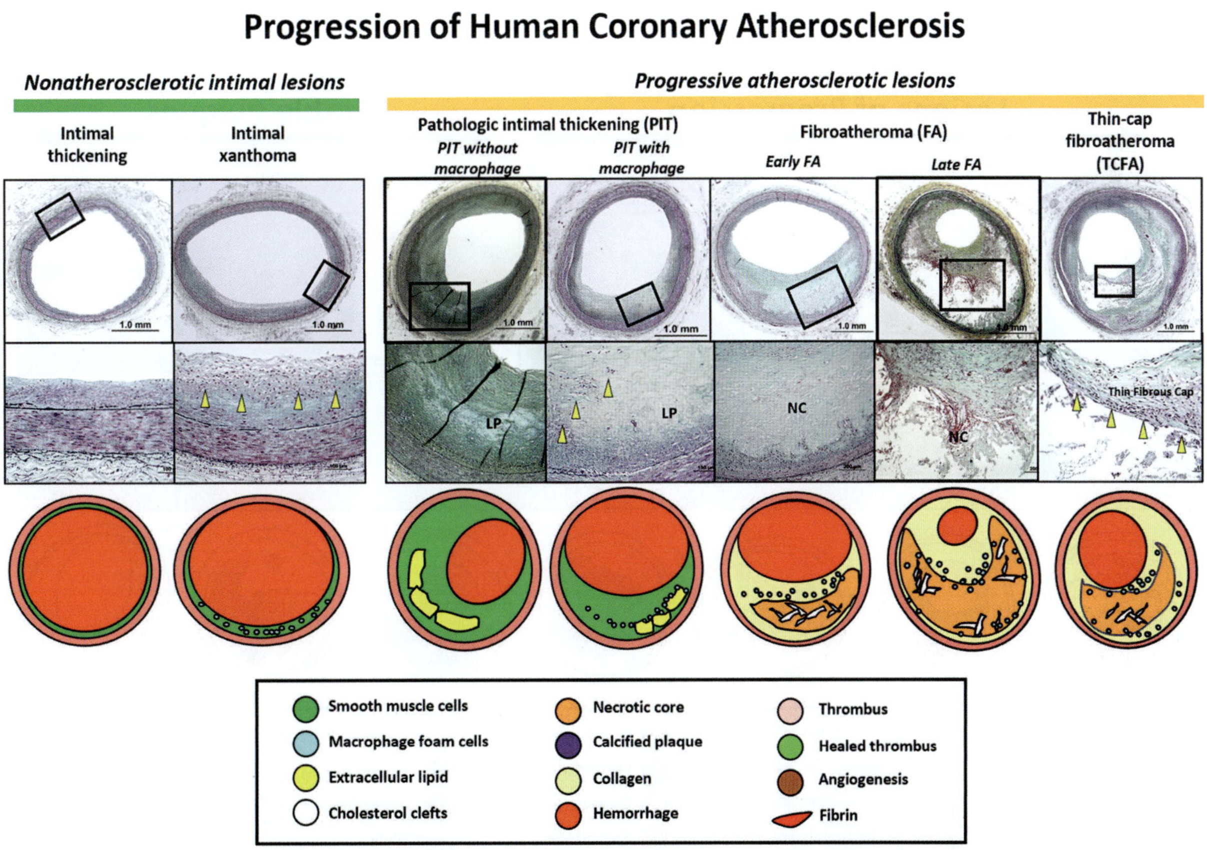

FIG. 12.1 Human Coronary Lesion Morphologies Categorized as Nonatherosclerotic Intimal Lesions, Progressive Atherosclerotic Lesions. Nonatherosclerotic intimal lesions, including intimal thickening and intimal xanthoma, while progressive atherosclerotic lesions beginning with pathologic intimal thickening (with and without macrophages) that go on to form fibroatheromas (early and late) and final phase prior to rupture is the thin-cap fibroatheroma. *LP*, Lipid pool; *NC*, necrotic core. (Reproduced and modified from Yahagi K, Kolodgie FD, Otsuka F, et al. Pathophysiology of native coronary, vein graft, and in-stent atherosclerosis. *Nat Rev Cardiol.* 2016;13:79–98.)

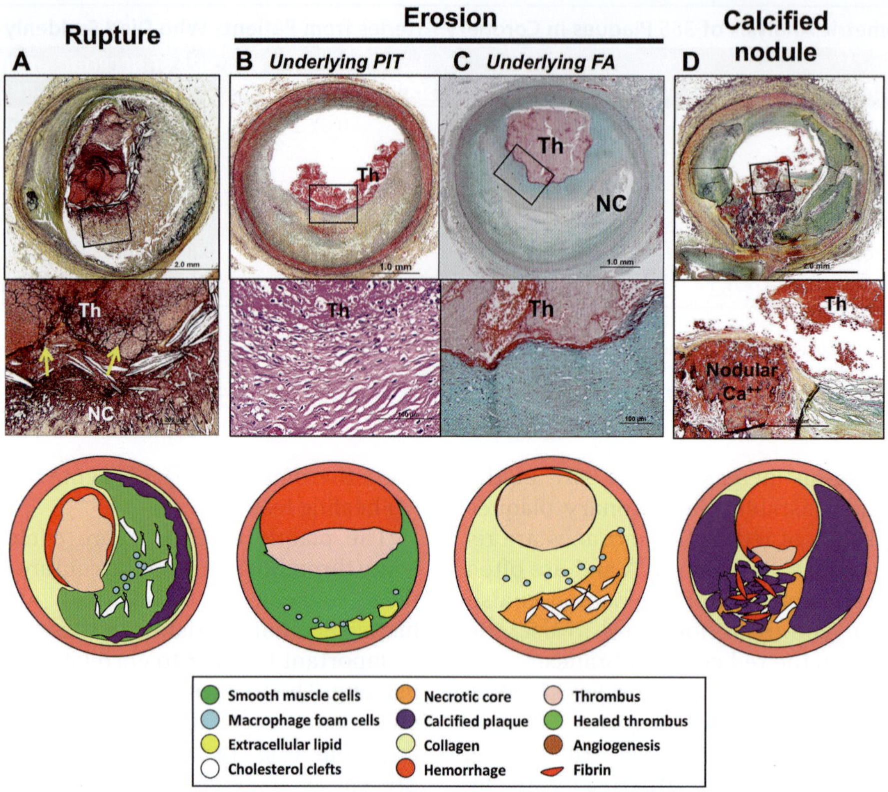

FIG. 12.2 Lesions of Acute Thrombosis. Histological and schematic images are shown for (A) plaque rupture, (B) plaque erosion with underlying pathological intimal thickening (PIT), and (C) with underlying fibroatheroma (FA). Least common is calcified nodule (D). Boxed area shows luminal thrombus with underlying nodular calcium. *NC*, Necrotic core; *Th*, thrombus. (A, B, and D were reproduced Falk E, Nakano M, Bentzon JF, Finn AV, Virmani R. Update on acute coronary syndromes: the pathologists' view. *Eur Heart J*. 2013;34:719–728; Other images were reproduced from Yahagi K, Kolodgie FD, Otsuka F, et al. Pathophysiology of native coronary, vein graft, and in-stent atherosclerosis. *Nat Rev Cardiol*. 2016;13:79–98.)

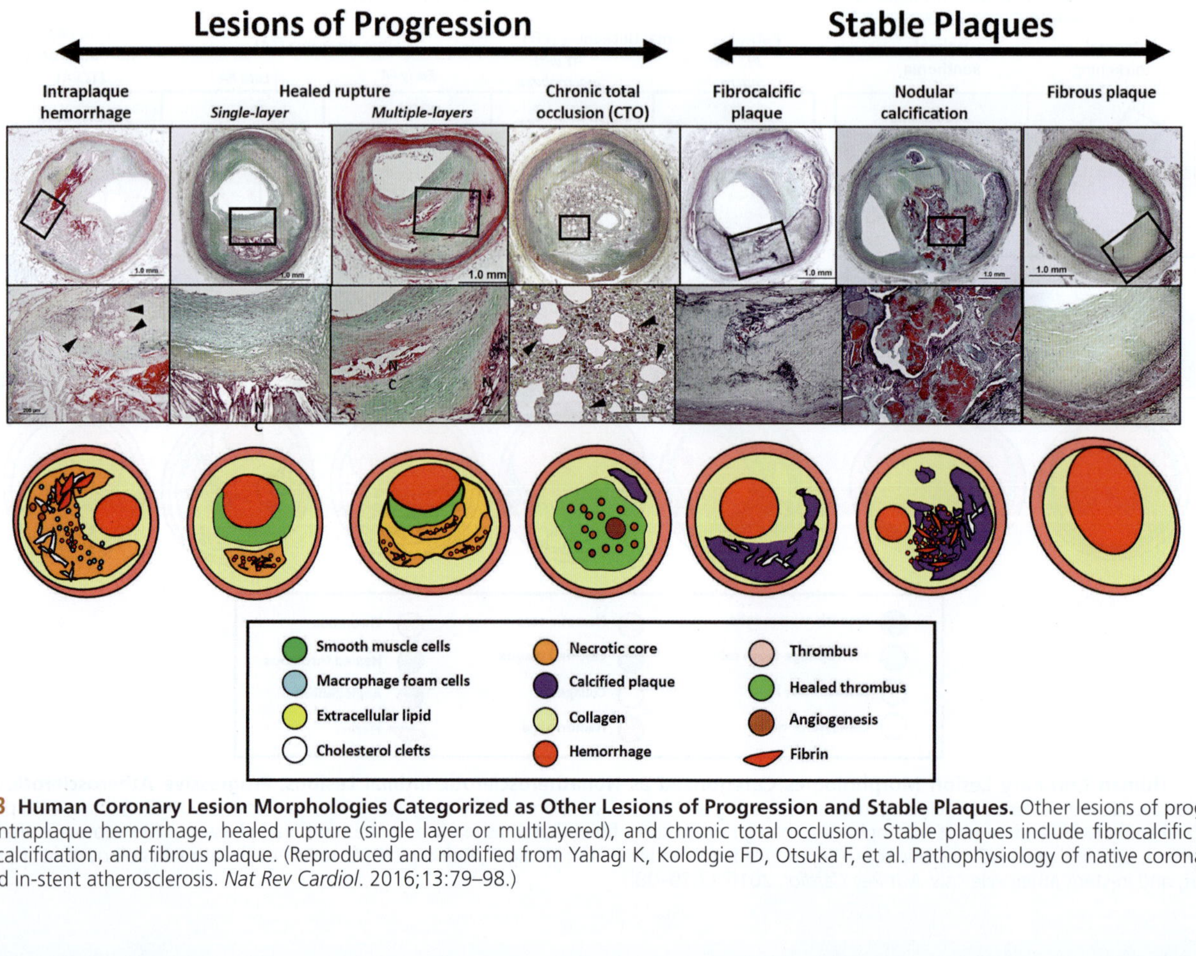

FIG. 12.3 Human Coronary Lesion Morphologies Categorized as Other Lesions of Progression and Stable Plaques. Other lesions of progression include intraplaque hemorrhage, healed rupture (single layer or multilayered), and chronic total occlusion. Stable plaques include fibrocalcific plaque, nodular calcification, and fibrous plaque. (Reproduced and modified from Yahagi K, Kolodgie FD, Otsuka F, et al. Pathophysiology of native coronary, vein graft, and in-stent atherosclerosis. *Nat Rev Cardiol*. 2016;13:79–98.)

NONATHEROSCLEROTIC INTIMAL LESIONS

Adaptive or Diffuse Intimal Thickening and Intimal Xanthoma

Intimal thickening is the earliest change in the arterial wall that can be detected using current imaging modalities such as intravascular imaging. Adaptive and diffuse intimal thickening is a physiological response to blood flow and can be observed in 30% of newborns. It is primarily composed of smooth muscle cells in a proteoglycan-rich matrix, which is a few cells thick. These intimal cell masses increase with age: 10% in the fetuses, 33.3% in infants, 17% in children, and 100% in adults. The IEL reduplicates and correlates with intimal thickening. The maximum changes occur at bifurcation sites of blood vessel where lipid accumulation is seen within intimal lesion that begin to form lipid pool of PIT lesions.[8] The same sites of intimal thickening are the sites where lipid pools form, leading to pathologic intimal thickening.

Intimal xanthoma, also known as fatty streaks, is primarily composed of focal accumulation of foamy macrophages within the intima, and even a few SMC may show presence of lipid droplets.[9,10] Intimal xanthomas are classified as nonatherosclerotic lesions, as these lesions have been shown to regress in PDAY (Pathobiological Determinants of Atherosclerosis in Youth Study) studies. Fatty streak lesions in 15- to 19-year-old adolescents occur predominantly in the thoracic aorta, whereas raised lesions (fibroatheromas) are seen mostly in the abdominal aorta in adults in their thirties. This suggests that fatty streak lesions regress with age and lesions of fibroatheromas have a different precursor.[11–13]

Progressive Atherosclerotic Lesions

PATHOLOGIC INTIMAL THICKENING

PIT is defined as the earliest atherosclerotic lesion leading to advanced atherosclerotic plaques. The classic histologic appearance shows an eccentric lesion rich in SMC with areas of lipid pools that are composed of several proteoglycans (biglycan and versican) and glycosaminoglycans (hyaluronan), without the presence of a necrotic core. The lipid pool proteoglycan-rich lesions have poorly delineated margins and show presence of circulating plasma lipids, apo B, and fibrin, which have been demonstrated by special stains.[3] We and others have shown that lipid pools contain remnants of SMC and PAS positive basement membranes of SMC undergoing apoptotic cell death.[14] Also, PIT is the earliest lesion to show calcification and microcalcifications (>0.5 µm, usually <15 µm) in the area of the lipid pool.[10,11] Early lesions of PIT do not show presence of macrophages; however, late phases show presence of foamy macrophages localized towards the lumen with or without lymphocytes.

FIBROATHEROMA

Fibroatheroma indicates a well-established atherosclerotic lesion composed of a necrotic core and an overlying fibrous cap.[15] The necrotic core, described as the "graveyard of macrophages," is histologically composed of macrophages that are infiltrating within the lipid pool and with matrix loss around the macrophages, leading to the formation of an early necrotic core.[16] Galis et al. showed that matrix metalloproteinases (MMPs) in foamy macrophages can digest the extracellular matrix and are likely responsible for the necrotic core formation and remodeling seen in atherosclerotic advanced lesions.[17] Schrijvers et al.[18] showed that phagocytosis of apoptotic cells (AC) is significantly impaired as compared to tonsil germinal centers. The ratio of free AC versus phagocytized AC is 19 times higher in atherosclerotic plaques, showing a severe defect.[18] The fibrous cap overlying the necrotic core consists of type I and type III collagen, proteoglycans, and SMC.[19] The size of the necrotic core and the thickness of the fibrous cap are strongly related to the plaque vulnerability to rupture. Fibroatheromas have been classified into two distinct stages: "early" or "late" depending on the relative extent of necrosis and persistent proteoglycan-rich matrix.[2] Late fibroatheromas shows a necrotic core with an absence of proteoglycan matrix that is rich in cholesterol crystals, showing presence of glycophorin A staining of erythrocyte membranes and presence of iron (from the breakdown of hemoglobin from red blood cells), thus suggesting that a fair amount of free cholesterol comes from intraplaque hemorrhage within the necrotic core. Also, surrounding the necrotic core, the plaque area is rich in vasa vasorum that are leaky, as shown by diffuse staining by von Willebrand factor, and the endothelial cells have poor intercellular junctions, as demonstrated by transmission electron microscopy.[5]

THIN-CAP FIBROATHEROMA

TCFA, classically called vulnerable plaques, are high-risk plaques that can result in an acute coronary syndrome.[20] Thin-cap fibroatheromas (vulnerable plaque) is a lesion with a large necrotic core (25% of plaque area) and a fibrous cap less than 65 mm thick with infiltration of macrophages (Table 12.2), without a plaque rupture (intact fibrous cap).[20a] The 65-mm thickness in cases without rupture was

TABLE 12.2 Morphologic Characteristics of Fibroatheroma, Thin-cap Fibroatheromas, and Plaque Rupture

PLAQUE TYPE	IEL AREA (mm²)	%STENOSIS (%)	NECROTIC CORE (%)	FIBROUS CAP THICKNESS (µm)	MACROPHAGE (%)	CALCIFICATION (%)
FA	10.1 ± 4.0	75.8 ± 14.2	17.7 ± 11.5	400 ± 190	1.8 ± 2.4	6.5 ± 13.5
TCFA	12.4 ± 5.5	70.8 ± 14.4	25.2 ± 15.7	40 ± 20	4.1 ± 4.5	5.3 ± 11.4
Rupture	14.2 ± 5.9	78.2 ± 14.0	35.9 ± 20.6	30 ± 10	5.7 ± 5.3	4.8 ± 7.7

Mean values are represented ± standard deviation.

FA, Fibroatheroma; *IEL*, internal elastic lamina, *TCFA*, thin-cap fibroatheroma.

Reproduced and modified from Narula J, Nakano M, Virmani R, et al. Histopathologic characteristics of atherosclerotic coronary disease and implications of the findings for the invasive and noninvasive detection of vulnerable plaques. *J Am Coll Cardiol*. 2013;61:1041–1051.

chosen as a criterion for vulnerability because in arteries with ruptured plaque, the mean (±SD) cap thickness was 23 ± 19 mm (95% of the caps measured less than 64 mm).[20] Although not all thin-cap fibroatheromas go on to rupture, it is likely that the lesions that rupture involve substantial mechanical stress. The thin fibrous cap is made up of type I collagen with sparse SMC, which provide tensile strength, and the cap is infiltrated by macrophages. Experimental studies of fibrous caps dissected from human atherosclerotic plaques have provided evidence of collagen breakdown when incubated with human macrophages release MMP-1 and MMP-2.[21] More recently, a mismatch of collagen and the presence of macrocalcifications in the fibrous cap have shown to behave as intensifiers of circumferential stress in the cap, causing an increase in the local stress that eventually leads to ruptures.[22]

Lesion With Thrombosis Relating Acute Coronary Syndrome

In cases of sudden death by coronary artery disease, the thrombosis rate is 68% in our CVPath Institute Registry that contains over 1200 cases. Of these, 23% had chronic total occlusion and the remaining all had no coronary thrombosis but had one or more major coronary arteries severely narrowed (>75% cross-sectional area narrowing) by an underlying atherosclerotic plaque. The main causes of thrombosis are plaque rupture in 63%, plaque erosion in 32%, and 5% by calcified nodule.[23] Patients dying from acute myocardial infarction at autopsy had plaque rupture in 75% of cases and erosion in 25%.[24] However, the mean age in our series of sudden deaths was 54 ± 16 years in women and 51 ± 12 years in men, whereas in acute myocardial infarction cases, the age of patients with plaque rupture was 68 ± 11 years and for erosion 70 ± 15 years, which is significantly different than those presenting for the first time as sudden coronary death. Therefore these differences in thrombosis rate are not surprising because erosions are more commonly observed in younger individuals (especially in women).

PLAQUE RUPTURE

Plaque rupture is the most frequent cause of acute coronary syndrome. Histologically, the ruptured plaques show a thin disrupted fibrous cap that is infiltrated by macrophages with an underlying large necrotic core that occupies approximately 36% of the plaque area; there is calcification, but the calcified area is small, occupying approximately 5% of the plaque area. At the site of disruption in the fibrous cap, the necrotic core is exposed to blood flow in the lumen, resulting in the activation of coagulation cascade, which consists predominately of platelet aggregation (Fig. 12.4). The thrombus is white in color at the site of plaque rupture, as it is rich in platelets that may results in occlusive or nonocclusive thrombus. The site of rupture of the fibrous cap usually occurs in the shoulder region, the weakest portion of the cap (this is especially true when rupture occurs during rest, at 36%). On the other hand, ruptures that occur during exercise are more frequent in the center of the cap (44%).[25] In the rest of the individuals rupture appeared circumferential (20%). Plaque hemorrhage was more frequent in individuals dying during exertion (72%) versus at rest (41%). Most plaques with rupture also show medial disruption, with a loss of IEL and medial thinning, and with a heavy inflammatory infiltrate consisting of T-lymphocytes and even plasma cells. These vessels with plaque rupture show positive remodeling. As mentioned above, MMPs secreted by macrophages are involved in thinning of the fibrous cap, and high shear and tensile stresses as hemodynamic factors also contribute to plaque rupture.[26–28] Microcalcification (>5 μm) and iron accumulation may potentially trigger for plaque rupture due to stress-induced disruption of the fibrous capsule.[15,29–31]

PLAQUE EROSION

Plaque erosion is the second most common cause of coronary thrombosis and has been shown to occur at a younger age, in less severely narrowed arteries, and with less calcifications as compared to plaque rupture. Plaque erosion is common in women, especially in women <50 years of age.[32–35] Morphologically, plaque erosion is characterized by the presence of a luminal thrombus with an underlying thick fibrous cap that is rich in smooth muscle cells in a proteoglycan matrix and has an absence of endothelial lining. Plaque erosion lesions have less inflammation as compared to rupture. The most common underlying plaque morphology in plaque erosion is early fibroatheroma (50%) followed by late fibroatheroma (34%), the least frequent being PIT (16%).[36] There is an absence of communication between the thrombus and the underlying necrotic core.[19,36] In contrast to plaque rupture, the culprit site of plaque erosion shows fewer macrophages and lymphocytes with an intact media, which is often negatively remodeled.[15,35,37]

Although distinct morphologic features of erosion prone plaques have not been identified, in fibroatheroma and in PIT lesions it is possible that vasospasm plays an important role because the artery wall is intact and is negatively remodeled.[19,38] The percentage of stenosis in erosion lesions is 70 ± 11% versus rupture 78 ± 12% ($P < .3$), calcification of plaque is significantly less frequent (23% versus 69%), and eccentricity of plaque is much higher (eccentric: concentric: erosion 82:18 and rupture 54:46).[33,36] The thrombus in erosion is more often organizing (>1 day in age, 88%) as compared to ruptures (54%).[39] Microemboli are more frequently observed in erosions than in ruptures (71% versus 42%, $P = .01$).[40]

CALCIFIED NODULE

Calcified nodule (CN) is the least common cause of coronary thrombosis, with an incidence varying from 2% to 5% reported in recent studies.[7,23] CN was first reported by us in 2000. Detailed morphologic findings indicate that it occurs usually in older individuals with a high prevalence of diabetes and chronic kidney disease. The thrombus is usually nonocclusive and consists of multiple, nodular fragments of calcium protruding and disrupting the overlying fibrous cap with loss of overlying endothelium.[41] The most frequent site of CN is usually the right coronary artery (61%), mostly in the mid-portion, followed by left main bifurcation (19%), the left circumflex (11%), and, least frequently, LAD (8%). We have described two types of calcifications: one that

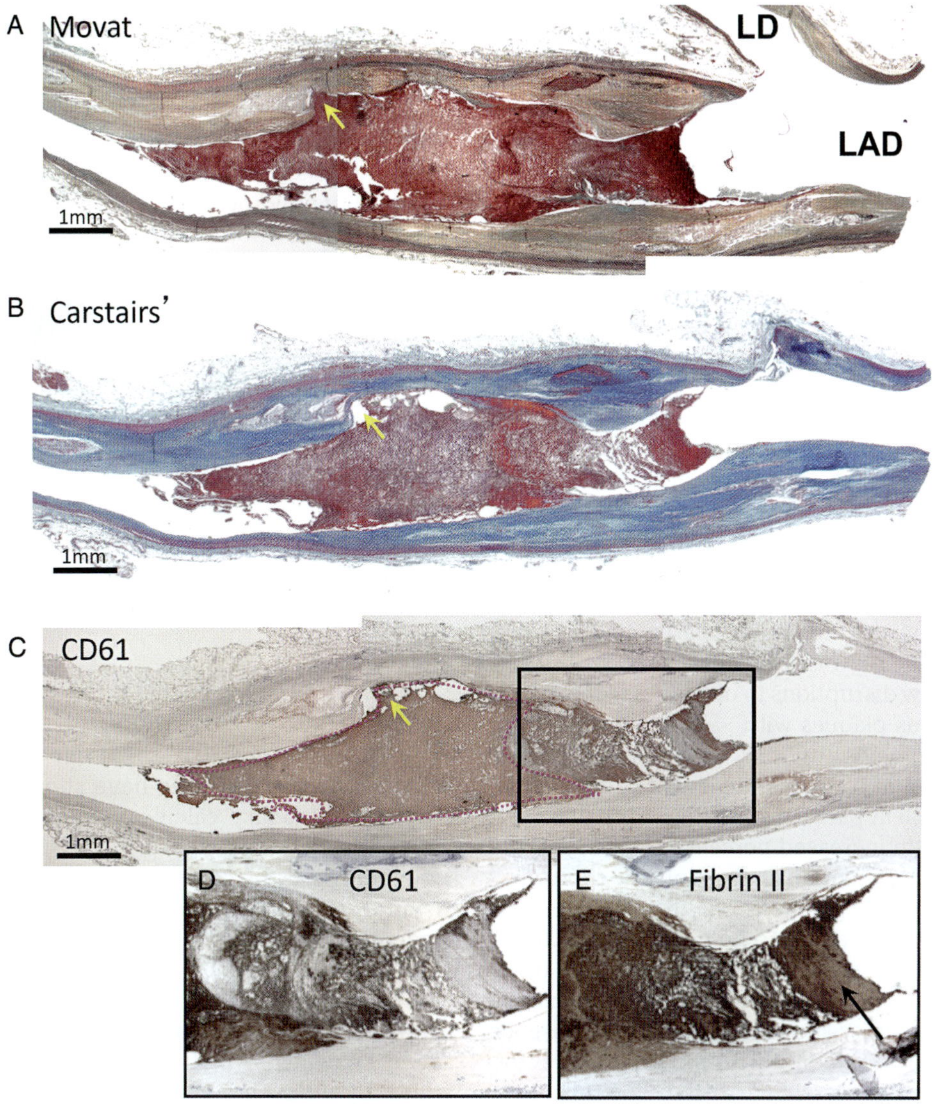

FIG. 12.4 Coronary Artery Occlusion Form Ruptured Plaque. Coronary artery with occlusive thrombus due to plaque rupture. Longitudinal histologic sections of LAD and LD stained by (A) Movat-Pentachrome, (B) Carstairs' stain, and CD61 Ab stain (C) note, the *yellow arrows* point to the site of plaque rupture and the *pink outline* in (C) shows the area of platelet-rich thrombus. *Black* boxed area is shown below at higher power in (D) (CD61 Ab) and (E) (fibrin II Ab) immunostained images demonstrating the region of the propagated thrombus that is rich in fibrin II (*black arrow*). *LAD*, Left anterior descending; *LD*, left diagonal branch (Reproduced and modified from Schwartz RS, Burke A, Farb A, et al. Microemboli and microvascular obstruction in acute coronary thrombosis and sudden coronary death: relation to epicardial plaque histopathology. *J Am Coll Cardiol*. 2009;54:2167–2173.)

occurs in necrotic cores (necrotic core calcium), the other being collagen calcification (also known as sheet calcium). We showed that the degree of circumferential sheet calcification was significantly less in the culprit section (89°) [interquartile range 54° to 177°] than in the adjacent proximal (206°) [interquartile 157° to 269°], and distal (240°) [interquartile range: 178° to 333°], ($P = .0004$) sections. It is important to note that plaque that underlies the area of the thrombus shows the presence of necrotic core calcification, which is sandwiched between the proximal and distal hard collagen-calcium. CN mostly forms in heavily calcified coronary segments—fibrocalcific plaque, the arc of calcification (90° to 270°) contains large amounts of rigid collagen calcification, lying directly adjacent to a more flexible (with less tensile strength; the arc of calcification is small) lesion containing necrotic core calcifications.[41] Calcified nodules are different from nodular calcifications that do not have surface thrombi and may remain within the fibrous cap in the intimal plaque. Clinically, these lesions have been reported to occur in highly calcified arteries; the incidence of CN varies from 4.2% of all lesions and is located more frequently in the ostial or mid-right coronary artery. Like our study, it is more frequently observed in patients on hemodialysis. In patients presenting with acute coronary syndrome (ACS), the incidence of CN in culprit lesion is reported as 5.3% and can be identified by OCT and by ultrasound.[42]

Stable Atherosclerotic Plaques (Healed Plaque Ruptures, Fibrocalcific Plaques, and Fibrous Plaques) (Fig. 12.3)

It is important to first understand what is labeled as stable plaques. These are lesions of fibroatheromas, healed plaque ruptures, fibrocalcific plaques, and fibrous plaques, and the lesion may or may not be severely narrowed. Stable angina pectoris patients usually have plaques that are severely narrowed (>75% cross-sectional area narrowing), resulting in a decrease in oxygen supply to the myocardium that usually occurs upon exercise and disappears with rest. The following describes the evolution of plaques that are positively remodeled to those that result in luminal compromise. Glagov et al. were the first to describe that luminal compromise does not occur until the artery is greater than 40% narrowed. They showed that the artery continues to enlarge as the plaque grows and the luminal stenosis may be delayed until the lesion occupies 40% of the internal elastic lamina.[43] Mann and Davies[44] reported on the mechanisms of plaque progression and showed that among men dying of ischemic heart disease, plaques that had <20% diameter stenosis had prior disruption in only 16% of sections. Plaque disruption is described as a discreet defect in the plaque's dense collagen (yellow white) and the defect area is filled by smooth muscle cells in loosely arrange collagen (green staining when utilizing Sirius red staining and visualized under polarized light) representing healed plaque rupture. However, plaques with 21% to 50% stenosis show disruptions in only a small fraction of cases (18%), whereas plaques with >51% narrowing show disruption more commonly (73%), thus suggesting that the main mechanism of plaque enlargement is through repeated ruptures.[44] Silent plaque rupture is a form of wound healing that results in increased percent stenosis, and the narrowing is less in healed than in acute plaque ruptures.[45]

Another type of stable plaque is one that is rich in collagen and calcium but has little to no necrotic core and is classified as fibrocalcified plaque. In patients dying of severe coronary disease the artery with fibrocalcific plaque is narrowed ≥75% in cross-sectional areas in the absence of acute thrombus. Also, plaques with the same characteristics may also be less severely narrowed. The third type of stable plaque is called fibrous plaque that forms from a healed propagated thrombus, and like wound healing, is rich in collagen type I.

Chronic Total Occlusion (Figure 12.3)

Chronic total occlusion (CTO) is another form of healed plaque rupture, except the lumen is totally occluded from a healed thrombus. CTO is a common finding among patients undergoing elective coronary angiography is reported to have a prevalence of 18%.[46] We have reported the prevalence of CTO in 23% in individuals without known coronary artery disease presenting with sudden coronary death. When comparing angiographic CTO with histologic findings, it has been reported that only 78% show complete occlusion and this is related to the presence of microchannels within the area of occlusion. We have reported histologic findings in CTOs of short and long duration. The short duration of CTO is characterized by abundant thrombus and necrotic core, and less negative remodeling, whereas long-duration CTO is characterized by negative remodeling and moderate calcifications.[47] The organized thrombus has neovascularization and early macrophage infiltration with areas of hemosiderin deposition and granulation tissue (eventually replaced by type I collagen).

Coronary Calcification and Atherosclerosis

Coronary artery calcifications in atherosclerosis have been recognized for more than a century. The process of coronary artery calcification begins as microcalcification (0.5 to 15 mm) and grows into larger fragments of calcium that eventually result in sheet-like deposits. Most PIT lesions show microcalcification, which we believe occur in areas of SMC apoptosis, whereas in early fibroatheroma, calcifications occurs in areas of macrophage infiltration within the lipid pool that undergo apoptosis, calcify, and appear as punctate (>15 mm) areas of calcifications. These areas progress to involve surrounding collagen matrix and coalesce to form fragments of calcification that are located near the media and vary in size from 1 to 3 mm. Eventually sheet calcifications (>3 mm diameter) can occur by extension of calcified areas into the necrotic core and or collagen. Fragmented calcium is more commonly observed in vulnerable and ruptured plaques, whereas sheet calcium is more common in healed plaque ruptures, stable plaques, and in calcified nodule and nodular calcification.

CCTA FOR THE DIAGNOSIS OF CORONARY MORPHOLOGY

Many pathologic studies have shown a good correlation between coronary calcifications and plaque burden but not with the lumen area.[31,48] It has been recognized for a long time that the coronary calcium score (see Chapter 3) is an excellent predictor of future cardiovascular events, independent of risk factors.[49] However, on an individual basis, it is not possible to predict by calcium score where the next cardiac event will occur in the coronary tree. To better predict which coronary plaques will rupture, it has been shown that high-risk plaque features can be identified by utilizing coronary CT angiography (CCTA). The high-risk plaques are classified as having positive remodeling, low-attenuation, and spotty calcifications.[50] Others have classified high-risk plaques as having positive remodeling, low-attenuation, or a napkin-ring sign (Fig. 12.5).[50a] The napkin ring sign refers to a qualitative plaque feature and can be defined in a noncalcified plaque cross-section by the presence of two features: a central area of low CT attenuation that is apparently in contact with the lumen, and a ring-like higher attenuation plaque tissue surrounding this central area.[51] Maurovich-Horvat et al. reported on plaque characteristics assessed by CCTA and histology utilizing 21 coronary arteries from seven donor hearts.[52] They classified CCTA findings into no plaque (NP) 22%, noncalcified plaques (NCP) 42%, mixed plaques (MP) 31%, and calcified plaques (CP) 5%. Among the NCP and MP, the pattern of the noncalcified portion of the plaque cross-section was assessed, and a homogenous pattern was described in 46% and a heterogenous pattern found in 53%. Among heterogenous plaques, 18% showed napkin-ring sign pattern. Histologically, all plaques were classified, and advanced lesions were considered as fibroatheroma (early and late) and thin-cap fibroatheromas. There was a good correlation between advanced lesions by histology and heterogenous plaques and napkin-ring sign by CCTA. This suggests that plaque attenuation pattern holds

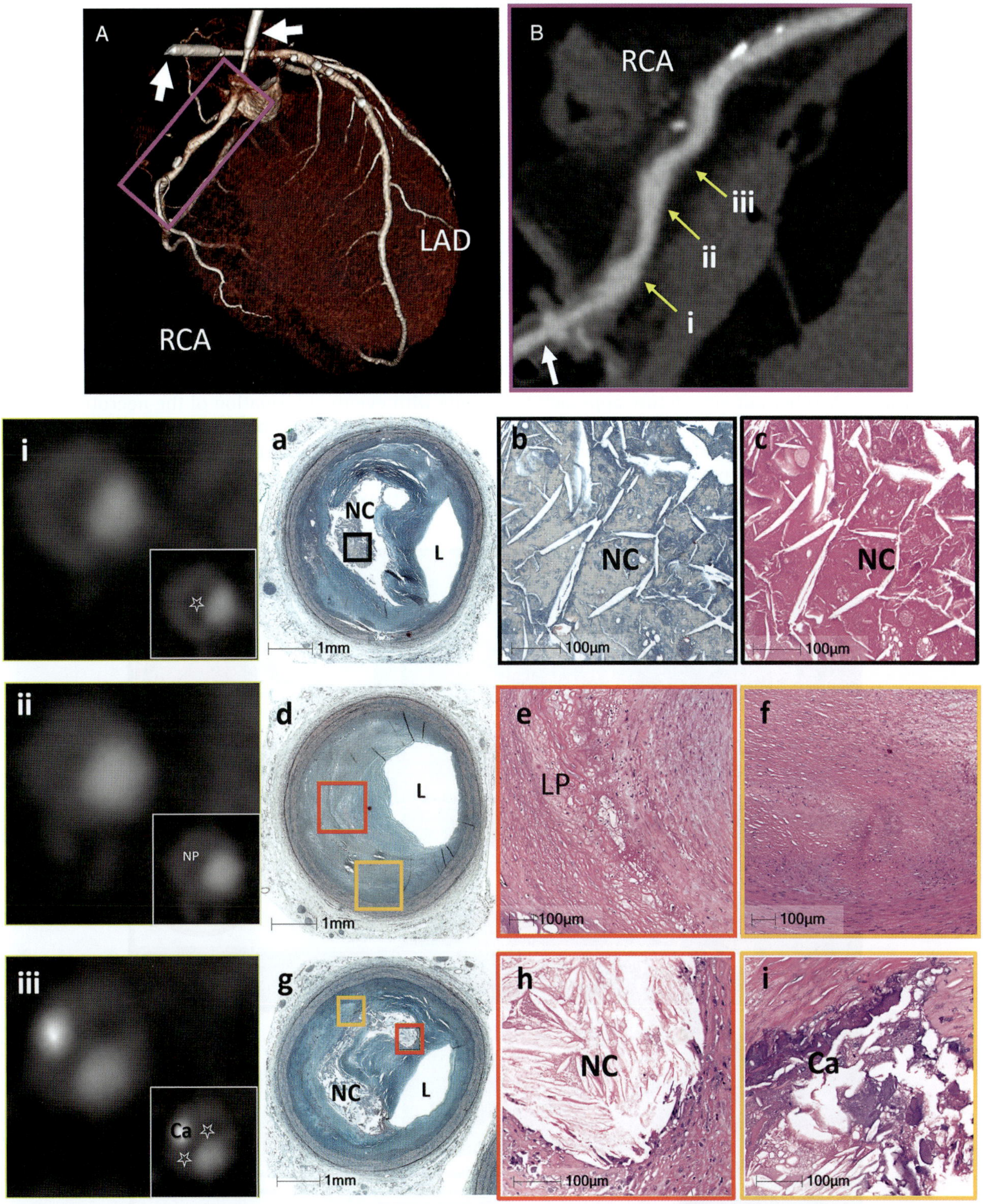

FIG. 12.5 Plaque With or Without Napkin-ring Sign as Assessed by CTA. (A) A volume-rendered coronary computed tomography angiography (CCTA) obtained from donor heart. The *white arrows* indicate coronary cannulas. (B) *Purple* boxed area shows curved multiplanar reformation of the RCA. The *white arrow* points to the canulated ostium of the RCA. *Yellow arrows* (i) to (iii) show corresponding cross-sections of CT and histology in the lower panels. (i) Cross-sectional CT image with napkin-ring sign. There is higher CT attenuation in the central of the cross-section (*star*). (a) The corresponding histopathologic section of a late fibroatheroma. Boxed area shows magnified images of necrotic core stained with Movat (b) and with H&E (c). (ii) Cross-sectional CT image of a noncalcified plaque without attenuation in the plaque in contrast-enhanced image. (d) The corresponding histopathologic section demonstrates PIT. *Red* boxed area shows presence of lipid pool in (e). *Yellow* boxed area shows homogeneous fibrous tissue (f). (iii) Cross-sectional CT image with the napkin-ring sign and calcified plaque (spotty calcification). Note, attenuation in central portion of the plaque (*stars*). (g) The corresponding histopathologic section demonstrates late fibroatheroma with calcification. *Red* boxed area shows presence of necrotic core (h). *Yellow* boxed area shows calcification in (i). *Ca*, Calcification; *L*, lumen; *LAD*, left anterior descending; *LP*, lipid pool; *NC*, necrotic core; *NP*, noncalcified homogenous plaque; *RCA*, right coronary artery; *star sign*, low attenuation region. (Reproduced and modified from Maurovich-Horvat P, Hoffmann U, Vorpahl M, Nakano M, Virmani R, Alkadhi H. The napkin-ring sign: CT signature of high-risk coronary plaques? *JACC Cardiovasc Imaging*. 2010;3:440–444.)

valuable information regarding plaque morphology and may improve plaque classification in CCTAs. The authors have further shown that in a subset of PROMISE (Prospective Multicenter Study for Evaluation of Chest Pain) trial that high-risk plaque found on CCTA is associated with future MACE (major adverse cardiovascular events).[53] CCTA done at autopsy has been shown in very few cases to correlate with histologic studies of plaque erosion (Fig. 12.6) and plaque rupture (Fig. 12.7).[53a]

To overcome the potential limitations of the spatial resolution of CCTA, recent advances have included improved detectors with better spatial resolution (Chapter 2), as well as the use of artificial intelligence and radiomics (Chapter 11) for plaque characterization.[54] These novel approaches could further improve the diagnostic accuracy of coronary CT angiography for identifying high-risk atherosclerotic lesions. Another potential future approach to image the evolution of plaques in vivo (Fig. 12.8)[41,55,56] is to use microCT (resolution in microns), which has better resolution when compared with conventional clinical CTA (resolution in millimeters) and thus may allow for more detailed visualization of plaque morphology. However, current microCT systems are most used for ex vivo imaging due to the larger radiation dose as well as limited temporal resolution.

CONCLUSION

This chapter summarizes the morphological evolution of atherosclerotic plaque progression, from early to advanced lesions, including thrombosis. The progression of coronary atherosclerosis begins with nonatherosclerotic lesions (adaptive intimal thickening, intimal xanthoma) and can progress to PIT, considered to be the earliest lesion of atherosclerosis. Macrophage infiltration into the lipid pool of this lesions converts PIT to fibroatheroma with eventual formation of the necrotic core devoid of matrix (the word *athero* comes from the Greek word meaning gruel or paste). The fibrous cap thins over time to eventually form a vulnerable lesion also called TCFA, which is the precursor lesion of plaque rupture. There are

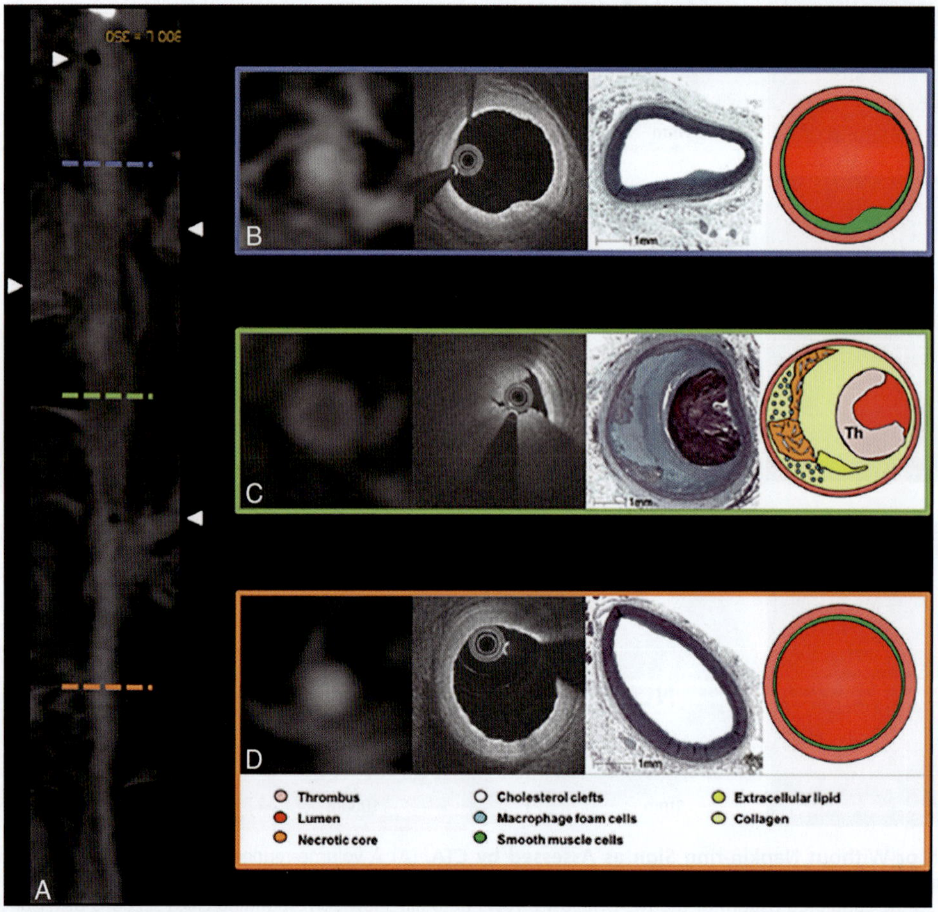

FIG. 12.6 Plaque Erosion by CCTA, OCT, and Histopathology. (A) Figure demonstrates a straight multiplanar reformat of the RCA by SECT. The RCA exhibits an occlusive luminal thrombus in the mid-segment. In each panel, every CCTA cross-section is coregistered from left to right with OCT, histopathology, and a schematic image, respectively. The ostial cannula, air bubbles, and extensive perivascular contrast extravasation (*white arrowheads*) are artifacts unique to postmortem CT scanning of explanted hearts. (B) Adaptive intimal thickening, characterized by the accumulation of smooth muscle cells. (C) Plaque erosion with an intact fibrous cap and an underlying early fibroatheroma. No communication is observed between luminal thrombus and necrotic core. CCTA demonstrates positive remodeling with a remodeling index of >1.1 and a napkin-ring sign–like appearance: hypo-attenuated core (127 ± 5 HU) surrounded by an external rim of higher attenuation (179 ± 7 HU). OCT demonstrates a massive thrombus with a strong attenuation behind it. (D) Minimal intimal thickening, which is still considered to be physiological. *CCTA*, Coronary computed tomography angiography; *HU*, Hounsfield units; *OCT*, optical coherence tomography; *RCA*, right coronary artery; *SECT*, single-energy computed tomography. (Reproduced from van den Hoogen IJ, Gianni U, Al Hussein Alawamlh O, et al. What atherosclerosis findings can CT see in sudden coronary death: plaque rupture versus plaque erosion. *J Cardiovasc Comput Tomogr*. 2020;14:214–218.)

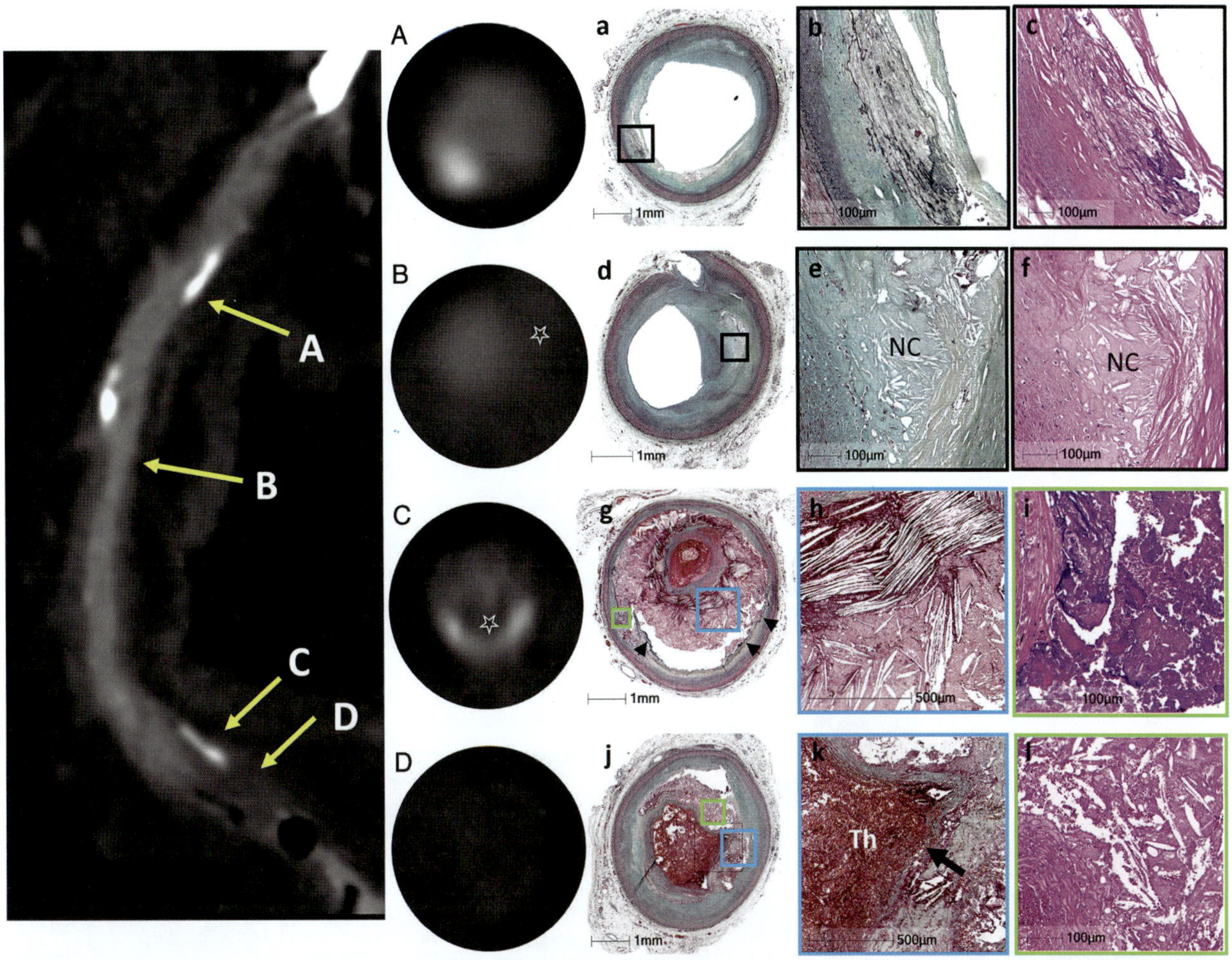

FIG. 12.7 Plaque Rupture Detected by CCTA and Corresponding Histopathology. Left panel shows curved proximal and mid-right RCA by DECT. The RCA exhibits diffuse nonobstructive CAD in (A) and (B) whereas (C) and (D) show the region of an occlusive luminal thrombus in the distal RCA segment. (A to D) *Yellow arrows* correspond to the location of each cross-section in right panels. (A) Cross-sectional image in the proximal RCA shows calcification. (a) Corresponding histology of (A) shows presence of fragment of calcification. In boxed area to the right, (b) and (c) show high-power images of the area of calcification stained with Movat (b) and H&E (c). (B) Low-attenuation plaque in the mid-segment. There is an eccentric attenuation lesion in the plaque area (*star*). (d) Shows the corresponding histology of a fibroatheroma with a necrotic core. Boxed area to the right shows high-power images of the necrotic core stained with Movat (e) and with H&E (f). (C) Low-attenuation lesion with calcification in the mid-RCA. There is an eccentric attenuated lesion in the plaque region (*star*) surrounded by semicircular calcification. (d) Corresponding histology on the right shows a late fibroatheroma with occlusive luminal thrombus. *Blue and green* boxed area show the presence of large necrotic core and calcified lesion at high power (h) and (i) stained with Movat and H&E, respectively. (D). CCTA cross-section of the culprit site in the mid-RCA segment. The coronary lumen is totally occluded with an underling napkin-ring sign of the hypo-attenuated core (HU104 ± 3). (j) Histology section corresponding to (D). The lumen is occluded by a thrombus with an underlying ruptured thin fibrous cap and an underlying necrotic core. *Blue* boxed area shows higher-power image of the area exhibit luminal thrombus (Th) and underlying rupture site (*arrow*) of the thin cap (k). *Green* boxed area shows underlying necrotic core (NC) (l). *CAD*, Coronary artery disease; *CCTA*, coronary computed tomography angiography; *DECT*, dual-energy computed tomography; *HU*, Hounsfield units; *RCA*, right coronary artery. (Reproduced and modified from van den Hoogen IJ, Gianni U, Al Hussein Alawamlh O, et al. What atherosclerosis findings can CT see in sudden coronary death: plaque rupture versus plaque erosion. *J Cardiovasc Comput Tomogr*. 2020;14:214–218.)

three main causes of coronary thrombosis, and the most common is plaque rupture, followed by plaque erosion and, least frequently, calcified nodule. Intraplaque hemorrhage also contributes significantly to the enlargement of the necrotic core and to the presence of cholesterol crystals that often dominate lesions that rupture. As plaque progresses, the vessel enlarges, but luminal compromise does not occur until the plaque occupies at least 40% of the cross-sectional area of the vessel. Plaque progression occurs from repeated healed plaque ruptures and plaque hemorrhage. Stable plaques are fibrocalcific plaques, which are healed plaque ruptures with a thick cap and fibrous plaques. Plaques may rupture silently and lead to chronic total occlusions. Coronary calcifications represent atherosclerosis and are easily identified by CT. The use of CCTA can detect the presence of high-risk plaques features that include positive remodeling, low-attenuated plaque, spotty calcifications, or a napkin-ring sign. These features of high-risk plaque are associated with a higher risk of future cardiovascular events.

DECLARATION OF INTERESTS

A.V. Finn has received consultant fees and honoraria from Abbott Vascular, Amgen, Biosensors, Boston Scientific, Celonova, Cook Medical, CSI, Lutonix Bard, Sinomed and Terumo Corporation. R. Virmani is a consultant of Abbott

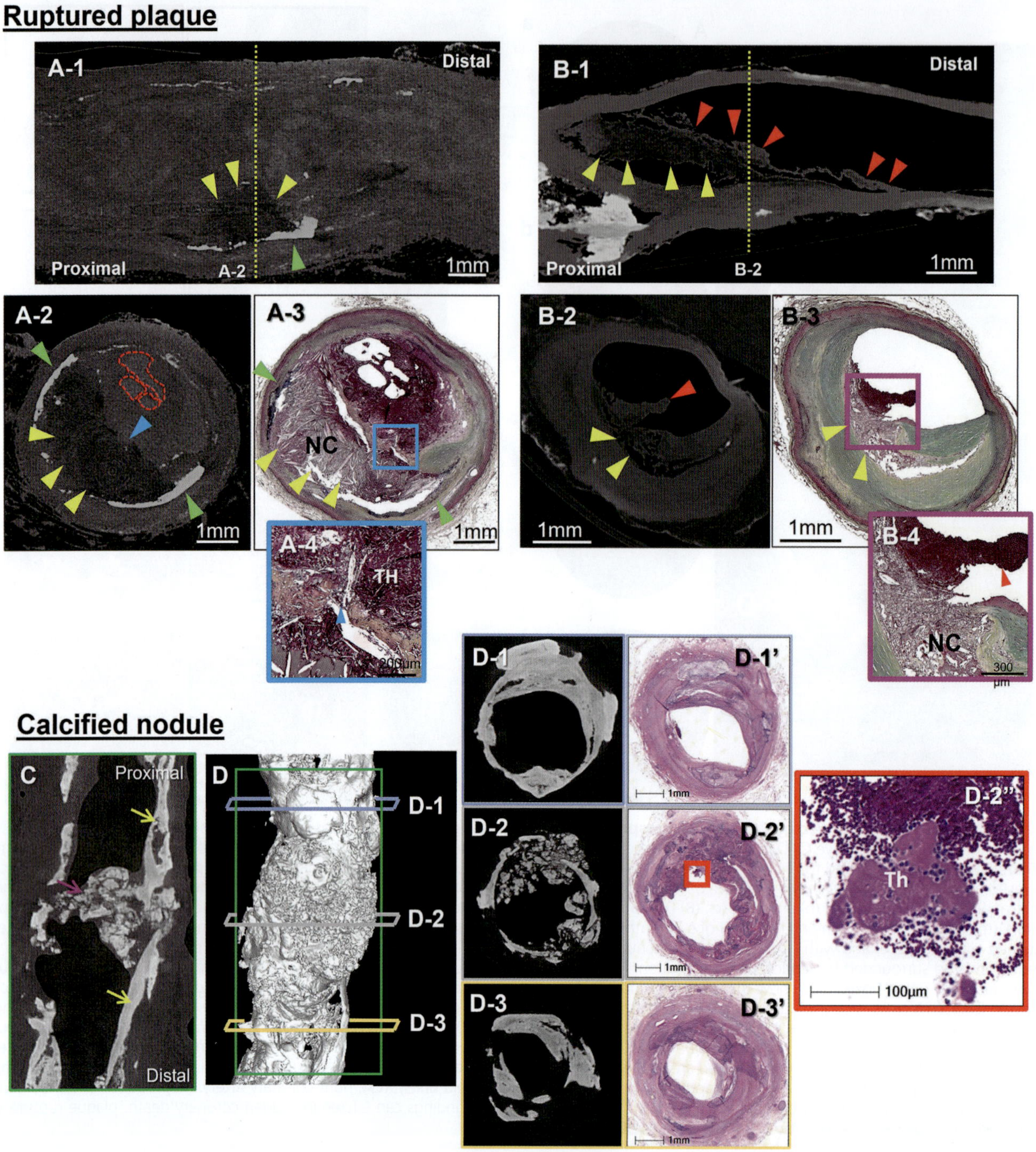

FIG. 12.8 Micro-CT Evaluation of the Ruptured Plaque With Occlusive Acute Thrombus. A-1, Longitudinal micro-CT image of the proximal RCA showing a low-intensity area, which corresponds to lipid core plaque (LCP) in A-2 (*yellow arrowheads*) and NC in A-3 (*yellow arrowheads*) with fragmented calcification (*green arrowheads*) toward the media at the site of total occlusion. A-2, The micro-CT cross-section image shows a low-intensity area (*yellow arrowheads*), indicating NC and underlying area of calcification (*green arrowheads*). A-3 and A-4, The matching histological image shows site of plaque rupture (*blue arrowhead*; rupture site highlighted in A-4) and underlying large NC (*yellow arrowheads*), which is marginated by calcification (*green arrowheads*). B-1 and B-2, Longitudinal and cross-section micro-CT images of the mid LCx showing irregularly dispersed luminal thrombus (*red arrowheads*) with underlying LCP (*yellow arrowheads* point to NC *while red arrowheads* show luminal thrombus). B-3, The histological image matching to the micro-CT image (B-2). B-4, A high-power image corresponding to a *pink* box in B-3, showing rupture site with overlying nonocclusive thrombus. (A-1 to B-4 are reproduced and modified from Jinnouchi H, Torii S, Kutyna M, et al. Micro-computed tomography demonstration of multiple plaque ruptures in a single individual presenting with sudden cardiac death. *Circ Cardiovasc Imaging*. 2018;11:e008331.) Calcified Nodule. Micro-CT of the longitudinally bisected half of the right coronary artery (C), and corresponding three-dimensional whole artery microCT showing only calcification (D). Lines D-1 to D-3 in D represent the sites of corresponding histological sections. D1 to D3 are microCT and the corresponding histological cross-sections (D-1′ to D-3′ H&E stained) from culprit sites (D-2, D-2′) and proximal (D-1, D-1′) and distal (D-3, D-3′). D-2″ is a high-power image of the red boxed area in D-2′, showing fibrin-platelet thrombus attached to the underlying calcified nodule at the culprit lesion. D-2. The culprit site in micro-CT shows both sheet calcium and necrotic core calcium (fragments of calcium) which protrude into the lumen. D1 and D3 show presence of only sheet collagen calcium. *CN*, Calcified nodule; *CT*, computed tomography; *LCP*, lipid core plaque; *LCx*, left circumflex artery; *NC*, necrotic core; *RCA*, right coronary artery; *Th*, thrombus. (C to D-2″ are reproduced and modified from Torii S, Sato Y, Otsuka F, et al. Eruptive calcified nodules as a potential mechanism of acute coronary thrombosis and sudden death. *J Am Coll Cardiol*. 2021;77:1599–1611.)

Vascular, Boston Scientific, Celonova, OrbusNeich Medical, Terumo Corporation, W. C. Gore, Edwards Lifesciences, Cook Medical, CSI, ReCor Medical, SinoMedical Sciences Technology, Surmodics, and Bard BD. K. Kawai, R. Virmani, and A.V. Finn are employees of the CVPath Institute that has received GranuResearch and Clinical Trial support from NIH-HL141425, Leducq Foundation Grant, 4C Medical, 4Tech, Abbott Vascular, Ablative Solutions. Absorption Systems, Advanced NanoTherapies, Aerwave Medical, Alivas, Amgen. Asahi Medical, Aurios Medical, Avantec Vascular, BD, Biosensors, Biotronik, Biotyx Medical, Bolt Medical, Boston Scientific, Canon USA, Cardiac Implants, Cardiawave, CardioMech, Celonova, Cerus EndoVascular, Chansu Vascular Technologies, Children's National Medical Center, Concept Medical, Cook Medical, Cooper Health, Cormaze Technologies GmbH, CRL/AccelLab, Croivalue, CSI, Dexcom, Edwards Lifesciences, Elucid Bioimaging, eLum Technologies, Emboline, Endotronix, Envision, Filterlex, Imperative Care, Innovalve, Innovative Cardiovascular Solutions, Intact Vascular, Interface Biolgics, Intershunt Techtnologies, Invatin Technologies, Lahav CRO, Limflow, L&J Biosciences, Lutonix, Lyra Therapeutics, Mayo Clinic, Maywell, MD Start, MedAlliance, Medanex, Medtronic, Mercator, Microport, Microvention, Neovasc, Nephronyx, Nova Vascular, Nyra Medical, Occultech, Olympus, Ohio Health, OrbusNeich, Ossio, Phenox, Pi-Cardia, Polares Medical, Polyvascular, Profusa, ProKidney LLC, Protembis, Pulse Biosciences, Qool Therapeutics, Recombinetics, ReCor Medical, Regencor, Renata Medical, Restore Medical, Ripple Therapeutics, Rush University, Sanofi, Shockwave, Sahajanand Medical Technologies, SoundPipe, Spartan Micro, Spectrawave, Surmodics, Terumo Corporation, The Jacobs Institute, Transmural Systems, Transverse Medical, TruLeaf Medical, UCSF, UPMC, Vesper, Vetex Medical, Whiteswell, WL Gore, and Xeltis.

The authors have no other relevant affiliations or financial involvement with any organization or entity with a financial interest in or financial conflict with the subject matter or materials discussed in the manuscript apart from those disclosed.

REFERENCES

1. Tsao CW, Aday AW, Almarzooq ZI, et al. Heart disease and stroke statistics-2022 update: a report from the American Heart Association. *Circulation*. 2022;145: e153–e639.
2. Yahagi K, Kolodgie FD, Otsuka F, et al. Pathophysiology of native coronary, vein graft, and in-stent atherosclerosis. *Nat Rev Cardiol*. 2016;13:79–98.
3. Nakagawa K, Nakashima Y. Pathologic intimal thickening in human atherosclerosis is formed by extracellular accumulation of plasma-derived lipids and dispersion of intimal smooth muscle cells. *Atherosclerosis*. 2018;274:235–242.
4. Otsuka F, Yasuda S, Noguchi T, Ishibashi-Ueda H. Pathology of coronary atherosclerosis and thrombosis. *Cardiovasc Diagn Ther*. 2016;6:396–408.
5. Sluimer JC, Kolodgie FD, Bijnens AP, et al. Thin-walled microvessels in human coronary atherosclerotic plaques show incomplete endothelial junctions relevance of compromised structural integrity for intraplaque microvascular leakage. *J Am Coll Cardiol*. 2009;53:1517–1527.
6. Kolodgie FD, Gold HK, Burke AP, et al. Intraplaque hemorrhage and progression of coronary atheroma. *N Engl J Med*. 2003;349:2316–2325.
7. Yahagi K, Davis HR, Arbustini E, Virmani R. Sex differences in coronary artery disease: pathological observations. *Atherosclerosis*. 2015;239:260–267.
8. Guerri-Guttenberg R, Castilla R, Cao G, Azzato F, Ambrosio G, Milei J. Coronary intimal thickening begins in fetuses and progresses in pediatric population and adolescents to atherosclerosis. *Angiology*. 2020;71:62–69.
9. Fan J, Watanabe T. Inflammatory reactions in the pathogenesis of atherosclerosis. *J Atheroscler Thromb*. 2003;10:63–71.
10. Aikawa M, Rabkin E, Okada Y, et al. Lipid lowering by diet reduces matrix metalloproteinase activity and increases collagen content of rabbit atheroma: a potential mechanism of lesion stabilization. *Circulation*. 1998;97:2433–2444.
11. Velican C. Relationship between regional aortic susceptibility to atherosclcrosis and macromolecular structural stability. *J Atheroscler Res*. 1969;9:193–201.
12. Velican C. A dissecting view on the role of the fatty streak in the pathogenesis of human atherosclerosis: culprit or bystander? *Med Interne*. 1981;19:321–337.
13. McGill Jr HC, McMahan CA, Herderick EE, et al. Effects of coronary heart disease risk factors on atherosclerosis of selected regions of the aorta and right coronary artery. Pday Research Group. Pathobiological determinants of atherosclerosis in youth. *Arterioscler Thromb Vasc Biol*. 2000;20: 836–845.
14. Kockx MM, De Meyer GR, Muhring J, Jacob W, Bult H, Herman AG. Apoptosis and related proteins in different stages of human atherosclerotic plaques. *Circulation*. 1998;97:2307–2315.
15. Virmani R, Kolodgie FD, Burke AP, Farb A, Schwartz SM. Lessons from sudden coronary death: a comprehensive morphological classification scheme for atherosclerotic lesions. *Arterioscler Thromb Vasc Biol*. 2000;20:1262–1275.
16. Tabas I. Macrophage death and defective inflammation resolution in atherosclerosis. *Nat Rev Immunol*. 2010;10:36–46.
17. Galis ZS, Sukhova GK, Kranzhöfer R, Clark S, Libby P. Macrophage foam cells from experimental atheroma constitutively produce matrix-degrading proteinases. *Proc Natl Acad Sci U S A*. 1995;92:402–406.
18. Schrijvers DM, De Meyer GR, Kockx MM, Herman AG, Martinet W. Phagocytosis of apoptotic cells by macrophages is impaired in atherosclerosis. *Arterioscler Thromb Vasc Biol*. 2005;25:1256–1261.
19. Sakakura K, Nakano M, Otsuka F, Ladich E, Kolodgie FD, Virmani R. Pathophysiology of atherosclerosis plaque progression. *Heart Lung Circ*. 2013;22:399–411.
20. Burke AP, Virmani R, Galis Z, Haudenschild CC, Muller JE. 34th Bethesda conference: task force #2—what is the pathologic basis for new atherosclerosis imaging techniques? *J Am Coll Cardiol*. 2003;41:1874–1886.
20a. Narula J, Nakano M, Virmani R, et al. Histopathologic characteristics of atherosclerotic coronary disease and implications of the findings for the invasive and noninvasive detection of vulnerable plaques. *J Am Coll Cardiol*. 2013;61:1041–1051.
21. Shah PK, Falk E, Badimon JJ, et al. Human monocyte-derived macrophages induce collagen breakdown in fibrous caps of atherosclerotic plaques. Potential role of matrix-degrading metalloproteinases and implications for plaque rupture. *Circulation*. 1995;92:1565–1569.
22. Cardoso L, Microcalcifications Weinbaum S. their genesis, growth, and biomechanical stability in fibrous cap rupture. *Adv Exp Med Biol*. 2018;1097:129–155.
23. Sato Y, Kawakami R, Sakamoto A, et al. Sex differences in coronary atherosclerosis. *Curr Atheroscler Rep*. 2022;24:23–32.
24. Arbustini E, Dal Bello B, Morbini P, et al. Plaque erosion is a major substrate for coronary thrombosis in acute myocardial infarction. *Heart (British Cardiac Society)*. 1999;82:269–272.
25. Burke AP, Farb A, Malcom GT, Liang Y, Smialek JE, Virmani R. Plaque rupture and sudden death related to exertion in men with coronary artery disease. *JAMA*. 1999;281:921–926.
26. Sukhova GK, Schönbeck U, Rabkin E, et al. Evidence for increased collagenolysis by interstitial collagenases-1 and -3 in vulnerable human atheromatous plaques. *Circulation*. 1999;99:2503–2509.
27. Gijsen FJ, Wentzel JJ, Thury A, et al. Strain distribution over plaques in human coronary arteries relates to shear stress. *Am J Physiol Heart Circ Physiol*. 2008;295:H1608–H1614.
28. Lenglet S, Mach F, Montecucco F. Role of matrix metalloproteinase-8 in atherosclerosis. *Mediators Inflamm*. 2013;2013:659282.
29. Kolodgie FD, Narula J, Burke AP, et al. Localization of apoptotic macrophages at the site of plaque rupture in sudden coronary death. *Am J Pathol*. 2000;157:1259–1268.
30. Vengrenyuk Y, Carlier S, Xanthos S, et al. A hypothesis for vulnerable plaque rupture due to stress-induced debonding around cellular microcalcifications in thin fibrous caps. *Proc Natl Acad Sci U S A*. 2006;103:14678–14683.
31. Otsuka F, Sakakura K, Yahagi K, Joner M, Virmani R. Has our understanding of calcification in human coronary atherosclerosis progressed? *Arterioscler Thromb Vasc Biol*. 2014;34:724–736.
32. Burke AP, Farb A, Malcom GT, Liang Y, Smialek J, Virmani R. Effect of risk factors on the mechanism of acute thrombosis and sudden coronary death in women. *Circulation*. 1998;97:2110–2116.
33. Farb A, Burke AP, Tang AL, et al. Coronary plaque erosion without rupture into a lipid core. A frequent cause of coronary thrombosis in sudden coronary death. *Circulation*. 1996;93:1354–1363.
34. Falk E, Nakano M, Bentzon JF, Finn AV, Virmani R. Update on acute coronary syndromes: the pathologists' view. *Eur Heart J*. 2013;34:719–728.
35. Burke AP, Kolodgie FD, Farb A, Weber D, Virmani R. Morphological predictors of arterial remodeling in coronary atherosclerosis. *Circulation*. 2002;105:297–303.
36. Yahagi K, Zarpak R, Sakakura K, et al. Multiple simultaneous plaque erosion in 3 coronary arteries. *JACC Cardiovasc Imaging*. 2014;7:1172–1174.
37. van der Wal AC, Becker AE, van der Loos CM, Das PK. Site of intimal rupture or erosion of thrombosed coronary atherosclerotic plaques is characterized by an inflammatory process irrespective of the dominant plaque morphology. *Circulation*. 1994;89:36–44.
38. Bentzon JF, Otsuka F, Virmani R, Falk E. Mechanisms of plaque formation and rupture. *Circ Res*. 2014;114:1852–1866.
39. Kramer MC, Rittersma SZ, de Winter RJ, et al. Relationship of thrombus healing to underlying plaque morphology in sudden coronary death. *J Am Coll Cardiol*. 2010;55:122–132.

40. Schwartz RS, Burke A, Farb A, et al. Microemboli and microvascular obstruction in acute coronary thrombosis and sudden coronary death: relation to epicardial plaque histopathology. *J Am Coll Cardiol*. 2009;54:2167–2173.
41. Torii S, Sato Y, Otsuka F, et al. Eruptive calcified nodules as a potential mechanism of acute coronary thrombosis and sudden death. *J Am Coll Cardiol*. 2021;77:1599–1611.
42. Vergallo R, Ren X, Yonetsu T, et al. Pancoronary plaque vulnerability in patients with acute coronary syndrome and ruptured culprit plaque: a 3-vessel optical coherence tomography study. *Am Heart J*. 2014;167:59–67.
43. Glagov S, Weisenberg E, Zarins CK, Stankunavicius R, Kolettis GJ. Compensatory enlargement of human atherosclerotic coronary arteries. *N Engl J Med*. 1987;316:1371–1375.
44. Mann J, Davies MJ. Mechanisms of progression in native coronary artery disease: role of healed plaque disruption. *Heart (British Cardiac Society)*. 1999;82:265–268.
45. Burke AP, Kolodgie FD, Farb A, et al. Healed plaque ruptures and sudden coronary death: evidence that subclinical rupture has a role in plaque progression. *Circulation*. 2001;103:934–940.
46. Fefer P, Knudtson ML, Cheema AN, et al. Current perspectives on coronary chronic total occlusions: the Canadian multicenter chronic total occlusions registry. *J Am Coll Cardiol*. 2012;59:991–997.
47. Sakakura K, Nakano M, Otsuka F, et al. Comparison of pathology of chronic total occlusion with and without coronary artery bypass graft. *Eur Heart J*. 2014;35:1683–1693.
48. Sangiorgi G, Rumberger JA, Severson A, et al. Arterial calcification and not lumen stenosis is highly correlated with atherosclerotic plaque burden in humans: a histologic study of 723 coronary artery segments using nondecalcifying methodology. *J Am Coll Cardiol*. 1998;31:126–133.
49. Budoff MJ, Achenbach S, Blumenthal RS, et al. Assessment of coronary artery disease by cardiac computed tomography: a scientific statement from the American Heart Association Committee on Cardiovascular Imaging and Intervention, Council on Cardiovascular Radiology and Intervention, and Committee on Cardiac Imaging, Council on Clinical Cardiology. *Circulation*. 2006;114:1761–1791.
50. Motoyama S, Kondo T, Sarai M, et al. Multislice computed tomographic characteristics of coronary lesions in acute coronary syndromes. *J Am Coll Cardiol*. 2007;50:319–326.
50a. Maurovich-Horvat P, Hoffmann U, Vorpahl M, Nakano M, Virmani R, Alkadhi H. The napkin-ring sign: CT signature of high-risk coronary plaques? *JACC Cardiovasc Imaging*. 2010;3:440–444.
51. Maurovich-Horvat P, Ferencik M, Voros S, Merkely B, Hoffmann U. Comprehensive plaque assessment by coronary CT angiography. *Nat Rev Cardiol*. 2014;11:390–402.
52. Maurovich-Horvat P, Schlett CL, Alkadhi H, et al. Differentiation of early from advanced coronary atherosclerotic lesions: systematic comparison of CT, intravascular us, and optical frequency domain imaging with histopathologic examination in ex vivo human hearts. *Radiology*. 2012;265:393–401.
53. Ferencik M, Mayrhofer T, Bittner DO, et al. Use of high-risk coronary atherosclerotic plaque detection for risk stratification of patients with stable chest pain: a secondary analysis of the promise randomized clinical trial. *JAMA Cardiol*. 2018;3:144–152.
53a. van den Hoogen IJ, Gianni U, Al Hussein Alawamlh O, et al. What atherosclerosis findings can CT see in sudden coronary death: plaque rupture versus plaque erosion. *J Cardiovasc Comput Tomogr*. 2020;14:214–218.
54. Kolossváry M, Karády J, Kikuchi Y, et al. Radiomics versus visual and histogram-based assessment to identify atheromatous lesions at coronary CT angiography: an ex vivo study. *Radiology*. 2019;293:89–96.
55. Kuntz SH, Jinnouchi H, Kutyna M, et al. Co-registration of peripheral atherosclerotic plaques assessed by conventional CT angiography, microct and histology in patients with chronic limb threatening ischaemia. *Eur J Vasc Endovasc Surg*. 2021;61:146–154.
56. Jinnouchi H, Torii S, Kutyna M, et al. Micro-computed tomography demonstration of multiple plaque ruptures in a single individual presenting with sudden cardiac death. *Circ Cardiovasc Imaging*. 2018;11:e008331.

13 Cardiac Computed Tomography Fractional Flow Reserve (CT-FFR) Current Clinical Evidence and Limitations

TIMOTHY ANDREW FAIRBAIRN, KAVITHA M. CHINNAIYAN, AND ROBERT D. SAFIAN

KEY POINTS

- The most widely used CT-derived fractional flow reserve (CT-FFR) technology utilizes the principles of computational fluid dynamics (CFD) to generate 3D anatomical and physiological models of the coronary arteries.
- CT-FFR improves the specificity for detecting myocardial ischemia when compared with coronary CT angiography (CCTA) alone and has higher diagnostic accuracy when compared with other noninvasive functional tests.
- CT-FFR reduces the frequency of unnecessary invasive coronary angiography (ICA) when compared with CCTA alone.
- A negative CT-FFR confers a low 5-year risk of cardiac events and revascularization, whereas a positive CT-FFR is associated with a higher risk of cardiac events and revascularization, that increase as CT-FFR values decrease.
- Optimal CT-FFR interpretation can change patient management and can be used to guide revascularization decisions.

PRINCIPLES OF CT-DERIVED FRACTIONAL FLOW RESERVE (CT-FFR)

In general, there are two types of CT-FFR, one that relies on computational fluid dynamics (CFD CT-FFR) and another that relies on machine learning and a reduced order CFD model (ML CT-FFR). CFD CT-FFR is commercially available and is widely used, whereas ML CT-FFR is not yet commercially available.

CFD CT-FFR

CFD CT FFR utilizes standard datasets from coronary CT angiography (CCTA) and applies CFD modeling to produce 3D anatomical and physiological models of the coronary arteries. The 3D physiological model is the result of a mathematical calculation of coronary flow, pressure, and resistance.[1] Pressure drop can be calculated by a fluid dynamic equation but is dependent on fluid viscosity and flow rate. Further, the flow rate is somewhat dependent on the distal microvasculature.[2] CFD modeling of FFR thus relies on the following assumptions[3]:

1. Total coronary blood flow at rest is directly proportional to myocardial mass.
2. Coronary microvascular resistance at rest is inversely proportional to the length and diameter of the epicardial coronary arteries.
3. There is a predictable decrease in microvascular resistance after the administration of sublingual nitroglycerin.
4. Flow and pressure in the coronary arteries can be calculated using supercomputers based on the Navier-Stokes equation.

Complex mathematical equations required for CFD CT-FFR require a supercomputer to generate the three-dimensional models of the coronary arteries from the segmented coronary CTA data. At present, the only FDA-approved method is HeartFlow CT-FFR (Redwood City, CA, USA), which is performed by off-site analysis. Coronary CTA data are transferred to a remote location via secure networks after deidentification of patient-specific data and then uploaded to a cloud-based server for generation of anatomical and physiological coronary models. Several point-of-care techniques for CT-derived FFR have been developed but are not commercially available. Several of these CT-FFR models utilize machine learning or deep learning rather than a CFD model approach.

ML CT-FFR

CFD CT-FFR are limited by the need for significant artificial intelligence–derived model simulations and the need for a technician to check the quality of the analysis. These deep learned models require a supercomputer that limits any onsite or immediate analysis and requires several hours for processing. In contrast, ML CT-FFR algorithms are trained on simulated coronary arteries using a reduced order CFD model to decrease the computational burden associated with CFD CT-FFR. Once the ML model has been trained and validated, it can simulate thousands of disease states that reduce the risk of variable performance and plateau effects. The ML CT-FFR models have good correlations with invasive FFR and CFD-FFR across a spectrum of stenosis severity[4,5] and varying degrees of coronary calcification.[6,7] The most important advantages of ML CT-FFR include a marked reduction in processing time, the possibility of point-of-care analysis, and reduction in costs compared with CFD CT-FFR.

Technical Factors and Rejection Rates

All techniques for CT-FFR require high-quality CTA images to allow the definition of lumen boundaries; CT-FFR is not a substitute for low-quality CTA images. Virtually any factors that degrade CTA image quality may adversely impact CT-FFR determination. Minimum CT requirements include a 64-slice scanner and optimal contrast opacification of the coronary arteries (HU >300). Sublingual nitroglycerin is required to achieve maximal coronary vasodilation, and heart rate control is essential. Heart rate is a key determinant of rejection rates, with acceptance much higher when heart rates <60 bpm.[8] Reported rejection rates for CFD CT-FFR range from 2.9% to 30%, with a realistic rejection rate of about 8%.[9] The most common causes of rejection relate to difficulties resolving lumen boundaries and are mostly associated with motion, misalignment, or blooming artifacts from calcium.[10] The length and circumferential distribution of calcium are more important than the calcium score; so-called "lead-pipe" calcification may be especially problematic for CT-FFR. For CFD CT-FFR, CTA image reconstruction can be optimized by the use of sharp kernels to improve detection of lumen boundaries. It is not possible to perform CT-FFR on stented vessels or on bypass grafts, but CT-FFR can be performed in nonstented vessels in patients with stents.

CT-FFR AS A PHYSIOLOGICAL TEST FOR ISCHEMIA

Coronary CTA is the only noninvasive technique that is more accurate than invasive coronary angiography (ICA) for plaque characterization, plaque burden, and extent of coronary artery disease (CAD). Studies of functional versus anatomic imaging for CAD suggest similar clinical outcomes at 2 years but better outcomes for CCTA at 5 years that are not related to more frequent percutaneous coronary intervention (PCI) or coronary artery bypass grafting (CABG).[11,12] CCTA enhances the ability to clarify the diagnosis of CAD in patients with chest pain and leads to more effective utilization of medications for primary prevention.[13]

The clinical premise for CT-FFR is based on its ability to improve the low specificity and positive predictive value of coronary CTA.[14] Clinical guidelines recommend CT-FFR in individuals with intermediate or indeterminate coronary stenosis (40–90% stenosis; CAD RADS 2–4) in vessels suitable for analysis (>1.8 mm diameter).[15] The broad range of stenosis severity for which physiological assessment is recommended is based on invasive and noninvasive data that suggest a poor correlation between visual assessment of stenosis severity and the presence of objective ischemia.[16] Reliance on visual assessments alone (by coronary CTA and by invasive angiography) can result in inappropriate revascularization.[17] In the cardiac catheterization laboratory, invasive techniques (fractional flow reserve [FFR] and various nonhyperemic pressure measurements such as instantaneous wave-free ratio [iFR]) are used to assess myocardial ischemia, reduce unnecessary revascularization, and improve clinical outcomes.[18,19] Just as invasive FFR improves the specificity of ICA, CT-FFR improves the specificity of CCTA (Fig. 13.1).

Diagnostic Accuracy Versus Invasive FFR

Three multicenter trials—DISCOVER FLOW, DeFACTO, and NXT—evaluated the accuracy of CT-FFR analysis compared with invasive FFR in a total of 609 patients and 1050 coronary vessels.[20–22] All three studies demonstrated that for the detection of ischemia, CT-FFR has higher specificity and accuracy compared with coronary CTA alone. The NXT Trial (Analysis of Coronary Blood Flow Using CT Angiography: Next Steps) reported per patient accuracy of 81% for CT-FFR and 53% for CTA and per-vessel accuracy of 86% for CT-FFR and 65% for CCTA. Another study has shown that there is a good correlation between CT-FFR and invasive FFR and iFR,[23] but accuracy is reduced in the "grey zone" of FFR values from 0.76 to 0.80, where there may be

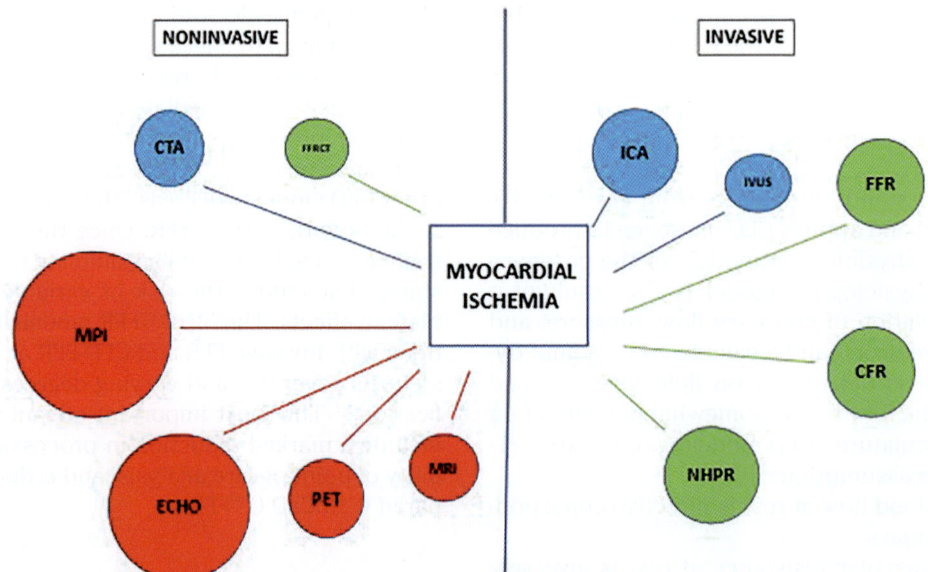

FIG. 13.1 Schematic Representation of Noninvasive and Invasive Tests for Evaluation of Myocardial Ischemia. Anatomical imaging, *blue*; functional imaging, *red*; physiological imaging, *green*. *CCTA*, Coronary computed tomography angiography; *CFR*, coronary flow reserve; *ECHO*, echocardiography; *FFR*, invasive fractional flow reserve; *CT-FFR*, CT-derived fractional flow reserve; *ICA*, invasive coronary angiography; *IVUS*, intravascular ultrasound; *MPI*, myocardial perfusion imaging; *MRI*, magnetic resonance imaging; *NHPR*, nonhyperemic pressure ratios; *PET*, positron emission tomography.

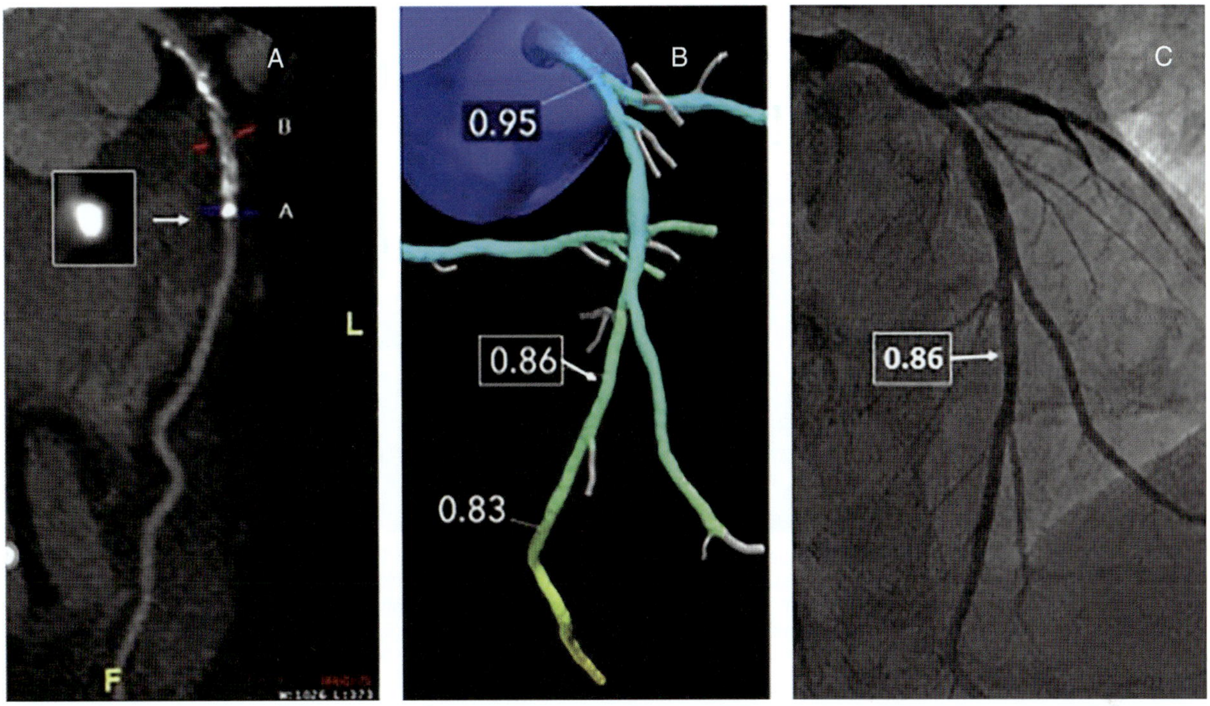

FIG. 13.2 CT-derived fractional flow reserve (CT-FFR) can improve the specificity of coronary computed tomography angiography (CCTA) even when calcification and blooming artifact obscure the lumen and preclude assessment of stenosis severity. CCTA shows dense calcified plaque and blooming artifact in the proximal left anterior descending (LAD), precluding assessment of stenosis severity (Panel A, *white arrow*). CT-FFR distal-to-the-lesion is 0.86, suggesting the absence of lesion-specific ischemia (Panel B). The referring physician was concerned about the proximal LAD and referred the patient for invasive coronary angiography (ICA), which confirmed calcified plaque and invasive fractional flow reserve of 0.86 (Panel C). The patient was managed with medical therapy; ICA could have been avoided.

up to 30% discordance.[24] This discordance may reflect the lack of precision associated with interpretation of continuous variables (such as CT-FFR and FFR) in the context of discrete cut points (such as positive [≤0.80] and negative [>0.80] FFR). Many cardiologists believe that invasive FFR is the gold standard for assessment of hemodynamic significance, but FFR values are also influenced by stenosis severity, site of measurement, errors related to pressure drift and dampening, and variability in individual responses to intravenous adenosine.[25,26] A reduction in specificity of CCTA to identify ischemic lesions is particularly apparent in heavily calcified coronary arteries. CT-FFR is readily performed in arteries with focal dense calcification and can increase the specificity of CCTA for identifying ischemia even in the presence of extensive blooming artifact (Fig. 13.2).[10]

CT-FFR Compared With Other Noninvasive Functional Tests

Functional testing (exercise/pharmacological radionuclide scintigraphy [SPECT], echocardiography, and magnetic resonance imaging) are frequently used to diagnose ischemia and drive management decisions. Several metaanalyses show that the diagnostic accuracy of CT-FFR is superior to other invasive and noninvasive tests for ischemia.[27] The PACIFIC CT-FFR substudy was a retrospective study of the diagnostic performance of CT-FFR with CT-FFR approach compared to CCTA alone, SPECT, and positron emission tomography (PET). PET had better diagnostic performance than SPECT and CTA alone, yet CT-FFR demonstrated the highest overall diagnostic performance.[28] A substudy showed a relationship between reduced CT-FFR, lower myocardial blood flow (MBF) during hyperemia and coronary flow reserve (CFR).[29] Small single studies have compared CT-FFR to SPECT, demonstrating a higher sensitivity for CT-FFR, higher specificity for SPECT, and similar overall diagnostic accuracy (Fig. 13.3). One study has compared CT-FFR to stress perfusion MRI, showing high sensitivity but lower specificity for CT-FFR, with no difference in overall accuracy to predict revascularization. The lower than expected CT-FFR specificity (42–55%) in these studies may be related to their use of distal vessel positivity.[30–32] Accordingly, current US guidelines indicate that CT-FFR should only be performed in proximal and mid-vessels in a "stenosis-specific" approach.[15]

CLINICAL APPLICATIONS OF CT-FFR

Many studies, including several large multicenter trials, have demonstrated that in patients with stable CAD, the use of CT-FFR analysis:

- Impacts clinical decisions compared with CTA alone
- Provides clinicians with data to discriminate between those coronary lesions that require revascularization versus those that do not
- Allows safe deferral of many patients away from ICA

Impact on Clinical Management

CT-FFR mitigates the need for additional testing with other modalities and is attractive as a "one-stop shop" for adjudication of the physiologic importance of intermediate degrees of stenoses, especially with respect to clinical

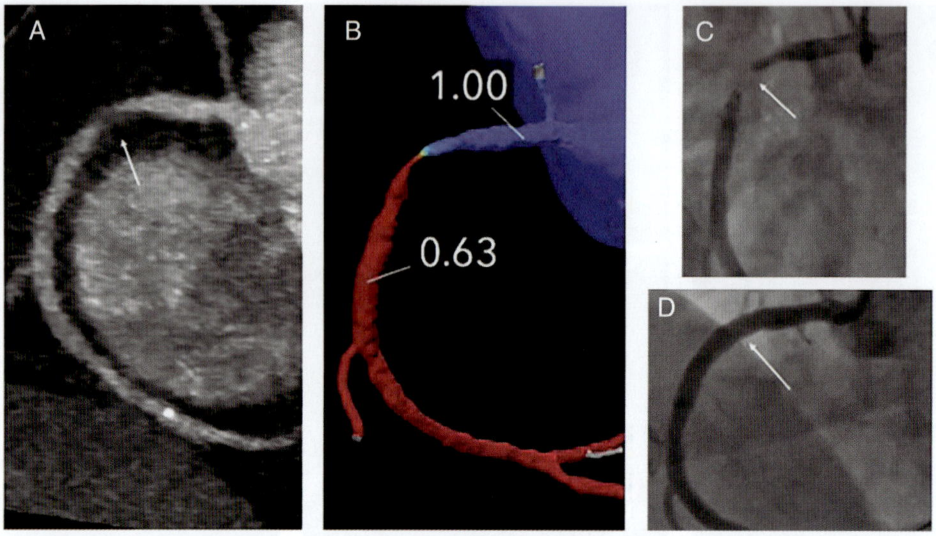

FIG. 13.3 A 56-year-old woman presents to the emergency department with exertional dyspnea. The initial ECG and cardiac biomarkers are normal. During stress myocardial perfusion imaging, she achieves 8.3 Metabolic Equivalents (METS) and 78% of age-predicted maximum heart rate. The test is negative for symptoms, and the ECG and perfusion scan are normal. Coronary computed tomography angiography (CCTA) shows >70% stenosis in the proximal right coronary artery (RCA) (Panel A, *white arrow*). CCTA-derived fractional flow reserve is 0.63, consistent with severe ischemia (Panel B). Invasive coronary angiography confirms subtotal occlusion of the RCA (Panel C, *white arrow*), managed by successful Percutaneous Coronary Intervention (PCI) (Panel D, *white arrow*).

decision-making regarding coronary revascularization. The ADVANCE registry was a real-world assessment of how a CT-FFR pathway impacts patient management. It showed that the addition of CT-FFR changed decision-making in 66% of cases, predominantly moving patients from requiring further tests to that of medical therapy. It also showed that when a CT-FFR was negative (value of >0.80), it was helpful in safely deferring ICA in one in four cases, thus functioning as an effective gatekeeper to the catheterization laboratory.[33]

What became clear was that patients with a lower CT-FFR were more likely to be referred for ICA (<0.71, 73%), have evidence of "obstructive," CAD and be revascularized compared to patients with a higher CT-FFR. Only a very small minority (3–6%) of negative CT-FFR actually received revascularization. Thus CT-FFR does improve the ability to discriminate lesions that are going to require treatment in the form of PCI or CABG. In the "grey-zone" territory of 0.75 to 0.80, a majority of patients (67%) were treated with medical therapy.

The safety of deferring ICA in patients with a negative CT-FFR has been examined in numerous studies (Table 13.1). In clinical trials, ICA is reduced by 83% compared to a straight to ICA strategy and by 22% when compared to a CCTA and "other" tests (principally functional tests such as stress echo) strategy.[34,35] This finding is consistent across countries and healthcare systems and appears unaffected by the type of "other" second-line functional tests used in a non-CT–FFR strategy. Importantly, there is not just a reduction in all ICA but a greater reduction (80% relative risk reduction) of ICA occurring without evidence of obstructive CAD (>50% diameter stenosis).[36]

Clinical Utility in Acute Chest Pain

Even though most CT-FFR studies are in patients with stable chest pain, there are emerging data for its use in acute chest pain in the emergency department: in one study there were no major adverse cardiac events (MACE) in patients with CT-FFR >0.80.[37] There is no support for CT-FFR in acute myocardial infarction, where abnormal volume-ratio may impact CFD modeling and reduce the specificity and accuracy of CT-FFR.[38]

CCT-FFR and Prognosis

Early studies of CT-FFR focused on diagnostic accuracy, but data on hard clinical outcomes are starting to emerge. In patients with stable CAD who are followed up to 5 years, CT-FFR >0.80 is associated with annual MACE rates of 0.2% to 0.5% (similar to patients with <30% stenosis), compared with annual MACE rates >1% in patients CT-FFR ≤0.80.[39–41] Similar to invasive FFR, there is a risk continuum of CT-FFR where lower values confer greater risk, and a reduction in CT-FFR of 0.05 increases the risk of MACE by 1.6-fold.[42] The Danish ADVANCE patients were followed up for 3 years' clinical outcomes, demonstrating that CT-FFR was able to independently and incrementally risk stratify patients for MI, cardiovascular death, and all-cause death to coronary artery calcium scoring.[43]

CT-FFR as a Gatekeeper to the Catheterization Laboratory

The "gatekeeper" concept refers to the need to identify patients who are referred for ICA with the ultimate objective of undergoing revascularization. Within this framework, the ratio of ICA/revascularization provides an index of the efficiency of ICA to identify patients who require revascularization. In PLATFORM, the revascularization/ICA ratio was 72% among patients randomized to the CTA and CT-FFR, and 32% in patients randomized to usual care, suggesting more efficient utilization of ICA in patients undergoing CT-FFR.[35] Observations were similar in the ADVANCE registry, where the revascularization/ICA ratio was 73%.[33]

TABLE 13.1 CT-FFR Clinical Utility Studies

STUDY NAME	INVESTIGATOR	PUBLICATION	CLINICAL UTILITY IMPLICATIONS
PLATFORM 90 Days	Douglas	*Eur Heart J* 2015	In this prospective study, 61% of planned ICAs were canceled based on CT-FFR guidance without adverse clinical consequences. HeartFlow CT-FFR reduced ICAs showing no significant stenosis by 83%.
PLATFORM 1 Year	Douglas	*J Am Coll Cardiol* 2016	No adverse clinical events at 1 year in 117 patients whose ICA was canceled based on CT-FFR results.
ADVANCE 90 days	Fairbairn	*Eur Heart J* 2018	In a prospective, 38-site, 5083-patient registry, use of CT-FFR resulted in changes in clinical management in 67% of patients compared to CCTA alone. Among those patients who went to ICA, 73% were revascularized. Negative CT-FFR (CT-FFR >0.80) was associated with low rates of ICA and zero MACE (major adverse cardiac events) at 90 days.
CT-FFR RIPCORD	Curzen	*JACC Card Imaging* 2016	CT-FFR data resulted in a change in treatment decision for 44% of patients. Of patients originally thought to require PCI, CT-FFR findings allowed for 30% to be reallocated to medical management and 18% to have their PCI target vessel changed.
PROMISE CT-FFR	Lu	*JACC Card Imaging* 2017	If used in the PROMISE trial, CT-FFR would have reduced the number of patients referred to ICA by 28% and decreased the number of ICAs showing no significant stenosis by 44%.
Aarhus CT-FFR Experience	Jensen	*Eur Heart J Card Imag* 2017	Use of CCTA and CT-FFR led to cancelation of 75% of planned ICAs in high-risk patients (use of CCTA alone would have canceled only 46%). The same clinical strategy safely kept 91% of low-to intermediate-risk patients from going to ICA.
Clinical Outcomes Following CT-FFR	Norgaard	*JACC* 2018	Prospective study of 3674 consecutive patients with stable chest pain who were evaluated with CTA and CT-FFR when needed. Results demonstrated that CT-FFR is effective for differentiating those patients with intermediate stenosis who could be managed medically versus those requiring ICA and possible stenting or CABG. Patients with intermediate stenosis by CCTA who had a negative CT-FFR had outcomes similar to patients who had no to minimal disease by CCTA.
FORECAST	Curzen	*EHJ* 2021	Prospective randomized trial of 1400 chest pain patients in the UK randomized 1:1 to a CTA + CT-FFR versus a usual testing strategy (mostly CTA + stress echo), There was a 22% reduction in ICA with no difference in MACE, HRQOL, or costs at 9 months.
PRECISE	Douglas	*JAMA Cardiol* 2023	Prospective randomized trial, international, of a precision strategy (PS: CTA+CT-FFR) versus usual testing (UT) strategy, and a deferred testing group for those with a low PROMISE risk score. Clinical efficacy was better in the PS group with a 76% reduction in ICA without obstructive CAD. Safety MI/death endpoint was similar between the groups, with higher statin and aspirin use in the PS group.

CABG, Coronary artery bypass grafting *CCTA*, coronary computed tomography angiography; *CT-FFR*, CT-derived fractional flow reserve; *HRQOL*, health-related quality of life *ICA*, invasive coronary angiography; *MACE*, major adverse cardiac events; *PCI*, percutaneous coronary intervention.

The PRECISE trial showed that a precision diagnostic strategy of CTA and CT-FFR increased clinical efficacy by primarily reducing ICA without obstructive disease by 80% compared to a usual testing strategy. Catheterizations with subsequent revascularization were subsequently higher (72% versus 31%) with no significant difference in hard clinical outcomes (MI, all death or fatal MI).[36]

Cost Savings

Several studies have documented that a CCTA plus selective CT-FFR analysis pathway can improve care and provide cost savings. Data from the PLATFORM clinical utility study determined the economic impact of incorporating CT-FFR into patient pathways. Utilizing Medicare national reimbursement rates and a $1500 price for CT-FFR, a 23% ($2481/patient) cost reduction at 90 days and a 26% cost reduction ($3109/patient) at 1 year was demonstrated.[44] The savings in PLATFORM came primarily from avoiding ICA based on physician interpretation of CT-FFR >0.80 as an absence of functionally significant disease. Additional savings resulted over time due to a lower rate of hospitalizations and medical office visits when CT-FFR was included in the patient care pathway.

The UK National Institute for Health and Care Excellence (NICE) performed a comprehensive cost-effectiveness assessment in 2017 modeling several different diagnostic pathways using different imaging modalities (echo, SPECT, MRI) and ICA. They concluded that a CCTA and CT-FFR pathway was the most cost effective and would save initially £214 per patient raising to £391 per patient on subsequent review in 2021. The FORECAST study investigated cost and clinical utility at 9 months in several UK hospitals where the technology was readily used. They demonstrated an insignificant 8% difference (higher costs for CT-FFR) at 9 months between an experimental CCTA/CT-FFR pathway and a standard-of-care CCTA pathway with other functional second-line tests when required.[34]

Cost effectiveness analyses based on incremental cost effectiveness ratio (ICERs) and quality adjusted life years (QALYs) show an anatomical pathway (CCTA+CT-FFR) consistently outperforms a functional pathway in different types of risk groups with stable chest pain. Noninvasive anatomic pathways are less costly and more effective. In most analyses a negative outcome is defined as an ICA where the patient did not have obstructive disease. Analyses suggest approximately 1.64 patients would need a CT-FFR diagnostic pathway to avoid an unnecessary

ICA, and that compared with CCTA alone, or CCTA plus other functional tests, a CT-FFR pathway still results in fewer unnecessary ICA.[45]

NUANCES OF INTERPRETATION OF CT-FFR FOR ISCHEMIA

The Impact of Site of Measurement on CT-FFR

Initial reporting of CT-FFR results relied on value measured from the distal vessel, but more recent studies confirm that values measured distal to the stenosis are more reliable for assessment of lesion-specific ischemia. In fact, some patients with normal coronary arteries or mild diffuse disease may have positive invasive or CT-FFR values when measured from the distal vessel and may explain "false-positive" tests in patients referred for ICA[46] (Fig. 13.4). Several studies show that CT-FFR measured distal to the stenosis has higher specificity, similar sensitivity, and higher diagnostic accuracy compared with CT-FFR values measured from the distal vessel. In fact, CT-FFR measured from distal to the lesion result in reclassification of 60% of CT-FFR values measured from the distal vessel. Similar observations apply to measurements of invasive FFR distal to the lesion compared with the distal vessel (Fig. 13.5).[47,48] This reclassification for CT-FFR is highest in the 50% to 69% stenosis. CT-FFR values should be measured 10 to 20 mm distal to the stenosis to achieve the highest accuracy, eliminate pressure recovery, and improve patient management.[49]

Indeed, CT-FFR and invasive FFR values decline from the ostium to the terminal vessel, regardless of FFR technique, even in normal coronary arteries.[50,51] Values obtained from the terminal vessel may overestimate lesion-specific ischemia and should be avoided. CT-FFR when measured 1 to 2 cm distal-to-the-lesion improves the diagnostic performance of CT-FFR relative to FFR, reducing the risk and cost of unnecessary ICA.

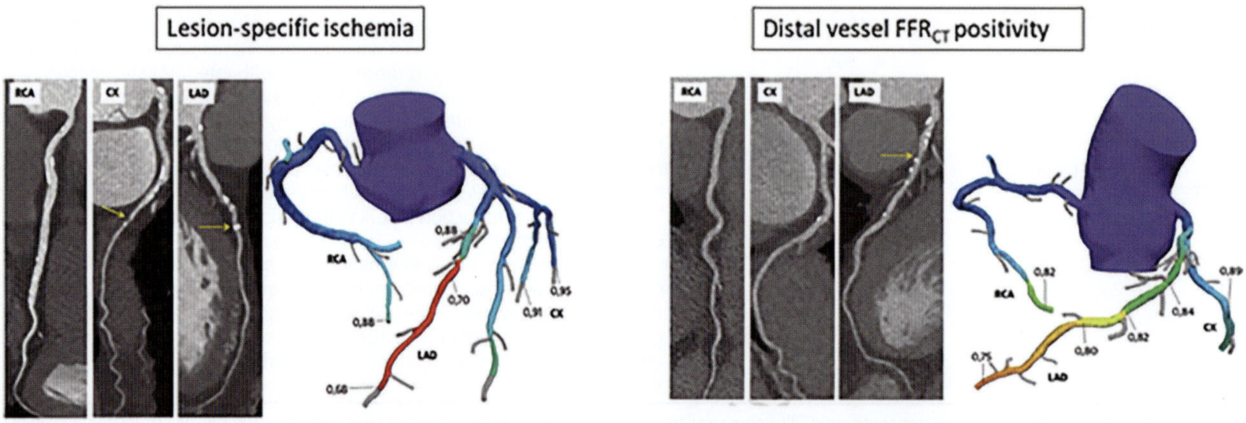

FIG. 13.4 Lesion-specific positive CT-derived fractional flow reserve (CT-FFR) versus a distal vessel positive CT-FFR. There is a focal drop in CT-FFR across a specific stenosis compared to a gradual decline across the whole vessel in distal vessel positivity.

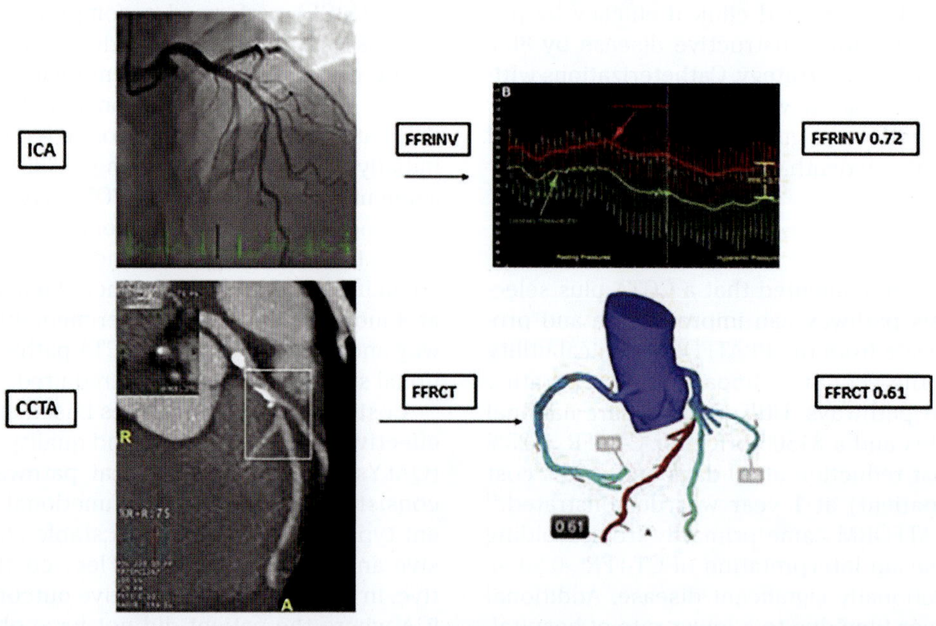

FIG. 13.5 Assessment of Lesion-specific Ischemia by Anatomical and Physiological Testing. Lesion-lesion specific ischemia is defined as CT-FFR ≤0.80 10 to 20 mm distal to the stenosis. *CCTA*, Coronary computed tomography angiography; *CT-FFR*, CT-derived fractional flow reserve (HeartFlow); *FFRINV*, invasive fractional flow reserve; *ICA*, invasive coronary angiography.

ΔCT-FFR

The invasive FFR peak pressure gradient (PPG) across a stenosis has been identified as a marker of benefit from revascularization, above simply using a lowest FFR value. A similar method can be applied in CT-FFR using the stenosis-specific value and a value immediately proximal to the stenosis to provide a trans-lesional gradient or "Delta" ΔCT-FFR. The EMERALD study assessed CCTA markers for predicting future plaque rupture and acute coronary syndrome (ACS) in 72 patients and 216 lesions.[52] They demonstrated that the strongest CCTA predicter of a future ACS was the ΔCT-FFR with a cutoff of ≥0.12, compared to conventional markers such as high-risk plaque, lowest CT-FFR value, lesion % stenosis, or even wall shear stress. The use of trans-lesional gradient while reporting CT-FFR was demonstrated to better identify patients who proceeded to undergo revascularization, especially in those with a CT-FFR 0.71 to 0.80. This indicates that the inclusion of this parameter may improve the accuracy of the test and appropriateness for any future referral to the catheterization lab.[49,53]

Impact of Volume to Mass Ratio, Gender, and Ethnicity on CT-FFR

The observation that normal or mildly diseased coronary arteries can have positive CT-FFR is consistent with mismatch between coronary artery volume (V) and left ventricular mass (M). Coronary flow normally has a linear relationship to coronary size and M. Normal physiology dictates that the greater the demand the greater the supply. Disruptions of the normal relationship between V and M is referred to as V/M mismatch, which can be computed by CFD CT-FFR. Low V/M ratio is associated with lower CT-FFR values even when significant CAD is absent and may be observed in patients with cardiomyopathy, microvascular dysfunction, and diabetes (Fig. 13.6). A low or high V/M

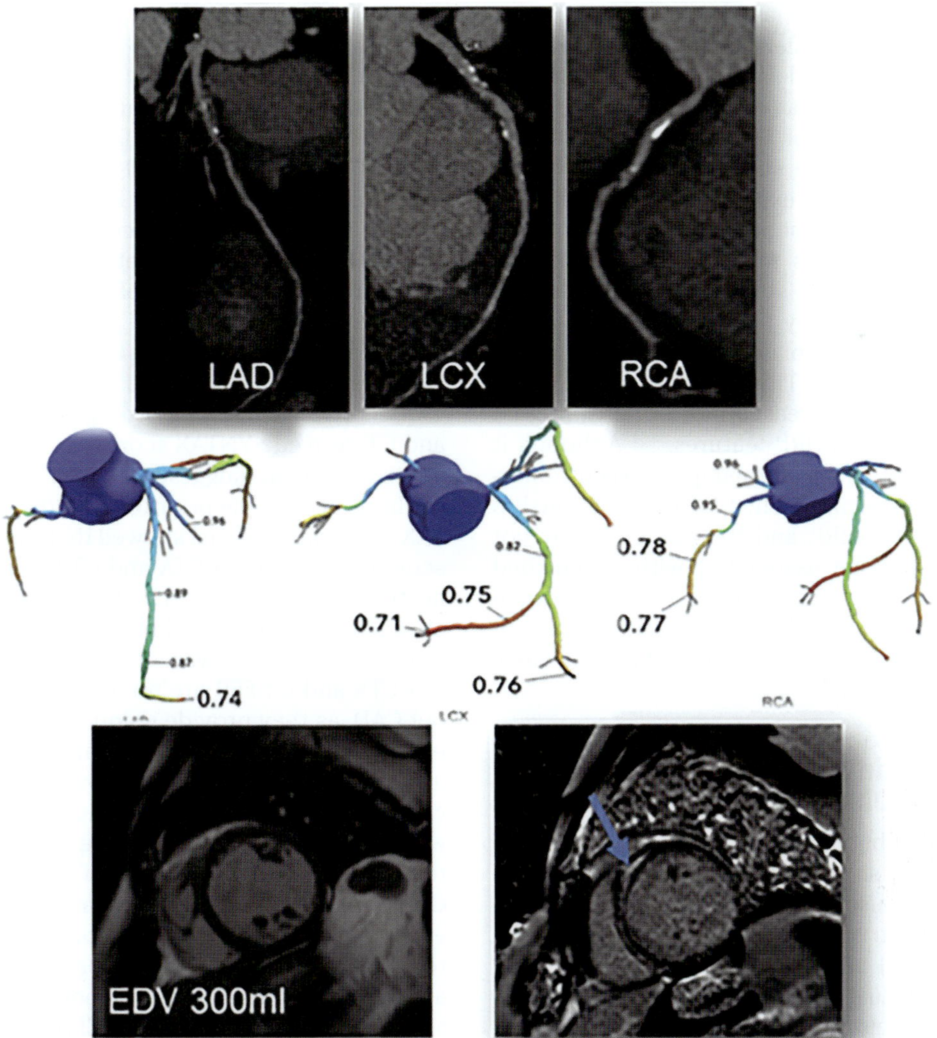

FIG. 13.6 A 45-year-old woman presents to the emergency department with possible ischemic chest pain. The initial ECG and cardiac biomarkers are normal. Coronary computed tomography angiography shows bulky noncalcified eccentric plaque in the proximal LAD (Panel A). Curved multiplanar reconstruction and cross-sectional imaging show positive remodeling and 50% to 70% stenosis (Panel B; REF, reference vessel), without low-attenuation plaque. CCTA-derived fractional flow reserve is 0.86, suggesting the absence of lesion-specific ischemia (Panel C). Medical therapy was advised, and the patient has remained stable for >4 years. *LAD*, Left anterior descending; *LCx*, left circumflex artery; *RCA*, right coronary artery. *EDV*, End Diastolic Volume.

may be predictive of a "positive" or "negative" invasive and noninvasive FFR and the likelihood of revascularization.

It is known from the invasive FFR literature that different sexes and ethnicities have different FFR values for the same degree of coronary stenosis. Women have a higher FFR and CT-FFR for the same degree of coronary stenosis and a higher V/M ratio. These factors independently predict a reduced likelihood of future revascularization.[54] Similarly, South Asian ethnicities have smaller coronary arteries and lower V/M compared with Caucasians and East Asians, which may result in lower CT-FFR for the same degree of coronary disease.[55]

Further study of V/M is needed to learn about how to utilize and interpret the test in different populations and presentations, but there is sufficient evidence to highlight the importance of test interpretation in the context of the individual patient.

CT-FFR AND INTERVENTIONAL CARDIOLOGY

Plaque Characterization, CT-FFR, and Ischemia

CCTA is widely acknowledged as the best noninvasive imaging tool for simple (calcified plaque) and advanced (high-risk plaque [HRP] defined as low attenuation plaque [LAP], positive remodeling, plaque burden) plaque characterization.[56] The presence of HRP, the relationship to ischemia, and risk of ACS are subjects of intense ongoing investigation and partially explain the enthusiasm for CCTA among patients with chest pain.[57]

Plaque volume by CCTA is strongly related to ischemia irrespective of diameter stenosis, and assessment of ischemia is strengthened by plaque characterization. LAP is also a strong predictor of ischemia, independent of other plaque characteristics. The likelihood of ischemia demonstrated by CT-FFR increases more than threefold in presence of 1 versus ≥2 HRP features.[58,59] Although it is easy to understand the relationship between abnormal FFR and lesion-specific ischemia, the relationship between abnormal FFR, HRP, and the risk of ACS is not so intuitive. LAP may be associated with diminished arteriolar vasodilator capacity, leading to an abnormal FFR. In other words, normal FFR suggests the absence of lesion-specific ischemia and the presence of normal vasodilator capacity.

Myocardial Ischemia and Myocardial Infarction in the Absence of Obstructive CAD

Patients may have abnormal invasive or noninvasive CT-FFR but do not have significant stenosis by angiography (anatomy-physiology mismatch). This mismatch could be due to diffuse nonobstructive atherosclerosis inducing a graded, continuous fall in pressure along the length of a coronary artery. A gradual decline in pressure in completely normal arteries vessels follows the relationship between changes in pressure, vessel length, and vessel diameter defined by Poiseuille's equation.[25,60] Some of these patients may have ischemia with nonobstructive CAD (INOCA). In fact, patients with INOCA may have ischemic symptoms that can be misdiagnosed. Accordingly, CCTA and CT-FFR may enable this diagnosis while excluding obstructive disease without ICA.[61,62]

Myocardial infarction in the absence of obstructive CAD (MINOCA) and INOCA are diseases on the spectrum of ischemic heart diseases in patients with minimal or no CAD. Potential etiologies for MINOCA include plaque instability, spontaneous coronary dissection, Takotsubo syndrome, myocarditis, coronary artery vasospasm, microvascular dysfunction, and supply-demand mismatch (Type 2 MI).[63] Although ICA and invasive coronary imaging may be appropriate in some patients, CCTA and CT-FFR may be useful to exclude obstructive CAD and identify nonatherosclerotic causes of MI.

CCTA and CT-FFR for Planning Revascularization

ICA has been the mainstay of decision-making regarding PCI and CABG, but several paradigm shifts have impacted revascularization decisions and cardiovascular outcomes. The first was a shift away from ICA alone to reliance on objective physiological measures of ischemia. The second was a shift away from qualitative lesion morphology to the application of more sophisticated risk prediction models such as the Synergy Between Percutaneous Coronary Intervention with Taxus and Cardiac Surgery (SYNTAX) score, the clinical SYNTAX score II, and the functional SYNTAX score.[64–67] The third was a shift away from unilateral decision-making by an interventional cardiologist to a shared-decision model incorporating a heart team, key stakeholders, and the patient and family.

We are now on the verge of another paradigm shift, characterized by integration of noninvasive anatomical and functional assessment using CCTA and CT-FFR to risk-stratify patients using CT-derived anatomic and functional SYNTAX scores.[68] There is a strong correlation between ICA- and CT-derived SYNTAX scores in patients with single and multivessel CAD, suggesting that a heart team consensus might be achievable prior to (or without) ICA.[66,69] The SYNTAX III Revolution Trial showed that the functional SYNTAX score derived from CCTA and CT-FFR resulted in reclassification of anatomical SYNTAX scores in 14% of patients, changed plans for CABG or PCI in 7% of patients, and altered target vessel revascularization in 12% of patients.[70]

CCTA and CT-FFR are no longer utilized to simply rule out CAD, as they provide unique information and a degree of empowerment that is not available with any other noninvasive technique. CCTA provides essential data about coronary artery anatomy, plaque characteristics, and, when coronary interventions are being planned, the ability to determine "normal to normal" vessel length (Fig. 13.7). CT-FFR provides detailed estimates of lesion-specific ischemia, and the newest application includes a PCI planning tool (Fig. 13.8) allowing cardiologists to plan stent location and sizing and use virtual remodeling of the lumen to assess the functional impact of PCI (Fig. 13.8).[71]

Studies utilizing this dedicated planning tool report early feasibility of assessing CT-FFR before and after virtual stenting in single and tandem lesions.[72] There is a good correlation between the CT-FFR and FFR before and after PCI and a high level of agreement between CT-FFR and Optical

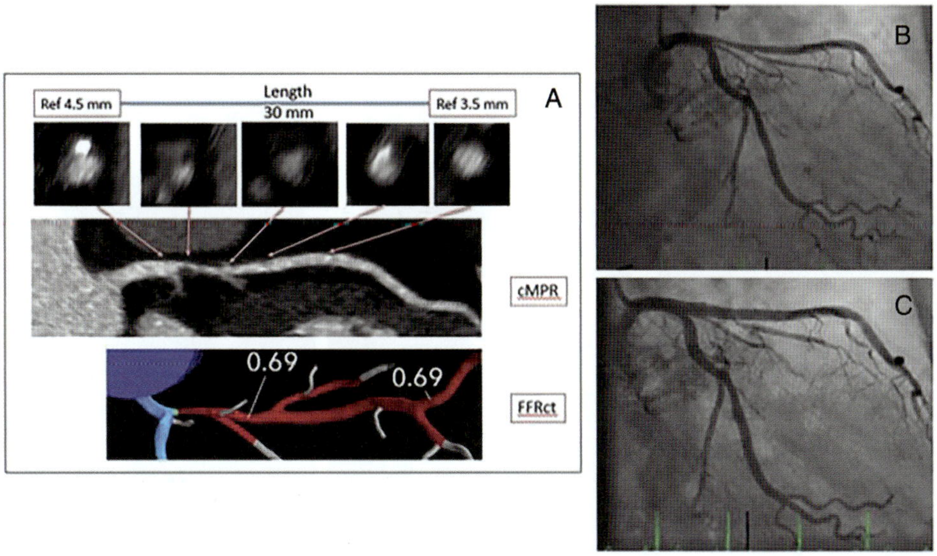

FIG. 13.7 A 55-year-old man develops typical low-threshold exertional angina 18 months after mechanical aortic valve replacement. Coronary computed tomography angiography (CCTA) shows mixed plaque and severe ostial left anterior descending (LAD) stenosis extending over a length of 30 mm from the left main to the mid LAD. The proximal (*left main*) and distal reference diameters are 4.5 mm and 3.5 mm, respectively. The CCTA-derived fractional flow reserve in the LAD is 0.69, consistent with severe ischemia (Panel A, cMPR [curved multiplanar reconstruction). These imaging data were used to plan percutaneous coronary intervention (PCI). Invasive coronary angiography (ICA) confirms severe proximal LAD stenosis (Panel B), managed by implantation of a 3.5 × 28 mm drug-eluting stent, dilated with a 3.5-mm noncompliant balloon distally and a 4.0-mm noncompliant balloon proximally. Final ICA shows an excellent result (Panel C), confirmed by intravascular ultrasound.

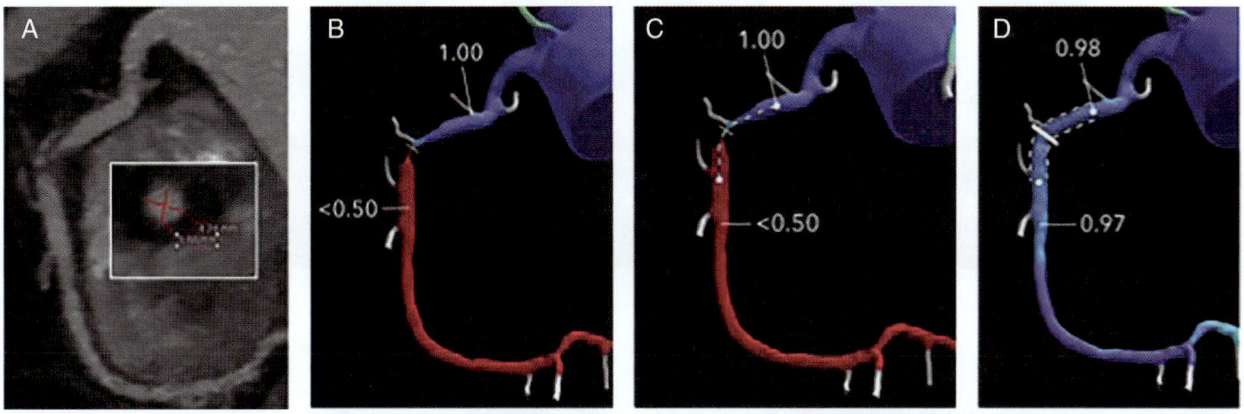

FIG. 13.8 A 55-year-old man presents to the emergency department with exertional chest pain at a low workload. Coronary computed tomography angiography shows severe stenosis in the proximal right coronary artery due to noncalcified plaque, with a reference diameter of 4.2 × 3.9 mm (Panel A); other coronary arteries are normal. The CT-derived fractional flow reserve (CT-FFR) <0.50 suggests severe ischemia (Panel B). The HeartFlow Planner suggests that a 4 × 23 mm drug eluting stent (DES) will cover the entire lesion (Panel C, *dotted white line*), and virtual remodeling of the lumen normalizes the CT-FFR distal to the stent (Panel D; final CT-FFR 0.97). Invasive coronary angiography (ICA) (not shown) confirmed severe stenosis, managed by implantation of a 4 × 24 mm DES; invasive fractional flow reserve is 0.96 after percutaneous coronary intervention (PCI).

Coherence Technology (OCT)–predicted luminal dimensions.[73] This signals a shift of CCTA and CT-FFR from a diagnostic tool to a therapeutic tool, enriching the cardiac catheterization laboratory for therapeutic interventions (Fig. 13.9). Further studies are planned to assess whether this CCTA/CT-FFR PCI planning approach can improve clinical outcomes compared to a standard invasive FFR approach.

Preoperative Evaluation for CAD

CCTA and CT-FFR have been incorporated into preoperative risk stratification prior to liver transplantation and vascular surgery to identify high-risk patients with silent myocardial ischemia.[74,75] This strategy was used to facilitate multidisciplinary care, improve perioperative management, identify patients who might benefit from postoperative revascularization, and decrease the 1-year risk of cardiovascular events.

Coronary Artery Anomalies

CCTA is superior to ICA for the diagnosis of coronary artery anomalies and for identifying the origin and course of anomalous arteries (Fig. 13.10). A large international registry is currently underway to study CCTA and CT-FFR in patients with anomalous coronary arteries (CT-FFR of Anomalous Coronary Arteries by Computed Tomography Study [FACTS]). Several observational studies suggest the value of CT-FFR for assessment of ischemia.[76,77]

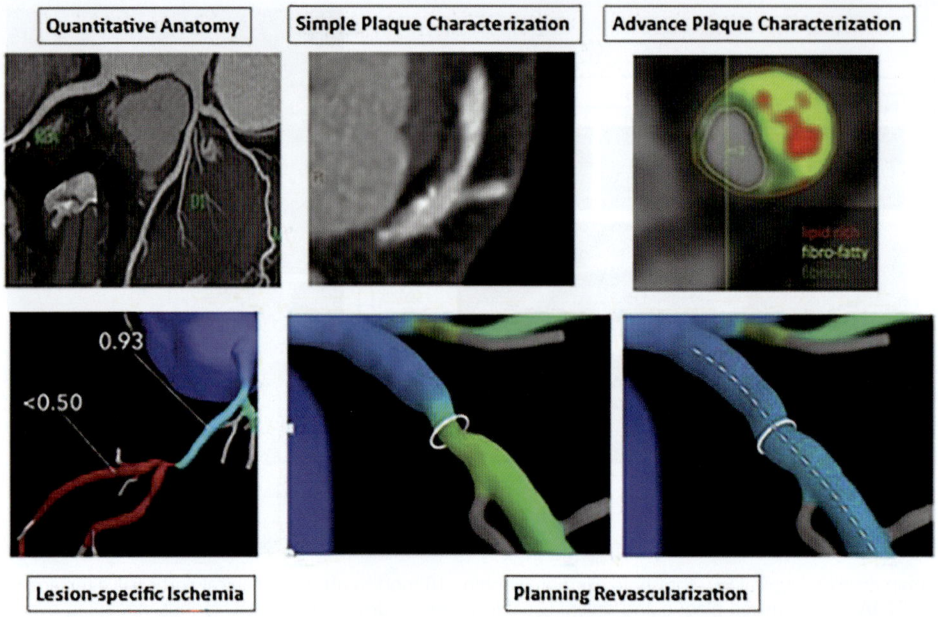

FIG. 13.9 Coronary computed tomography angiography (CCTA) and CT-derived fractional flow reserve (CT-FFR) as the gatekeeper to the cardiac catheterization laboratory. CCTA and CT-FFR provide essential information about coronary artery anatomy, simple and advanced plaque characterization, lesion-specific ischemia, and planning revascularization. These data allow derivation of anatomic and functional SYNTAX scores, without invasive coronary artery.

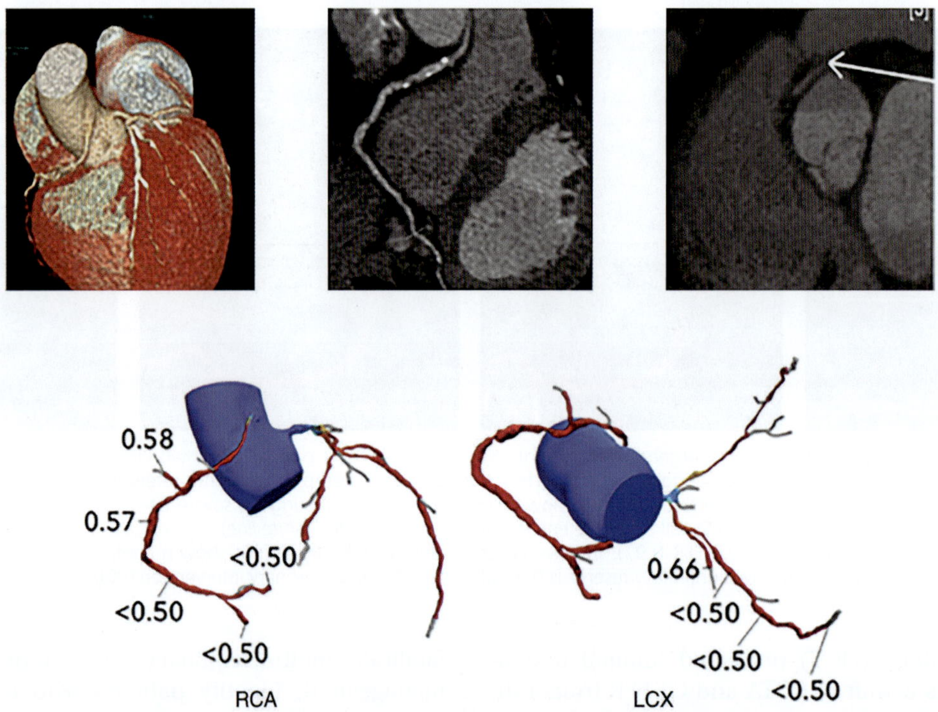

FIG. 13.10 An anomalous right coronary artery (RCA) arising superior to the sinus and from the left traveling anterior with an intramural course (*arrow*). The left anterior descending and left circumflex had severe stenosis in the proximal segments with only mild coronary artery disease in the RCA. The proximal RCA was narrowed with acute angle, intramural course, and the CCTA-derived fractional flow reserve was positive across this narrowing. The patient went for a coronary artery bypass grafting (CABG).

FUTURE APPLICATIONS

Our understanding of fluid dynamics in the coronary arteries is mostly derived from invasive data, but CTA and CFD have provided additional insight into wall shear stress (WSS), axial plaque stress (APS), and localization and progression of atherosclerotic plaque.[76] In Exploring the Mechanism of Plaque Rupture in Acute Coronary Syndrome Using Coronary CT Angiography and Computational Fluid Dynamic (EMERALD), CT-FFR, WSS, and APS were more predictive of subsequent ACS compared with diameter stenosis alone or diameter stenosis plus HRP features.[52]

REFERENCES

1. Jaquet C, Najman L, Talbot H, et al. Generation of patient-specific cardiac vascular networks: a hybrid image-based and synthetic geometric model. *IEEE Trans Biomed Eng.* 2019;66(4):946–955. https://doi.org/10.1109/TBME.2018.2865667.
2. Papamanolis L, Kim HJ, Jaquet C, et al. Myocardial perfusion simulation for coronary artery disease: a coupled patient-specific multiscale model. *Ann Biomed Eng.* 2021;49(5):1432–1447. https://doi.org/10.1007/s10439-020-02681-z.
3. Taylor CA, Fonte TA, Min JK, City R, Angeles L. Computational fluid dynamics applied to cardiac computed tomography for noninvasive quantification of fractional flow reserve scientific basis. *J Am Coll Cardiol.* 2013;61(22):2233–2241. https://doi.org/10.1016/j.jacc.2012.11.083.
4. Itu L, Rapaka S, Passerini T, et al. A machine-learning approach for computation of fractional flow reserve from coronary computed tomography. *J Appl Physiol.* 2016;121:42–52. https://doi.org/10.1152/japplphysiol.00752.2015.-Frac.
5. Hu X, Yang M, Han L, Du Y. Diagnostic performance of machine-learning-based computed fractional flow reserve (FFR) derived from coronary computed tomography angiography for the assessment of myocardial ischemia verified by invasive FFR. *Int J Cardiovasc Imaging.* 2018;34(12):1987–1996. https://doi.org/10.1007/s10554-018-1419-9.
6. Coenen A, Kim YH, Kruk M, et al. Diagnostic accuracy of a machine-learning approach to coronary computed tomographic angiography–based fractional flow reserve result from the MACHINE consortium. *Circ Cardiovasc Imaging.* 2018;11(6):e007217. https://doi.org/10.1161/CIRCIMAGING.117.007217.
7. Yeri A, Shah RV. Comparison of computational fluid dynamics and machine learning–based fractional flow reserve in coronary artery disease. *Circ Cardiovasc Imaging.* 2018;11(6):e007950. https://doi.org/10.1161/CIRCIMAGING.118.007950.
8. Leipsic J, Yang TH, Thompson A, et al. CT angiography (CTA) and diagnostic performance of noninvasive fractional flow reserve: results from the determination of fractional flow reserve by anatomic CTA (DeFACTO) study. *Am J Roentgenol.* 2014;202(5):989–994. https://doi.org/10.2214/AJR.13.11441.
9. Pontone G, Weir-McCall JR, Baggiano A, et al. Determinants of rejection rate for coronary CT angiography fractional flow reserve analysis. *Radiology.* 2019;292(3):597–605. https://doi.org/10.1148/radiol.2019182673.
10. Nørgaard BL, Gaur S, Leipsic J, et al. Influence of coronary calcification on the diagnostic performance of CT angiography derived FFR in coronary artery disease a substudy of the NXT trial. *JACC Cardiovasc Imaging.* 2015;8(9):1045–1055. https://doi.org/10.1016/j.jcmg.2015.06.003.
11. Douglas PS, Hoffmann U, Patel MR, et al. Outcomes of anatomical versus functional testing for coronary artery disease. *N Engl J Med.* 2015;372(14):1291–1300. https://doi.org/10.1056/NEJMoa1415516.
12. Scot-Heart InvestigatorsNewby DE, Adamson PD, et al. Coronary CT angiography and 5-year risk of myocardial infarction. *N Engl J Med.* 2018;379(10):924–933. https://doi.org/10.1056/NEJMoa1805971.
13. Williams MC, Hunter A, Shah ASV, et al. Use of coronary computed tomographic angiography to guide management of patients with coronary disease. *J Am Coll Cardiol.* 2016;67(15):1759–1768. https://doi.org/10.1016/j.jacc.2016.02.026.
14. Nakazato R, Park HB, Berman DS, et al. Noninvasive fractional flow reserve derived from computed tomography angiography for coronary lesions of intermediate stenosis severity results from the DeFACTO study. *Circ Cardiovasc Imaging.* 2013;6(6):881–889. https://doi.org/10.1161/CIRCIMAGING.113.000297.
15. Gulati M, Levy PD, Mukherjee D, et al. 2021 AHA/ACC/ASE/CHEST/SAEM/SCCT/SCMR guideline for the evaluation and diagnosis of chest pain: a report of the American college of cardiology/American Heart Association Joint Committee on clinical practice guidelines. *Circulation.* 2021;144(22):e368–e454. https://doi.org/10.1161/CIR.0000000000001029.
16. Williams MC, Golay SK, Hunter A, et al. Observer variability in the assessment of CT coronary angiography and coronary artery calcium score: substudy of the Scottish COmputed Tomography of the HEART (SCOT-HEART) trial. *Open Heart.* 2015;2(1):e000234. https://doi.org/10.1136/openhrt-2014-000234.
17. Inohara T, Kohsaka S, Miyata H, et al. Appropriateness ratings of percutaneous coronary intervention in Japan and its association with the trend of noninvasive testing. *JACC Cardiovasc Interv.* 2014;7(9):1000–1009. https://doi.org/10.1016/j.jcin.2014.06.006.
18. Lotfi A, Jeremias A, Fearon WF, et al. Expert consensus statement on the use of fractional flow reserve, intravascular ultrasound, and optical coherence tomography: a consensus statement of the society of cardiovascular angiography and interventions. *Catheter Cardiovasc Interv.* 2014;83(4):509–518. https://doi.org/10.1002/ccd.25222.
19. Desai NR, Bradley SM, Parzynski CS, et al. Appropriate use criteria for coronary revascularization and trends in utilization, patient selection and appropriateness of percutaneous coronary intervention: trends in appropriateness of PCI HHS public access. *JAMA.* 2015;17(31419):2045–2053. https://doi.org/10.1001/jama.2015.13764.
20. Koo BK, Erglis A, Doh JH, et al. Diagnosis of ischemia-causing coronary stenoses by noninvasive fractional flow reserve computed from coronary computed tomographic angiograms: results from the prospective multicenter DISCOVER-FLOW (Diagnosis of Ischemia-Causing Stenoses Obtained Via Noninvasive Fractional Flow Reserve) study. *J Am Coll Cardiol.* 2011;58(19):1989–1997. https://doi.org/10.1016/j.jacc.2011.06.066.
21. Min JK, Leipsic J, Pencina MJ, et al. Diagnostic accuracy of fractional flow reserve from anatomic CT angiography. *J Am Med Assoc.* 2012;308(12):1237–1245. https://doi.org/10.1001/2012.jama.11274.
22. Nørgaard BL, Leipsic J, Gaur S, et al. Diagnostic performance of noninvasive fractional flow reserve derived from coronary computed tomography angiography in suspected coronary artery disease. *J Am Coll Cardiol.* 2014;63(12):1145–1155. https://doi.org/10.1016/j.jacc.2013.11.043.
23. Cook CM. Diagnostic accuracy of computed tomography–derived fractional flow reserve a systematic review. *J Am Med Assoc.* 2017;2(7):803–810. https://doi.org/10.1001/jamacardio.2017.1314.
24. Nørgaard BL, Hjort J, Gaur S, et al. Clinical use of coronary CTA-derived FFR for decision-making in stable CAD. *JACC Cardiovasc Imaging.* 2017;10(5):541–550. https://doi.org/10.1016/j.jcmg.2015.11.025.
25. Crystal G, Klein L. Fractional flow reserve: physiological basis, advantages and limitations, and potential gender differences. *Curr Cardiol Rev.* 2015;11(3):209–219. https://doi.org/10.2174/1573403X10666141020113318.
26. Kolli KK, Min JK, Ha S, Soohoo H, Xiong G. Effect of varying hemodynamic and vascular conditions on fractional flow reserve: an in vitro study. *J Am Heart Assoc.* 2016;5(7):1–13. https://doi.org/10.1161/JAHA.116.003634.
27. Driessen RS, Danad I, Stuijfzand WJ, et al. Comparison of coronary computed tomography angiography, fractional flow reserve, and perfusion imaging for ischemia diagnosis. *J Am Coll Cardiol.* 2019;73(2):161–173. https://doi.org/10.1016/j.jacc.2018.10.056.
28. Danad I, Van Rossum AC, Knaapen P, et al. 1185Head-to-head comparison of FFR-CT against coronary CT angiography and myocardial perfusion imaging for the diagnosis of ischaemia. *Eur Heart J.* 2018;39(suppl_1). https://doi.org/10.1093/eurheartj/ehy565.1185.
29. van Diemen PA, Schumacher SP, Bom MJ, et al. The association of coronary lumen volume to left ventricle mass ratio with myocardial blood flow and fractional flow reserve. *J Cardiovasc Comput Tomogr.* 2019;13(4):179–187. https://doi.org/10.1016/j.jcct.2019.06.016.
30. Nørgaard BL, Gormsen LC, Bøtker HE, et al. Myocardial perfusion imaging versus computed tomography angiography-derived fractional flow reserve testing in stable patients with intermediate-range coronary lesions: influence on Downstream Diagnostic workflows and invasive angiography findings. *J Am Heart Assoc.* 2017;6(8):e005587. https://doi.org/10.1161/JAHA.117.005587.
31. Rønnow Sand NP, Nissen L, Winther S, et al. Prediction of coronary revascularization in stable angina: comparison of FFRCT with CMR stress perfusion imaging. *JACC Cardiovasc Imaging.* 2020;13(4):994–1004. https://doi.org/10.1016/j.jcmg.2019.06.028.
32. Sand NPR, Veien KT, Nielsen SS, et al. ProspEctive comparison of FFR derived from coronary CT angiography with SPECT perfusion imaging in stable coronary artery disease. *JACC Cardiovasc Imaging.* 2018;11(11):1640–1650. https://doi.org/10.1016/j.jcmg.2018.05.004.
33. Fairbairn TA, Nieman K, Akasaka T, et al. Real-world clinical utility and impact on clinical decision-making of coronary computed tomography angiography-derived fractional flow reserve: lessons from the ADVANCE registry. *Eur Heart J.* 2018;39(41):3701–3711. https://doi.org/10.1093/eurheartj/ehy530.
34. Curzen N, Nicholas Z, Stuart B, et al. Fractional flow reserve derived from computed tomography coronary angiography in the assessment and management of stable chest pain: the FORECAST randomized trial. *Eur Heart J.* 2021;42(37):3844–3852. https://doi.org/10.1093/eurheartj/ehab444.
35. Douglas PS, Pontone G, Hlatky MA, et al. Clinical outcomes of fractional flow reserve by computed tomographic angiography-guided diagnostic strategies vs. usual care in patients with suspected coronary artery disease: the prospective longitudinal trial of FFRct: outcome and resource impacts stud. *Eur Heart J.* 2015;36(47):3359–3367. https://doi.org/10.1093/eurheartj/ehv444.
36. Douglas PS, Nanna MG, Kelsey MD, et al. Comparison of an initial risk-based testing strategy vs usual testing in stable symptomatic patients with suspected coronary artery disease: the PRECISE randomized clinical trial. *JAMA Cardiol.* 2023;8(10):904–914. https://doi.org/10.1001/jamacardio.2023.2595.
37. Chinnaiyan KM, Safian RD, Gallagher ML, et al. Clinical use of CT-derived fractional flow reserve in the emergency department. *JACC Cardiovasc Imaging.* 2020;13(2):452–461. https://doi.org/10.1016/j.jcmg.2019.05.025.
38. Gaur S, Taylor CA, Jensen JM, et al. FFR derived from coronary CT angiography in nonculprit lesions of patients with recent STEMI. *JACC Cardiovasc Imaging.* 2017;10(4):424–433. https://doi.org/10.1016/j.jcmg.2016.05.019.
39. Patel MR, Norgaard BL, Fairbairn TA, et al. One-year impact on medical practice and clinical outcomes of FFR_{CT}: the ADVANCE registry. *JACC Cardiovasc Imaging.* 2020;13(1 Pt 1):97–105. https://doi.org/10.1016/j.jcmg.2019.03.003.
40. Nørgaard BL, Terkelsen CJ, Mathiassen ON, et al. Coronary CT angiographic and flow reserve-guided management of patients with stable ischemic heart disease. *J Am Coll Cardiol.* 2018;72(18):2123–2134. https://doi.org/10.1016/j.jacc.2018.07.043.
41. Ihdayhid AR, Norgaard BL, Gaur S, et al. Prognostic value and risk continuum of noninvasive fractional flow reserve derived from coronary CT angiography. *Radiology.* 2019;292(2):343–351. https://doi.org/10.1148/radiol.2019182264.
42. Nørgaard BL, Gaur S, Fairbairn TA, et al. Prognostic value of coronary computed tomography angiographic derived fractional flow reserve: a systematic review and meta-analysis. *Heart.* 2022;108(3):194–202. https://doi.org/10.1136/heartjnl-2021-319773.
43. Madsen KT, Nørgaard BL, Øvrehus KA, et al. Prognostic value of coronary CT angiography–derived fractional flow reserve on 3-year outcomes in patients

with stable angina. *Radiology*. 2023;308(3):e230524. https://doi.org/10.1148/radiol.230524.

44. Hlatky MA, de Bruyne B, Pontone G, et al. Quality-of-life and economic outcomes of assessing fractional flow reserve with computed tomography angiography: PLATFORM. *J Am Coll Cardiol*. 2015;66(21):2315–2323. https://doi.org/10.1016/j.jacc.2015.09.051.
45. Karády J, Mayrhofer T, Ivanov A, et al. Cost-effectiveness analysis of anatomic vs functional index testing in patients with low-risk stable chest pain. *JAMA Netw Open*. 2020;3(12):e2028312. https://doi.org/10.1001/jamanetworkopen.2020.28312.
46. Kueh SH, Mooney J, Ohana M, et al. Fractional flow reserve derived from coronary computed tomography angiography reclassification rate using value distal to lesion compared to lowest value. *J Cardiovasc Comput Tomogr*. 2017;11(6):462–467. https://doi.org/10.1016/j.jcct.2017.09.009.
47. Kitabata H, Leipsic J, Patel MR, et al. Incidence and predictors of lesion-specific ischemia by FFRCT: learnings from the international ADVANCE registry. *J Cardiovasc Comput Tomogr*. 2018;12(2):95–100. https://doi.org/10.1016/j.jcct.2018.01.008.
48. Cami E, Tagami T, Raff G, et al. Assessment of lesion-specific ischemia using fractional flow reserve (FFR) profiles derived from coronary computed tomography angiography (FFRCT) and invasive pressure measurements (FFRINV): importance of the site of measurement and implications for patient referral for invasive coronary angiography and percutaneous coronary intervention. *J Cardiovasc Comput Tomogr*. 2018;12(6):480–492. https://doi.org/10.1016/j.jcct.2018.09.003.
49. Takagi H, Leipsic JA, McNamara N, et al. Trans-lesional fractional flow reserve gradient as derived from coronary CT improves patient management: ADVANCE registry. *J Cardiovasc Comput Tomogr*. 2022;16(1):19–26. https://doi.org/10.1016/j.jcct.2021.08.003.
50. Achenbach S, Rudolph T, Rieber J, et al. Performing and interpreting fractional flow reserve measurements in clinical practice: an expert consensus document. *Interv Cardiol Rev*. 2017;12(2):97–109. https://doi.org/10.15420/icr.2017:13:2.
51. Pijls NH, De Bruyne B. Coronary pressure measurement and fractional flow reserve. *Heart*. 1998;80(6):539–542. http://www.ncbi.nlm.nih.gov/pubmed/10065019%5Cnhttp://www.ncbi.nlm.nih.gov/pmc/articles/PMC1728867/pdf/v080p00539.pdf.
52. Lee JM, Choi G, Koo BK, et al. Identification of high-risk plaques destined to cause acute coronary syndrome using coronary computed tomographic angiography and computational fluid dynamics. *JACC Cardiovasc Imaging*. 2019;12(6):1032–1043. https://doi.org/10.1016/j.jcmg.2018.01.023.
53. Cury RC, Leipsic J, Abbara S, et al. CAD-RADS™ 2.0 –2022 coronary artery disease-reporting and data system: an expert consensus document of the Society of Cardiovascular Computed Tomography (SCCT), the American College of Cardiology (ACC), the American College of Radiology (ACR), and the North America Society of Cardiovascular Imaging (NASCI). *J Cardiovasc Comput Tomogr*. 2022;16(6):536–557. https://doi.org/10.1016/j.jcct.2022.07.002.
54. Fairbairn TA, Dobson R, Hurwitz-Koweek L, et al. Sex differences in coronary computed tomography angiography–derived fractional flow reserve: lessons from ADVANCE. *JACC Cardiovasc Imaging*. 2020;13(12):2576–2587. https://doi.org/10.1016/j.jcmg.2020.07.008.
55. Ihdayhid AR, Thakur U, Yap G, et al. Ethnic differences in coronary anatomy, left ventricular mass and CT-derived fractional flow reserve. *J Cardiovasc Comput Tomogr*. 2021;15(3):249–257. https://doi.org/10.1016/j.jcct.2020.09.004.
56. Shaw LJ, Blankstein R, Bax JJ, et al. Society of cardiovascular computed tomography /North American society of cardiovascular imaging—expert consensus document on coronary CT imaging of atherosclerotic plaque. *J Cardiovasc Comput Tomogr*. 2021;15(2):93–109. https://doi.org/10.1016/j.jcct.2020.11.002.
57. Motoyama S, Ito H, Sarai M, et al. Plaque characterization by coronary computed tomography angiography and the likelihood of acute coronary events in mid-term follow-up. *J Am Coll Cardiol*. 2015;66(4):337–346.
58. Doris MK, Otaki Y, Arnson Y, et al. Non-invasive fractional flow reserve in vessels without severe obstructive stenosis is associated with coronary plaque burden. *J Cardiovasc Comput Tomogr*. 2018;12(5):379–384. https://doi.org/10.1016/j.jcct.2018.05.003.
59. Yang S, Koo BK, Hoshino M, et al. CT angiographic and plaque predictors of functionally significant coronary disease and outcome using machine learning. *JACC Cardiovasc Imaging*. 2021;14(3):629–641. https://doi.org/10.1016/j.jcmg.2020.08.025.
60. Corcoran D, Hennigan B, Berry C. Fractional flow reserve: a clinical perspective. *Int J Cardiovasc Imaging*. 2017;33(7):961–974. https://doi.org/10.1007/s10554-017-1159-2.
61. Schuijf JD, Matheson MB, Ostovaneh MR, et al. Ischemia and no obstructive stenosis (INOCA) at CT angiography, CT myocardial perfusion, invasive coronary angiography, and SPECT: the CORE320 study. *Radiology*. 2020;294(1):61–73. https://doi.org/10.1148/radiol.2019190978.
62. Noel Bairey Merz C, Pepine CJ, Walsh MN, Fleg JL. Ischemia and No Obstructive Coronary Artery Disease (INOCA): developing evidence-based therapies and research agenda for the next decade. *Circulation*. 2017;135(11):1075–1092. https://doi.org/10.1161/CIRCULATIONAHA.116.024534.
63. Ford TJ, Yii E, Sidik N, et al. Ischemia and no obstructive coronary artery disease: prevalence and correlates of coronary vasomotion disorders. *Circ Cardiovasc Interv*. 2019;12(12):e008126. https://doi.org/10.1161/CIRCINTERVENTIONS.119.008126.
64. Papadopoulou SL, Girasis C, Dharampal A, et al. CT-SYNTAX score. *JACC Cardiovasc Imaging*. 2013;6(3):413–415. https://doi.org/10.1016/j.jcmg.2012.09.013.
65. Sianos G, Morel MA, Kappetein AP, et al. The SYNTAX score: an angiographic tool grading the complexity of coronary artery disease. *EuroIntervention*. 2005;1(2):219–227.
66. Nam CW, Mangiacapra F, Entjes R, et al. Functional SYNTAX score for risk assessment in multivessel coronary artery disease. *J Am Coll Cardiol*. 2011;58(12):1211–1218. https://doi.org/10.1016/j.jacc.2011.06.020.
67. Farooq V, van Klaveren D, Steyerberg EW, et al. Anatomical and clinical characteristics to guide decision making between coronary artery bypass surgery and percutaneous coronary intervention for individual patients: development and validation of SYNTAX score II. *Lancet*. 2013;381(9867):639–650. https://doi.org/10.1016/S0140-6736(13)60108-7.
68. Collet C, Onuma Y, Miyazaki Y, Morel MA, Serruys PW. Integration of non-invasive functional assessments with anatomical risk stratification in complex coronary artery disease: the non-invasive functional SYNTAX score. *Cardiovasc Diagn Ther*. 2017;7(2):151–158. https://doi.org/10.21037/cdt.2017.03.19.
69. Nørgaard BL, Leipsic J, Achenbach S. Coronary CT angiography to guide treatment decision making: lessons from the SYNTAX II trial *. *J Am Coll Cardiol*. 2018;71(24):2770–2772. https://doi.org/10.1016/j.jacc.2018.02.052.
70. Andreini D, Modolo R, Katagiri Y, et al. Impact of fractional flow reserve derived from coronary computed tomography angiography on heart team treatment decision-making in patients with multivessel coronary artery disease: insights from the SYNTAX III REVOLUTION trial. *Circ Cardiovasc Interv*. 2019;12(12):e007607. https://doi.org/10.1161/CIRCINTERVENTIONS.118.007607.
71. Feldmann K, Cami E, Safian RD. Planning percutaneous coronary interventions using computed tomography angiography and fractional flow reserve-derived from computed tomography: a state-of-the-art review. *Catheter Cardiovasc Interv*. 2019;93(2):298–304. https://doi.org/10.1002/ccd.27817.
72. Sonck J, Miyazaki Y, Mandry D, Andreini D. Non-invasive treatment planning of tandem coronary artery lesions using an interactive planner for PCI. *EuroIntervention*. 2018;14(8):924–925. https://doi.org/10.4244/eij-d-17-00815.
73. Collet C, Sonck J, Leipsic J, et al. Implementing coronary computed tomography angiography in the catheterization laboratory. *JACC Cardiovasc Imaging*. 2021;14(9):1846–1855. https://doi.org/10.1016/j.jcmg.2020.07.048.
74. Krievins D, Zellans E, Latkovskis G, et al. Coronary revascularization of patients with silent coronary ischemia may reduce the risk of myocardial infarction and cardiovascular death after carotid endarterectomy. *J Vasc Surg*. 2022;76:750–759. https://doi.org/10.1016/j.jvs.2022.05.004.
75. Budde RPJ, Nous FMA, Roest S, et al. CT-derived fractional flow reserve (FFRct) for functional coronary artery evaluation in the follow-up of patients after heart transplantation. *Eur Radiol*. 2022;32(3):1843–1852. https://doi.org/10.1007/s00330-021-08246-5.
76. Gijsen F, Katagiri Y, Barlis P, et al. Expert recommendations on the assessment of wall shear stress in human coronary arteries: existing methodologies, technical considerations, and clinical applications. *Eur Heart J*. 2019;40(41):3421–3433. https://doi.org/10.1093/eurheartj/ehz551.
77. Adjedj J, Hyafil F, du Fretay XH, et al. Physiological evaluation of anomalous aortic origin of a coronary artery using computed tomography–derived fractional flow reserve. *J Am Heart Assoc*. 2021;10(7):e018593. https://doi.org/10.1161/JAHA.120.018593.

14 Evaluating Coronary Inflammation Using the Fat Attenuation Index

CHARALAMBOS ANTONIADES AND ALEXIOS S. ANTONOPOULOS

KEY POINTS

- Inflammatory changes in the composition of perivascular adipose tissue (PVAT) can be visualized by using pericoronary fat attenuation index (FAI) maps from the postprocessing of routine coronary CT angiography (CCTA) scans.
- FAI Score quantifies the inflammatory load of each coronary artery, is interpreted in nomograms and captures the residual inflammatory risk.
- FAI Score can be interpreted as a standalone metric of risk, or it can be used in combination with plaque characteristics or patient's risk factor profile to determine the patient's absolute risk for future cardiovascular events via an AI enabled algorithm (AI Risk Score) FAI Score and AI Risk Score can be used in clinical practice to enhance cardiovascular risk stratification and guide personalized administration of preventive treatments.

INTRODUCTION

Coronary CT angiography (CCTA) is increasingly used as a diagnostic modality for assessing coronary anatomy with a class I indication in the latest US and European clinical guidelines for the evaluation of patients with stable chest pain.[1,2] Classic CCTA interpretation can provide important information on the presence of nonobstructive plaques, the quantification of atherosclerosis extent[3] or non-calcified plaque burden,[4] plaque phenotyping for anatomical high-risk plaque (HRP) features, and the assessment of the hemodynamic significance of lesions by myocardial perfusion CT or fractional flow reserve computed tomography (CT-FFR).[5]

However, prevention of cardiovascular events relies not only on the detection of obstructive, flow-limiting coronary lesions that cause symptoms but also on the early identification of plaques at risk for rupture, a process which is driven by vascular inflammation.[6] The causal relationship between inflammation and cardiovascular disease (CVD) is strengthened by the findings of recent randomized clinical trials that showed for the first time that lowering of inflammation by antiinflammatory agents such as canakinumab[7] or colchicine[8,9] reduces the risk for cardiovascular events. The notion of "residual inflammatory risk"[10] has been therefore coined to describe the cardiovascular risk related to inflammatory burden despite optimal management of traditional cardiovascular risk factors.[10] Detection of arterial inflammation could identify vulnerable patients at risk for cardiovascular events and guide targeted deployment of novel therapeutics.[11] However, the direct quantification of coronary inflammation has remained an unattainable goal in cardiovascular medicine until recently.

A recently developed imaging biomarker extracted from conventional CCTA images, the Fat Attenuation Index (FAI), allows detection and quantification of the inflammation-related changes in pericoronary fat CT attenuation and can be used as a metric of the arterial inflammatory burden.[12] FAI overcomes many of the limitations inherent to common biomarkers of vascular inflammation, is prognostic of future cardiovascular events and can track dynamic changes in coronary inflammatory burden.[13] Thus pericoronary FAI allows the detection of vulnerable patients at high residual inflammatory risk and can guide the therapeutic management to prevent cardiovascular events.

In this chapter we discuss the science behind the discovery and clinical validation of FAI, its diagnostic and prognostic value, and we compare it with other commonly used biomarkers for the detection of vascular inflammation. Finally, we explain how pericoronary FAI is used in everyday clinical practice to enhance cardiovascular risk stratification and guide personalized administration of preventive treatments.

THE INTERPLAY BETWEEN ADIPOSE TISSUE AND THE CARDIOVASCULAR SYSTEM

Adipose tissue beyond energy storage: Adipose tissue is a term used to collectively refer to body fat depots and subtypes with distinct properties. A basic distinction of adipose tissue is dividing it into white and brown adipose tissue, the latter being predominantly found in mammals during infant life and being responsible for the uncoupling of mitochondrial oxidation to produce heat, that is, nonshivering thermogenesis.[14] In adult life, most of human adiposity consists of white adipose tissue with minimal amounts of brown fat, which is found mainly in the upper back, above the clavicles, around the vertebrae, and in the mediastinum. The browning of white adipocytes may induce the expression of an intermediate phenotype between that of white and brown adipose tissue, a process termed "beiging,"[15] and therefore islets of beige adipose tissue can be found within white adipose tissue mass. To overcome the complexities related to adipose tissue subtypes (which lie outside the scope of the present chapter), any reference made herein to adipose tissue implies the white adipose tissue.

Human adipose tissue had for years been considered responsible for the storage of excess caloric intake in the form of triglycerides in lipid droplets. However, this traditional concept of adipose tissue as a depot for passive energy storage has been recently overturned.[15] It is now well understood that adipose tissue is an active endocrine organ whose function determines systemic metabolic status and insulin resistance, vasomotor function and arterial hypertension, atherosclerosis development, and risk of atrial fibrillation and heart failure.[16–18] This is achieved by the release of active adipokines in the circulation that can exert endocrine effects on the cardiovascular system. In addition, local adipose tissue depots exert paracrine or even vasocrine effects on nearby organs.[14]

Biological differences between distinct adipose tissue depots: The anatomical location of human AT defines its phenotype, biology, and secretory profile.[14] Visceral AT (thoracic or abdominal), which surrounds the visceral organs, contains smaller, less differentiated adipocytes with a rich stroma-vascular matrix, and a higher content of fibroblasts, residing and infiltrating immune cells compared to the subcutaneous depot.[19] Visceral AT is a rich source of adipokines, and its secretory profile is strongly associated with cardiometabolic risk (e.g., insulin resistance, arterial hypertension, diabetes, and metabolic syndrome). Ectopic visceral adiposity (such as epicardial, intrahepatic, intramuscular) is also positively associated with CVD risk.[14] On the other hand, subcutaneous depot contains larger, more well-differentiated adipocytes, has a lower secretory activity, and its relationship with CVD risk is weak or neutral.[20] Among these AT depots, perivascular adipose tissue (PVAT) plays a pivotal role in the physiology of the cardiovascular system given its direct, anatomical proximity to the arterial wall.

The role of PVAT in the cardiovascular system physiology: PVAT is the layer of adipose tissue surrounding an artery, consisting of (pre)adipocytes, fibroblasts, residing inflammatory cells, and a rich a stroma-vascular matrix. In contrast to other fat depots that influence cardiovascular physiology in an endocrine manner, PVAT exerts paracrine effects on the adjacent artery (outside-in signaling), affecting vascular biology given the absence of any anatomical barrier (e.g., separating fascia).[17,21,22] PVAT actively secretes numerous bioactive mediators such as adipokines, miRNAs, lipid mediators, and gaseous molecules that affect vascular physiology, relaxation, vascular wall oxidative stress and inflammation.[23] Adipokines in PVAT secretome (e.g., adiponectin, omentin, apelin, and adipocyte-derived relaxing factor, etc.) and gaseous molecules such as nitric oxide and hydrogen sulfide can induce vasodilation through the opening of K^+ channels in smooth muscle cells (SMC).[24] The effect of PVAT adipokines such as adiponectin on vascular endothelial NO bioavailability can also enhance vasodilation. These effects are mitigated under inflammatory conditions, such as obesity leading to a proinflammatory PVAT profile and thus to vasoconstriction, SMC migration, and endothelial dysfunction.[25]

Inside-out signaling from the vascular wall to PVAT: In contrast to the classical concept of an one-way communication from PVAT to the vascular wall, evidence supports that a constant bidirectional communication takes place between the two structures.[23] The vascular wall can influence PVAT through paracrine signals ("inside-out" signaling) that drive changes in PVAT biology, phenotype, and secretory profile.[23] In our previous studies on human arteries it was shown that oxidative stress in the vascular wall leads to the release of lipid peroxidation products (such as 4-hydroxynonenal) that diffuse to PVAT, driving an upregulation in adiponectin gene expression and secretion.[17] Adiponectin exerts antioxidant effects on the adjacent vascular wall possibly as a local defense mechanism in response to increased vascular oxidative stress.[17] In a similar manner, proinflammatory cytokines (such as interleukin-6, tumor necrosis factor-α, and interferon-γ) secreted from the inflamed vascular wall or atheromatous plaques are diffused to the surrounding PVAT and change its phenotype; inflammatory cytokines prevent the differentiation of preadipocytes to mature adipocytes (i.e., decrease the expression of differentiation markers) and inhibit lipid droplet accumulation in PVAT adipocytes.[12] These findings suggest that in contrast to the traditional concept of PVAT as a driver of vascular disease, changes in PVAT biology may be the result of vascular disease (i.e., vascular inflammation), and therefore PVAT may serve as an internal "sensor" of vascular disease. The concept of the cross-talk between PVAT and the vascular wall is summarized in the illustration of Fig. 14.1.

Defining perivascular adipose tissue: PVAT[13,26,27] around the coronary arteries has distinct biological properties compared to the rest of Epicardial adipose tissue (EAT), far from the arterial wall.[12] Given that there is no fascia separating PVAT from non-PVAT and that the effects of the arterial wall are more potent closer to the vessel, there is a gradual transition between PVAT and non-PVAT within EAT. The most widely accepted definition of PVAT is that of a layer of adipose tissue located within a radial distance from the vascular wall equal to the luminal diameter of the adjacent artery.[28–34] This definition applies to the PVAT surrounding any artery in the human body up to a luminal diameter of 20 mm. For example, around arteries of a larger caliber (e.g., the aorta), PVAT extends up to 20 mm from the outer surface of the vessel by convention.

THE SCIENCE BEHIND THE FAT ATTENUATION INDEX AND CLINICAL VALIDATION

PVAT Imaging as a Sensor of Vascular Inflammation

The discovery of the "inside-out" signaling from the vascular wall to its surrounding PVAT led to the discovery that mediators released from the vascular wall have direct effects on PVAT's phenotype, particularly on adipocytes biology.[17,21,23] Following the discovery of this cross-talk between the vascular wall and PVAT, we have shown that experimentally induced inflammation in the vascular wall leads to rapid changes in PVAT phenotype; perivascular adipocytes lose their differentiation status, and their capacity for intracellular storage of lipid droplets and become smaller.[12] These changes at molecular level result in a change in perivascular tissue phenotype, which in the presence, and because of, vascular inflammation has a lower lipid content and a respective decrease in its lipid:water ratio.[12] In addition, because the diffusion and the effect of inflammatory mediators on the surrounding PVAT is attenuated with increasing distance from the vascular wall, there is a gradient in adipocyte size with smaller adipocytes close to an inflamed artery and larger, lipid-laden adipocytes at increased radial distance from the arterial wall.[12,23] The respective gradient in the lipid:water content of perivascular tissue in the presence of arterial inflammation can be easily detected by imaging as a gradient in the

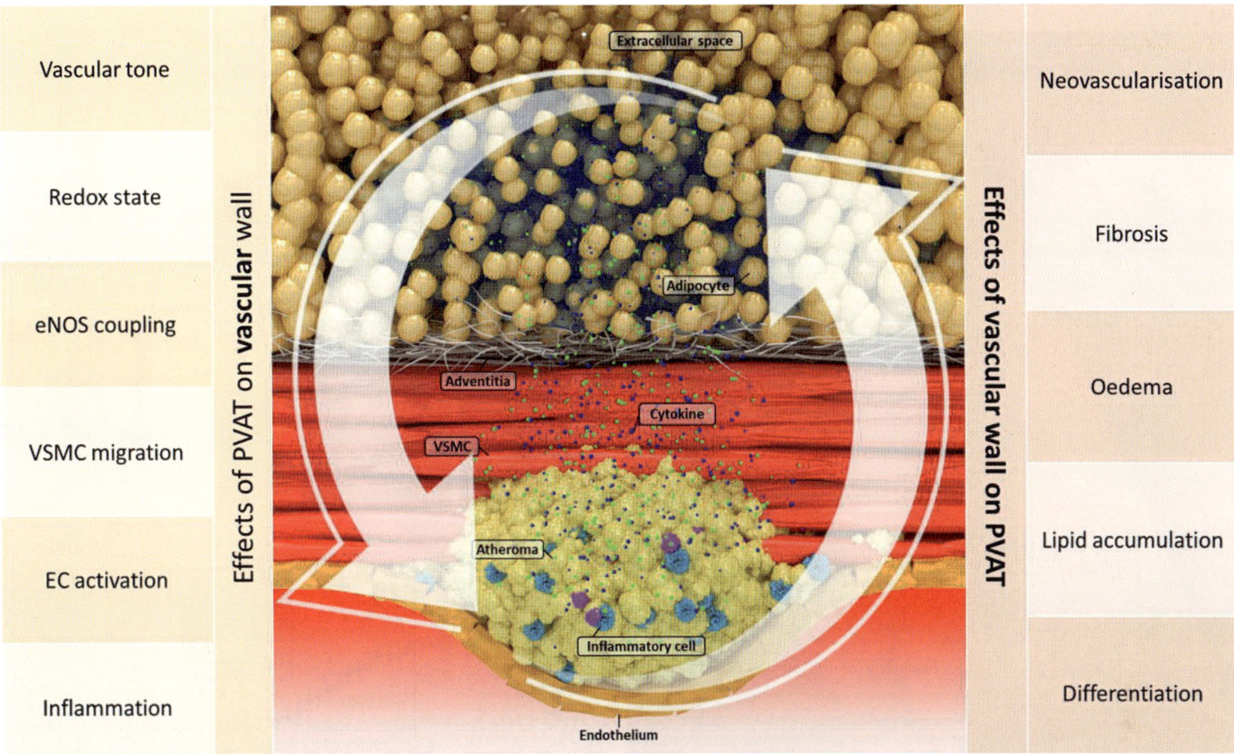

FIG. 14.1 Illustration of the bidirectional interplay between the vascular wall and perivascular adipose tissue and its major components. An animated video presenting how the cross-talk between PVAT and the vascular wall leads to changes in PVAT's texture and composition, visible with computed tomography can be found in the above reference. *EC*, Endothelial cell; *eNOS*, endothelial NOS; *PVAT*, perivascular adipose tissue; *VSMC*, vascular smooth muscle cell. (Reused from Kotanidis CP, Antoniades C. Perivascular fat imaging by computed tomography (CT): a virtual guide. *Br J Pharmacol*. 2021;178:4270–4290.)

CT attenuation: perivascular tissue closer to an inflamed artery has a CT attenuation towards the −30 Hounsfield unit (HU) spectrum range, with its attenuation dropping to more negative values, towards the −190 HU range, with increasing radial distance from the vascular wall. The greater the effect of vascular inflammation, the higher the PVAT attenuation close to the artery, and the steeper the observed 3D gradient in CT attenuation with increasing distance from the arterial wall.[12] These changes in the phenotypic appearance of PVAT close to an artery can be readily detected on routine CT datasets by appropriate image post processing. Therefore the imaging phenotype of PVAT may serve as an internal "thermometer" of vascular inflammation. This is schematically represented in Fig. 14.2.

Visualizing Vascular Inflammation by Perivascular FAI Heat Maps

In the original study that introduced FAI as an imaging biomarker of vascular inflammation, FAI was biologically validated in ex vivo scans of AT explants and in vivo clinical scans.[12] Both in the in vivo scans of human AT and ex vivo scans of AT explants from the epicardial, thoracic and subcutaneous AT depots of the same patients, FAI (i.e., the metric of attenuation gradients within the AT within a region of interest corrected for technical scanning parameters) was inversely correlated with the expression of adipocyte differentiation markers and adipocyte size.[12] In addition, FAI was validated against 18F-fluorodeoxyglucose (^{18F}FDG) positron emission tomography (PET) imaging, and a strong positive correlation between FAI and ^{18F}FDG uptake was observed in subcutaneous AT.[12] In the same original study, adipocytes of coronary PVAT were smaller in size and less differentiated with decreasing radial distance from the right coronary artery (RCA). These histological observations were followed by respective changes in FAI around the RCA on clinical CCTA scans.[12] FAI was measured in sequential cylindrical layers of 1 mm thickness up to a radial distance of 20 mm from the coronary artery wall in a 40 mm-long segment of the proximal RCA (10–50 mm from its origin). Perivascular tissue layers closer to the coronary artery wall, where adipocytes are smaller, less differentiated, and contain a lower lipid:water ratio, had higher FAI values. The RCA was used as a model to validate the ex vivo findings, given the absence of any major side branches and the ability to discriminate PVAT from non-PVAT, as well as the abundant amount of adipose tissue surrounding RCA, which can easily be harvested without any major bleeding risk, in contrast to the other coronary arteries. These findings suggest that changes in FAI, calculated from CT images, are directly proportional to the degree of vascular inflammation inside the human coronary arteries measured in vivo.[12]

The first clinical validation of this new biomarker by its application in clinically indicated CCTA scans suggested that patients with advanced atherosclerosis have higher FAI values around their proximal RCA.[12] Pericoronary FAI was also positively associated with atherosclerotic plaque burden in all major epicardial coronary arteries. These findings were independent of traditional cardiovascular risk factors, age, gender, and coronary calcium

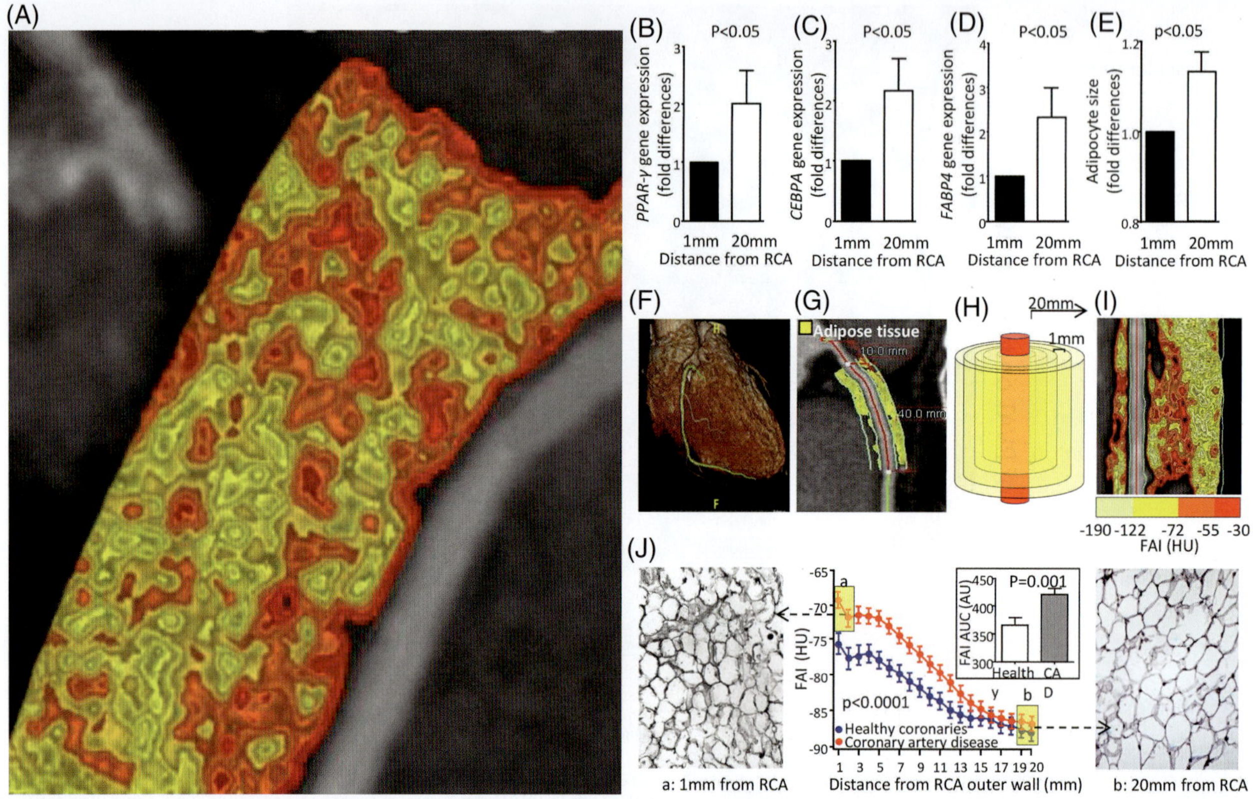

FIG. 14.2 (A) Example of a coronary CT angiography (CCTA) scan and pericoronary fat attenuation index (FAI) mapping showing the gradient in CT attenuation around a coronary artery. (B) PPAR-g, (C) CEBPA, and (D) CEBPA4 gene expression and (E) adipocyte size in pericoronary adipose tissue samples attached to the right coronary artery (RCA) and paired samples ~20 mm away from it. (F–H) The attenuation readings around the RCA of patients undergoing CCTA was calculated for each cylindrical 1-mm-thick layer of pericoronary tissue in a radial distance 1 to 20 mm from RCA wall, to generate the necessary attenuation gradients captured by fat attenuation index (FAI). (I) FAI mapping of perivascular adipose tissue (PVAT) around the RCA. (J) FAI and radial distance from vascular wall in patients with CAD (n = 149) versus healthy individuals (n = 117). (Reproduced with permission from Antonopoulos AS, Sanna F, Sabharwal N, et al. Detecting human coronary inflammation by imaging perivascular fat. *Sci Transl Med.* 2017;9:eaal2658.)

score.[12] In addition, FAI measured around culprit and nonculprit lesions in patients with acute coronary syndromes and stable coronary artery disease (CAD) patients had excellent diagnostic accuracy for identifying unstable plaques.[12] Specifically, pericoronary FAI was measured around culprit plaques and compared to FAI around a segment proximal to the lesion in patients with recent (<3 days) acute myocardial infarction.[12] Culprit lesions had significantly higher FAI values compared with nonculprit lesions from the same patients or lesions from stable CAD patients. The increase in FAI around culprit lesions was independent of stent implantation in the ruptured lesion, and FAI had an excellent ability to discriminate between culprit and nonculprit plaques (area under the curve [AUC] of 0.91).[12]

External validation of these findings by independent research groups has subsequently yielded similar results, confirming the diagnostic value of coronary PVAT attenuation as a metric of coronary inflammation.[34–38] In a study involving intravascular ultrasound and measurements of coronary PVAT attenuation by CT, it was shown that coronary segments with atherosclerosis had higher (i.e., less negative) values of coronary PVAT attenuation compared to coronary segments without any visible plaques.[35] Subsequent studies also reported significant differences in average pericoronary fat attenuation of culprit versus nonculprit lesions of patients with acute coronary syndrome (ACS) and lesions of patients with stable CAD.[34,36–38] A metaanalysis of all published evidence on the diagnostic value of FAI as a marker of unstable plaques showed a significant difference of 4.5 HU (95%CI 1.1–7.9) in coronary PVAT attenuation around stable and unstable plaques.[39] Coronary PVAT attenuation as a biomarker of coronary inflammation has been also validated against 18F-sodium fluoride (^{18F}NaF) PET imaging of coronary plaques, which tracks active microcalcification and plaque inflammation.[40] Simultaneous assessment of coronary PVAT on CT and plaque inflammation on PET suggested a strong positive correlation between ^{18F}NaF uptake by plaques with high-risk anatomical features and coronary PVAT attenuation.[40] In line with these observations, higher coronary PVAT attenuation values have been reported in Myocardial Infarction with Non-Obstructive Coronary Arteries (MINOCA) patients compared with healthy controls,[36] patients with vasospastic angina,[41] or myocarditis and Takotsubo syndrome.[42] These findings suggest that ongoing inflammatory processes in the coronary arteries or the human heart can be detected by analyzing images of PVAT or epicardial AT, whereas local CT attenuation metrics of PVAT around coronary lesions (e.g., unweighted measurements such as the mean attenuation of PVAT or weighted measurements such as FAI) can serve as a valuable biomarker of plaque inflammation and instability. The reported association of coronary PVAT attenuation with hemodynamically significant lesions as assessed by fractional flow reserve[43,44] or PET-derived coronary flow reserve[45] are less readily explainable and may be driven by the presence of vascular inflammation in advanced atherosclerosis. Coronary PVAT attenuation is not and should not be interpreted as a metric of luminal stenosis but rather as a metric of the underlying atherosclerotic disease activity, driven by vascular inflammation.

Changes in FAI in Response to Therapeutic Interventions

Interventions that lower vascular wall inflammation are associated with a reduction in pericoronary FAI.[30,46] In the original clinical validation study of FAI,[12] a significant increase in FAI around culprit lesions in patients with acute myocardial infarction was observed that returned to control group levels 5 weeks after the index myocardial infarction event. A similar finding was observed post ACS in another study, where there was both "cooling down" of the culprit lesion as well as the overall coronary tree over a 6-month period, measured by peri-lesion FAI and proximal RCA FAI measurements, respectively.[12] This could reflect both a time-dependent resolution of plaque/vascular inflammation as well as the effects of optimal treatment (e.g., antiinflammatory effects of statins, aspirin, and other medication initiated post ACS). The effect of statins on FAI was confirmed in an observational clinical study that involved a follow-up CCTA scan at 1 to 1.5 years interval after initiation of statin treatment, where there was a significant reduction in lesion-specific pericoronary FAI around noncalcified and mixed coronary plaques but not around calcified plaques,[30] a finding that was also confirmed in stable CAD patients who underwent serial CCTA scans.[47] Consequently, statins may exert an antiinflammatory effect on coronary atherosclerosis, which can be detected by pericoronary FAI, even before these changes can be identified by CCTA as a decrease in plaque burden.

In a prospective clinical study involving patients with psoriasis, which is characterized by systemic low-grade inflammation, patients were scanned at baseline and 1 year after allocation to treatment with either biologic antiinflammatory agents (i.e., anti–tumor necrosis factor α therapy or anti–interleukin (IL) 12/23 and anti–IL-17 therapies) or no biologic agents or topical/light therapy (control group). Perivascular FAI around major epicardial arteries was significantly reduced at 1 year with biologic antiinflammatory agents, irrespectively of the presence or not of coronary plaques.[48] This evidence suggests that in contrast to other potential imaging biomarkers of coronary plaques, such as coronary calcium score or HRP features, the biological information captured by FAI offers a method to monitor fluctuations in coronary inflammatory burden either due to a plaque rupture event or in response to treatment. Notably, FAI can offer both lesion-specific information (when applied around a certain coronary lesion) or information on the background inflammation of the coronary arterial tree (when applied to the proximal segments of epicardial coronary arteries) even in the absence of any visible plaques. This could be particularly relevant as a soft clinical endpoint for the design of randomized clinical trials testing the effects of novel antiinflammatory treatments before investigating their effects on hard clinical outcomes (i.e., cardiovascular mortality, nonfatal myocardial infarction).

Pericoronary FAI and Cardiovascular Risk Prediction

The prognostic value of FAI was originally explored in the Cardiovascular RISk Prediction using Computed Tomography (CRISP-CT) study.[49] In CRISP-CT, a total of 3912 individuals undergoing clinically indicated CCTA were followed up prospectively for a mean of 8 years for cardiovascular events; CCTA imaging datasets were manually analyzed, and FAI maps around the proximal segments (10–50 mm from their origin) of the three major epicardial coronary arteries were generated. In both the derivation cohort (n = 1872) and the validation cohort (n = 2040), pericoronary FAI around the proximal RCA and left anterior descending (LAD) were associated with cardiac mortality.[49] A cutoff value in pericoronary FAI of −70.1 HU identified a high-risk patient subgroup with increased risk for cardiac mortality (ninefold in the European derivation and 5.7-fold in the USA validation cohort). The prognostic value of FAI was independent of age, sex, traditional cardiovascular risk factors, coronary atherosclerosis extent, coronary calcium score (CCS), and presence of HRP features (i.e., low-attenuation plaque, napkin-ring sign, spotty calcification, and positive remodeling).[49] Moreover, FAI enhanced both all-cause and cardiac mortality risk discrimination and stratification. Adding FAI on top of a model including age, sex, CVD risk factors, CAD extent, and number of HRP features yielded significant incremental prognostic value ($\Delta_{AUC} = 0.049$ in the derivation cohort and $\Delta_{AUC} = 0.075$ in the validation cohort).[49] FAI retained its incremental prognostic value even after inclusion of CCS in the prognostic model for both endpoints. However, it lost its predictive value for cardiac mortality in patients who started statin or aspirin treatment after CCTA, whereas it remained predictive value among patients who did not change their treatment after CCTA. This likely indicates that the CVD risk detected by FAI may be modified with optimal medical therapy.[49] After subgroup analyses, FAI remained positively associated with cardiac and all-cause mortality endpoints in both primary and secondary prevention. FAI values above the cutoff were also associated with a fivefold risk of acute myocardial infarction, which directly links coronary inflammation with plaque instability and acute plaque rupture events prospectively.[49]

Consequently, the CRISP-CT findings suggest that pericoronary FAI predicts all-cause and cardiac mortality above traditional CVD risk factors, CCS, and CCTA-derived anatomical information and may be useful in risk discrimination and reclassification in both primary and secondary prevention, as well as identifying patients with residual vascular inflammatory risk. The role of CCTA in CVD prevention has been already highlighted by the Scottish Computed Tomography of the Heart (SCOT-HEART) trial,[50] in which CCTA imaging in patients with stable chest pain was associated with initiation of more preventive measures. This may have contributed to the significantly decreased risk for death from CAD or nonfatal myocardial infarction in patients with stable chest pain referred for CCTA compared with those who received standard care.[50] In contrast to anatomical assessment of the coronary tree, FAI provides information on vascular inflammation, representing a novel imaging biomarker that can identify vulnerable patients at increased risk of cardiac mortality, even before the formation of visible coronary plaques. Pericoronary FAI mapping offers a novel approach for the identification of vulnerable patients at risk for events. Pericoronary FAI could also drive the initiation or intensification of preventive treatment; as evidenced from the CRISP-CT study, the risk identified by FAI might be modifiable by treatment such as statin or aspirin.[49]

Subsequent studies have also confirmed the predictive ability of coronary PVAT attenuation for cardiovascular events. In a study of 539 patients undergoing CCTA for CAD diagnosis, coronary PVAT attenuation around the RCA was associated with a composite outcome consisting of death and nonfatal myocardial infarction, even after adjustment for clinical risk factors, CCS, HRP features, plaque volume, and ischemia.[51] In a another cohort of 333 type 2 diabetes patients, coronary PVAT attenuation around the LAD was independently associated with the risk for major adverse cardiovascular events after adjustment for significant stenoses and HRP features and offered significant incremental prognostic value on top of the baseline model.[52] A third independent study also reported a significant association of coronary PVAT attenuation around RCA with major adverse cardiovascular events after adjustment for traditional risk factors, atherosclerosis extent on CCTA, and presence of ischaemia on single-photon emission computed tomography myocardial perfusion imaging.[29] This association was lost after adjustment for CCS, in contrast to CRISP-CT study findings, although this was a study with relatively small sample size (n = 356) and limited number of cardiovascular events.[53] Another source of heterogeneity between studies in the field is the use of unweighted measurements of the mean attenuation of PVAT by most studies, which may perform less well for prognostication of events compared to FAI (which captures the attenuation gradients of PVAT, adjusted for technical/scanning and anatomical parameters that can influence the reading).[53,54] Despite the different methodological approaches employed by each study, when all available published evidence was included in a metaanalysis, coronary PVAT attenuation/FAI (measured around the RCA) was associated with increased risk for major adverse cardiovascular events.[39] The findings of the CRISP-CT and subsequent smaller studies were also confirmed by a post-hoc analysis of 1697 patients from the SCOT-HEART study,[55] where coronary PVAT attenuation had independent and incremental value for the prediction of fatal or nonfatal myocardial infarction on top of plaque burden, obstructive coronary disease, and clinical risk profile.[55] Therefore to date accumulated evidence strongly suggests that coronary PVAT attenuation is an imaging biomarker with independent prognostic value for coronary events in patients undergoing a clinically-indicated CCTA.

CARDIOVASCULAR RISK STRATIFICATION BY USE FAI MAPPING AND HIGH-RISK PLAQUE FEATURES BY CCTA

The combination of anatomical HRP features with the biological information offered by pericoronary FAI measurements is an efficient strategy to improve the risk stratification of patients undergoing CCTA.[32] In the CRISP-CT study, it was demonstrated that the subgroup of patients with both high pericoronary FAI and the presence of HRP features had a sevenfold increased risk for cardiac mortality compared with patients with low pericoronary FAI and no HRP. Notably the increased risk was mainly attributable to the high coronary inflammatory burden, because even in the absence of HRP features, patients with high FAI had a 5.6-fold higher risk for cardiac mortality, whereas the subgroup of patients with HRP but with low FAI did not have increased risk for cardiac events.[32] These observations are similar to the findings derived from the post-hoc analysis of SCOT-HEART study. The addition of coronary PVAT attenuation measurements in a prognostic model on top of low-attenuation plaque (LAP) significantly increased the prognostic performance of the model in CRISP-CT. Compared to the subgroup of patients without LAP or high-coronary PVAT attenuation, the subgroup of patients with LAP had a 4.9-fold increased risk for major adverse cardiac events (MACE), whereas patients with both LAP and high-coronary PVAT attenuation had an 11.7-fold increased risk for cardiac events (Fig. 14.3).[55]

COMPARATIVE PERFORMANCE OF FAI VERSUS ESTABLISHED BIOMARKERS OF VASCULAR INFLAMMATION

An imaging-guided detection of vascular inflammation offers advantages over conventional risk stratification based on plasma biomarkers of inflammation.[11] Indeed, plasma biomarkers such as high-sensitivity C-reactive protein (hs-CRP) or proinflammatory mediators such as IL-6, IL-1b, and tumor necrosis factor-α have been widely tested in clinical research[11] as they have certain advantages (e.g., low cost and ease of measurement from a single blood sample). However, plasma biomarkers also come with certain limitations, the most important one being their limited vascular specificity, as plasma inflammatory biomarkers are increased in the case of any ongoing inflammatory process in the human body.[13] For example, it has been demonstrated that almost 50% of patients with established vascular disease would be considered to be at residual inflammatory risk based on plasma C-reactive protein (CRP) measurements.[10] Vascular imaging can overcome this limitation by providing specific information on the arterial wall. CCS, the most widely used imaging biomarker in the primary prevention setting, informs on the extent of coronary atherosclerosis; however, although CCS provides a robust measure of risk, it is not modifiable and does not respond to interventions that lower vascular inflammation. Similarly to CCS, HRP features on CCTA flag rupture-prone coronary plaques, but this anatomical information is

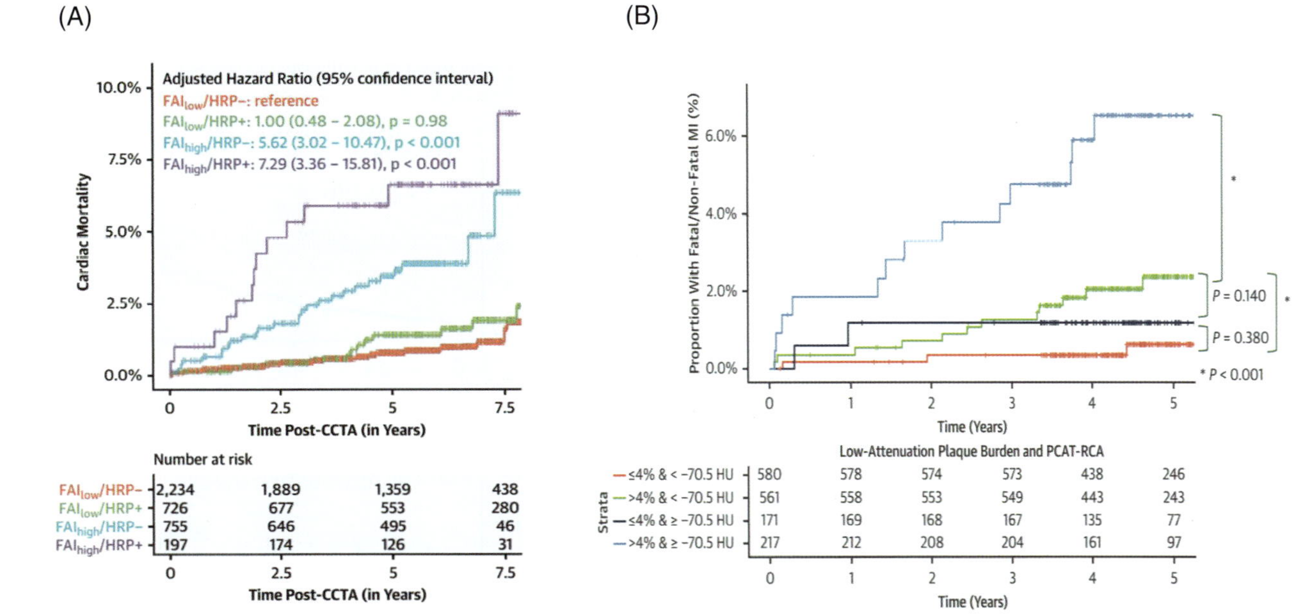

FIG. 14.3 Combining pericoronary attenuation and high-risk plaque metrics. (A) Patients with elevated fat attenuation index (FAI) and high-risk plaque features had striking increase of their risk for cardiac mortality in the CRISP-CT study, whereas patients with high FAI but no high-risk plaque also had a 5.6-fold increase of their risk for a fatal cardiac event.[32] Similar results were observed when measuring FAI in any epicardial vessel (left or right coronary artery). (B) Patients with low-attenuation plaque volume >4% had an approximately fourfold increase in their risk for fatal or nonfatal myocardial infarction (MI) in SCOT-HEART trial, but that was increased to >11-fold when unadjusted pericoronary fat attenuation was added into the model.[55] The incremental value of perivascular adipose tissue (PCAT) could only be demonstrated for the right coronary artery. Both images reproduced with permission.[32,55]

only weakly associated with plaque metabolic activity/inflammation.[40] PET/CT imaging can detect in vivo tissue inflammation. The most common radioactive tracer, ^{18F}FDG, is absorbed by metabolically active cells and is useful in detecting the inflammatory burden in carotid arteries or the aorta, but its utility for the imaging of coronary arterial inflammation is limited because of increased background noise and significant radiotracer uptake by the myocardium. Other radiotracers more specific for coronary inflammation such as sodium fluoride ^{18F}NaFor Gallium 68 (68Ga)-DOTATATE are promising but their prognostic value remains less well studied.[56]

A recent metaanalysis explored the added prognostic value of systemic inflammatory biomarkers and PVAT-determined vascular inflammation, on top of the clinical risk profile and/or atherosclerosis extent for major adverse cardiovascular events.[57] Circulating plasma biomarkers such as CRP and IL-6 significantly, albeit marginally, improved CVD risk prognostication (Δ_{AUC} of 1.8% and 1.7%, respectively). Conversely, CCTA-derived biomarkers offered the highest incremental prognostic value for the composite outcome, and this was maximized when coronary PVAT attenuation mapping was added to high-risk plaque features (Δ_{AUC} of 8.2%). The findings of this metaanalysis are not unexpected and related to the low specificity of plasma biomarkers for vascular inflammation. Therefore CCTA imaging of PVAT for coronary inflammation quantification should be considered the best currently available biomarker of vascular inflammation, with diagnostic and independent prognostic value (Fig. 14.4), which if implemented in clinical practice has the potential to enhance CVD prognostication and guide patient selection for antiinflammatory treatment.[58]

TRANSLATING FAI IN CLINICAL PRACTICE: INTRODUCTION OF FAI SCORE

STANDARDIZATION OF THE REPORTING OF CORONARY PVAT ATTENUATION

Coronary PVAT attenuation measurements can be applied around coronary plaques to get information about the presence of local vascular inflammation[12] or around proximal epicardial segments of the three major epicardial coronary arteries as a metric of the global inflammatory burden in the coronary tree for risk stratification purposes.[49] The original method of FAI analysis over a 40 mm-long epicardial coronary segment (10–50 mm from its origin) extending to a radial distance in perivascular tissue equal to the diameter of the coronary vessel analyzed has been adopted by the majority of studies in the field.[29,30,48,54,55] However, the use of unadjusted mean attenuation measurements of PVAT has not performed as well as FAI for the prediction of clinical outcomes in CRISP-CT study.[54] For example, FAI has superior prognostic value for MACE compared with unadjusted coronary PVAT attenuation measurements (Fig. 14.4D). Although high unadjusted PCAT measurements have been associated with a 2.5-fold increase in the risk of MACE,[39] high FAI was associated with up to ninefold increased risk for cardiac mortality and fivefold increase of the risk for nonfatal MI in the CRISP-CT study.[49] Therefore coronary PVAT attenuation gradient measurements need to undergo a series of adjustments for technical factors (e.g., tube voltage and other image-acquisition/scanner parameters as well as corrections related with the local anatomy and biological characteristics of the perivascular space) to reflect the degree of inflammation inside the adjacent artery.

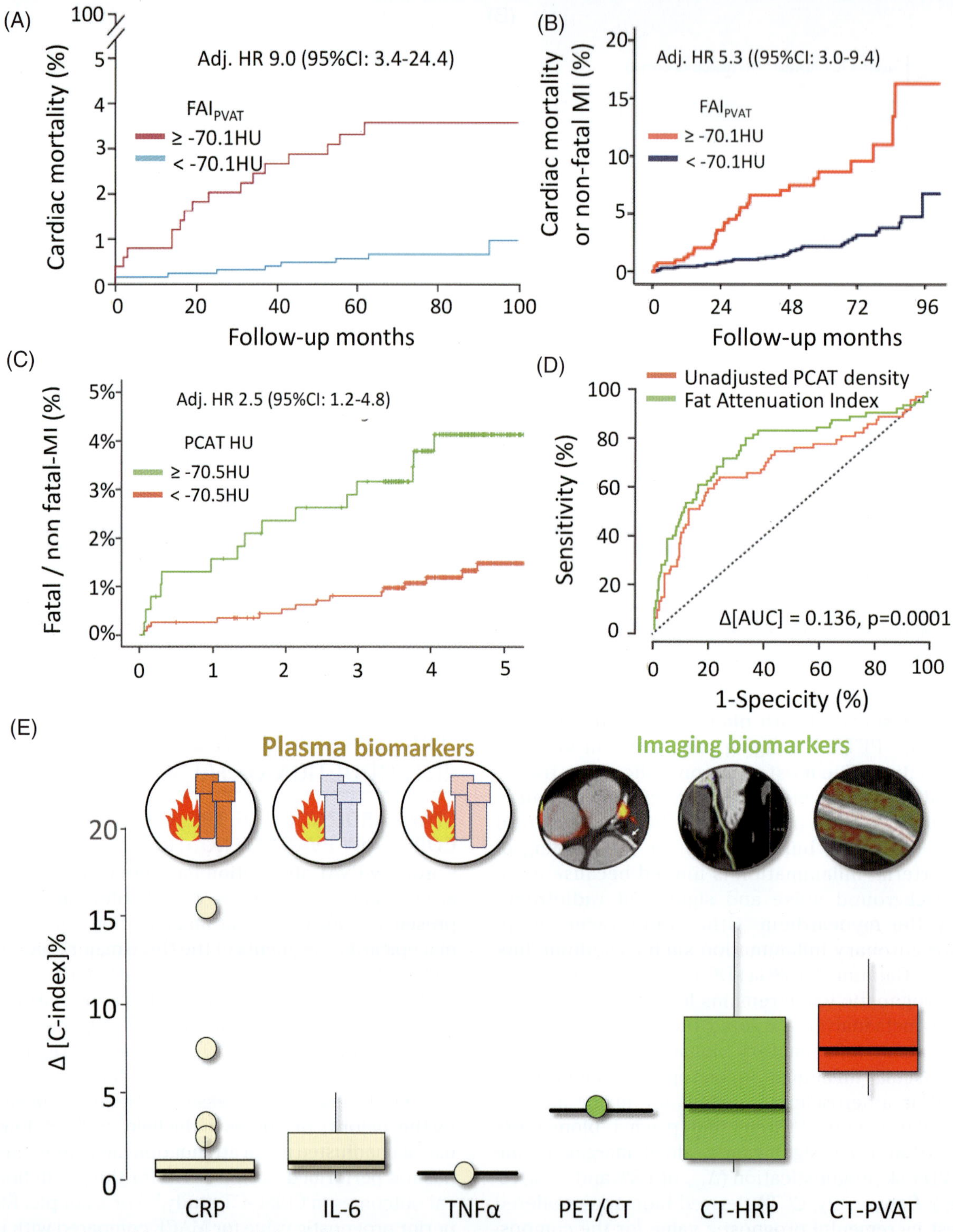

FIG. 14.4 Prognostic value of fat attenuation index (FAI) in prospective outcomes studies. (A) Prognostic value of FAI for cardiac mortality (A) or nonfatal myocardial infarction (B) in CRISP-CT study.[49] (C) Prognostic value of unadjusted coronary perivascular adipose tissue (PVAT) attenuation values in SCOT-HEART trial.[55] (D) The superior performance of fully weighted FAI versus unadjusted PVAT density; unadjusted PVAT density had borderline predictive value for cardiac mortality, whereas fully weighted FAI leads to improved risk prediction by 13.6%.[54] (E) The added prognostic value of vascular inflammation biomarkers for major adverse cardiovascular events on top of patient risk profile and coronary atherosclerosis extent is greater than that of plasma biomarkers according to a metaanalysis (n = 351,628 individuals). PVAT imaging by CT was associated with the maximum added prognostic information among the studied vascular inflammation biomarkers.[57]

To overcome this limitation and standardize the reporting of coronary inflammation in clinical CCTA interpretation, the FAI Score was developed,[59] that is, the FAI value of PVAT around each major epicardial coronary artery adjusted for age, gender, technical, and biological/anatomical parameters. The FAI Score value of each one of the three epicardial coronary arteries (RCA, LAD, and left circumflex [LCx]) can be projected upon age-specific and sex-specific nomograms to get a metric of the inflammatory burden of each coronary artery in relation to individuals of a similar sex and age group (Fig. 14.5). FAI Score (expressed in percentiles) is reflective of the relevant risk for cardiovascular

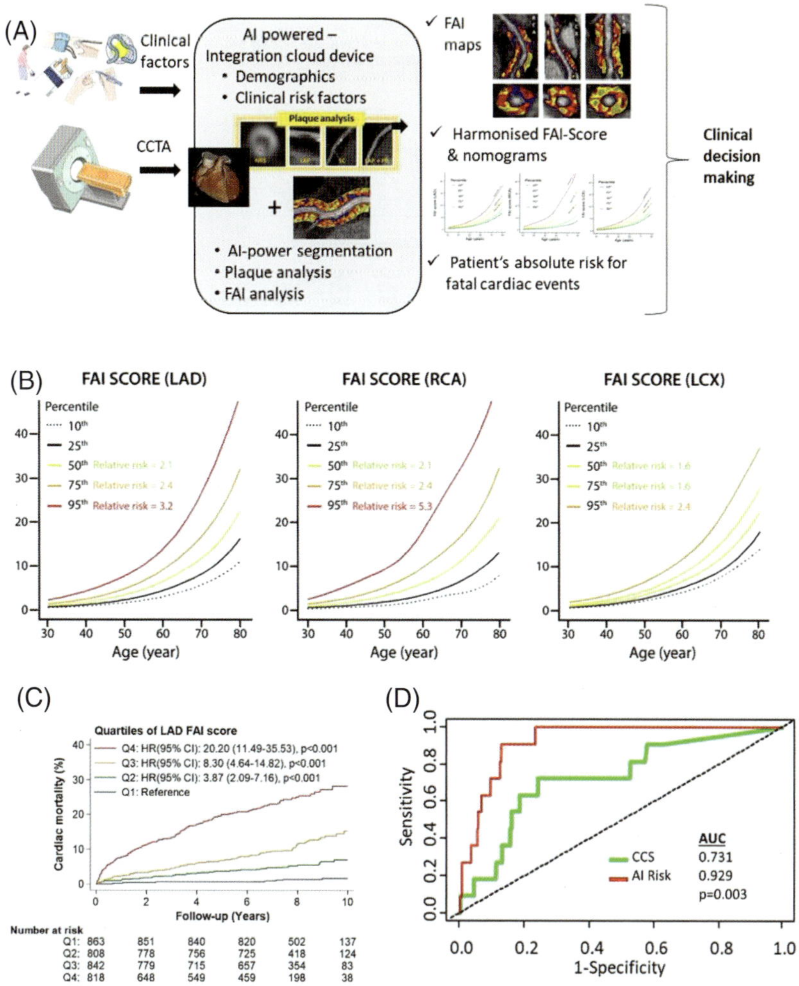

(E) Cardiac mortality –whole population

QRISK3	AI-Risk Classification Low/ mid	High	Very high	Total	Reclassified upwards		Reclassified downwards	
Low/ mid	1458 (36)	342 (20)	265 (11)	2065	607	29.4%	-	-
High	293 (26)	265 (38)	421 (116)	979	421	43.0%	293	29.9%
Very high	26 (2)	50 (4)	221 (67)	297	-	-	76	25.6%
Total	1777	657	907	3341	1028	30.8%	369	11.0%

Cardiac mortality – no obstructive CAD

QRISK3	AI-Risk Classification Low/ mid	High	Very high	Total	Reclassified upwards		Reclassified downwards	
Low/ mid	1362 (28)	293 (13)	224 (8)	1879	517	27.5%	-	-
High	233 (22)	169 (17)	203 (36)	605	203	33.6%	233	38.5%
Very high	18 (1)	28 (1)	94 (20)	140	-	-	46	32.9%
Total	1613	190	521	2624	720	27.4%	279	10.6%

FIG. 14.5 Personalized Cardiovascular Risk Prediction by AI Risk Score. (A) AI Risk Score is an automated cloud-based medical device that has been trained through deep learning to automate the segmentation of heart structures, identify the perivascular adipose tissue (PVAT), calculate the fat attenuation index (FAI), and integrate its value with scan technical details and patient demographics to provide metrics of atherosclerotic/inflammatory effects around each coronary vessel (FAI Score), as well as an integrated cardiac risk stratification tool (AI Risk Score, modified). (B) Standardization of coronary perivascular FAI and nomograms for age (FAI Score) for left anterior descending artery (LAD), right coronary artery (RCA), and left circumflex coronary artery (LCx). FAI Score informs on the coronary vessel–specific inflammation burden and the associated relative risk for a fatal cardiac event compared to the age group of reference. For instance, a young individual with no traditional risk factors may be at low absolute risk for a fatal cardiac event; however, a high FAI Score may indicate increased relative risk for cardiac events in the long term as a result of subclinical vascular inflammation. All figure panels were reproduced from the authors/publishers. (C) Kaplan-Meier curves for the prognostic value of FAI Score in the LAD evaluated over a median 7.7 years for cardiac mortality (B) in a nested analysis of 3393 patients from ORFAN study. (D) Receiver operating characteristics (ROC) curve analysis for the prognostic value of coronary calcium score (CCS) and AI Risk score (modified) in CRISPT-CT. (E) Reclassification table for discrete cardiac risk groups in the ORFAN study based on AI Risk–based risk stratification against a baseline clinical risk prediction model (QRISK3). Number of patients are reported for each category and cardiac mortality events are reported in brackets. Patients reclassified to a higher risk category by AI Risk Score appear in red color–shaded cells, whereas those reclassified to a lower risk category by AI Risk Score in green color–shaded cells. (Figures derived from Oikonomou EK, Antonopoulos AS, Schottlander D, et al. Standardized measurement of coronary inflammation using cardiovascular computed tomography: integration in clinical care as a prognostic medical device. *Cardiovasc Res*. 2021;117:2677–2690.)

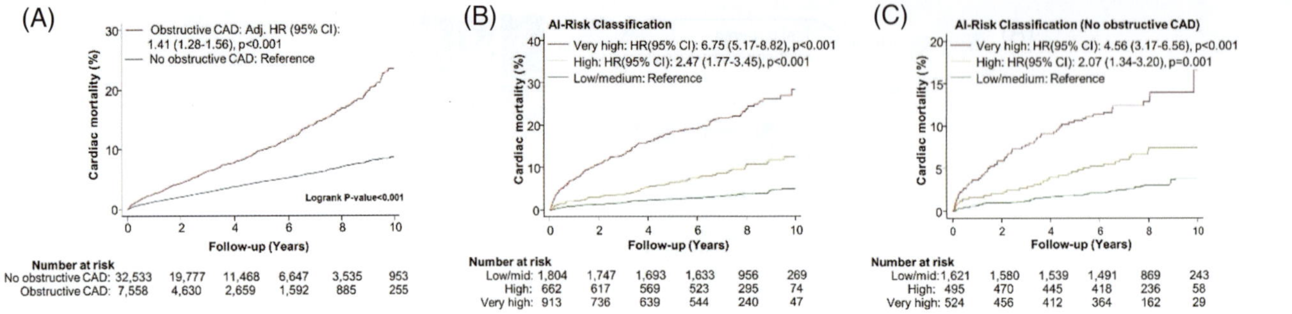

FIG. 14.6 Cardiovascular Risk Prediction in the Presence or Absence of Obstructive CAD. Kaplan-Meier curve for (A) cardiac mortality in 40,091 patients from the ORFAN study undergoing diagnostic coronary CT angiography (CCTA). Kaplan-Meier curves for the prognostic value of FAI Score in the LAD evaluated over a median 7.7 years for cardiac mortality (B) in a nested analysis of 3393 patients and (C) patients with no obstructive CAD. *CAD*, Coronary artery disease. HR adjusted for age, sex, and cardiovascular risk factors including diabetes, hypertension, hyperlipidaemia, and smoking status.

events of an individual compared with his/her peer group. For example, a young individual without any major cardiovascular risk factors may be at low absolute cardiovascular risk (a representative case of the typical low-risk population of patients undergoing CCTA) but at high relative risk in comparison to his/her peers due to the presence of vascular inflammation. A cutoff in FAI Score above the 75th centile for LAD or RCA (or ≥95th centile for LCx) is used to define intermediate cardiac mortality risk, whereas a FAI Score value equal of greater than the 90th centile for LAD or RCA defines a high-risk subgroup. When clinical risk factors and coronary plaque–related information is added on top of the FAI Score, an AI risk score can be calculated, which is an individual's absolute risk for cardiac mortality over the next 8 years. The AI risk score reclassified ~16% of patients undergoing CCTA to a higher risk category and ~17% to lower risk category compared to a clinical risk factor–based model, that is, nearly a third of the total population (Fig. 14.5).

In a recent analysis of 40,091 patients undergoing CCTA in seven UK Hospitals and prospective follow-up, it was demonstrated that the absolute number of MACE were more than twofold higher in patients without obstructive CAD compared to patients with obstructive CAD (n = 3124 vs. n = 1453, respectively). This finding highlights the unmet need for improved management and risk stratification of patients with mild or no coronary atheromatosis. In the same study, in a nested analysis of 3393 patients, the prognostic value of FAI Score and performance of AI Risk were evaluated over a median (IQR) follow-up of 7.7 (6.4–9.1) years (Fig. 14.6). Patients with FAI Score in the LAD above the 75th percentile, as compared with those below the 25th percentile, had 6.7-fold higher risk of MACE and 20-fold higher risk for cardiac mortality, whereas among those without obstructive CAD, the risk of MACE and cardiac mortality were 4.8-fold and 10.5-fold higher, respectively. Similar results were observed for FAI Score in the LCx and RCA. Patients identified as high/very high risk by AI Risk had significantly higher risk of MACE independently from the presence of obstructive CAD. The better prognostic performance of the AI Risk Score for LCx compared to the CRISP-CT study results is probably due to the improved proprietary algorithms used in the recent version of the AI-Risk platform, as well as the better mechanisms of outcomes data collection in the UK-arm of the ORFAN study (which utilizes nationwide databases). Overall, AI Risk Score significantly reclassified patients compared to a clinical risk factors–based risk prediction model (QRISK3) in the whole cohort and those without obstructive CAD. Furthermore, in a real-world evaluation cohort of 744 consecutive patients undergoing CCTA for chest pain investigation in four UK hospitals, AI Risk Score resulted in change of management in 45% of the patients, by triggering statin initiation (24%), statin dose intensification (13%), or addition of further treatments (e.g., colchicine, 8%). These data provide the first robust evidence on the value of this AI-assisted absolute risk prediction algorithm (AI Risk) as a precision medicine tool, which resulted in reclassification and change of management in a substantial proportion of patients undergoing routine CCTA. A proposed[59] therapeutic algorithm for management of patients based on FAI Score and the AI Risk Score estimation is presented in Fig. 14.7.

BEYOND THE FAT ATTENUATION INDEX: BUILDING RADIOTRANSCRIPTOMIC SIGNATURES OF VASCULAR DISEASE

The inflamed vascular wall secretes a variety of molecules with paracrine effect on the surrounding perivascular space.[12,23,60] Depending on the type of inflammatory molecules generated by the inflamed coronary artery, the vascular secretome triggers different degrees of perivascular lipolysis, edema, angiogenesis and fibrosis.[23,28,59,61,62] The proportional changes of these different components in the perivascular space give a characteristic texture of the perivascular space, which can be captured by its higher-order or texture radiomic profile.[23,28,61,62] If the ground truth for these changes is defined using histology or even better transcriptomic information for tissue biopsies, then powerful radiomic signatures of perivascular space can be created, tailored around specific type of vascular inflammation we may wish to capture.[28,61–64] Indeed, artificial intelligence or machine learning methods have been used to link the radiomic phenotyping of perivascular space with distinct biological processes, such as adipose tissue inflammation vascularity, fibrosis, and lipolysis by examining relevant changes in the

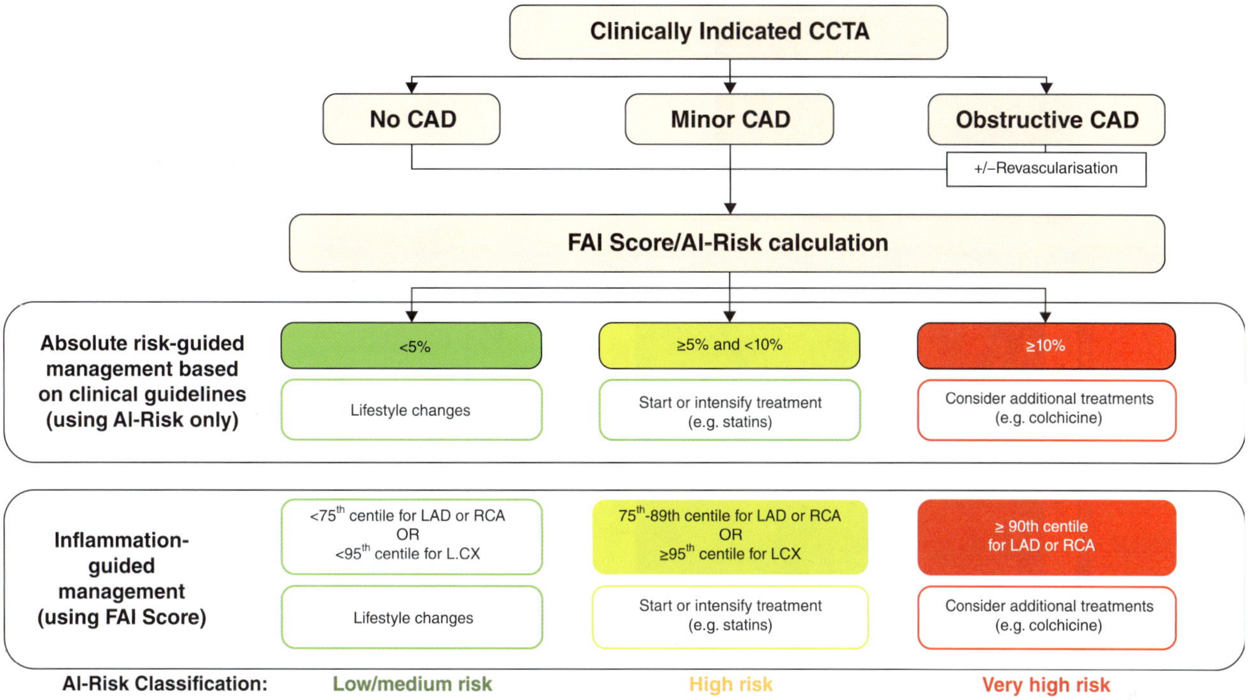

FIG. 14.7 Proposed Algorithm for Implementation of FAI Score and AI Risk Score in Clinical Practice. A proposed algorithm for the management of patients based on the level of risk and/or the degree of coronary inflammation, as presented in Oikonomou et al.[61] *AUC*, Area under the curve; *CAD*, coronary artery disease; *CCTA*, coronary CT angiography; *FAI*, fat attenuation index; *LAD*, left anterior descending; *LCx*, left circumflex coronary artery; *RCA*, right coronary artery; *95% CI*, 95% confidence interval. (All figures derived from Oikonomou EK, Antonopoulos AS, Schottlander D, et al. Standardized measurement of coronary inflammation using cardiovascular computed tomography: integration in clinical care as a prognostic medical device. *Cardiovasc Res*. 2021;117:2677–2690.)

transcriptomic profile of the tissue, to build complex radiotranscriptomic signatures. The Fat Radiomic Profile (FRP) of coronary PVAT when first trained in nested case-control cohort of patients with major adverse cardiovascular events and then tested in the SCOT-HEART population improved prediction for major adverse cardiovascular events beyond traditional risk factors, CCS, coronary stenosis, and HRP features on CCTA (Δ_{AUC} = 0.126, *P* 0.001) (Fig. 14.8).

This radiotranscriptomic platform allows for various medical hypotheses to be tested and may ultimately enable a more personalized approach to disease management. For example, by using this radiotranscriptomic platform, based on CT imaging/radiomics and tissue transcriptomic profile, a radiotranscriptomic signature of cytokine-driven vascular inflammation has been developed (C19-RS) (Fig. 14.8).[62] That signature was trained to track cytokine-driven inflammation in the aorta and the internal mammary arteries, and it was then tested in gated CCTCAS as well as nongated CTA of the pulmonary arteries of patients with COVID-19, a condition that is known to trigger cytokine-induced vascular inflammation.[62] Indeed, in paired scans of patients pre- and post-COVID-19, C19RS was strikingly increased within 6 months postinfection, whereas patients with high C19-RS during their hospital admission, had eightfold higher risk to die in the hospital, a relative risk that was eliminated by the use of dexamethasone (Fig. 14.6).[62] This kind of radiotranscriptomic platforms offer unique opportunities for the development of novel imaging biomarkers tailored around the biology of interest and is expected to transform the field of imaging-based risk stratification in primary and secondary prevention. These radiotranscriptomic platforms offer potential opportunities for the development of custom-made imaging biomarkers that will support the development and eventually guide the deployment of novel therapeutics targeting vascular inflammation.

CONCLUSIONS

PVAT is now considered as a "sensor" of paracrine inflammatory signals coming from the vascular wall, given that its texture and composition changes in response to these signals. These changes can be visualized by using perivascular tissue attenuation maps. The inflammatory load of the coronary arteries can be quantified in a standardized way by using the FAI Score of each coronary artery, which is then interpreted in nomograms that can provide a percentile score. FAI Score changes in response to antiinflammatory treatments or statins and captures the residual inflammatory risk, which can be interpreted as a standalone metric of risk, or it can be used in combination with plaque characteristics and patient's risk factor profile to determine AI Risk Score, which is the patient's absolute risk for future cardiovascular events. In a real-world cohort of patients undergoing routine CCTA, AI Risk Score reclassified and led to change in clinical management of a substantial proportion

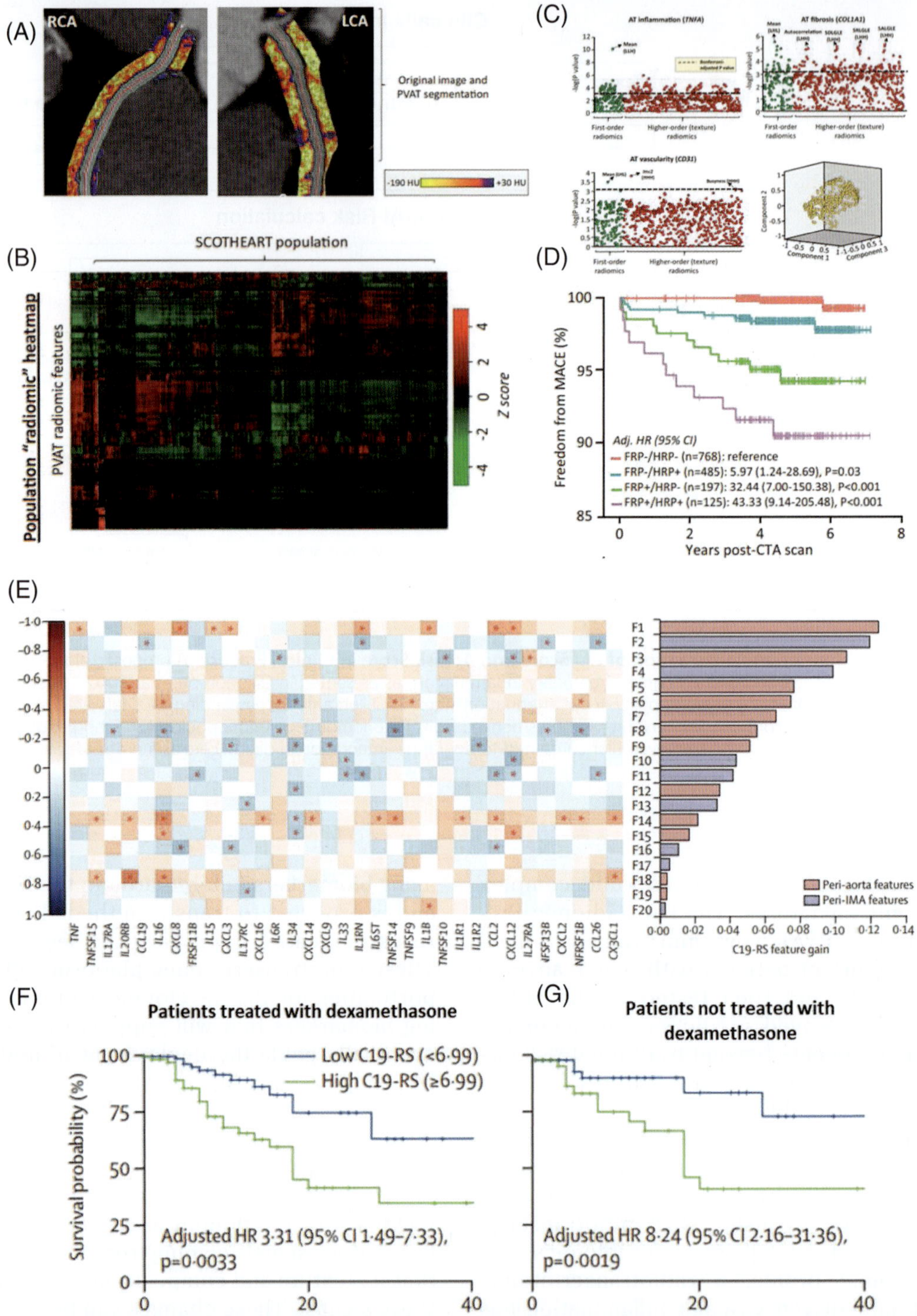

FIG. 14.8 A Radiotranscriptomic Platform to Create Custom Signatures of Vascular Inflammation. (A) Coronary perivascular adipose tissue (PVAT) imaging features can be used to extract a high number of shape-, attenuation-, and texture-related statistics (i.e., radiomics). (B) Heat map of scaled radiomic features (*right*) of all stable radiomic features in the SCOT-HEART population. (C) Extracted radiomic features can be tested against the transcriptome profile of PVAT to identify features informing on distinct biological processes such as adipose tissue inflammation, vascularity, and fibrosis. (D) Selected radiomic features can form distinct radiomic signatures of PVAT, in this case fat radiomic profile adipose tissue inflammation, vascularity, and fibrosis, which had strong independent predictive value for major adverse cardiac events (MACE) in the SCOT-HEART population (reproduced with permission[28]). (E) A custom radiotranscriptomic signature of cytokine-driven vascular inflammation (C19-RS); feature importance of the top 20 radiomic features of perivascular tissue around internal mammary arteries (IMA) and their correlation with cpm (count per million) values with key inflammatory genes from IMAs in patients undergoing cardiac surgery. (F) A high C19-RS was associated with increased risk for in-hospital death in patients with COVID-19. (G) Kaplan-Meier curve and adjusted HR for in-hospital death for high versus low C19-RS groups in the COVID-19-positive patients that did not receive dexamethasone treatment. *FRP*, Fat Radiomic Profile; *HRP*, high-risk plaque; *LAD*, left anterior descending; *RCA*, right coronary artery. (Reproduced with permission from Kotanidis CP, Xie C, Alexander D, et al. Constructing custom-made radiotranscriptomic signatures of vascular inflammation from routine CT angiograms: a prospective outcomes validation study in COVID-19. *Lancet Digit Health*. 2022;4[10]:e705–e716. https://doi.org/10.1016/S2589-7500(22)00132-7.)

of patients. Beyond FAI Score, novel radiotranscriptomic platforms allow sophisticated phenotyping of the perivascular tissue and may allow quantification of specific types of inflammatory signals coming from the vascular wall.

DISCLOSURES

C.A is founder, shareholder and director of Caristo Diagnostics Ltd., a CT image analysis company. A.A. has served as consultant of Caristo Diagnostics Ltd. The technologies described in this work are subject to patent US10,695,023B2 and patent applications PCT/GB2017/053262, GB2018/1818049.7, GR20180100490 and GR20180100510, licensed through exclusive license to Caristo Diagnostics. C.A. has received honoraria/consulting fees from Amarin, Covance, Silence Therapeutics, AMGEN, Abcentra, Nodthera, Novartis and Lilly and Caristo Diagnostics, while he has received research grant from Sanofi, Novo Nordisk, Astra Zeneca, Caristo and Lexicon

C.A. acknowledges support for the specific work discussed here, from the Oxford British Heart Foundation (CH/F/21/90009, TG/19/2/34831 and RG/F/21/110040), the Oxford BHF Centre of Research Excellence (RE/18/3/34214), the Oxford NIHR Biomedical Research Centre and Innovate UK.

REFERENCES

1. Knuuti J, Wijns W, Saraste A, et al. 2019 ESC guidelines for the diagnosis and management of chronic coronary syndromes. *Eur Heart J*. 2020;41:407–477. https://doi.org/10.1093/eurheartj/ehz425.
2. Writing Committee M, Gulati M, Levy PD, et al. 2021 AHA/ACC/ASE/CHEST/SAEM/SCCT/SCMR guideline for the evaluation and diagnosis of chest pain: a report of the American College of Cardiology/American Heart Association Joint Committee on clinical practice guidelines. *J Am Coll Cardiol*. 2021;78:e187–e285. https://doi.org/10.1016/j.jacc.2021.07.053.
3. Min JK, Shaw LJ, Devereux RB, et al. Prognostic value of multidetector coronary computed tomographic angiography for prediction of all-cause mortality. *J Am Coll Cardiol*. 2007;50:1161–1170. https://doi.org/10.1016/j.jacc.2007.03.067.
4. Hell MM, Motwani M, Otaki Y, et al. Quantitative global plaque characteristics from coronary computed tomography angiography for the prediction of future cardiac mortality during long-term follow-up. *Eur Heart J Cardiovasc Imaging*. 2017;18:1331–1339. https://doi.org/10.1093/ehjci/jex183.
5. Coenen A, Rossi A, Lubbers MM, et al. Integrating CT myocardial perfusion and CT-FFR in the work-up of coronary artery disease. *JACC Cardiovasc Imaging*. 2017;10:760–770. https://doi.org/10.1016/j.jcmg.2016.09.028.
6. Hansson GK. Inflammation, atherosclerosis, and coronary artery disease. *N Engl J Med*. 2005;352:1685–1695. https://doi.org/10.1056/NEJMra043430.
7. Ridker PM, Everett BM, Thuren T, et al. Antiinflammatory therapy with canakinumab for atherosclerotic disease. *N Engl J Med*. 2017;377(12):1119–1131. https://doi.org/10.1056/NEJMoa1707914.
8. Tardif JC, Kouz S, Waters DD, et al. Efficacy and safety of low-dose colchicine after myocardial infarction. *N Engl J Med*. 2019;381:2497–2505. https://doi.org/10.1056/NEJMoa1912388.
9. Nidorf SM, Fiolet ATL, Mosterd A, et al. Colchicine in patients with chronic coronary disease. *N Engl J Med*. 2020;383(19):1838–1847. https://doi.org/10.1056/NEJMoa2021372.
10. Ridker PM. How common is residual inflammatory risk? *Circ Res*. 2017;120:617–619. https://doi.org/10.1161/CIRCRESAHA.116.310527.
11. Antoniades C, Antonopoulos AS, Deanfield J. Imaging residual inflammatory cardiovascular risk. *Eur Heart J*. 2020;41(6):748–758. https://doi.org/10.1093/eurheartj/ehz474.
12. Antonopoulos AS, Sanna F, Sabharwal N, et al. Detecting human coronary inflammation by imaging perivascular fat. *Sci Transl Med*. 2017;9(398):eaal2658. https://doi.org/10.1126/scitranslmed.aal2658.
13. Antoniades C, Antonopoulos AS, Deanfield J. Imaging residual inflammatory cardiovascular risk. *Eur Heart J*. 2020;41:748–758. https://doi.org/10.1093/eurheartj/ehz474.
14. Antonopoulos AS, Tousoulis D. The molecular mechanisms of obesity paradox. *Cardiovasc Res*. 2017;113:1074–1086. https://doi.org/10.1093/cvr/cvx106.
15. Rosen ED, Spiegelman BM. What we talk about when we talk about fat. *Cell*. 2014;156:20–44. https://doi.org/10.1016/j.cell.2013.12.012.
16. Margaritis M, Antonopoulos AS, Digby J, et al. *The Interplay Between Perivascular Adipose Tissue and the Arterial Wall Regulates NADPH-Oxidase Activity in Human Vessels*. Lippincott Williams & Wilkins; 2013.
17. Margaritis M, Antonopoulos AS, Digby J, et al. Interactions between vascular wall and perivascular adipose tissue reveal novel roles for adiponectin in the regulation of endothelial nitric oxide synthase function in human vessels. *Circulation*. 2013;127:2209–2221. https://doi.org/10.1161/CIRCULATIONAHA.112.001133.
18. Sacks HS, Fain JN. Human epicardial adipose tissue: a review. *Am Heart J*. 2007;153:907–917. https://doi.org/10.1016/j.ahj.2007.03.019.
19. Iacobellis G. Epicardial adipose tissue in contemporary cardiology. *Nat Rev Cardiol*. 2022;19(9):593–606. https://doi.org/10.1038/s41569-022-00679-9.
20. Antonopoulos AS, Margaritis M, Coutinho P, et al. Reciprocal effects of systemic inflammation and brain natriuretic peptide on adiponectin biosynthesis in adipose tissue of patients with ischemic heart disease. *Arterioscler Thromb Vasc Biol*. 2014;34:2151–2159. https://doi.org/10.1161/ATVBAHA.114.303828.
21. Antonopoulos AS, Margaritis M, Coutinho P, et al. Adiponectin as a link between type 2 diabetes and vascular NADPH oxidase activity in the human arterial wall: the regulatory role of perivascular adipose tissue. *Diabetes*. 2015;64:2207–2219. https://doi.org/10.2337/db14-1011.
22. Chang L, Garcia-Barrio MT, Chen YE. Perivascular adipose tissue regulates vascular function by targeting vascular smooth muscle cells. *Arterioscler Thromb Vasc Biol*. 2020;40:1094–1109. https://doi.org/10.1161/ATVBAHA.120.312464.
23. Oikonomou EK, Antoniades C. The role of adipose tissue in cardiovascular health and disease. *Nat Rev Cardiol*. 2019;16:83–99. https://doi.org/10.1038/s41569-018-0097-6.
24. Akoumianakis I, Tarun A, Antoniades C. Perivascular adipose tissue as a regulator of vascular disease pathogenesis: identifying novel therapeutic targets. *Br J Pharmacol*. 2017;174:3411–3424. https://doi.org/10.1111/bph.13666.
25. Kim HW, Shi H, Winkler MA, Lee R, Weintraub NL. Perivascular adipose tissue and vascular perturbation/atherosclerosis. *Arterioscler Thromb Vasc Biol*. 2020;40:2569–2576. https://doi.org/10.1161/ATVBAHA.120.312470.
26. Turaihi AH, Serne EH, Molthoff CFM, et al. Perivascular adipose tissue controls insulin-stimulated perfusion, mitochondrial protein expression, and glucose uptake in muscle through adipomuscular arterioles. *Diabetes*. 2020;69:603–613. https://doi.org/10.2337/db18-1066.
27. Costa RM, Neves KB, Tostes RC, Lobato NS. Perivascular adipose tissue as a relevant fat depot for cardiovascular risk in obesity. *Front Physiol*. 2018;9:253. https://doi.org/10.3389/fphys.2018.00253.
28. Oikonomou EK, Williams MC, Kotanidis CP, et al. A novel machine learning-derived radiotranscriptomic signature of perivascular fat improves cardiac risk prediction using coronary CT angiography. *Eur Heart J*. 2019;40:3529–3543. https://doi.org/10.1093/eurheartj/ehz592.
29. Bengs S, Haider A, Warnock GI, et al. Quantification of perivascular inflammation does not provide incremental prognostic value over myocardial perfusion imaging and calcium scoring. *Eur J Nucl Med Mol Imaging*. 2021;48:1806–1812. https://doi.org/10.1007/s00259-020-05106-0.
30. Dai X, Yu L, Lu Z, Shen C, Tao X, Zhang J. Serial change of perivascular fat attenuation index after statin treatment: insights from a coronary CT angiography follow-up study. *Int J Cardiol*. 2020;319:144–149. https://doi.org/10.1016/j.ijcard.2020.06.008.
31. Antonopoulos AS, Antoniades C. Perivascular fat attenuation index by computed tomography as a metric of coronary inflammation. *J Am Coll Cardiol*. 2018;71:2708–2709. https://doi.org/10.1016/j.jacc.2018.03.511.
32. Oikonomou EK, Desai MY, Marwan M, et al. Perivascular fat attenuation index stratifies cardiac risk associated with high-risk plaques in the CRISP-CT study. *J Am Coll Cardiol*. 2020;76:755–757. https://doi.org/10.1016/j.jacc.2020.05.078.
33. Mazurek T, Kobylecka M, Zielenkiewicz M, et al. PET/CT evaluation of ^{18}F-FDG uptake in pericoronary adipose tissue in patients with stable coronary artery disease: independent predictor of atherosclerotic lesions' formation? *J Nucl Cardiol*. 2017;24(3):1075–1084. https://doi.org/10.1007/s12350-015-0370-6.
34. Goeller M, Achenbach S, Cadet S, et al. Pericoronary adipose tissue computed tomography attenuation and high-risk plaque characteristics in acute coronary syndrome compared with stable coronary artery disease. *JAMA Cardiol*. 2018;3:858–863. https://doi.org/10.1001/jamacardio.2018.1997.
35. Marwan M, Hell M, Schuhback A, et al. CT Attenuation of pericoronary adipose tissue in normal versus atherosclerotic coronary segments as defined by intravascular ultrasound. *J Comput Assist Tomogr*. 2017;41:762–767. https://doi.org/10.1097/RCT.0000000000000589.
36. Gaibazzi N, Martini C, Botti A, Pinazzi A, Bottazzi B, Palumbo AA. Coronary inflammation by computed tomography pericoronary fat attenuation in MINOCA and tako-tsubo syndrome. *J Am Heart Assoc*. 2019;8:e013235. https://doi.org/10.1161/jaha.119.013235.
37. Sugiyama T, Kanaji Y, Hoshino M, et al. Determinants of pericoronary adipose tissue attenuation on computed tomography angiography in coronary artery disease. *J Am Heart Assoc*. 2020;9:e016202. https://doi.org/10.1161/jaha.120.016202.
38. Lin A, Kolossvary M, Yuvaraj J, et al. Myocardial infarction associates with a distinct pericoronary adipose tissue radiomic phenotype: a prospective case-control study. *JACC Cardiovasc Imaging*. 2020;13:2371–2383. https://doi.org/10.1016/j.jcmg.2020.06.033.
39. Sagris M, Antonopoulos AS, Simantiris S, et al. Pericoronary fat attenuation index-a new imaging biomarker and its diagnostic and prognostic utility: a systematic review and meta-analysis. *Eur Heart J Cardiovasc Imaging*. 2022;23(12):e526–e536. https://doi.org/10.1093/ehjci/jeac174.

40. Kwiecinski J, Dey D, Cadet S, et al. Peri-coronary adipose tissue density is associated with (18)F-sodium fluoride coronary uptake in stable patients with high-risk plaques. *JACC Cardiovasc Imaging*. 2019;12:2000–2010. https://doi.org/10.1016/j.jcmg.2018.11.032.
41. Ohyama K, Matsumoto Y, Takanami K, et al. Coronary adventitial and perivascular adipose tissue inflammation in patients with vasospastic angina. *J Am Coll Cardiol*. 2018;71:414–425. https://doi.org/10.1016/j.jacc.2017.11.046.
42. Pergola V, Previtero M, Cecere A, et al. Clinical value and time course of pericoronary fat inflammation in patients with angiographically nonobstructive coronaries: a preliminary report. *J Clin Med*. 2021;10(8):1786. https://doi.org/10.3390/jcm10081786.
43. Yu M, Dai X, Deng J, Lu Z, Shen C, Zhang J. Diagnostic performance of perivascular fat attenuation index to predict hemodynamic significance of coronary stenosis: a preliminary coronary computed tomography angiography study. *Eur Radiol*. 2020;30:673–681. https://doi.org/10.1007/s00330-019-06400-8.
44. Hoshino M, Yang S, Sugiyama T, et al. Peri-coronary inflammation is associated with findings on coronary computed tomography angiography and fractional flow reserve. *J Cardiovasc Comput Tomogr*. 2020;14:483–489. https://doi.org/10.1016/j.jcct.2020.02.002.
45. Nomura CH, Assuncao Jr AN, PO Guimaraes, et al. Association between perivascular inflammation and downstream myocardial perfusion in patients with suspected coronary artery disease. *Eur Heart J Cardiovasc Imaging*. 2020;21:599–605. https://doi.org/10.1093/ehjci/jeaa023.
46. Elnabawi Y, Oikonomou E, Dey A, et al. Treatment with biologic therapy in psoriasis is associated with a reduction in coronary artery inflammation, assessed by perivascular Fat Attenuation Index. *J Am Coll Cardiol*. 2019;73:87. https://doi.org/10.1016/S0735-1097(19)30695-3.
47. Goeller M, Tamarappoo BK, Kwan AC, et al. Relationship between changes in pericoronary adipose tissue attenuation and coronary plaque burden quantified from coronary computed tomography angiography. *Eur Heart J Cardiovasc Imaging*. 2019;20:636–643. https://doi.org/10.1093/ehjci/jez013.
48. Elnabawi YA, Oikonomou EK, Dey AK, et al. Association of biologic therapy with coronary inflammation in patients with psoriasis as assessed by perivascular fat attenuation index. *JAMA Cardiol*. 2019;4(9):885–891. https://doi.org/10.1001/jamacardio.2019.2589.
49. Oikonomou EK, Marwan M, Desai MY, et al. Non-invasive detection of coronary inflammation using computed tomography and prediction of residual cardiovascular risk (the CRISP CT study): a post-hoc analysis of prospective outcome data. *Lancet*. 2018;392:929–939. https://doi.org/10.1016/S0140-6736(18)31114-0.
50. Investigators S-H, Newby DE, Adamson PD, et al. Coronary CT angiography and 5-year risk of myocardial infarction. *N Engl J Med*. 2018;379:924–933. https://doi.org/10.1056/NEJMoa1805971.
51. van Diemen PA, Bom MJ, Driessen RS, et al. Prognostic value of RCA pericoronary adipose tissue CT-attenuation beyond high-risk plaques, plaque volume, and ischemia. *JACC Cardiovasc Imaging*. 2021;14:1598–1610. https://doi.org/10.1016/j.jcmg.2021.02.026.
52. Ichikawa K, Miyoshi T, Osawa K, et al. High pericoronary adipose tissue attenuation on computed tomography angiography predicts cardiovascular events in patients with type 2 diabetes mellitus: post-hoc analysis from a prospective cohort study. *Cardiovasc Diabetol*. 2022;21:44. https://doi.org/10.1186/s12933-022-01478-9.
53. Antonopoulos AS, Antoniades C. Reply to: quantification of perivascular inflammation does not provide incremental prognostic value over myocardial perfusion imaging and calcium scoring. *Eur J Nucl Med Mol Imaging*. 2021;48:1707–1708. https://doi.org/10.1007/s00259-020-05171-5.
54. Antoniades C, Shirodaria C. Detecting coronary inflammation with perivascular fat attenuation imaging: making sense from perivascular attenuation maps. *JACC Cardiovasc Imaging*. 2019;12:2011–2014. https://doi.org/10.1016/j.jcmg.2018.12.024.
55. Tzolos E, Williams MC, McElhinney P, et al. Pericoronary adipose tissue attenuation, low-attenuation plaque burden, and 5-year risk of myocardial infarction. *JACC Cardiovasc Imaging*. 2022;15:1078–1088. https://doi.org/10.1016/j.jcmg.2022.02.004.
56. Marchesseau S, Seneviratna A, Sjoholm AT, et al. Hybrid PET/CT and PET/MRI imaging of vulnerable coronary plaque and myocardial scar tissue in acute myocardial infarction. *J Nucl Cardiol*. 2018;25:2001–2011. https://doi.org/10.1007/s12350-017-0918-8.
57. Antonopoulos AS, Angelopoulos A, Papanikolaou P, et al. Biomarkers of vascular inflammation for cardiovascular risk prognostication: a meta-analysis. *JACC Cardiovasc Imaging*. 2022;15:460–471. https://doi.org/10.1016/j.jcmg.2021.09.014.
58. Visseren FLJ, Mach F, Smulders YM, et al. 2021 ESC guidelines on cardiovascular disease prevention in clinical practice. *Eur Heart J*. 2021;42:3227–3337. https://doi.org/10.1093/eurheartj/ehab484.
59. Oikonomou EK, Antonopoulos AS, Schottlander D, et al. Standardized measurement of coronary inflammation using cardiovascular computed tomography: integration in clinical care as a prognostic medical device. *Cardiovasc Res*. 2021;117:2677–2690. https://doi.org/10.1093/cvr/cvab286.
60. Akoumianakis I, Polkinghorne M, Antoniades C. Non-canonical WNT signalling in cardiovascular disease: mechanisms and therapeutic implications. *Nat Rev Cardiol*. 2022;19(12):783–797. https://doi.org/10.1038/s41569-022-00718-5.
61. Oikonomou EK, Siddique M, Antoniades C. Artificial intelligence in medical imaging: a radiomic guide to precision phenotyping of cardiovascular disease. *Cardiovasc Res*. 2020;116:2040–2054. https://doi.org/10.1093/cvr/cvaa021.
62. Kotanidis CP, Xie C, Alexander D, et al. Constructing custom-made radiotranscriptomic signatures of vascular inflammation from routine CT angiograms: a prospective outcomes validation study in COVID-19. *Lancet Digit Health*. 2022;4(10):e705–e716. https://doi.org/10.1016/S2589-7500(22)00132-7.
63. Antonopoulos AS, Angelopoulos A, Tsioufis K, Antoniades C, Tousoulis D. Cardiovascular risk stratification by coronary computed tomography angiography imaging: current state-of-the-art. *Eur J Prev Cardiol*. 2022;29:608–624. https://doi.org/10.1093/eurjpc/zwab067.
64. Kluner LV, Oikonomou EK, Antoniades C. Assessing cardiovascular risk by using the fat attenuation index in coronary CT angiography. *Radiol Cardiothorac Imaging*. 2021;3:e200563. https://doi.org/10.1148/ryct.2021200563.
65. Kotanidis CP, Antoniades C. Perivascular fat imaging by computed tomography (CT): a virtual guide. *Br J Pharmacol*. 2021;178:4270–4290. https://doi.org/10.1111/bph.15634.

15 Myocardial Perfusion Imaging

KOEN NIEMAN AND AMIT R. PATEL

KEY POINTS

- CT myocardial perfusion imaging identifies hemodynamically significant coronary disease, with incremental value over CCTA.
- The diagnostic performance of CT myocardial perfusion imaging was shown to be equivalent to other stress imaging techniques and CT-based fractional flow reserve.
- Dynamic perfusion protocols allow for calculation of quantitative measures of myocardial blood flow.
- As opposed to CT-based fractional flow reserve, CT myocardial perfusion imaging is not limited by CCTA quality and can be performed after PCI, CABG, and in patients with chronic total occlusions or prior infarcts.

BACKGROUND

The primary indication for coronary CT angiography (CCTA) is to determine if angina-like symptoms are due to the presence of coronary disease. The mechanism of angina is a mismatch between the oxygen delivered to and the oxygen demanded by the myocardium. It is well established that the degree of coronary stenosis does not reliably predict the myocardial perfusion responsible for oxygen delivery[1,2]; thus there is a need to understand the downstream impact of a coronary stenosis on myocardial perfusion to best understand whether a patient's angina is due to a coronary stenosis and whether revascularization is likely to improve their symptoms. Additionally, angina can also occur in the absence of epicardial coronary artery disease (CAD) due to conditions such as coronary microvascular dysfunction that too is associated with reduced myocardial perfusion. Although historically myocardial blood flow radiotracers that can be imaged using single-photon emission computed tomography (SPECT) have been most commonly utilized, iodinated contrast agents can also perfuse into the tissue[3] and attenuate CT x-rays proportionately to its concentration and thus has the potential to detect variations in myocardial blood flow. The clinical utility of CT myocardial perfusion imaging was first evident when the presence of resting myocardial perfusion defects could be detected using iodinated contrast agents in the setting of a recent acute myocardial infarction.[4,5] Initial validation of stress CT perfusion using the first-pass technique was performed against the gold standard of microsphere-derived myocardial blood flow in the canine model of obstructive CAD and revealed a very strong correlation of perfusion measurements during resting and hyperemic conditions derived using the two techniques.[6] These initial findings were translated into humans using CT perfusion technique in which a single CT acquisition performed following the administration of a vasodilator and timed to be acquired once the iodinated contrast agent had arrived into the myocardium.[7] Since these initial developments, stress CT perfusion has been extensively validated by multiple clinical investigators and in a wide range of clinical scenarios. Several technological advancements now allow for absolute quantification of myocardial blood flow during resting and stress conditions while maintaining clinically acceptable radiation doses.

STRESS IMAGING

The myocardium extracts nearly 80% of the oxygen from the blood; therefore increased oxygen supply can only be achieved by increasing blood flow. Autoregulatory systems alter coronary blood flow through vascular resistance. During intense exercise, coronary flow can be increased fivefold by releasing resistance in the small coronary arteries and arterioles. Narrowing of the epicardial coronary arteries adds resistance to flow. Not until a stenosis is very severe, sufficient flow can be maintained at rest through autoregulated vasodilation of the peripheral vascular bed. However, when demand increases during exercise, yet the vasodilatory reserve has been partially spent, insufficient blood supply can result in symptoms of anginal pectoris. The objective of stress myocardial perfusion imaging is to demonstrate absolute or relatively reduced myocardial blood flow during hyperemia.

Myocardial hyperemia can be achieved through physical exercise, inotropic drugs (dobutamine), or vasodilators. For practical reasons, CT myocardial perfusion imaging is typically performed using intravenous vasodilators. Adenosine acts as a direct coronary vasodilator by binding and activating all known adenosine receptors. Adenosine induces maximal coronary vasodilation primarily though relaxation of the vascular smooth muscle cells in the resistance vessels (A_{2A} receptor). Adenosine is a short-acting drug, dosed based on weight and administered continuously for 3 to 5 minutes using an infusion pump. Side effects are common but often limited to flushing, chest pressure, and dyspnea, which rapidly normalize after the infusion is discontinued. Significant but rare side effects include atrioventricular block and bronchoconstriction (A_{2B} and A_3 receptors). Aminophylline and caffeine reverse adverse effects but are rarely needed due to the short half-life of the adenosine. Contraindications to adenosine include bronchospastic lung disease, second- or third-degree atrioventricular block, and sick sinus syndrome. Caffeine, chocolate, aminophylline, and theophylline should be avoided at least 12 to 18 hours before the exam. Regadenoson selectively

TABLE 15.1 Absolute and Relative Contraindications to Stress CT Myocardial Perfusion Imaging

ABSOLUTE CONTRAINDICATION	RELATIVE CONTRAINDICATION
High-risk unstable angina	Known left main stenosis >50%
Uncontrolled congestive heart failure	LV outflow tract obstruction
Uncontrolled hypertension (BP >200/110 mmHg)	Electrolyte abnormalities
Hypotension (SBP <90 mmHg)	Significant tachyarrhythmia or bradyarrhythmia
Allergy to contrast medium or stress agent	Recent stroke
Uncontrolled cardiac arrhythmias	Recent seizure
Severe aortic stenosis	Moderate renal insufficiency (GFR 30–60 ml/min/m^2)
Bronchospastic lung disease	Body mass index >40 kg/m^2
Active myocardial infarction, pulmonary embolism, myocarditis, pericarditis, aortic dissection, or other acute illness.	
Severe pulmonary hypertension	
Severe renal insufficiency (GFR <30 ml/min/m^2)	
High-degree atrioventricular block	
Unable to cooperate with breathhold instructions	

GFR, Glomerular filtration rate; *SBP,* systolic blood pressure.
Adapted from Patel AR, Bamberg F, Branch K, et al. Society of cardiovascular computed tomography expert consensus document on myocardial computed tomography perfusion imaging. *J Cardiovasc Comput Tomogr*. 2020;14:87–100.

binds to the A_{2A} receptor and thereby has fewer side effects that are typically associated with the other adenosine receptors. Contrary to adenosine, regadenoson may be considered in patients with bronchospastic lung disease but no active wheezing. A standard dose is injected as a slow bolus and maximum hyperemia is reached after approximately 30 seconds. Aminophylline and caffeine reverse the effect of regadenoson and can be helpful to normalize the heart rate if a coronary CT scan is planned after the perfusion study. Dipyridamole, which blocks the cellular reuptake of adenosine, and adenosine-triphosphate are less frequently used vasodilators for CT myocardial perfusion imaging (MPI_{CT}). Vasodilator-mediated hyperemia generally does not cause absolute myocardial ischemia, and severe complications such as myocardial infarction or ventricular arrhythmia are very rare. The only exception are patients with completely occluded coronary arteries with blood supply dependent on collateral flow, in which case decreased perfusion pressure can drop blood flow below resting conditions (steal phenomenon). Absolute and relative contraindications of MPI_{CT} are summarized in Table 15.1. Heart rate and blood pressure are monitored at regular intervals during and after the procedure. Vasodilators cause a moderately increased heart rate, which can be helpful to indicate response to the drug.

STATIC PERFUSION IMAGING

Hardware and Scan Protocol

Stress CT perfusion images can be acquired either at a single time point when the contrast agent has maximally perfused into the myocardium (static CT perfusion) or repetitively as the contrast agent transits through the chambers of the heart and the myocardium (dynamic CT perfusion). The major advantage of static CT perfusion imaging is that it minimizes the radiation exposure to the patient. Although, static CT perfusion imaging can be performed on most contemporary multidetector CT scanners with at least 64 detector rows and electrocardiogram gating capabilities, the use of dual-source or wide-detector CT systems is preferred for optimal image quality.

As with any diagnostic test, patient selection with a focus on pretest probability and a careful consideration of risk and benefit is paramount to obtaining clinically meaningful results. Peak myocardial enhancement and peak coronary enhancement occur nearly simultaneously. Thus any well-performed coronary CTA using either a manual or automated bolus tracking algorithm to trigger the scan will typically result in diagnostic quality resting myocardial perfusion images without the need for any significant adjustments in the acquisition protocol. Either manual or automated bolus tracking can be used to obtain stress CT perfusion images during peak myocardial enhancement. Similar to coronary imaging, the region of interest for bolus tracking is placed in the ascending aorta. Once the Hounsfield units (HU) in the region of interest have increased 50 to 100 HU above baseline, the scan is triggered with a delay that accounts for the faster transit time of contrast media that occurs during hyperemic conditions.

DATA INTERPRETATION

Interpretation of static CT perfusion images[8] is typically performed by reconstructing images into the short-axis, horizontal-long-axis, and vertical-long-axis planes using 5 to 8 mm slice thickness and using a narrow window width of 200 to 300 HU with a level around 100 to 150 HU. Image analysis can be aided by using both minimum- and average-intensity projections. During hyperemia, ischemic myocardial segments will appear darker and have a lower attenuation than ischemic segments. The perfusion defect will be in a coronary distribution and be more pronounced along the subendocardium and may often spare the subepicardium (Figs. 15.1 and 15.2). The degree of hypoattenuation and the transmurality of the perfusion defect are markers of the severity of ischemia, whereas the number of myocardial segments that are involved represents the extent of myocardial ischemia. Defects that are present during hyperemic conditions but not resting conditions are interpreted as secondary to ischemia, whereas the presence of a defect during both hyperemic and resting conditions likely represents myocardial infarction or scar. The interpretation of perfusion images should be performed in

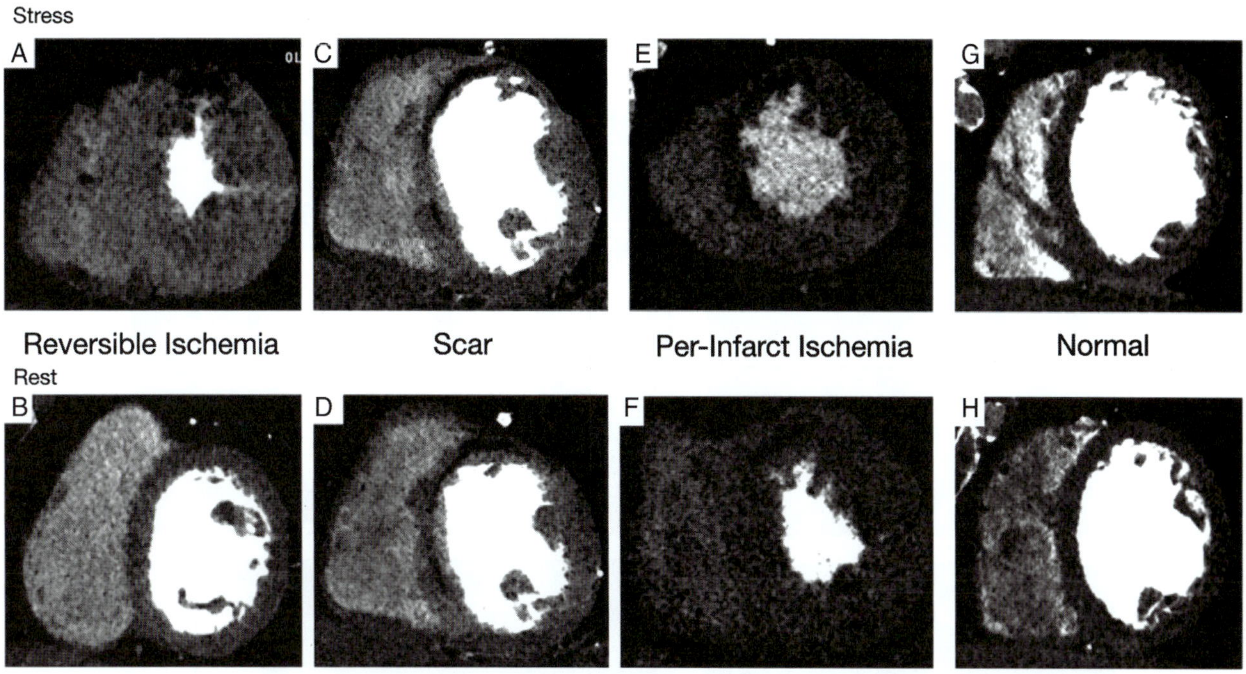

FIG. 15.1 Different behaviors of the myocardial perfusion defects in stress and rest CT scans. Hypoperfusion during stress with normal perfusion at rest is indicative of reversible ischemia (Panels A–B); hypoperfusion during stress that persists with same extension at rest is indicative of scar (Panels C–D); hypoperfusion during stress that persists at rest but with less extension than during stress is indicative of peri-infarct reversible ischemia (Panels E–F). Panels G and H show normal myocardial perfusion at stress and rest CT scans. Of note, Panels A, E, and F are acquired during systole as evidenced by the thicker myocardium. The remainder of images are acquired during diastole. (Adopted from Mushtaq S, Conte E, Pontone G, et al. State-of-the-art-myocardial perfusion stress testing: static CT perfusion. *J Cardiovasc Comput Tomogr.* 2020;14[4]:294–302.)

the context of the coronary anatomy. The presence of a perfusion defect in a myocardium territory distal to a stenotic coronary artery likely signifies that the coronary stenosis is hemodynamically significant. Conversely, the absence of a perfusion defect distal to a coronary stenosis suggests that the coronary stenosis is not hemodynamically significant. Alternatively, the presence of a perfusion defect in the absence of a coronary stenosis suggests that there may be abnormal function of the coronary microvasculature or the presence of a primary myocardial pathology.

DIAGNOSTIC PERFORMANCE

Static stress CT perfusion has been validated against other noninvasive stress perfusion imaging tests, invasive coronary angiography, and invasive fractional flow reserve (Table 15.2).[9] Low specificity is often cited as a limitation of CCTA. The addition of static stress CT perfusion to CCTA in patients with intermediate to high risk of CAD has been shown to improve the specificity for detecting hemodynamically significant CAD from 54% to 83% and the accuracy from 76% to 91%, while maintaining the sensitivity at 98%.[10] Similarly, when compared to CCTA, static stress CT perfusion improved the diagnostic accuracy of detecting significant coronary obstruction in patients with coronary stents from 77% to 87% on a per-patient basis, with the combination of CCTA and stress perfusion having the highest diagnostic accuracy at 91%.[11] Indeed, because of its improved specificity, the addition of static stress CTP to CCTA has been shown to reduce the need for downstream invasive testing in patients with acute chest pain.[12]

CHALLENGES, CONTRAINDICATIONS

The primary advantage of static CT perfusion is that it can be performed using a relatively low radiation dose. However, image interpretation can be challenging. Because static CT stress perfusion images are acquired during a single phase of the cardiac cycle, there can be uncertainty with whether an apparent perfusion defect represents a true perfusion defect or an imaging artifact, in particular those related to cardiac motion.[13] A particularly challenging artifact to resolve is the beam hardening artifact that can occur due to attenuation created by remote structures such as a bone or neighboring structures such as the contrast-enhanced aorta. In some cases, beam hardening can be recognized by reviewing several phases, as such artifacts may disappear when a different phase is selected. Additionally, because only a single set of images are acquired, the images should ideally be acquired during peak myocardial enhancement; however, there is no systematic way to ensure optimal timing of the acquisition during contrast perfusion. Several imaging artifacts and acquisition problems are shown in Fig. 15.3. Finally, assessment of static stress CT perfusion are primarily reliant of qualitative assessment, although semiquantitative approaches such as transmyocardial perfusion ratio have shown promise.[8]

DYNAMIC PERFUSION IMAGING

Hardware and Scan Protocol

Dynamic CT myocardial perfusion imaging involves acquisition of a temporal series of images of the myocardium as

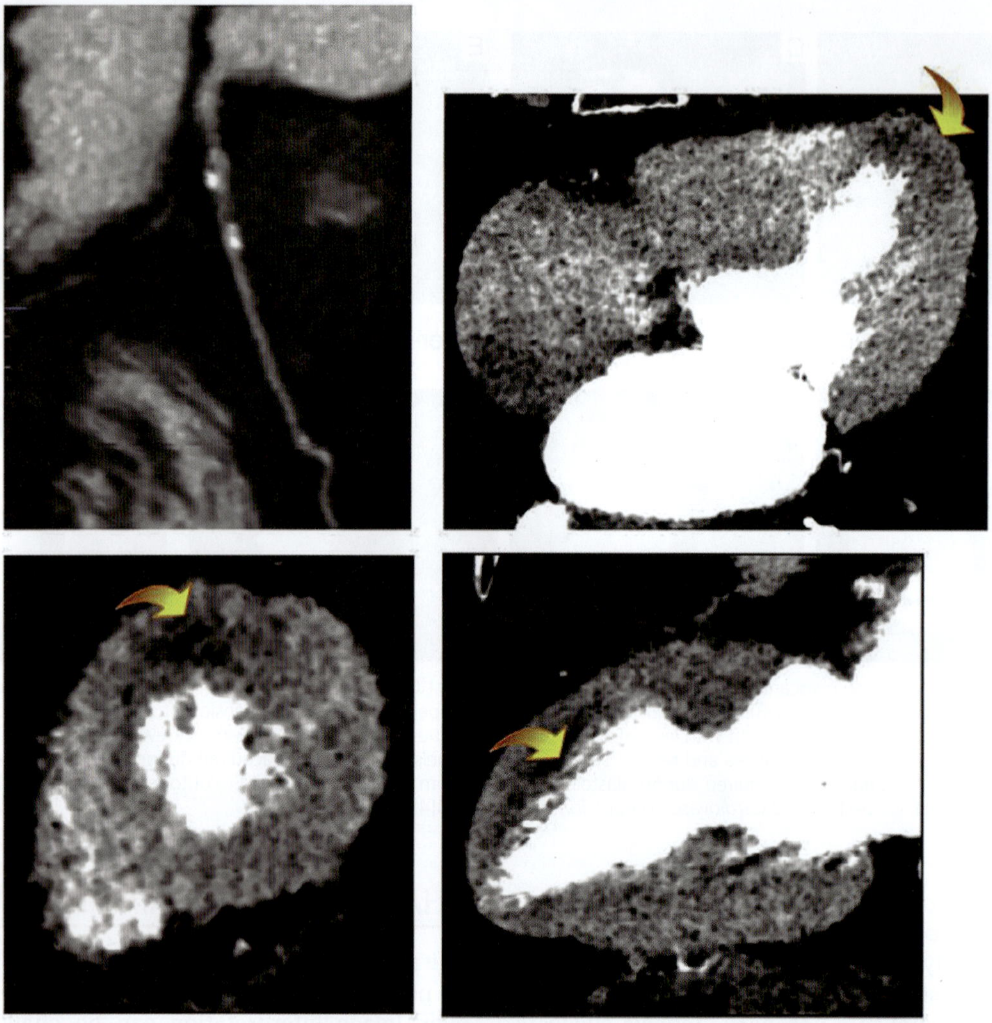

FIG. 15.2 Stress myocardial perfusion imaging. Images obtained under conditions of vasodilator stress in a patient with significant stenosis in the proximal left anterior descending (LAD) coronary artery: multi-planar reconstruction showing heavy calcification of the artery (*top left*) and CT perfusion images depicting a subendocardial defect in the LAD territory (*arrows*), visible in both long-axis (*right*) and short-axis (*bottom left*) views. (Reproduced from Singh A, Mor-Avi V, Patel AR. The role of computed tomography myocardial perfusion imaging in clinical practice. *J Cardiovasc Comput Tomogr*. 2020;14:185–194.)

contrast medium passing through the myocardium. Serial imaging requires a wide-detector CT system to cover the entire heart in a single or two acquisitions. If the detector array allows for complete coverage of the myocardium, then complete samples can be acquired every heart cycle, although in clinical practice the sampling rate will be lowered to limit dose. Second- and third-generation dual-source CT scanners have a narrower detector array, which requires acquisition of the top and bottom half of the heart in an alternating fashion (shuttle mode), and for most common heart rates sample one complete dataset every four heart cycles. To limit overall exposure, the individual samples are acquired using a low tube output and have a relatively noisy appearance (Figs. 15.4 and 15.5).

Contrast medium with a high iodine concentration is administrated as a short bolus at a high injection rate, followed by a saline bolus chaser, preferably through a large antecubital vein on the right side. The imaging sequence starts just before the contrast medium reaches the right ventricle and continues for approximately 30 seconds. Depending on the type of scanner, images will be acquired every beat, every other beat, or at a variable rate during the transit of contrast medium. The scan is typically performed during a long breathhold. To compensate for gradual displacement of the heart during the acquisition, the images need to be realigned using motion or displacement correction software. Dedicated reconstruction algorithms decrease beam hardening at the interface of the contrast-filled ventricular cavity and the myocardium.

IMAGE PROCESSING AND INTERPRETATION

What differentiates dynamic from static MPI_{CT} is the ability to quantify myocardial perfusion. Absolute parameters of myocardial perfusion are calculated using deconvolution analysis of tracer kinetics based on a two-compartment model of the intravascular and interstitial space, applied to the arterial input function (time-attenuation curve for the aorta) and the time-resolved enhancement of the myocardium.[14] For shuttle-mode operated dual-source CT, a hybrid model combines a simplified deconvolution algorithm with the maximum-slope method.[15] Myocardial blood flow (MBF) is calculated by dividing the maximum slope of the

TABLE 15.2 Diagnostic Performance of Static MPI_{CT}

AUTHOR/ YEAR	STUDY POPULATION	CT PROTOCOL	REFERENCE STANDARD	PER PATIENT ANALYSIS *PER VESSEL ANALYSIS SENS	SPEC	POSITIVE PREDICTIVE VALUE.(PPV)	NEGATIVE PREDICTIVE VALUE (NPV)
Cury[36]	Abnormal SPECT (n = 26)	Stress CTP	SPECT	94	78	89	87
George[37]	Abnormal SPECT (n = 40)	CTCA + Stress CTP	SPECT	86	92	92	85
George[38]	Abnormal SPECT (n = 50)	Stress CTP	SPECT	50	89	55	87
Cury[66]	Abnormal SPECT (n = 124)	Stress CTP	SPECT	90	84	36	99
Bettencourt[39]	Symptomatic with suspected CAD (n = 150)	CTCA + Stress CTP	Cardiac perfusion MRI	90	81	80	90
Feuchtner[40]	Intermediate-high risk for CAD (n = 30)	Stress CTP	Cardiac perfusion MRI	96*	88*	93*	94*
Blankstein[7]	Previous SPECT (n = 34)	Dual-source Stress CTP	Invasive coronary angiography	92	67	89	75
Ladeiras-Lopes[41]	Suspected CAD (n = 95)	CTCA + Stress CTP	Invasive coronary angiography	67	93	88	78
CORE-320[42]	Suspected CAD (n = 381)	CTCA + Stress CTP	Invasive coronary angiography	78	73	85	64
Nasis[43]	Abnormal SPECT (n = 20)	CTCA + Stress CTP	Invasive coronary angiography	94	98	94	98
Reif[44]	Known CAD with stents (n = 91)	CTCA + Stress CTP	Invasive coronary angiography	82	88	61	96
Rocha-Filho[45]	Suspected CAD (n = 36)	CTCA + Dual-source Stress CTP	Invasive coronary angiography	96	100	100	91
Rochitte[46]	Suspected or known CAD (n = 391)	Stress CTP	Invasive coronary angiography	80	74	65	76
Greif[47]	Chest pain symptoms (n = 65)	CTCA + Stress CTP	Invasive FFR	97	69	76	96
Ko[48]	Documented >50% stenosis (n = 42)	CTCA + Stress CTP	Invasive FFR	76*	84*	82*	79*
Ko[49]	Symptomatic patients (n = 40)	CTCA + Stress CTP	Invasive FFR	74*	66*	56*	81*
Wong[50]	Symptomatic patients with known or suspected CAD (n = 75)	CTCA + stress CTP	Invasive FFR	76	89	78	88

*only reported data at per vessel level and not at per person level *CAD*, Coronary artery disease; *CT*, computed tomography; *CTCA*, computed tomography coronary angiography; *CTP*, computed tomography perfusion; *FFR*, fractional flow reserve; *SPECT*, single photon emission computed tomography.
Modified from Singh A, Mor-Avi V, Patel AR. The role of computed tomography myocardial perfusion imaging in clinical practice. *J Cardiovasc Comput Tomogr*. 2020;14:185–194.

fit model curve by the peak of the arterial input function in milliliter per minute per volume of myocardial tissue. Other parameters such as the perfused blood volume and first-pass distribution volume may also be calculated but have not been extensively investigated.[16] Hyperemic MBF values by CT are typically reported in the range of 1 to 2.5 ml/min/ml for patients or myocardial territories without obstructive coronary artery disease. The MBF measured by CT is lower than some other perfusion imaging techniques. In addition, there are substantial differences in MBF between individuals that cannot be fully explained by differences in disease severity alone. Postulated causes

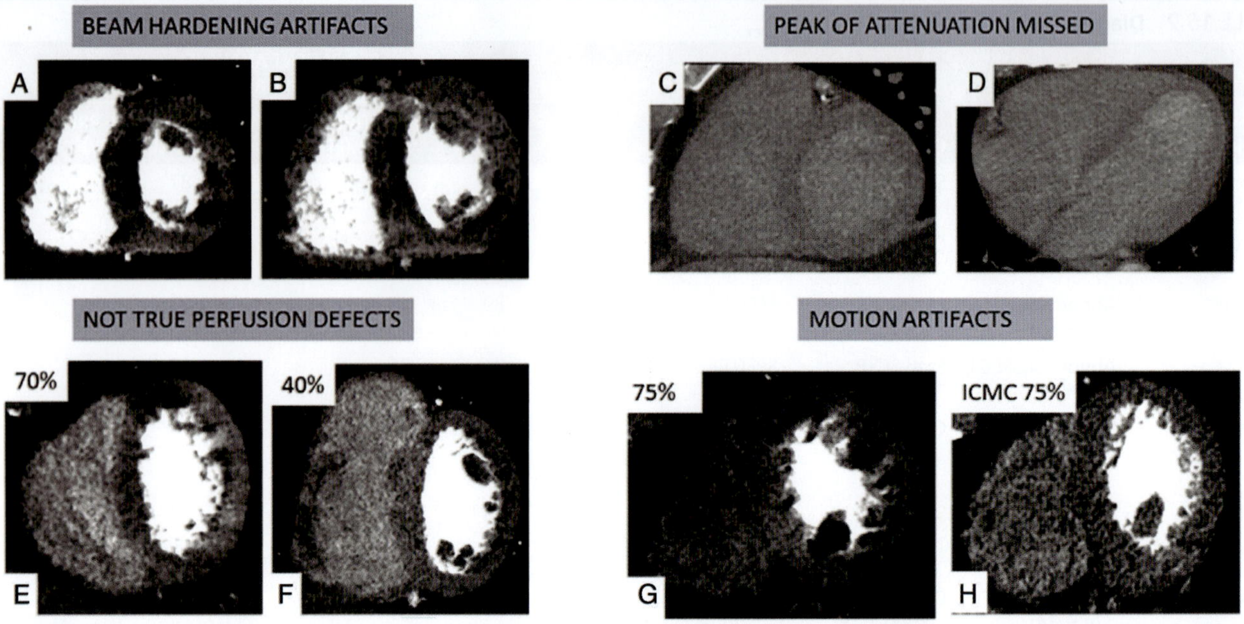

FIG. 15.3 Main artifacts of static CT perfusion. Panels A and B show an example of beam hardening artifacts on septum and posterolateral wall that could be misinterpreted as perfusion defects. Panels C and D show a case of uninterpretable myocardial perfusion due to late acquisition of the images. Panels E and F show a case of nontrue perfusion defect in anteroseptal wall present at diastolic phase (70%) but not in systolic phase (40%). Panels G and H show motion artifacts due to high heart rate during the stress phase that could be misinterpreted as perfusion defects (Panel G). The defect is confirmed to be an artifact because it is not preset after application of an intracycle motion correction algorithm (Panel H). Intravenous (IV); contrast medium (CM); arterial input function (AIF); myocardial blood flow (MBF). (Reproduced from Mushtaq S, Conte E, Pontone G, et al. State-of-the-art-myocardial perfusion stress testing: static CT perfusion. *J Cardiovasc Comput Tomogr*. 2020;14[4]:294–302.)

for this include a variable response to vasodilator, the low sampling rate of dual-source CT perfusion protocols, the nonlinear extraction rate of iodine, as well as the accuracy of the models used for MBF calculation. A practical solution to the variability of the baseline MBF values is the calculation of indexed MBF values. MBF values in a myocardial region of possible hypoperfusion can be divided by MBF values sampled in a territory without obstructive CAD.[17] As an alternative approach that is less observer dependent, the sampled MBF values can be divided by a measure of global blood flow such as the 75th percentile of MBF values throughout the myocardial volume.[18] Although the threshold for myocardial ischemia varies substantially between technical validation studies (0.75–1.64 ml/min/ml), the range is narrower for a MBF indexed by the 75th percentile of the global MBF (0.71–0.80) (Table 15.3). Although visual assessment of MBF maps and indexed MBF values generally suffice for the identification of hemodynamically significant CAD, further research is needed to improve the reproducibility of absolute MBF values derived by dynamic MPI_{CT} and expand its utility for assessment of diffuse CAD or microvascular CAD.

Myocardial blood flow and other perfusion parameters can be reviewed as color-coded, 3D image datasets. Multiplanar reformations can be created to display specific territories. Alternatively, polar maps can be created by averaging the transmural values and reduce the perfusion data to a 2D scale. When the results are further averaged per myocardial segment, so-called bullseye maps can be created. Finally, software applications have been developed for projection of the coronary arteries onto the 2D or 3D perfusion maps for direct correlation of angiographic and perfusion imaging results.

DIAGNOSTIC PERFORMANCE

The diagnostic performance of dynamic MPI_{CT} has been compared to invasive fractional flow reserve (FFR) and other noninvasive perfusion techniques in single- and several multicenter studies (Table 15.4). These studies consistently demonstrated improved diagnostic accuracy by MPI_{CT} for the detection of hemodynamically significant CAD compared to CCTA alone. Substantial improvement in specificity, potentially at the expense of a small loss in sensitivity, result from reclassification of angiographically significant coronary lesions (typically >50% diameter stenosis) that are not hemodynamically significant. In the larger studies the sensitivity and specificity of MPI_{CT} are around 80% with a fairly wide range of performance between studies (70–90%) (Table 15.2). Myocardial perfusion imaging and catheter-based FFR are associated by their ability to detect inducible myocardial ischemia; however, they do not measure identical physiological phenomena. FFR measures the hemodynamic severity of obstructions in the epicardial conduit vessels, whereas perfusion imaging techniques capture disease in the microvasculature as well. Discordant results in technical validation studies may also be related to technical challenges and patient characteristics. Dynamic perfusion imaging using CT relies on spatial consistency between the samples, therefore arrhythmia or gross displacement from breathing can interfere with algorithms for MBF calculation. Ideally myocardial enhancement is rapid, short, and intense, but in patients with heart failure, severe valvular regurgitation, or when there are other reasons for prolonged circulation time, the contrast enhancement curve flattens out.

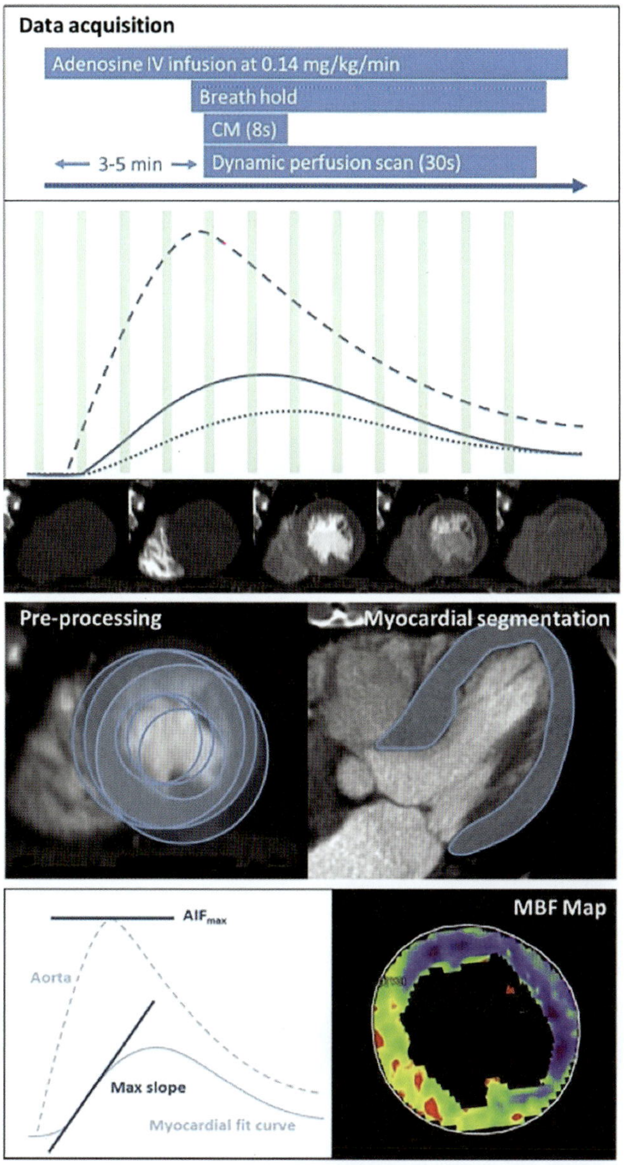

FIG. 15.4 Dynamic Myocardial Perfusion Imaging Methods. After 3 to 5 minutes of adenosine infusion the dynamic CT data is acquired over 30 seconds following a short, high-rate contrast medium while breath-holding. A series of images are acquired as the contrast medium passes through the cardiac cavities and the myocardium. Preprocessing includes displacement correction of the myocardium. The myocardium is semiautomatically segmented. After deconvolution the maximum slope method is applied to the fit curve to calculate the myocardial blood flow. Color-coded myocardial blood flow map indicates low perfusion (*blue*) in the anterolateral wall.

DIFFERENTIATION OF REVERSIBLE ISCHEMIA AND PERMANENT SCAR

There are several ways to differentiate reversible ischemia from permanent scar by MPI_{CT} alone or in combination with other acquisitions. A CCTA performed at rest provides an impression of the resting myocardial perfusion. Low attenuation values in the range of nonenhanced myocardium indicate reduced perfusion; however, lower attenuation values may indicate the presence of fatty replacement in chronic scar. Other phenomena such as wall thinning and calcifications may be seen in chronic scar.[19] Dynamic perfusion protocols can be performed both at rest and during hyperemia, but this is not common practice because of cumulative dose considerations. Very low MBF values, combined with a thin wall, on the stress perfusion scan suggests prior myocardial infarction.[20] Similar to MRI, myocardial scar can be detected by visualizing the slow washout of iodine contrast medium on images acquired 5 to 7 minutes after contrast injection (late-enhancement imaging). Finally, availability of the CT coronary angiogram will provide further clues whether myocardial territories are infarcted or not.[21–23]

INNOVATION

There are several hardware-based innovations occurring in the field of CT that are likely to benefit stress CT perfusion imaging. The use of dual-energy CT has the potential to improve CT perfusion by not only reducing imaging artifact such as beam hardening but also improving quantification of myocardial contrast enhancement though determination of the iodine concentration present in the myocardium as the contrast agent perfuses through it. The underlying concept of dual-energy CT (DECT) imaging entails the concomitant application of two different photon energy levels (typically one high energy ~140kV, and one low energy ~80kV), capitalizing on the inherent differences in x-ray attenuation properties of different materials and tissues. The iodine content of the myocardium can be translated into a color-coded map, which allows for a quantitative surrogate for perfusion as it represents the pattern of blood volume distribution.[9] Although there is minimal experience with the use of photon-counting CT (see Chapter 13) for performing stress CT perfusion imaging, it is likely that the technology will improve the quantification of myocardial blood flow and allow the use of lower amounts of iodinated contrast and radiation dose. Finally, machine-learning and other computational techniques are likely to impact the performance and interpretation of myocardial perfusion scans in the future.[24,25]

CT PERFUSION IMAGING IN CLINICAL PRACTICE

One of the potential advantages of MPI_{CT} compared to other perfusion techniques is that it can be performed in conjunction with CCTA, thereby providing a comprehensive examination of anatomy and function in a single session. Dynamic MPI_{CT} provides quantitative measures of myocardial perfusion with unparalleled spatial resolution covering the entire left ventricle. This allows for direct correlation between the coronary anatomy, angiographic disease burden, and blood flow in the dependent myocardial territories. There are also drawbacks and practical challenges to MPI_{CT}, as well as safety considerations related to the exposure of x-rays, contrast media, and stress agents. Overall, the data from single-center and multicenter studies show that CTP is technically feasible in experienced as well as less experienced centers and that it has incremental value over CCTA for the identification of hemodynamically significant coronary artery disease. A published

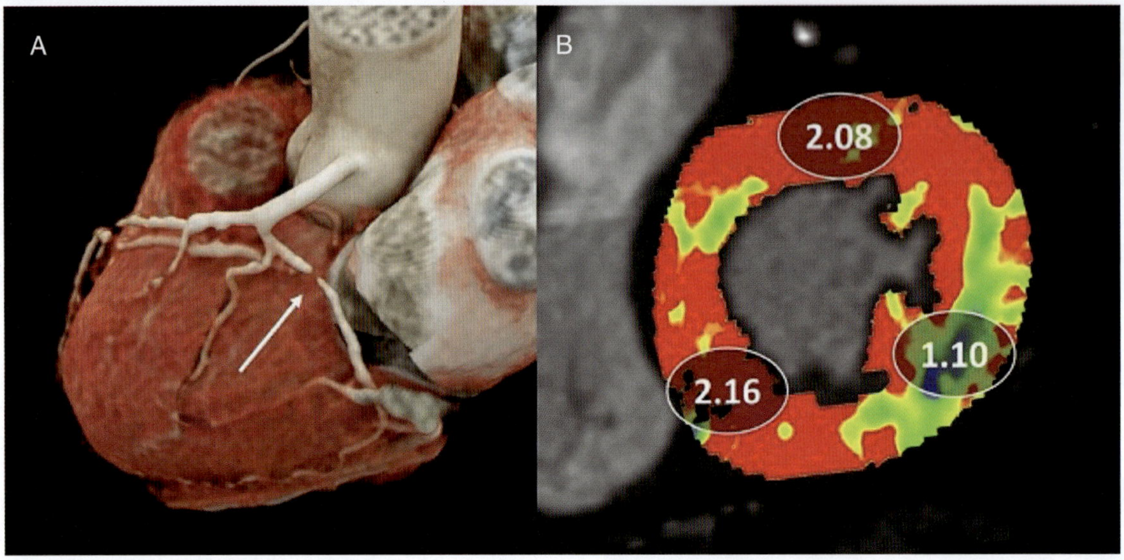

FIG. 15.5 **Dynamic Myocardial Perfusion Case.** Patient with a severe proximal left circumflex stenosis on coronary CT angiography (A). The myocardial perfusion map of the vasodilator-stress, dynamic myocardial perfusion scan shows a perfusion defect in the posterolateral wall (B). Manual samples in the posterolateral wall confirm low blood flow values compared to remote territories.

TABLE 15.3 Absolute and Relative MBF Thresholds to Identify Myocardial Ischemia

AUTHOR, YEAR	MBF (ML/ML/MIN)	MBF INDEX	REFERENCE MBF (DENOMINATOR)
Bamberg[51]	0.75		
Huber[52]	1.64		
Greif[47]	0.75		
Rossi[18]	0.78		
Kono[17]	1.03	0.85	Manually sampled remote myocardium
Bamberg[20]	0.88		
Coenen[29]	0.91	0.71	75th percentile of LV volume
Rossi[16]	1.06	0.73	75th percentile of LV volume
Li[53]	0.99		
Pontone[54]	1.01		
De Knegt[55]		0.72	75th percentile of LV volume
Kitagawa[56]	1.16	0.71	75th percentile of LV volume
Nous[57]	1.42	0.80	75th percentile of LV volume

Summary of reported absolute myocardial blood flow (MBF) threshold derived for diagnostic validation studies. *MBF index*, MBF values normalized against a reference MBF value, often the 75th percentile of the MBF values throughout the entire LV myocardium. Although the range in thresholds for absolute MBF values is more than twofold, the range is narrower for the normalized MBF thresholds.

metaanalysis suggests that dynamic MPI_{CT} is superior to static MPI_{CT}[26] for the identification of hemodynamically significant coronary artery disease, although data were derived from separate studies, and dynamic MPI_{CT} studies were of a more recent date. Sparse data from head-to-head comparisons between static and dynamic MPI_{CT} do not indicate significant differences in diagnostic accuracy.[27] Other metaanalyses indicate that the diagnostic performance of MPI_{CT} is equivalent or better compared with other perfusion imaging modalities.[28] CT-based fractional flow reserve (CT-FFR), which represents an alternative approach to assess the hemodynamic significance of coronary disease on CCTA (see Chapter 13), does not require an additional scan or administration of vasodilators. Several studies that directly compared CTP and CT-FFR in the same patients, using invasive FFR as reference, demonstrated equivalent performance.[29–31] However, because of the practical advantages, CT-FFR is more frequently performed in regions where this technology is available for clinical use. However, when CT-FFR cannot be performed because of technical reasons (prior stenting or bypass graft surgery, prior myocardial infarction, severe calcification, insufficient CCTA quality) or is not available, MPI_{CT} can be a valuable alternative.[11]

The most optimal sequence of examination, CCTA followed by MPI_{CT} or vice versa, remains a topic of debate and may partially depend on the clinical context. When the presence of coronary disease is unknown, and particularly when the pretest probability is relatively low, it is more efficient to perform MPI_{CT} after CCTA. In such cases MPI_{CT} will only be required if significant coronary disease is detected. Based on the low observed prevalence of CAD in

TABLE 15.4 Diagnostic Performance of Dynamic MPI_{CT}

AUTHOR (YEAR)	N	CT SYSTEM	DOSE (mSv)	MBF THRESHOLD (mL/g/min)	REFERENCE	CTA			MPI_{CT}		
						Se (%)	Sp (%)	AUC	Se (%)	Sp (%)	AUC
Bamberg[20]	33	128-slice DSCT	NR	0.75	ICA/FFR_{cath}	100	51		93	87	
Wang[58]	30	128-slice DSCT	9.5 ± 1.3	NR	MPI_{SPECT}	90	51		100	76	
Huber[52]	32	256 SSCT	9.5	1.64	ICA >75% FFR_{cath} ≤ 0.75				76	100	0.86
Rossi[18]	99	128-slice DSCT		0.78	FFR_{cath} ≤0.75	61	77		85	89	0.95
Kono[17]	42	128-slice DSCT	9.4	0.85 (indexed)	FFR_{cath} ≤0.80				98	70	0.85
Kikuchi[59]	32	320-slice SSCT	12.8 ± 2.9	2.97 (CFR)	PET				86	92	0.90
Tanabe[60]	53	256 SSCT	10.5–10.6	0.92	SPECT (n = 25)				95	72	0.87
				0.98	MRI (n = 28)				78	80	0.89
Coenen[29]	74	128-slice DSCT	9.3–1.8	0.71 (indexed)	ICA/FFR_{cath} ≤0.80	78	49	0.70	73	68	0.75
Rossi[16]	115	128/192-DSCT	6.0–10.3	75 (indexed)	ICA/FFR_{cath} ≤0.80	35	95	0.65	89	73	0.85
Pontone[54]	85	256-slice SSCT	5.3 ± 0.7	1.01	ICA/FFR_{cath}	83	66	0.83	73	86	0.88
Nishiyama[61]	38	256-slice SSCT	10.2 ± 1.2	1.26	ICA/FFR_{cath} <0.75	96	57	0.84	83	93	0.96
Alessio[62]	34	256-slice SSCT	8.4 ± 1.1	1.26	82-Rb PET				75	83	NR
De Knegt[55]	93	128-slice DSCT	19[a]	0.72 (indexed)	ICA/FFR_{cath} ≤0.80	82	76	0.79	84	89	0.86
Kuwahara[63]	27	256-slice SSCT	10.2 1.3	1.7	ICA/FFR_{cath}				95	90	0.79
				(0.8)					95	90	0.94
Oleksiak[64]	56	192-slice DSCT									
Kitagawa[56]	157	128-slice DSCT	4.9 1.2			93	36	0.65	72	75	0.74
Nous[57]	132	192-slice DSCT	4.4 (3.3–6.3)	142 (0.80)	ICA/FFR_{cath} ≤0.80	96	72	NR	84	89	0.82

[a]K factor, 0.026.

Summary of selected studies comparing dynamic stress CT myocardial perfusion imaging (MPI) against invasive coronary angiography (ICA) with fractional flow reserve (FFR_{cath}) or other noninvasive functional tests. Sensitivity (Se), specificity (Sp), area under the curve (AUC), not reported (NR), myocardial blood flow (MBF, ml/min/100 cc myocardium), single/dual-source computed tomography (SSCT/DSCT), coronary flow rate (CFR).

all comers with chest pain, only a minority would require a stress perfusion scan.[32–34] For example, in the aforementioned CRESCENT 2 trial, only 22% of patients with stable chest pain and no history of CAD required a MPI_{CT} scan.[35] Practical drawbacks of the CCTA-MPI_{CT} strategy is the requirement for immediate interpretation of the CCTA, and flexibility in the cardiac CT service to perform ad hoc stress testing. A delay between CCTA, and perfusion imaging of at least 15 minutes is recommended to allow for washout of contrast medium. If the stress perfusion scan is performed first, then no contrast wash out is required and CCTA pre-medication will not interfere with the stress scan. The major drawback of first doing the stress CT scan is the redundancy of the stress perfusion scan if the CCTA turns out negative. Therefore the MPI_{CT}-CCTA sequence will be more efficient, at least from the patient's perspective, if the probability of CAD is high.

To date, the clinical utility of MPI_{CT} has been prospectively investigated in a number of small studies. The CRESCENT 2 trial randomized stable, symptomatic patients with suspected coronary disease between a tiered cardiac CT evaluation, including dynamic MPI_{CT} for patients with >50% stenosis on CCTA and standard care based on conventional stress tests. The cardiac CT approach resulted in a significantly higher yield for invasive angiography for the identification of coronary artery disease with an ESC class 1 indication for revascularization. The CATCH 2 trial investigated the utility of static MPI_{CT} in patients who recently presented in the ED with chest pain and were ruled out for an acute coronary syndrome and showed that CCTA with MPI safely reduced the need for invasive angiography and revascularizations.[12] In the United States, clinical implementation of MPI_{CT} has been hindered by lack of reimbursement. At the present, there are no specific recommendations, either for or against MPI_{CT} in clinical practice guidelines by the major cardiology societies.

REFERENCES

1. Uren NG, Melin JA, De Bruyne B, Wijns W, Baudhuin T, Camici PG. Relation between myocardial blood flow and the severity of coronary-artery stenosis. *N Engl J Med*. 1994;330:1782–1788.
2. Berne RM. Regulation of coronary blood flow. *Physiol Rev*. 1964;44:1–29.
3. Axel L. Cerebral blood flow determination by rapid-sequence computed tomography: theoretical analysis. *Radiology*. 1980;137:679–686.
4. Hoffmann U, Millea R, Enzweiler C, et al. Acute myocardial infarction: contrast-enhanced multi-detector row CT in a porcine model. *Radiology*. 2004;231:697–701.
5. Mahnken AH, Koos R, Katoh M, et al. Assessment of myocardial viability in reperfused acute myocardial infarction using 16-slice computed tomography in comparison to magnetic resonance imaging. *J Am Coll Cardiol*. 2005;45:2042–2047.
6. George RT, Silva C, Cordeiro MAS, et al. Multidetector computed tomography myocardial perfusion imaging during adenosine stress. *J Am Coll Cardiol*. 2006;48:153–160.

7. Blankstein R, Shturman LD, Rogers IS, et al. Adenosine-induced stress myocardial perfusion imaging using dual-source cardiac computed tomography. *J Am Coll Cardiol.* 2009;54:1072–1084.
8. Patel AR, Bamberg F, Branch K, et al. Society of cardiovascular computed tomography expert consensus document on myocardial computed tomography perfusion imaging. *J Cardiovasc Comput Tomogr.* 2020;14:87–100.
9. Singh A, Mor-Avi V, Patel AR. The role of computed tomography myocardial perfusion imaging in clinical practice. *J Cardiovasc Comput Tomogr.* 2020;14:185–194. https://doi.org/10.1016/j.jcct.2019.05.011.
10. Gianluca P, Andreini D, Guaricci AI, et al. Incremental diagnostic value of stress computed tomography myocardial perfusion with whole-heart coverage CT scanner in intermediate- to high-risk symptomatic patients suspected of coronary artery disease. *JACC Cardiovasc Imaging.* 2019;12:338–349.
11. Andreini D, Mushtaq S, Pontone G, et al. CT perfusion versus coronary CT angiography in patients with suspected in-stent restenosis or CAD progression. *JACC Cardiovasc Imaging.* 2020;13:732–742.
12. Sørgaard MH, Linde JJ, Kühl JT, et al. Value of myocardial perfusion assessment with coronary computed tomography angiography in patients with recent acute-onset chest pain. *JACC Cardiovasc Imaging.* 2018;11:1611–1621.
13. Blankstein R, Rogers IS, Cury RC. Practical tips and tricks in cardiovascular computed tomography: diagnosis of myocardial infarction. *J Cardiovasc Comput Tomogr.* 2009;3:104–111.
14. George RT, Jerosch-Herold M, Silva C, et al. Quantification of myocardial perfusion using dynamic 64-detector computed tomography. *Invest Radiol.* 2007;42(12):815–822. http://nsr.bioeng.washington.
15. Mahnken AH, Klotz E, Pietsch H, et al. Quantitative whole heart stress perfusion CT imaging as noninvasive assessment of hemodynamics in coronary artery stenosis preliminary animal experience. *Invest Radiol.* 2010;45(6):298–305. www.investigativeradiology.com.
16. Rossi A, Wragg A, Klotz E, et al. Dynamic computed tomography myocardial perfusion imaging. *Circ Cardiovasc Imaging.* 2017;10:e005505.
17. Kono AK, Coenen A, Lubbers M, et al. Relative myocardial blood flow by dynamic computed tomographic perfusion imaging predicts hemodynamic significance of coronary stenosis better than absolute blood flow. *Invest Radiol.* 2014;49(12):801–807. www.investigativeradiology.com.
18. Rossi A, Dharampal A, Wragg A, et al. Diagnostic performance of hyperaemic myocardial blood flow index obtained by dynamic computed tomography: does it predict functionally significant coronary lesions? *Eur Heart J Cardiovasc Imaging.* 2014;15:85–94.
19. Nieman K, Cury RC, Ferencik M, et al. Differentiation of recent and chronic myocardial infarction by cardiac computed tomography. *Am J Cardiol.* 2006;98:303–308.
20. Bamberg F, Hinkel R, Marcus RP, et al. Feasibility of dynamic CT-based adenosine stress myocardial perfusion imaging to detect and differentiate ischemic and infarcted myocardium in an large experimental porcine animal model. *Int J Cardiovasc Imaging.* 2014;30:803–812.
21. Adams DF, Hessel SJ, Judy PF, Stein JA, Abrams HL. Computed tomography of the normal and infarcted myocardium. *AJR Am J Roentgenol.* 1976;126:786–791.
22. Lardo AC, Cordeiro MAS, Silva C, et al. Contrast-enhanced multidetector computed tomography viability imaging after myocardial infarction: characterization of myocyte death, microvascular obstruction, and chronic scar. *Circulation.* 2006;113:394–404.
23. Hamdy A, Kitagawa K, Goto Y, et al. Comparison of the different imaging time points in delayed phase cardiac CT for myocardial scar assessment and extracellular volume fraction estimation in patients with old myocardial infarction. *Int J Cardiovasc Imaging.* 2019;35:917–926.
24. Kim Y-C, Choe YH. Automated identification of myocardial perfusion defects in dynamic cardiac computed tomography using deep learning. *Phys Med.* 2023;107:102555.
25. Michallek F, Nakamura S, Kurita T, et al. Fractal analysis of dynamic stress CT-perfusion imaging for detection of hemodynamically relevant coronary artery disease. *JACC Cardiovasc Imaging.* 2022;15:1591–1601.
26. Danad I, Szymonifka J, Schulman-Marcus J, Min JK. Static and dynamic assessment of myocardial perfusion by computed tomography. *Eur Heart J Cardiovasc Imaging.* 2016;17:836–844.
27. Lee JW, Choe YH, Kim SM, et al. Comparison of diagnostic performance between dynamic versus static adenosine-stress myocardial CT perfusion to detect hemodynamically significant coronary artery stenosis: a prospective multicenter study. *Medicine.* 2022;101:e30477.
28. Takx RAP, Blomberg BA, Aidi HE, et al. Diagnostic accuracy of stress myocardial perfusion imaging compared to invasive coronary angiography with fractional flow reserve meta-analysis. *Circ Cardiovasc Imaging.* 2015;8(1):e002666.
29. Coenen A, Rossi A, Lubbers MM, et al. Integrating CT myocardial perfusion and CT-FFR in the work-up of coronary artery disease. *JACC Cardiovasc Imaging.* 2017;10:760–770.
30. Yang DH, Kim Y-H, Roh JH, et al. Diagnostic performance of on-site CT-derived fractional flow reserve versus CT perfusion. *Eur Heart J Cardiovasc Imaging.* 2017;18:432–440.
31. Pontone G, Baggiano A, Andreini D, et al. Stress computed tomography perfusion versus fractional flow reserve CT derived in suspected coronary artery disease: the PERFECTION study. *JACC Cardiovasc Imaging.* 2019;12:1487–1497.
32. Dedic A, Rossi A, Kate GJRT, et al. First-line evaluation of coronary artery disease with coronary calcium scanning or exercise electrocardiography. *Int J Cardiol.* 2013;163:190–195.
33. Douglas PS, Hoffmann U, Patel MR, et al. Outcomes of anatomical versus functional testing for coronary artery disease. *N Engl J Med.* 2015;372: 1291–1300.
34. SCOT-HEART Investigators. CT coronary angiography in patients with suspected angina due to coronary heart disease (SCOT-HEART): an open-label, parallel-group, multicentre trial. *Lancet.* 2015;385:2383–2391.
35. Lubbers M, Coenen A, Kofflard M, et al. Comprehensive cardiac CT with myocardial perfusion imaging versus functional testing in suspected coronary artery disease: the multicenter, randomized CRESCENT-II trial. *JACC Cardiovasc Imaging.* 2018;11:1625–1636.
36. Cury RC, Magalhães TA, Paladino AT, et al. Dipyridamole stress and rest transmural myocardial perfusion ratio evaluation by 64 detector-row computed tomography. *J Cardiovasc Comput Tomogr.* 2015;5:443–448.
37. George RT, Arbab-Zadeh A, Miller JM, et al. Adenosine stress 64- and 256-row detector computed tomography angiography and perfusion imaging: a pilot study evaluating the transmural extent of perfusion abnormalities to predict atherosclerosis causing myocardial ischemia. *Circ Cardiovasc Imaging.* 2009;2:174–182.
38. George RT, Arbab-Zadeh A, Miller JM, et al. Computed tomography myocardial perfusion imaging with 320-row detector computed tomography accurately detects myocardial ischemia in patients with obstructive coronary artery disease. *Circ Cardiovasc Imaging.* 2012;5:333–340.
39. Bettencourt N, Ferreira ND, Leite D, et al. CAD detection in patients with intermediate-high pre-test probability: low-dose CT delayed enhancement detects ischemic myocardial scar with moderate accuracy but does not improve performance of a stress-rest CT perfusion protocol. *JACC Cardiovasc Imaging.* 2013;6:1062–1071.
40. Feuchtner G, Goetti R, Plass A, et al. Adenosine stress high-pitch 128-slice dual-source myocardial computed tomography perfusion for imaging of reversible myocardial ischemia: comparison with magnetic resonance imaging. *Circ Cardiovasc Imaging.* 2011;4:540–549.
41. Ladeiras-Lopes R, Bettencourt N, Ferreira N, et al. CT myocardial perfusion and coronary CT angiography: influence of coronary calcium on a stress-rest protocol. *J Cardiovasc Comput Tomogr.* 2016;10:215–220.
42. Magalhães TA, Kishi S, George RT, et al. Combined coronary angiography and myocardial perfusion by computed tomography in the identification of flow-limiting stenosis—the CORE320 study: an integrated analysis of CT coronary angiography and myocardial perfusion. *J Cardiovasc Comput Tomogr.* 2015;9:438–445.
43. Nasis A, Ko BS, Leung MC, et al. Diagnostic accuracy of combined coronary angiography and adenosine stress myocardial perfusion imaging using 320-detector computed tomography: pilot study. *Eur Radiol.* 2013;23: 1812–1821.
44. Rief M, Zimmermann E, Stenzel F, et al. Computed tomography angiography and myocardial computed tomography perfusion in patients with coronary stents: prospective intraindividual comparison with conventional coronary angiography. *J Am Coll Cardiol.* 2013;62:1476–1485.
45. Rocha-Filho JA, Blankstein R, Shturman LD, et al. Incremental value of adenosine-induced stress myocardial perfusion imaging with dual-source CT at cardiac CT angiography. *Radiology.* 2010;254:410–419.
46. Rochitte CE, George RT, Chen MY, et al. Computed tomography angiography and perfusion to assess coronary artery stenosis causing perfusion defects by single photon emission computed tomography: the CORE320 study. *Eur Heart J.* 2014;35:1120–1130.
47. Greif M, von Ziegler F, Bamberg F, et al. CT stress perfusion imaging for detection of haemodynamically relevant coronary stenosis as defined by FFR. *Heart.* 2013;99:1004–1011.
48. Ko BS, Cameron JD, Meredith IT, et al. Computed tomography stress myocardial perfusion imaging in patients considered for revascularization: a comparison with fractional flow reserve. *Eur Heart J.* 2012;33:67–77.
49. Ko BS, Cameron JD, Leung M, et al. Combined CT coronary angiography and stress myocardial perfusion imaging for hemodynamically significant stenoses in patients with suspected coronary artery disease: a comparison with fractional flow reserve. *JACC Cardiovasc Imaging.* 2012;5:1097–1111.
50. Wong DTL, Ko BS, Cameron JD, et al. Comparison of diagnostic accuracy of combined assessment using adenosine stress computed tomography perfusion + computed tomography angiography with transluminal attenuation gradient + computed tomography angiography against invasive fractional flow reserve. *J Am Coll Cardiol.* 2014;63:1904–1912.
51. Bamberg F, Becker A, Schwarz F, et al. Detection of hemodynamically significant coronary artery stenosis: incremental diagnostic value of dynamic CT-based myocardial perfusion imaging. *Radiology.* 2011;260:689–698.
52. Huber AM, Leber V, Gramer BM, et al. Myocardium: dynamic versus single-shot CT perfusion imaging. *Radiology.* 2013;269:378–386.
53. Li Y, Yu M, Dai X, et al. Detection of hemodynamically significant coronary stenosis: CT myocardial perfusion versus machine learning CT fractional flow reserve. *Radiology.* 2019;293:305–314.
54. Pontone G, Baggiano A, Andreini D, et al. Dynamic stress computed tomography perfusion with a whole-heart coverage scanner in addition to coronary computed tomography angiography and fractional flow reserve computed tomography derived. *JACC Cardiovasc Imaging.* 2019;12:2460–2471.
55. de Knegt MC, Rossi A, Petersen SE, et al. Stress myocardial perfusion with qualitative magnetic resonance and quantitative dynamic computed tomography: comparison of diagnostic performance and incremental value over coronary computed tomography angiography. *Eur Heart J Cardiovasc Imaging.* 2020:jeaa270. http://doi.org/10.1093/ehjci/jeaa270.

56. Kitagawa K, Nakamura S, Ota H, et al. Diagnostic performance of dynamic myocardial perfusion imaging using dual-source computed tomography. *J Am Coll Cardiol*. 2021;78:1937–1949.
57. Nous FMA, Geisler T, Kruk MBP, et al. Dynamic myocardial perfusion CT for the detection of hemodynamically significant coronary artery disease. *JACC Cardiovasc Imaging*. 2022;15:75–87.
58. Wang Y, Qin L, Shi X, et al. Adenosine-stress dynamic myocardial perfusion imaging with second-generation dual-source CT: comparison with conventional catheter coronary angiography and SPECT nuclear myocardial perfusion imaging. *AJR Am J Roentgenol*. 2012;198:521–529.
59. Kikuchi Y, Oyama-Manabe N, Naya M, et al. Quantification of myocardial blood flow using dynamic 320-row multi-detector CT as compared with $^{15}O\text{-}H_2O$ PET. *Eur Radiol*. 2014;24:1547–1556.
60. Tanabe Y, Kido T, Uetani T, et al. Differentiation of myocardial ischemia and infarction assessed by dynamic computed tomography perfusion imaging and comparison with cardiac magnetic resonance and single-photon emission computed tomography. *Eur Radiol*. 2016;26:3790–3801.
61. Nishiyama H, Tanabe Y, Kido T, et al. Incremental diagnostic value of whole-heart dynamic computed tomography perfusion imaging for detecting obstructive coronary artery disease. *J Cardiol*. 2019;73:425–431.
62. Alessio AM, Bindschadler M, Busey JM, Shuman WP, Caldwell JH, Branch KR. Accuracy of myocardial blood flow estimation from dynamic contrast-enhanced cardiac CT compared with PET. *Circ Cardiovasc Imaging*. 2019;12:e008323.
63. Kuwahara N, Tanabe Y, Kido T, et al. Coronary artery stenosis-related perfusion ratio using dynamic computed tomography myocardial perfusion imaging: a pilot for identification of hemodynamically significant coronary artery disease. *Cardiovasc Interv Ther*. 2020;35:327–335.
64. Oleksiak A, Kruk M, Pugliese F, et al. Regadenoson dynamic computed tomography myocardial perfusion using low-dose protocol for evaluation of the ischemic burden. ULYSSES study. *J Cardiovasc Comput Tomogr*. 2020;14:428–436.
65. Mushtaq S, Conte E, Pontone G, et al. State-of-the-art-myocardial perfusion stress testing: static CT perfusion. *J Cardiovasc Comput Tomogr*. 2020;14:294–302. https://doi.org/10.1016/j.jcct.2019.09.002.
66. Cury RC, Kitt TM, Feaheny K, et al. A randomized, multicenter, multivendor study of myocardial perfusion imaging with regadenoson CT perfusion vs single photon emission CT. *J Cardiovasc Comput Tomogr*. 2015;9(2). 103–112. e1-2. http://doi.org/10.1016/j.jcct.2015.01.002.

16 Cardiac Computed Tomography in Patients With Diabetes

RHANDERSON CARDOSO AND MARCIO S. BITTENCOURT

KEY POINTS

- The risk of ASCVD events in patients with diabetes is heterogeneous. The coronary artery calcium (CAC) score can predict ASCVD events in individuals with diabetes independently of atherosclerotic risk factors.
- Individuals with diabetes and a CAC score ≥300 AU have a risk similar to that of secondary prevention cohorts.
- An elevated CAC score in patients with type 1 or type 2 diabetes is a more robust marker of increased ASCVD risk than disease-specific risk factors, including duration of diabetes.
- In patients with diabetes and suspected chronic coronary syndrome without established coronary artery disease, coronary CT angiography may be preferred over functional imaging to identify coronary stenosis and estimate plaque burden.
- Plaque burden, assessed by coronary CT angiography, is a major predictor of future atherosclerotic adverse events. The estimated plaque burden in patients with diabetes may guide the need and intensity of preventive pharmacotherapy.

INTRODUCTION

Diabetes is one of the leading causes of death worldwide. In contrast to other cardiovascular risk factors, the incidence and prevalence of diabetes continues to increase in both developing and developed countries.[1] According to the International Diabetes Federation, there are 537 million individuals worldwide with diabetes, the majority of whom are in low- and middle-income countries, and this number is expected to increase to 783 million in the next two decades.[2]

Cardiovascular disease (CVD), which includes atherosclerotic cardiovascular disease (ASCVD) and heart failure, represents the leading cause of morbidity and mortality among those with diabetes. More than half of deaths in patients with type 2 diabetes are due to CVD.[3] In a pooled analysis of nearly 5 million individuals with type 2 diabetes, the overall prevalence of clinical coronary heart disease (CHD) was 21%.[3] In addition to being an independent risk factor for coronary artery disease (CAD), diabetes is associated with many comorbidities that also increase cardiovascular risk, such as hypertension, obesity, and metabolic syndrome. The reduction in the risk of atherosclerotic endpoints in patients with diabetes requires adequate risk stratification and tailoring the intensity of medical therapies accordingly. In the following sections, we discuss how cardiac CT can help guide risk assessment, diagnosis of coronary atherosclerosis, and, ultimately, the management of CHD in patients with diabetes mellitus. The discussion will also include specific aspects of the use of cardiac CT in patients with diabetes, such as the use of iodinated contrast media (ICM) in this population.

IODINATED CONTRAST MEDIA USE IN PATIENTS WITH DIABETES

Both type 1 and type 2 diabetes mellitus are independently associated with the development of acute kidney injury after the use of ICM.[4] However, the development of contrast-induced acute kidney injury (CI-AKI) with the use of ICM, formerly known as contrast-induced nephropathy, is much less frequent than previously thought (see Chapter 1 Image Acquisition Protocols for Different Types of Cardiac CT). Earlier studies on the incidence of CI-AKI yielded conflated numbers due to selection bias and lack of a control group.[5]

A more contemporary large study of 12,508 individuals who underwent contrast-enhanced and unenhanced scans, with propensity score matching to minimize confounding, found no difference in the incidence of AKI between contrast-enhanced and unenhanced studies across all subgroups of estimated glomerular filtration rate (eGFR), including in those with eGFR <30 mL/min/1.73 m^2 (OR 0.97; 95% CI 0.72–1.30).[6] Another propensity-matched study, however, including over 20,000 CT examinations, showed an increase in AKI following contrast-enhanced studies compared with unenhanced exams in patients with an eGFR <30 mL/min/1.73 m^2.[7]

The American College of Radiology (ACR) recommends an assessment of renal function with serum creatinine and eGFR prior to administration of ICM in patients with significant risk factors for CI-AKI, including those with known chronic kidney disease, prior AKI, or albuminuria. A history of diabetes mellitus is an optional criterion to evaluate renal function.[5]

However, for those patients taking metformin, an evaluation of renal function is recommended prior to the use of ICM. Although metformin itself is not associated with AKI, the development of AKI in a patient taking metformin is associated with the rare, but serious, adverse event of lactic acidosis.[8] Currently, there is no recommendation to discontinue metformin prior to or after the administration of iodinated contrast media in patients on metformin with an eGFR ≥30 mL/min/1.73 m^2 and without AKI. In contrast,

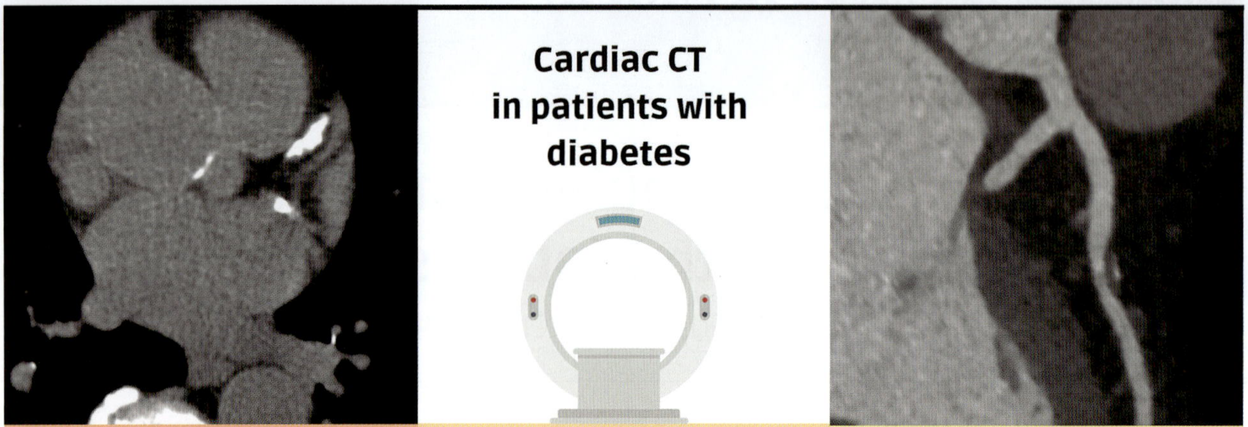

Young patients	Warranty period of CAC = 0	CCTA use in stable chest pain
• Age 20-30 years: up to 1/3 of patients with diabetes and other CV risk factors have CAC > 0. • CAC is an independent risk predictor for CHD and mortality in the young (< 40 years old).	• The average time of conversion from CAC = 0 to CAC > 0 in patients with diabetes is 3-5 years.	• Total plaque burden is a key prognostic factor in stable CHD. • CCTA reduces MACE in patients with diabetes and no known CHD relative to functional testing. • CCTA leads to more targeted initiation of preventive therapies relative to functional testing.
Intravenous contrast administration	**CAC use for escalation of preventive therapies**	**CCTA use in low-risk acute chest pain**
• Assess renal function before CT if: albuminuria, CKD, prior AKI, or metformin use. • Hold metformin if eGFR < 30 mL/min/1.73 m2. • Resume metformin after ⩾ 48 hours once renal function is reassessed and stable.	• Advanced risk stratification with CAC may guide use of multiple preventive therapies: 1. Aspirin; 2. Statin & non-statin lipid therapy 3. Icosapent ethyl; 4. GLP1-RA or SGLT2i	• In patients without ECG changes or positive biomarkers, CCTA use may reduce hospital admissions relative to functional testing. • Diagnosis of subclinical non-obstructive CAD may lead to increased preventive therapies.
CAC score	**CCTA for risk stratification in asymptomatic patients**	**CCTA use in high-risk acute chest pain**
• CAC provides robust ASCVD risk stratification in type 2 and type 1 diabetes. • CAC may be considered in type 2 or type 1 diabetes if it would guide patient care	• Limited incremental benefit over CAC. • Requires contrast use, with increased cost, radiation, and time relative to CAC. • CCTA is not routinely indicated in this scenario.	• If ischemic ECG changes and/or elevated biomarkers, nearly 80% of patients with diabetes have ⩾ 50% coronary stenosis. • No routine indication for CCTA use in this scenario.

FIG. 16.1 Role of cardiac CT in asymptomatic and symptomatic patients with diabetes. *AKI,* Acute kidney infection; *CAC,* coronary artery calcium; *CAD,* coronary CT angiography; *CCTA,* coronary CT angiography; *CHD,* coronary heart disease; *CKD, eGFR,* estimated glomerular filtration rate; *GLP1-RA,* glucagon-like peptide-1 receptor agonists; *MACE,* major adverse cardiovascular events; *SGLT2i,* sodium-glucose cotransporter-2 inhibitors.

those with AKI or chronic kidney disease with an eGFR <30 mL/min/1.73 m^2 who are undergoing a CT with ICM should withhold metformin prior to the procedure. Per ACR recommendations, metformin should only be resumed in these patients 48 hours after administration of contrast and after renal function has been reevaluated (Fig. 16.1).[5]

CARDIOVASCULAR RISK IN PATIENTS WITH DIABETES

Older studies suggested that adults with diabetes have similar risk for future myocardial infarction (MI) as adults with prior MI and no diabetes, leading to the concept of diabetes as a "CHD risk equivalent."[9] However, this concept has been proven incorrect. A large metaanalysis found a 43% lower risk of CHD events in individuals with diabetes and no prior MI as compared with those who had a prior MI but no diabetes.[10]

The cardiovascular risk in patients with diabetes is quite heterogeneous. A large Swedish study found that those with optimal control of five specific risk factors had little or no excess CHD risk compared with matched nondiabetic controls, whereas those with three or more uncontrolled risk factors had an increase in CHD risk. The five risk factors were elevated glycated hemoglobin, elevated low-density lipoprotein cholesterol level, albuminuria, smoking, and elevated blood pressure. Of note, most patients with diabetes who lacked these additional risk factors were treated with statins and antihypertensives.[11]

Accurate risk stratification is a core principle of cardiovascular prevention. The expected absolute risk reduction with different preventive pharmacotherapies is highly dependent on baseline risk.[12] Therefore numerous clinical practice guidelines have endorsed risk-based goals or risk-related thresholds for therapy initiation, including in the management of lipids, blood pressure, and aspirin.[13–15] The American College of Cardiology and American Heart Association recommend the use of the Pooled Cohort Equations for risk estimation in primary prevention.[16] Although this calculator does not incorporate diabetes-specific risk factors beyond the presence versus absence of diabetes, the American Diabetes Association endorses its use, citing that overall risk prediction with this tool does not differ in those with versus without diabetes.[17]

The 2021 European Society Guidelines on Cardiovascular Disease Prevention stratifies patients with diabetes and without established ASCVD into three risk categories, using diabetes-specific risk factors: (1) moderate risk: short-standing diabetes (<10 years) without target-organ damage; (2) high risk: patients with diabetes who are not moderate risk but do not have severe target-organ damage; and (3) very high risk: patients with diabetes and severe target-organ damage, defined as eGFR <45 mL/min/1.73 m^2, microalbuminuria with eGFR 45 to 59 mL/min/1.73 m^2, proteinuria, or microvascular disease in at least three sites.[18]

Importantly, risk stratification based on risk factors alone has several shortcomings. First, risk scores tend to overestimate risk in modern populations. For example, the treatment of diabetes has improved substantially since the inception of the cohorts included in the Pooled Cohort Equations.[19] Second, among patients with diabetes, the duration of disease, presence of albuminuria, and involvement of other target organs are independently associated with higher cardiovascular risk, and these factors are generally not accounted for in risk prediction tools. Finally, the tools for risk estimation are generally validated for a specific age range, such as the Pooled Cohort Equations, which is valid only for individuals aged 40 to 79 years old. Therefore there is a need for advanced risk stratification strategies to be used in selective patients with diabetes, in circumstances where precise risk assessment could change patient management.

CORONARY ARTERY CALCIUM FOR RISK STRATIFICATION IN PATIENTS WITH DIABETES

Coronary artery calcium (CAC), a quantitative measure of calcified coronary plaque, is a well-established, guideline-recommended tool for advanced risk stratification in asymptomatic individuals at borderline and intermediate risk (see Chapter 3 Coronary Artery Calcium Scanning: Indications and Patient Management).[19] The power of CAC for personalized risk stratification can be leveraged to guide preventive care in patients with diabetes, particularly in light of the growing gamut of pharmacotherapies with the potential to reduce cardiovascular risk, which now includes aspirin, statins, non-statin lipid-lowering therapy, icosapent ethyl, glucagon-like peptide-1 receptor agonists (GLP-1RA), and sodium-glucose cotransporter-2 (SGLT2) inhibitors.

The ASCVD event rate in individuals with diabetes is directly proportional to the burden of atherosclerosis as measured by the CAC score (Fig. 16.2). Studies have shown that CAC predicts cardiovascular mortality in patients with diabetes independently of traditional risk factors, glycated hemoglobin, and duration of diabetes.[20] Among patients with type 2 diabetes, a doubling of the CAC score is associated with a 32% increase in the risk of cardiovascular events.[21] Moreover, in the Multi-Ethnic Study of Atherosclerosis (MESA) study, asymptomatic patients with diabetes and an elevated CAC >400 AU had a 10-year ASCVD event rate >30%, which is similar to that of individuals with prior ASCVD (secondary prevention).[22,23] In other words, diabetes, if associated with a CAC score >300 AU, may truly be a "CHD risk equivalent," with a risk similar to that of secondary prevention.

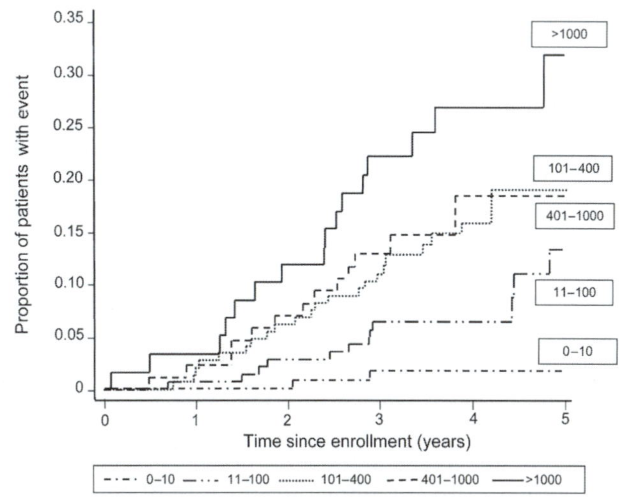

FIG. 16.2 Kaplan-Meier curve of 589 asymptomatic patients with type 2 diabetes, median age of 63.1 years, and median diabetes duration of 7 years. The figure shows the proportion of patients with a coronary heart disease event or stroke over a median follow-up of 4 years, stratified by categories of coronary artery calcium (CAC). CAC remained predictive of a first cardiovascular event in a model fully adjusted for age, sex, ethnicity, smoking, duration of diabetes, lipid levels, blood pressure, antihypertensive therapy, and lipid-lowering therapy. (Reproduced from Elkeles RS, Godsland IF, Feher MD, et al. Coronary calcium measurement improves prediction of cardiovascular events in asymptomatic patients with type 2 diabetes: the predict study. *Eur Heart J.* 2008;29:2244–2251.)

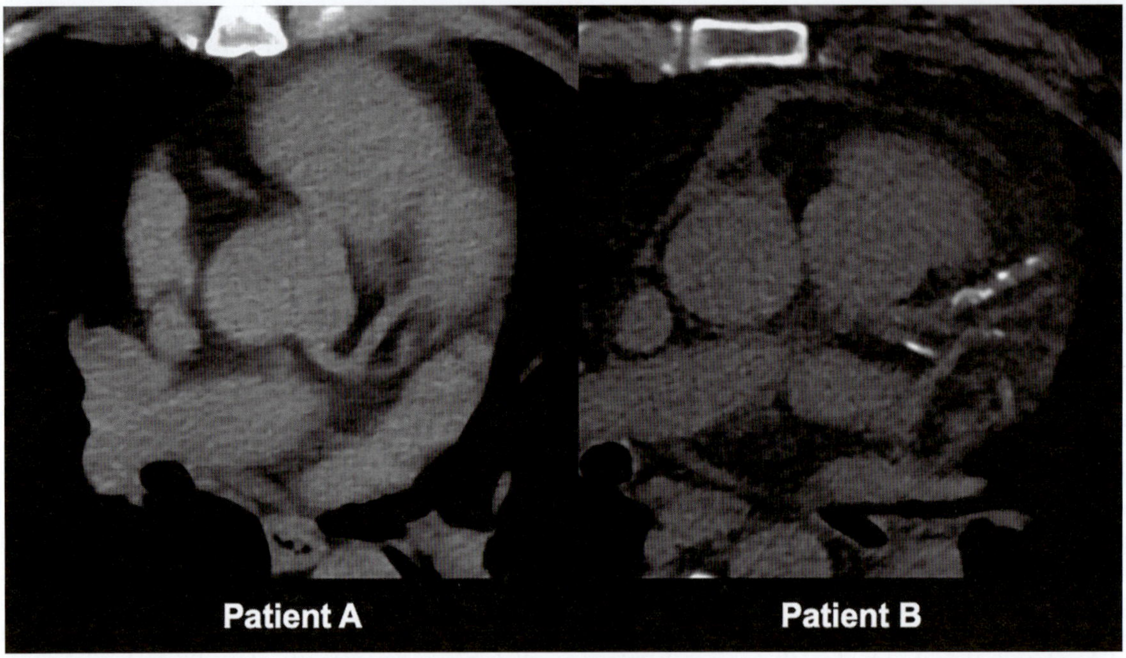

FIG. 16.3 The figure illustrates the coronary artery calcium (CAC) score of two asymptomatic patients with diabetes who had similar age and comorbidities. Patient A was a 62-year-old woman. Patient B was a 54-year-old man. Both individuals had a history of hypertension and type 2 diabetes on oral agents with glycated hemoglobin of approximately 7%. Patient A had a CAC score of 0, whereas Patient B had severe CAC with a score of 576 Agatston units. The 10-year risk of coronary heart disease events for Patient A was estimated at 5.6% without the CAC score and reclassified to 2.4% with the CAC score of 0. The 10-year risk of coronary heart disease events for patient B was estimated at 9.6% without the CAC score and reclassified to 19.6% after incorporating the CAC score. Risk calculator available at https://www.mesa-nhlbi.org/CAC-Tools.aspx.

TABLE 16.1 **Prevalence of Calcium Score of 0 in Cohorts of Patients With Type 2 Diabetes**

STUDY	NUMBER OF PATIENTS	AGE, YEARS (MEAN ± SD)	MEN, %	STATIN USE, %	PROPORTION WITH CAC = 0	10-YEAR EVENT RATE IN CAC = 0	FOLLOW-UP (YEARS)
Valenti[24]	810	54.7 ± 10.8	59.4%	NA	34%	All-cause mortality, 8.7%	15 years
Mitchell[25]	928	54.3 ± 8.8	64.4%	74%	53.7%	NA	NA
Kowall[26]	223	61.5 ± 7.3[a]	55.2%	11.6%	18.4%	NA	NA
Malik[22]	881	64.7 ± 9.5	52%	25.5%	37.3%	ASCVD, 7.5%	11.1 years

[a]Among patients with glycated hemoglobin ≥7.0%.
ASCVD, Atherosclerotic cardiovascular disease; *CAC*, coronary artery calcium; *NA*, not available; *SD*, standard deviation.

In contrast, adult patients with type 2 diabetes and a CAC of 0 may be at a low 10-year risk of ASCVD endpoints. In the MESA study, among 881 participants with diabetes, 37% had a CAC of 0. In those with diabetes and a baseline 10-year ASCVD risk of <15% as calculated by the Pooled Cohort Equations, a CAC of 0 was associated with a 10-year ASCVD event rate of 5%.[22] In a single center cohort of the Tennessee Heart and Vascular Institute, the 5-year mortality rate in individuals with a CAC of 0 was similar between those with diabetes versus without, albeit higher at 15 years in patients with diabetes.[24] The CAC score can be incorporated with traditional risk factors to compute the 10-year risk of CHD events with the MESA risk score calculator, available at https://www.mesa-nhlbi.org/CAC-Tools.aspx (Fig. 16.3).

When considering the use of CAC to downgrade the predicted ASCVD risk in individuals with diabetes, one must consider two aspects: (1) what is the likelihood of a CAC of 0 in this population? and (2) will a CAC of 0 impact patient care in any way?

The second point will be discussed in the next section. As for the first question, multiple studies have confirmed that a considerable proportion of adult patients with type 2 diabetes do indeed have a CAC score of 0. In the previously mentioned study from Tennessee, one-third of patients with diabetes had a CAC of 0 (mean age 54.7 years).[24] In the Walter Reed Army Medical Center population, among 928 patients with diabetes and a mean age of 54.2 years, 499 (53.7%) had a CAC of 0.[25] In the Heinz Nixdorf Recall Study, a population-based cohort in Germany, among 337 patients with diabetes at baseline, with a mean age of 61 years old, the prevalence of CAC of 0 was 22% and 14% in those with glycated hemoglobin <7.0% and ≥7.0%, respectively (Table 16.1).[26]

YOUNG INDIVIDUALS

Early-onset type 2 diabetes is associated with more rapid progression of disease when compared with those who develop diabetes later in life.[27] Identification of subclinical atherosclerosis in young adults (<40 years old) portents a high lifetime risk for future ASCVD events and provides a unique opportunity to intervene on modifiable risk factors and reduce long-term risk. However, less is known about risk stratification in this age group compared with middle-aged and older individuals.

In a cohort of 86 asymptomatic individuals with type 2 diabetes aged 30 to 39 years old, the prevalence of any CAD as identified by CCTA was 58%.[28] After multivariate adjustments, those with diabetes were 25% more likely to have CAC than age- and sex-matched individuals without diabetes.[28] In a population of 1156 individuals with type 1 diabetes with a mean age of 42.8 years, 29% had a CAC > 0.[29]

Even in the very young, aged 20 to 30 years, the prevalence of CAC >0 in those with diabetes has been reported at 13%.[30] In the CAC Consortium, the prevalence of CAC >0 among individuals 20 to 30 years old reached 34.4% among those with three or more risk factors (including diabetes), despite the young age of the group.[30] Similar findings were reported in the Western Denmark Heart Registry. In a group of 3691 individuals aged 18 through 45 years old, 511 (13.8%) had a CAC >0. Diabetes mellitus was associated with an increased prevalence of CAC >0 relative to those without diabetes, with a multivariable-adjusted odds ratio of 2.5.[31]

The discriminatory ability of CAC for predicting ASCVD events is maintained in young patients. Among 22,346 individuals aged 30 to 49 years old who underwent CAC testing in the CAC Consortium, the rate of CHD mortality was 10-fold higher in individuals with CAC >100 AU relative to those with a CAC of 0. A CAC >100 AU was identified in 7% of the group. In multivariable analyses, the adjusted hazards ratio of CHD mortality and all-cause mortality for those with CAC >100 remained significant and were 5.6 and 2.6, respectively.[32]

So when might CAC be clinically useful in this young patient population? Ultimately, it depends on whether the results of CAC testing would influence patient care in a meaningful way. The implications of potential test results on management should be discussed a priori with patients in the context of a shared decision-making process. Among young individuals with diabetes and multiple other risk factors, an elevated CAC may guide escalation of preventive therapies, despite the young age.

CAC USE IN PATIENTS WITH TYPE 1 DIABETES

The relationship between CAC and ASCVD event rates also holds true in patients with type 1 diabetes. Among 1156 patients with type 1 diabetes from the DCCT (Diabetes Control and Complications Trial)/EDIC (Epidemiology of Diabetes Interventions and Complications) trials, with a mean age of 42.8 years, 71% had a CAC score of zero, which was associated with a low rate of nonfatal MI, nonfatal stroke, or cardiovascular death (2.5 per 1000 patient-years) over a follow-up of 10 to 13 years, whereas those with a CAC score >300 AU had an event rate of 18.2 per 1000 patient-years, despite the relatively young age of the cohort. Patients with moderate CAC (101–300 AU) had an intermediate risk of major adverse cardiovascular events (MACE), at 13.9 per 1000 patient-years (Fig. 16.4). However, there was no significant improvement in discrimination of ASCVD event rates with CAC when added to a model that included traditional cardiovascular risk factors.[29]

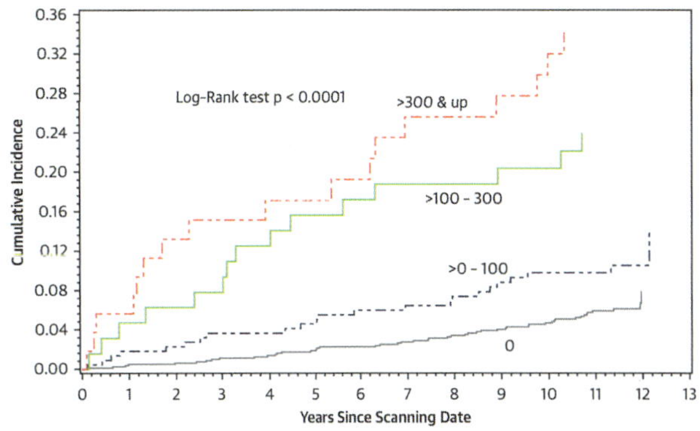

No. at Risk			
0	817	786	730
>0-100	221	206	185
>100-300	65	54	47
>300	53	40	32

FIG. 16.4 Cumulative incidence of first cardiovascular events by categories of coronary artery calcium (CAC) in patients with type 1 diabetes from the Diabetes Control and Complications Trial (DCCT) and Epidemiology of Diabetes Intervention and Complications (EDIC) cohorts. (Reproduced from Budoff M, Backlund J-YC, Bluemke DA, et al. The association of coronary artery calcification with subsequent incidence of cardiovascular disease in type 1 diabetes: the DCCT/EDIC trials. *JACC Cardiovasc Imaging*. 2019;12:1341–1349.)

The 2018 AHA/ACC/Multisociety Cholesterol Clinical Practice Guidelines recommend at least moderate-intensity statin for adults 40 to 75 years of age with diabetes mellitus and high-intensity statin therapy in those with multiple ASCVD risk factors, followed by ezetimibe, if needed, to lower LDL-C by ≥50% in those with ASCVD risk of 20% or higher. The CAC score could be used as a risk enhancer to identify patients with diabetes at need for higher-intensity lipid-lowering therapy. Similarly, for patients aged 20 to 39 years of age, statin therapy is recommended if there are particular risk factors, such as ≥10 years of type 2 diabetes or ≥20 years of type 1 diabetes, albuminuria, impaired kidney function, neuropathy, retinopathy, or reduced ankle-brachial index. An elevated CAC score, in patients with type 1 or type 2 diabetes, is a more robust marker of increased ASCVD risk than disease-specific risk factors, including duration of diabetes.[15,22]

MANAGEMENT OF PATIENTS WITH DIABETES AND NO CORONARY ARTERY CALCIUM

The 2019 ACC/AHA Guideline on Primary Prevention of Cardiovascular Disease recommends selective use of CAC for additional risk stratification in intermediate-risk adults (7.5 to <20% 10-year ASCVD risk). If the CAC is zero in this group, clinicians may consider to defer statin therapy, with the notable exception of individuals who smoke, those with a family history of premature CHD, and patients with diabetes.[15,16] Indeed, despite the evidence of a lower risk of ASCVD events in patients with diabetes who have no coronary artery calcification, there is limited evidence to support withholding of lipid-lowering therapy based on a CAC score of 0 in patients with diabetes as some of the cohorts that demonstrated a low risk among individuals with diabetes and a CAC of 0 had a large proportion of participants treated with statin therapy.[22]

One notable study supporting the safety of no statin use in patients with diabetes and a CAC of 0 was a retrospective study from Walter Reed Army Medical Center. Among 928 patients with diabetes followed for a median of 9.4 years, the use of statin therapy was associated with a reduction in the risk of MACE in those with a CAC >0 (adjusted hazard ratio 0.33; 95% CI 0.19–0.56) but not in individuals with a CAC score of 0 (n = 499). The adjusted hazard ratio for MACE with statin versus no statin use in patients with diabetes and a CAC of 0 was 0.90 (95% CI 0.35–2.31) over a median follow-up of 9.4 years.[25]

If a clinical decision is made to withhold statin therapy in patients with type 2 diabetes based on the absence of coronary artery calcifications, it is important to monitor the patient for the development of incident CAC. In adult patients with diabetes, the average time of conversion to CAC >0 has been estimated at 3.1 years and 4.3 years for men and women, respectively. This interval is 35% to 40% shorter than that for people without diabetes.[33] A strategy of repeating CAC testing before the average period of conversion to CAC >0 would lead to repeat imaging prior to an event in approximately 80% of patients who go on to have a coronary event within 10 years from the baseline CAC of 0.[33]

In summary, it is not recommended to withhold statin therapy in patients with type 2 diabetes and a CAC of 0. In patients with a CAC of 0 who are not initiated on statins, whether due to reluctance to initiate statins or if statin intolerant, then it may be reasonable to repeat CAC testing within 3 to 5 years to assess for the development of incident CAC.

Of note, the rate of CAC progression in patients with CAC >0 on the baseline exam also has independent value in risk stratification.[34] However, there is no recommendation for repeating CAC routinely in this population due to added cost, concerns about repeated exposure to radiation, uncertainties on how to define CAC progression and, most importantly, limited actionable value.[35]

CAC SCORE TO GUIDE ESCALATION OF PREVENTIVE THERAPIES

The CAC score, in addition to other risk factors, can help guide the allocation of a growing number of preventive pharmacotherapies available for patients with diabetes without established ASCVD. With an increasing array of options for preventive therapies in this population, spanning from antiplatelets to lipid-lowering and cardiometabolic agents, the use of CAC may inform the estimated absolute risk of individual patients and, therefore, the expected net benefit from specific preventive pharmacotherapies (Fig. 16.5).

For example, aspirin has been shown to have limited benefit in patients with diabetes who do not have established cardiovascular disease. In the Study of Cardiovascular Events in Diabetes (ASCEND) trial, such patients had a 1.1% absolute risk reduction in the incidence of serious vascular events over a mean follow-up of 7.4 years with aspirin (8.5%) relative to placebo (9.6%). However, the increase in major bleeding events with aspirin (4.1%) relative to placebo (3.2%) was also of similar magnitude, calling into question the net benefit of aspirin in this group.[36] It would appear logical that identifying patients at higher risk of cardiovascular events could potentiate the absolute risk reduction of aspirin. A CAC score ≥100 AU can consistently identify patients who would experience a net benefit of aspirin use in primary prevention, provided the bleeding risk is low.[37,38] In fact, in the MESA cohort, a CAC score ≥100 was superior to a high ASCVD risk score to identify a net benefit for aspirin use in primary prevention.[38] Conversely, epidemiologic models indicate that individuals with a CAC of 0 in primary prevention have a number needed to treat with aspirin to prevent a cardiovascular event higher than the number needed to harm in causing a major bleeding episode, even in those with an ASCVD risk score >20%.[38]

The same concept of using absolute risk to individualize expected magnitude of net benefit from preventive therapies can be applied to lipid-lowering therapies, such as ezetimibe, proprotein convertase subtilisin/kexin type 9 (PCSK9) inhibitors, icosapent ethyl, and cardiometabolic agents, including GLP-1 receptor agonists and SGLT-2 inhibitors.

The key concept is that patients with type 2 diabetes and a CAC score ≥300 to 400 AU have an event rate similar to that of individuals with prior MI, that is, ≥30 ASCVD events/1000 patient-years.[22,23,39] Therefore the magnitude of benefit from preventive therapies in this population is expected to be similar to the magnitude of benefit of these agents in secondary prevention cohorts. Take LDL-C therapy, for instance. Though outcome trials with PCSK9 inhibitors and inclisiran are still lacking in high-risk primary prevention, it may be reasonable to use these therapies in patients with diabetes and a CAC score ≥300 to 400 AU who fail to reach aggressive LDL-C targets despite the use of maximally tolerated statin therapy, similar to how these therapies are used in secondary prevention. The Effect of Evolocumab in Patients at High Cardiovascular Risk Without Prior Myocardial Infarction or Stroke (VESALIUS-CV) trial is examining the use of evolocumab in high-risk patients without prior ASCVD events. Diabetes mellitus with a CAC ≥100 AU as well as sufficient burden of CAD on CCTA are among the inclusion criteria for enrollment.[40]

In the Reduction of Cardiovascular Events with Icosapent Ethyl-Intervention Trial (REDUCE-IT), icosapent ethyl was associated with a 25% relative risk reduction and a 4.8% absolute risk reduction in the primary endpoint of cardiovascular death, nonfatal MI, stroke, revascularization, or unstable angina. This trial enrolled 8179 individuals with fasting triglyceride levels of 135 to 499 mg/dL and either established cardiovascular disease (secondary prevention) or diabetes plus other risk factors (primary prevention). The magnitude of absolute risk reduction in the secondary prevention cohort (6.2%) was substantially higher than that of the primary prevention group (1.4%). Given the

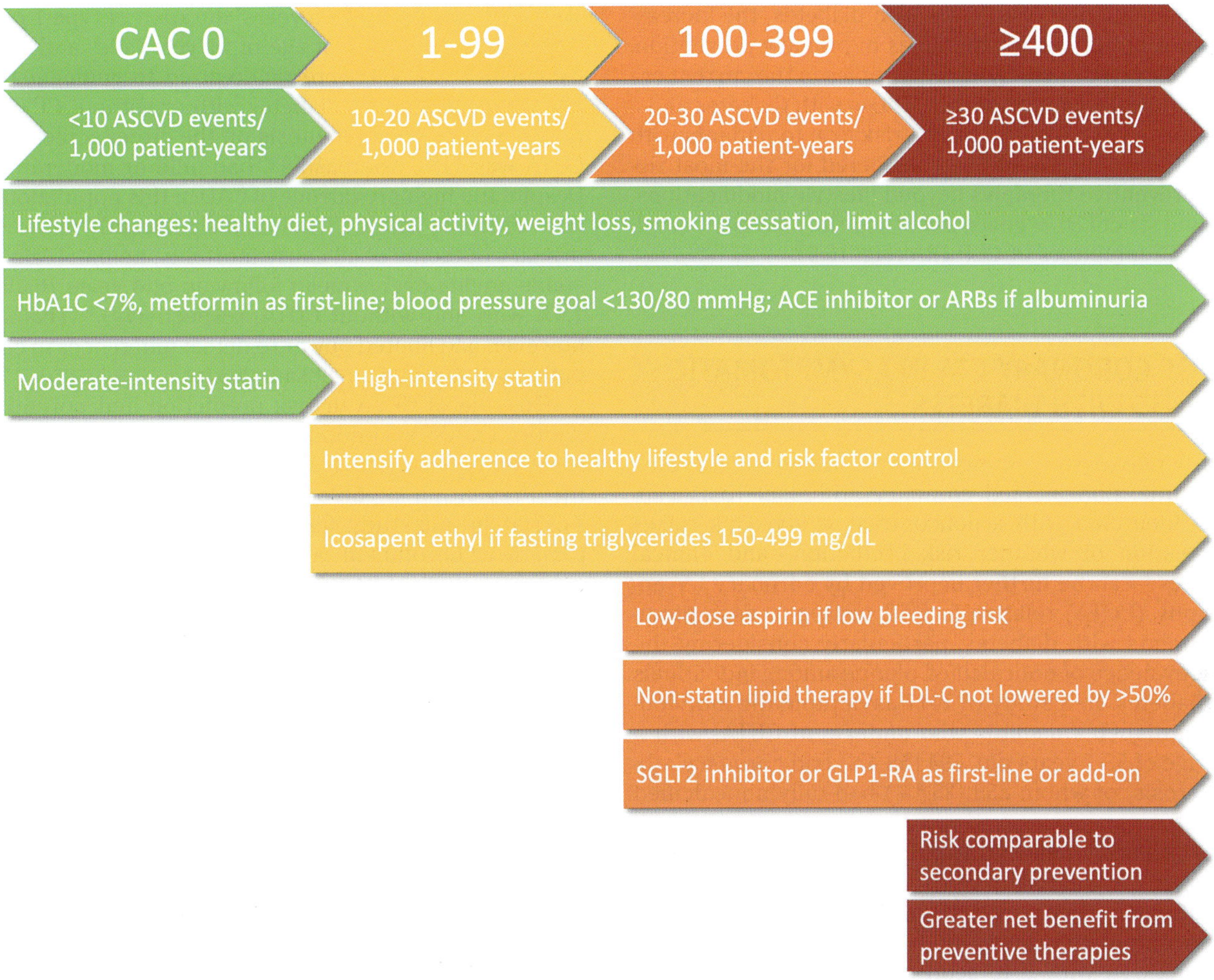

FIG. 16.5 Potential framework for risk stratification in patients with type 2 diabetes who undergo Angiotensin Receptor Blockers (ARB), coronary artery calcium (CAC) testing. The incorporation of CAC results to other risk factors and patient preferences may guide allocation of preventive pharmacotherapies. *ASCVD*, Atherosclerotic cardiovascular disease; *GLP1-RA*, glucagon-like peptide-1 receptor agonists; *SGLT2*, sodium-glucose cotransporter-2. (Reproduced from Cardoso R, Dudum R, Ferraro RA, et al. Cardiac computed tomography for personalized management of patients with type 2 diabetes mellitus. *Circ Cardiovasc Imaging*. 2020;13:e011365.)

medication costs and potential risks of polypharmacy, clinicians and patients considering the use of icosapent ethyl for primary prevention in patients with diabetes may want to perform advanced risk stratification with a CAC score. In those with a CAC score ≥300 to 400 AU, the net benefit with icosapent ethyl would be expected to be more favorable and closer to that of the secondary prevention cohort in the REDUCE-IT trial.

These concepts can also apply to the use of SGLT2 inhibitors and GLP-1 receptor agonists, as these agents have shown to have a larger net benefit among patients with diabetes who have had prior atherosclerotic events (secondary prevention) as compared to individuals without prior events (primary prevention). In a metaanalysis of randomized trials of SGLT2 inhibitors versus placebo in patients with diabetes, the event rate in primary versus secondary prevention cohort was 15 and 40 events per 1000 patient-years, respectively. The magnitude of absolute risk reduction with SGLT2 inhibitors relative to placebo was not significant in the primary prevention group, but was significant at 5 events per 1000 patient-years in the secondary prevention group.[41] Under the premise of similar risk to that of secondary prevention, those with diabetes and a CAC score ≥300 to 400 AU may have a greater benefit from an SGLT2 inhibitor for ASCVD risk reduction, although this has not been tested prospectively.

This hypothesis is corroborated by a recent analysis of the data from MESA, CARDIA (Coronary Artery Risk Development in Young Adults), and the Dallas Heart Study, modeling the predicted number needed to treat to prevent one composite endpoint of cardiovascular death, nonfatal MI, or nonfatal stroke over 5 years with the use of GLP-1RA. Using a 10% relative reduction over 5 years, patients with a CAC of 0 were estimated to have a 5-year number needed to treat to prevent one cardiovascular event that was 3.3-fold higher than those with CAC >100 AU (NNT 280 versus 85, respectively).[42]

In summary, the allocation of preventive therapies for patients with diabetes must go beyond the dichotomy of primary versus secondary prevention. Within the group of patients who do not have known atherosclerotic events, the CAC score, in addition to other risk factors, can provide further risk stratification that, in turn, may guide therapy. This is of particular importance in the context of the growing population of patients with diabetes, the increasing gamut of options for therapies in primary prevention, and the elevated costs of some therapies in the current era of limited healthcare resources. Those with diabetes and a CAC score ≥300 to 400 AU have a risk akin to patients with prior MI and thus should be considered for the most rigorous preventive therapies beyond lifestyle modifications, including strict LDL-C goals, use of aspirin, icosapent ethyl, and SGLT2 inhibitors or GLP-1RA (Fig. 16.5).

USE OF CORONARY CTA IN ASYMPTOMATIC PATIENTS WITH DIABETES

Notwithstanding the strength of CAC in identifying calcified plaque, noncalcified coronary atherosclerosis cannot be identified with a noncontrast study. This raises the question of whether risk prediction—and clinical outcomes—can be further improved by coronary CT angiography (CCTA) relative to CAC testing in asymptomatic patients with diabetes, particularly considering the high prevalence of noncalcified plaque among individuals with diabetes. In a study of 1017 asymptomatic individuals with diabetes mellitus who underwent CCTA, with a mean age of 55.7 years old, 594 (58.4%) had coronary atherosclerosis, of whom 255 (25.1%) had only noncalcified plaque.[43]

It is generally believed that CCTA has an incremental value over CAC testing in risk stratification of asymptomatic patients, albeit small.[44,45] In a South Korean study, 591 asymptomatic individuals with type 2 diabetes underwent CCTA with CAC score and were followed for a median of 5.3 years. The c-statistic for a prediction model including traditional risk factors plus CAC was 0.724, which improved to 0.784 by adding the severity of CAD by CCTA ($P = 0.005$).[45] Of note, these results may reflect, in part, the fact that the presence of obstructive CAD on CCTA is associated with incident downstream coronary revascularization, which was included as part of the composite endpoint. Nevertheless, as previously discussed, CAC testing has robust data for risk stratification, despite its inability to detect noncalcified plaque, even in patients with diabetes. Therefore any incremental value of advanced risk stratification with CCTA relative to CAC must be weighed against the added cost, increased time, need for intravenous contrast, and higher radiation dose. When all these factors are considered, the conclusion is that CAC testing may be sufficient for risk stratification in asymptomatic patients with diabetes who are being considered for further testing for risk stratification. However, the use of quantitative coronary plaque analysis may further enhance the value of CCTA, and thus the net befit of CCTA versus CAC will require further investigation as our technology and clinical data expand.

Moreover, the use of CCTA for routine screening of obstructive and nonobstructive CAD in patients with diabetes has not been shown to improve clinical outcomes. In the Effect of Screening for Coronary Artery Disease Using CT Angiography on Mortality and Cardiac Events in High-Risk Patients with Diabetes (FACTOR-64) study, 900 patients with at least 3 to 5 years' duration of type 1 or type 2 diabetes, with a mean age of 61 years old, and without established ASCVD, were randomized to guideline-directed preventive care in diabetes with or without CCTA. The prevalence of severe stenosis on the group screened with CCTA was 11%, whereas 58% had mild or moderate CAD. Despite the high prevalence of CAD in this population, routine screening with CCTA did not significantly improve the primary outcome of all-cause mortality, nonfatal MI, or unstable angina over a mean follow-up of 4 years (6.2% and 7.6% with and without CCTA, respectively).[46] This study, however, had limited power to detect differences in clinical outcomes given its small sample size.

The role of CCTA in risk prediction and potential reduction in ASCVD endpoints is being further explored in the Computed Tomography Coronary Angiography for the Prevention of Myocardial Infarction (SCOT-HEART 2) Trial. In this study, 6000 participants, who are asymptomatic at enrollment, aged 40 to 70 years old, and with one or more risk factors (including diabetes), will be randomized to cardiovascular risk prediction with or without CCTA for a primary endpoint of CHD death or MI.[47] Until the results are available, CCTA is not recommended for routine screening of subclinical CAD or risk stratification in patients with diabetes who are asymptomatic (Fig. 16.1).

CARDIAC CT USE IN PATIENTS WITH DIABETES AND STABLE CHEST PAIN

It is well established with invasive coronary angiography that the distribution and extent of coronary artery stenoses are associated with adverse cardiovascular outcomes.[48] The advent of CCTA has confirmed this paradigm and extended it beyond the notion of obstructive plaque. As discussed in Chapters 4 and 9, the total burden of coronary atherosclerosis by CCTA, including obstructive and nonobstructive, is *the* key determinant of ASCVD risk.[49–51]

Whether identification of obstructive or nonobstructive coronary atherosclerosis with CCTA in patients with stable chest pain syndromes can improve outcomes relative to no CCTA or functional testing was the subject of two randomized controlled trials: the Scottish Computed Tomography of the Heart (SCOT-HEART) and the Prospective Multicenter Imaging Study for Evaluation of Chest Pain (PROMISE). Although there is some discrepancy in the overall findings of these studies, a meta-analysis found that, compared with usual care, CCTA reduced MI at the cost of an increase in the incidence of coronary revascularization.[52]

Among patients with diabetes, both SCOT-HEART and PROMISE showed favorable outcomes with CCTA over functional testing alone. In the SCOT-HEART trial, 4146 patients with chest pain were randomized to standard care, predominantly with exercise treadmill testing, with or without CCTA. In a subgroup study of 444 patients with diabetes who were followed over a 5-year period, there was a substantially lower rate of the primary endpoint of death from CHD or nonfatal MI in individuals who underwent CCTA (3.1%) relative to standard care (7.7%) (HR 0.36; 95% CI 0.15–0.87).[53]

The PROMISE trial, in contrast, randomized 10,003 symptomatic patients to CCTA or functional testing. In the functional testing group, nuclear stress imaging was used in two-thirds of patients. Although the overall results of the trial showed no significant difference between groups, in patients with diabetes (n = 1908) there was a significant reduction in the incidence of cardiovascular death or MI over a 2-year period with CCTA (1.1%) as compared with functional testing (2.6%), with an effect estimate nearly identical to that of the SCOT-HEART trial (HR 0.38; 95% CI 0.18–0.79; $P = 0.01$) (Fig. 16.6).[54,55]

Both studies showed that the use of CCTA in patients with stable chest pain symptoms leads to higher use of medical therapy capable of reducing atherosclerotic events. Among the subgroup of patients with diabetes in the PROMISE trial, the proportion of patients who were using statin medications 60 days after testing was higher in the CCTA group (65%) compared with the functional testing group (58%).[54] Even more importantly, CCTA allowed for a more *targeted* use of medical therapy, as treatment was more likely to be allocated to individuals with a higher burden of CAD. In the SCOT-HEART trial, preventive treatment was altered within 6 weeks of the initial visit in only 5% of patients in the standard care arm, whereas in the CCTA arm, 45% of those with nonobstructive or obstructive CAD had a modification in preventive therapy.[56] In patients with no evidence of CAD on CCTA, <1% had any modification in preventive therapy at the follow-up visit.[56]

Altogether, these data suggest that patients with diabetes and stable chest pain syndromes *without known CAD* may benefit from a testing strategy of CCTA over functional testing (Fig. 16.7). Such an approach can identify clinical or subclinical atherosclerosis and can lead to an intensification of preventive therapies and ultimately to a reduction in atherosclerotic cardiovascular events.

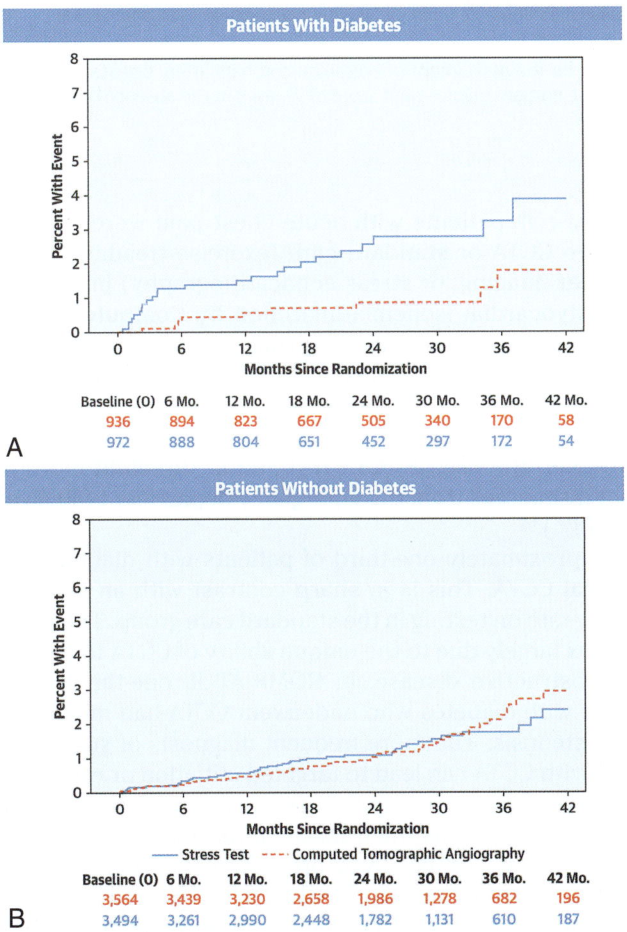

FIG. 16.6 Among 1908 patients with diabetes from the Prospective Multicenter Imaging Study for Evaluation of Chest Pain (PROMISE) trial, there was a significant reduction in the risk of cardiovascular death or myocardial infarction in those randomized to coronary CT angiography (CCTA) compared with functional stress testing (OR 0.38; 95% CI 0.18–0.79; $P = 0.01$), whereas there was no significant difference between both groups among patients without diabetes. (Reproduced from Sharma A, Coles A, Sekaran NK, et al. Stress testing versus CT angiography in patients with diabetes and suspected coronary artery disease. *J Am Coll Cardiol.* 2019;73:893–902.)

PLAQUE CHARACTERIZATION

In addition to the total burden of CAD, there are certain plaque characteristics that portent higher risk of atherosclerotic events (see Chapters 11 and 12). These features include (1) low-attenuation plaque, with a noncalcified component of <30 HU; (2) positive remodeling; (3) spotty calcifications; and (4) the napkin-ring sign, which consists of a peripheral rim of high attenuation around a central area of low-attenuation plaque. Notably, in the SCOT-HEART trial, the total burden of low-attenuation plaque was the strongest predictor of incident MI in patients with stable chest pain, even after adjustment for CAC score, severity of stenosis, and cardiovascular risk score.[57]

Patients with diabetes have a higher volume and progression of low-attenuation plaque on CCTA relative to individuals without diabetes, adjusted for risk factors and extent of baseline plaque burden.[58] These data correspond to findings from optical coherence tomography on invasive coronary angiography, demonstrating a higher prevalence of lipid-rich plaque and macrophage accumulation in both culprit and nonculprit plaques of patients with diabetes who develop acute coronary syndromes relative to patients without diabetes.[59] The inflammatory component of coronary atherosclerosis, as assessed by the novel CT marker of pericoronary fat attenuation (see Chapter 14), is also associated with the incidence of adverse cardiovascular events in patients with diabetes, after adjustment for stenosis and other features of high-risk plaque.[60]

The clinical applicability of these findings, however, still warrants further investigations. Whether any specific therapies or interventions are warranted based on findings of plaque inflammation or other high-risk features remains to be determined. Specifically, there are three challenges that relate to the implementation of therapies based on plaque characterization. First, high-risk plaque features have a low positive predictive value for identifying future events. In patients with diabetes followed for a median of 9.2 years, a culprit plaque event occurred in only 3.5% of plaques

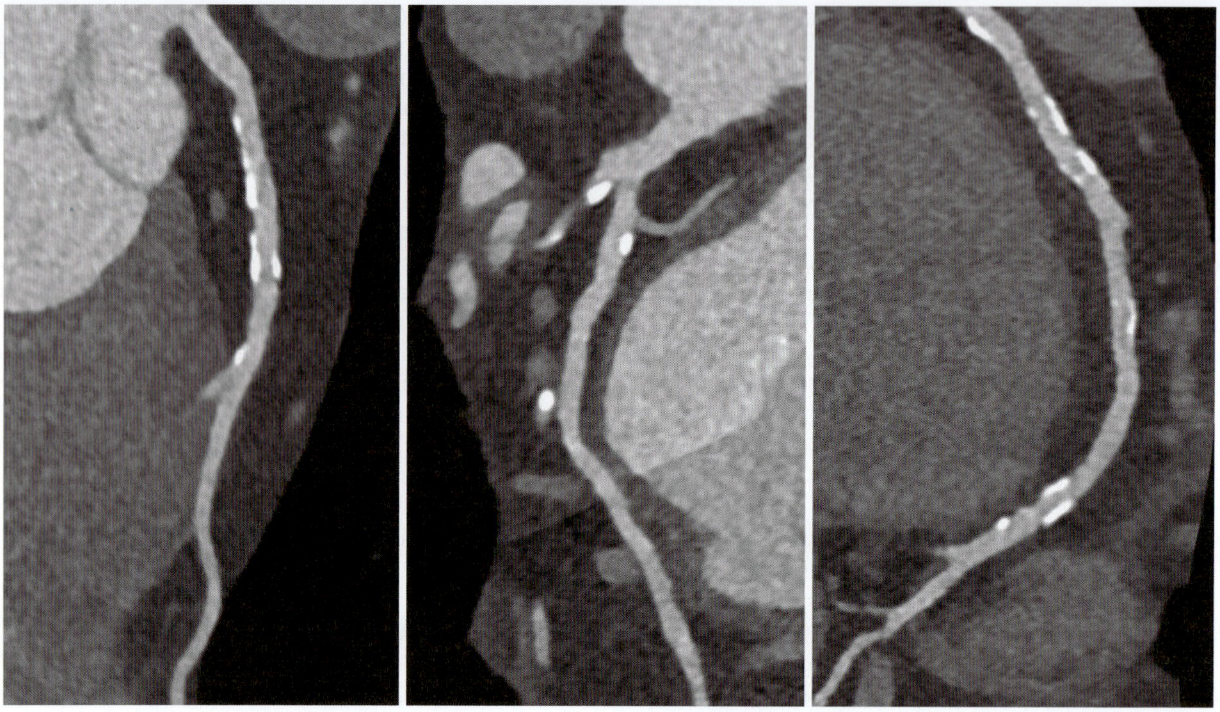

FIG. 16.7 In a 54-year-old man with diabetes and without known atherosclerotic disease presenting with chest pain suspicious for chronic coronary syndrome, coronary CT angiography (CCTA) may be preferred over functional imaging for the assessment of epicardial coronary artery disease, due to the evaluation of plaque burden with CCTA. The visualization of a severe amount of plaque (segment involvement score of 7), even in the absence of significant stenosis, has implications for preventive pharmacotherapies.

with two or more high-risk plaque features.[61] The second challenge is the mutability of high-risk plaque. Plaque characteristics are dynamic. In a study including patients with 425 high-risk plaque lesions who underwent repeat CCTA with an interval ≥2 years, 100 lesions (23.5%) had lost the features of high risk.[62] And, finally, most studies of high-risk plaque features have not adjusted for total plaque burden. In the SCOT-HEART trial, adverse plaque features were not independent of CHD death or MI when adjusted for CAC, which served as a measure of overall coronary plaque burden.[63]

Given these challenges and limited data for any specific interventions for high-risk plaque, how may clinicians use these findings when encountered in CCTA of patients with diabetes? For now, by providing high-intensity preventive therapies to this patient population, including both pharmacological therapy and lifestyle interventions. Patients with diabetes and high-risk plaque features on CCTA require the most aggressive preventive therapy.

CARDIAC CT USE IN PATIENTS WITH DIABETES AND LOW-RISK ACUTE CHEST PAIN

CCTA has also been studied in patients presenting acutely with chest pain. This includes those with low-risk chest pain, characterized by negative troponins and no definitive electrocardiographic changes of ischemia, and those with high-risk chest pain or confirmed acute coronary syndrome, with elevated biomarkers of cardiac injury or ischemic findings on electrocardiogram.

Low-risk patients with acute chest pain were randomized to CCTA or standard care (exercise treadmill study, nuclear imaging, or stress echocardiography) in the Rule Out Myocardial Ischemia/Infarction by Computer Assisted Tomography (ROMICAT II) trial.[64] When examining the 173 patients with diabetes in this trial, the median overall length of stay was similar between those who underwent CCTA (23.9 hours) versus standard care (27.2 hours). However, the use of CCTA resulted in threefold more direct discharges from the emergency department (40% versus 14%).[64]

Approximately one-third of patients with diabetes had normal CCTA. This is in sharp contrast with an 83% normalcy rate on testing in the standard care group. The difference is largely due to the unique ability of CCTA to identify nonobstructive disease. In ROMICAT II, one-third of patients with diabetes who underwent CCTA had minimal or mild stenosis. The more frequent diagnosis of subclinical CAD with CCTA can lead to targeted initiation or escalation of preventive therapy in this group, although it is still unknown whether this will translate into a reduction in future ASCVD events, especially as preventive therapies are often not implemented in this population.[65] This study suggests that, in individuals with diabetes and low-risk acute chest pain, CCTA can be used as a quick adjudicator of patients with (1) no coronary atherosclerosis; (2) minimal or mild disease, who would benefit from preventive therapy; (3) severe stenosis, who need invasive treatment in the context of acute chest pain; and (4) intermediate lesions, for whom additional workup may be considered, either with noninvasive functional testing or fractional flow reserve computed tomography (CT-FFR).[64]

CARDIAC CT USE IN PATIENTS WITH DIABETES AND HIGH-RISK ACUTE CHEST PAIN

The role of CCTA in patients with non-ST-segment elevation acute coronary syndrome (ACS) was studied in the Very Early Versus Deferred Invasive Evaluation Using Computerized Tomography in Patients with Acute Coronary Syndromes (VERDICT) trial. In this study, 1023 patients with a clinical suspicion of ACS with ischemic ECG changes and/or elevated troponin were randomized to either very early (≤12 hours) or standard (48–72 h) invasive coronary angiography. Both arms had a clinically blinded CCTA prior to invasive angiography. Among 130 patients with diabetes, the prevalence of ≥50% coronary stenosis on CCTA was 79%. Given the high prevalence of obstructive disease in this population of patients with diabetes and suspicion of ACS, the role of a noninvasive anatomic evaluation with CCTA is probably limited. Moreover, the negative predictive value was approximately 85%, which is also suboptimal. Therefore most of these patients may be better suited with invasive coronary angiography, not CCTA.[66]

SUMMARY AND FUTURE DIRECTIONS

Cardiac CT is a powerful tool for advanced stratification of cardiovascular risk and for diagnosis of CHD in patients with diabetes. In asymptomatic patients, cardiac CT can be used to identify individuals with an elevated CAC score, who may benefit from intense preventive pharmacotherapies and lifestyle interventions. In contrast, a substantial proportion of patients with diabetes have a CAC of 0, and these individuals are at lower risk of atherosclerotic events. If therapeutic decisions are made based on a CAC of 0, a follow-up test could be considered in 3 to 5 years, which is the average period of conversion to CAC >0 in patients with diabetes. Finally, in patients with diabetes who have anginal symptoms suggestive of chronic CHD or low-risk acute chest pain (i.e., negative biomarkers of cardiac injury and no ischemic ECG changes), CCTA is a robust diagnostic tool that can accurately identify coronary plaque and stenosis. The total plaque burden is a major determinant of the risk of future atherosclerotic adverse events. Future studies are warranted on how to incorporate information from coronary plaque characteristics and plaque burden for deciding on the role and intensity of preventive pharmacotherapies in this population.

REFERENCES

1. Lin X, Xu Y, Pan X, et al. Global, regional, and national burden and trend of diabetes in 195 countries and territories: an analysis from 1990 to 2025. *Sci Rep*. 2020;10:14790.
2. https://diabetesatlas.org/.
3. Einarson TR, Acs A, Ludwig C, Panton UH. Prevalence of cardiovascular disease in type 2 diabetes: a systematic literature review of scientific evidence from across the world in 2007–2017. *Cardiovasc Diabetol*. 2018;17:83.
4. Davenport MS, Khalatbari S, Dillman JR, Cohan RH, Caoili EM, Ellis JH. Contrast material-induced nephrotoxicity and intravenous low-osmolality iodinated contrast material. *Radiology*. 2013;267:94–105.
5. American College of Radiology. ACR Manual on Contrast Media. 2022. https://www.acr.org/-/media/ACR/files/clinical-resources/contrast_media.pdf.
6. McDonald JS, McDonald RJ, Carter RE, Katzberg RW, Kallmes DF, Williamson EE. Risk of intravenous contrast material-mediated acute kidney injury: a propensity score-matched study stratified by baseline-estimated glomerular filtration rate. *Radiology*. 2014;271:65–73.
7. Davenport MS, Khalatbari S, Cohan RH, Dillman JR, Myles JD, Ellis JH. Contrast material-induced nephrotoxicity and intravenous low-osmolality iodinated contrast material: risk stratification by using estimated glomerular filtration rate. *Radiology*. 2013;268:719–728.
8. Lazarus B, Wu A, Shin J-I, et al. Association of metformin use with risk of lactic acidosis across the range of kidney function: a community-based cohort study. *JAMA Intern Med*. 2018;178:903–910.
9. Haffner SM, Lehto S, Rönnemaa T, Pyörälä K, Laakso M. Mortality from coronary heart disease in subjects with type 2 diabetes and in nondiabetic subjects with and without prior myocardial infarction. *N Engl J Med*. 1998;339:229–234.
10. Bulugahapitiya U, Siyambalapitiya S, Sithole J, Idris I. Is diabetes a coronary risk equivalent? Systematic review and meta-analysis. *Diabet Med*. 2009;26:142–148.
11. Rawshani A, Rawshani A, Franzén S, et al. Risk factors, mortality, and cardiovascular outcomes in patients with type 2 diabetes. *N Engl J Med*. 2018;379:633–644.
12. Cardoso R, Blumenthal RS, Kopecky S, Lopez-Jimenez F, Martin SS. How low to go with lipid-lowering therapies in a cost-effective and prudent manner. *Mayo Clin Proc*. 2019;94:660–669.
13. Hecht H, Blaha MJ, Berman DS, et al. Clinical indications for coronary artery calcium scoring in asymptomatic patients: expert consensus statement from the society of cardiovascular computed tomography. *J Cardiovasc Comput Tomogr*. 2017;11:157–168.
14. Whelton PK, Carey RM, Aronow WS, et al. 2017 ACC/AHA/AAPA/ABC/ACPM/AGS/APhA/ASH/ASPC/NMA/PCNA Guideline for the prevention, detection, evaluation, and management of high blood pressure in adults: a report of the American College of Cardiology/American Heart Association task force on clinical practice guidelines. *J Am Coll Cardiol*. 2018;71:e127–e248.
15. Grundy SM, Stone NJ, Bailey AL, et al. 2018 AHA/ACC/AACVPR/AAPA/ABC/ACPM/ADA/AGS/APhA/ASPC/NLA/PCNA Guideline on the management of blood cholesterol: a report of the American College of Cardiology/American Heart Association task force on clinical practice guidelines. *Circulation*. 2019;139:e1082–e1143.
16. Arnett DK, Blumenthal RS, Albert MA, et al. 2019 ACC/AHA Guideline on the primary prevention of cardiovascular disease: a report of the American College of Cardiology/American Heart Association task force on clinical practice guidelines. *J Am Coll Cardiol*. 2019;74:e177–e232.
17. American Diabetes Association Professional Practice Committee. 10. Cardiovascular disease and risk management: standards of medical care in diabetes-2022. *Diabetes Care*. 2022;45:S144–S174.
18. Visseren FLJ, Mach F, Smulders YM, et al. 2021 ESC Guidelines on cardiovascular disease prevention in clinical practice. *Eur Heart J*. 2021;42:3227–3337.
19. Nasir K, Cainzos-Achirica M. Role of coronary artery calcium score in the primary prevention of cardiovascular disease. *BMJ*. 2021;373:n776.
20. Agarwal S, Cox AJ, Herrington DM, et al. Coronary calcium score predicts cardiovascular mortality in diabetes: diabetes heart study. *Diabetes Care*. 2013;36:972–977.
21. Elkeles RS, Godsland IF, Feher MD, et al. Coronary calcium measurement improves prediction of cardiovascular events in asymptomatic patients with type 2 diabetes: the predict study. *Eur Heart J*. 2008;29:2244–2251.
22. Malik S, Zhao Y, Budoff M, et al. Coronary artery calcium score for long-term risk classification in individuals with type 2 diabetes and metabolic syndrome from the multi-ethnic study of atherosclerosis. *JAMA Cardiol*. 2017;2:1332–1340.
23. Marso SP, Bain SC, Consoli A, et al. Semaglutide and cardiovascular outcomes in patients with type 2 diabetes. *N Engl J Med*. 2016;375:1834–1844.
24. Valenti V, Hartaigh BÓ, Cho I, et al. Absence of coronary artery calcium identifies asymptomatic diabetic individuals at low near-term but not long-term risk of mortality: a 15-year follow-up study of 9715 patients. *Circ Cardiovasc Imaging*. 2016;9:e003528.
25. Mitchell JD, Fergestrom N, Gage BF, et al. Impact of statins on cardiovascular outcomes following coronary artery calcium scoring. *J Am Coll Cardiol*. 2018;72:3233–3242.
26. Kowall B, Lehmann N, Mahabadi A-A, et al. Progression of coronary artery calcification is stronger in poorly than in well controlled diabetes: results from the heinz nixdorf recall study. *J Diabetes Complications*. 2017;31:234–240.
27. Barrett T, Jalaludin MY, Turan S, Hafez M, Shehadeh N. Novo Nordisk Pediatric Type 2 Diabetes Global Expert Panel. Rapid progression of type 2 diabetes and related complications in children and young people—a literature review. *Pediatr Diabetes*. 2020;21:158–172.
28. Nezarat N, Budoff MJ, Luo Y, et al. Presence, characteristics, and volumes of coronary plaque determined by computed tomography angiography in young type 2 diabetes mellitus. *Am J Cardiol*. 2017;119:1566–1571.
29. Budoff M, Backlund J-YC, Bluemke DA, et al. The association of coronary artery calcification with subsequent incidence of cardiovascular disease in type 1 diabetes: the DCCT/EDIC trials. *JACC Cardiovasc Imaging*. 2019;12:1341–1349.
30. Osei AD, Uddin SMI, Dzaye O, et al. Predictors of coronary artery calcium among 20-30-year-olds: the coronary artery calcium consortium. *Atherosclerosis*. 2020;301:65–68.
31. Mortensen MB, Dzaye O, Bødtker H, et al. Interplay of risk factors and coronary artery calcium for CHD risk in young patients. *JACC Cardiovasc Imaging*. 2021;14:2387–2396.
32. Miedema MD, Dardari ZA, Nasir K, et al. Association of coronary artery calcium with long-term, cause-specific mortality among young adults. *JAMA Netw Open*. 2019;2:e197440.

33. Dzaye O, Dardari ZA, Cainzos-Achirica M, et al. Warranty period of a calcium score of zero: comprehensive analysis from MESA. *JACC Cardiovasc Imaging.* 2021;14:990–1002.
34. Budoff MJ, Young R, Lopez VA, et al. Progression of coronary calcium and incident coronary heart disease events: MESA (Multi-Ethnic Study of Atherosclerosis). *J Am Coll Cardiol.* 2013;61:1231–1239.
35. Paixao ARM, Chakravorty R, Khera A, et al. Disagreement between different definitions of coronary artery calcium progression. *JACC Cardiovasc Imaging.* 2015;8:743–744.
36. Study Collaborative Group ASCEND, Bowman L, Mafham M, et al. Effects of aspirin for primary prevention in persons with diabetes mellitus. *N Engl J Med.* 2018;379:1529–1539.
37. Ajufo E, Ayers CR, Vigen R, et al. Value of coronary artery calcium scanning in association with the net benefit of aspirin in primary prevention of atherosclerotic cardiovascular disease. *JAMA Cardiol.* 2021;6:179–187.
38. Cainzos-Achirica M, Miedema MD, McEvoy JW, et al. Coronary artery calcium for personalized allocation of aspirin in primary prevention of cardiovascular disease in 2019: the MESA study (Multi-Ethnic Study of Atherosclerosis). *Circulation.* 2020;141:1541–1553.
39. Cardoso R, Dudum R, Ferraro RA, et al. Cardiac computed tomography for personalized management of patients with type 2 diabetes mellitus. *Circ Cardiovasc Imaging.* 2020;13:e011365.
40. https://www.clinicaltrials.gov/ct2/show/NCT03872401.
41. Zelniker TA, Wiviott SD, Raz I, et al. SGLT2 Inhibitors for primary and secondary prevention of cardiovascular and renal outcomes in type 2 diabetes: a systematic review and meta-analysis of cardiovascular outcome trials. *Lancet.* 2019;393:31–39.
42. Cainzos-Achirica M, Patel KV, Quispe R, et al. Coronary artery calcium for the allocation of GLP-1RA for primary prevention of atherosclerotic cardiovascular disease. *JACC Cardiovasc Imaging.* 2021;14:1470–1472.
43. Park G-M, Lee J-H, Lee S-W, et al. Comparison of coronary computed tomographic angiographic findings in asymptomatic subjects with versus without diabetes mellitus. *Am J Cardiol.* 2015;116:372–378.
44. Min JK, Labounty TM, Gomez MJ, et al. Incremental prognostic value of coronary computed tomographic angiography over coronary artery calcium score for risk prediction of major adverse cardiac events in asymptomatic diabetic individuals. *Atherosclerosis.* 2014;232:298–304.
45. Kang SH, Park G-M, Lee S-W, et al. Long-term prognostic value of coronary CT angiography in asymptomatic type 2 diabetes mellitus. *JACC Cardiovasc Imaging.* 2016;9:1292–1300.
46. Muhlestein JB, Lappé DL, Lima JAC, et al. Effect of screening for coronary artery disease using CT angiography on mortality and cardiac events in high-risk patients with diabetes: the FACTOR-64 randomized clinical trial. *JAMA.* 2014;312:2234–2243.
47. https://clinicaltrials.gov/ct2/show/NCT03920176. https://www.nature.com/articles/s41598-020-71908-9.pdf.
48. Fihn SD, Gardin JM, Abrams J, et al. 2012 ACCF/AHA/ACP/AATS/PCNA/SCAI/STS Guideline for the diagnosis and management of patients with stable ischemic heart disease: a report of the American College of Cardiology Foundation/American Heart Association task force on practice guidelines, and the American College of Physicians, American Association for Thoracic Surgery, preventive cardiovascular nurses association, society for cardiovascular angiography and interventions, and society of thoracic surgeons. *J Am Coll Cardiol.* 2012;60:e44–e164.
49. Shaw LJ, Blankstein R, Bax JJ, et al. Society of cardiovascular computed Tomography/North American society of cardiovascular imaging - expert consensus document on coronary CT imaging of atherosclerotic plaque. *J Cardiovasc Comput Tomogr.* 2021;15:93–109.
50. Bittencourt MS, Hulten E, Ghoshhajra B, et al. Prognostic value of nonobstructive and obstructive coronary artery disease detected by coronary computed tomography angiography to identify cardiovascular events. *Circ Cardiovasc Imaging.* 2014;7:282–291.
51. Mortensen MB, Dzaye O, Steffensen FH, et al. Impact of plaque burden versus stenosis on ischemic events in patients with coronary atherosclerosis. *J Am Coll Cardiol.* 2020;76:2803–2813.
52. Bittencourt MS, Hulten EA, Murthy VL, et al. Clinical outcomes after evaluation of stable chest pain by coronary computed tomographic angiography versus usual care: a meta-analysis. *Circ Cardiovasc Imaging.* 2016;9:e004419.
53. Scot-Heart InvestigatorsNewby DE, Adamson PD, et al. Coronary CT angiography and 5-year risk of myocardial infarction. *N Engl J Med.* 2018;379:924–933.
54. Sharma A, Coles A, Sekaran NK, et al. Stress testing versus CT angiography in patients with diabetes and suspected coronary artery disease. *J Am Coll Cardiol.* 2019;73:893–902.
55. Douglas PS, Hoffmann U, Patel MR, et al. Outcomes of anatomical versus functional testing for coronary artery disease. *N Engl J Med.* 2015;372:1291–1300.
56. Adamson PD, Williams MC, Dweck MR, et al. Guiding therapy by coronary CT angiography improves outcomes in patients with stable chest pain. *J Am Coll Cardiol.* 2019;74:2058–2070.
57. Williams MC, Kwiecinski J, Doris M, et al. Low-attenuation noncalcified plaque on coronary computed tomography angiography predicts myocardial infarction: results from the multicenter scot-heart trial (Scottish Computed Tomography of the HEART). *Circulation.* 2020;141:1452–1462.
58. Lakshmanan S, Budoff MJ. Effect of diabetes mellitus on coronary plaque characteristics and progression by serial Coronary Computed Tomography Angiography (CCTA). https://academic.oup.com/eurheartj/article/42/Supplement_1/ehab724.0162/6392426.
59. Sugiyama T, Yamamoto E, Bryniarski K, et al. Coronary plaque characteristics in patients with diabetes mellitus who presented with acute coronary syndromes. *J Am Heart Assoc.* 2018;7:e009245.
60. Ichikawa K, Miyoshi T, Osawa K, et al. High pericoronary adipose tissue attenuation on computed tomography angiography predicts cardiovascular events in patients with type 2 diabetes mellitus: post-hoc analysis from a prospective cohort study. *Cardiovasc Diabetol.* 2022;21:44.
61. Halon DA, Lavi I, Barnett-Griness O, et al. Plaque morphology as predictor of late plaque events in patients with asymptomatic type 2 diabetes: a long-term observational study. *JACC Cardiovasc Imaging.* 2019;12:1353–1363.
62. Lee S-E, Sung JM, Andreini D, et al. Differences in progression to obstructive lesions per high-risk plaque features and plaque volumes with CCTA. *JACC Cardiovasc Imaging.* 2020;13:1409–1417.
63. Williams MC, Moss AJ, Dweck M, et al. Coronary artery plaque characteristics associated with adverse outcomes in the scot-heart study. *J Am Coll Cardiol.* 2019;73:291–301.
64. Truong QA, Schulman-Marcus J, Zakroysky P, et al. Coronary CT angiography versus standard emergency department evaluation for acute chest pain and diabetic patients: is there benefit with early coronary CT angiography? Results of the randomized comparative effectiveness Romicat II trial. *J Am Heart Assoc.* 2016;5:e003137.
65. Honigberg MC, Lander BS, Baliyan V, et al. Preventive management of nonobstructive CAD after coronary CT angiography in the emergency department. *JACC Cardiovasc Imaging.* 2020;13:437–448.
66. Linde JJ, Kelbæk H, Hansen TF, et al. Coronary CT angiography in patients with non-ST-segment elevation acute coronary syndrome. *J Am Coll Cardiol.* 2020;75:453–463.

17 CCTA in Chronic Inflammatory Diseases

NIDHI H. PATEL AND NEHAL N. MEHTA

KEY POINTS

- Chronic inflammatory diseases such as systemic lupus erythematosus (SLE), rheumatoid arthritis (RA), psoriasis, and human immunodeficiency virus (HIV) heighten the risk of cardiometabolic diseases such as diabetes, high-risk coronary artery disease, myocardial infarction, and stroke.
- Large studies reveal the residual risk of inflammation on cardiovascular disease beyond traditional risk factors. Targeted studies in those with chronic inflammatory disease show antiinflammatory therapies influence plaque characteristics assessed on CCTA.
- Integrating CCTA into care for patients with chronic inflammatory disease offers avenues to identify vulnerable plaques, understand pathophysiology of inflammation of cardiometabolic disease, and assess treatment response.

INTRODUCTION

Systemic inflammation is a well-known contributor to development of atherosclerosis. Chronic inflammatory diseases in humans confer an increased risk of cardiovascular diseases including myocardial infarction, stroke, and accelerated development of high-risk, rupture-prone coronary plaques. Coronary computed tomography angiography (CCTA) has aided in the identification of such plaques to better understand pathophysiology and treatment options to guide mitigating this risk in clinical practice. This chapter will cover chronic inflammatory diseases and how CCTA-associated technologies have evolved our understanding of inflammatory atherogenesis.

EPIDEMIOLOGY

Chronic inflammatory disease states such as systemic lupus erythematosus (SLE), rheumatoid arthritis (RA), psoriasis, and human immunodeficiency virus (HIV) account for 3% to 7% of the population and are associated with increased cardiovascular morbidity and mortality.[1,2] Patients with these conditions develop cardiovascular disease almost a decade earlier than the general population and are at increased risk for myocardial infarction, cerebrovascular events, and heart failure. For example, patients with HIV are twice as likely to develop cardiovascular disease or have a myocardial infarction (MI)[3] and three times as likely to suffer a stroke[4] compared with the general population. Some studies estimate patients with these conditions have a decreased life expectancy of 6 to 10 years.[5,6] Excessive immune activation in these conditions also predisposes patients to cardiometabolic disease including dyslipidemia, metabolic syndrome, and obesity. The interplay between systemic inflammation and cardiometabolic disease is thought to accelerate atherosclerosis and coronary disease in these diseases.

ATHEROSCLEROSIS AND INFLAMMATION

Inflammation is critical in the initiation and progression of all stages of atherosclerosis.[7] Atherogenesis is thought to begin when lipoproteins (e.g., low-density lipoproteins [LDL] and very-low-density lipoproteins [VLDL]) accumulate in the subendothelial space and undergo oxidation. The presence of inflammation increases the uptake of these oxidized lipids into macrophages, leading to formation of foamy, lipid-laden macrophages that compromise the plaque core. Oxidized lipids are also atherogenic and further induce the expression of proinflammatory cytokines, chemokines, and adhesion molecules.[7] Adhesion molecules allow leukocytes, which normally cannot attach to the endothelial wall, to attach and further propagate inflammation. Increased inflammatory signaling within the atheroma then leads to migration of leukocytes into the intima, recruitment of circulating monocytes and neutrophils, and interaction between these cell types to promote plaque formation.[8] The growing plaque is prone to rupture and can interrupt coronary blood flow, resulting in myocardial infarction.

Chronic inflammatory diseases like psoriasis (Fig. 17.1) heighten all stages of the atherosclerotic process. Metabolic derangement and dyslipidemia associated with these diseases contribute to increased oxidation of lipids and decrease the atheroprotective function of high-density lipoprotein (HDL).[9,10] Endothelial dysfunction leads to vascular injury and increased infiltration of immune cells in the intima.[7] Systemic inflammation upregulates proinflammatory mediators within the plaque and vessel wall contributing to accelerated plaque development.[11] Given that chronic inflammatory diseases and atherogenesis share several common pathways, studying these diseases has enhanced our pathophysiological understanding of atherosclerosis.

RESIDUAL INFLAMMATORY RISK: PRIMARY AND SECONDARY PREVENTION TRIALS

Several large studies in the general population underscore the residual risk of inflammation on cardiovascular disease (CVD) beyond traditional risk factors and hyperlipidemia. The Anti-inflammatory Therapy with Canakinumab for Atherosclerotic disease (CANTOS)[11] trial in 2017 provided first proof of concept that inhibiting inflammation reduces

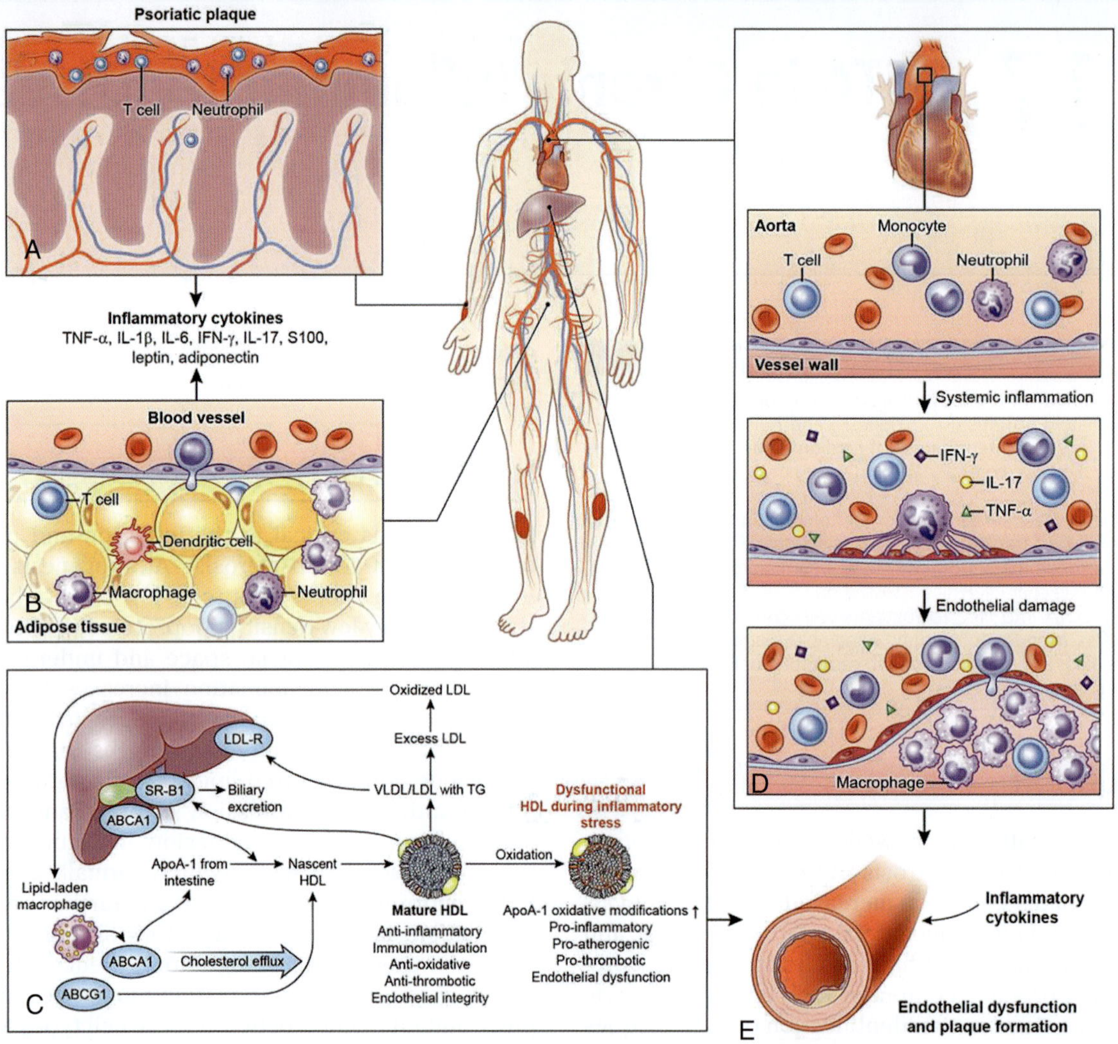

FIG. 17.1 Systemic effects of chronic low-grade inflammation in psoriasis. (A) Psoriasis is associated with increased circulating proinflammatory cytokines. (B) Chronic inflammation is associated with adipose tissue dysfunction characterized by proinflammatory cytokines and adipokines associated with endothelial dysfunction. (C) Psoriasis exhibits a deranged lipid profile and impaired HDL function, which in combination with chronic inflammation accelerate atherosclerotic vascular disease. (D) The vessel wall is infiltrated through a complex interplay of proinflammatory cellular components, cholesterol crystals, and various lipoproteins. (E) Psoriasis and upregulates T-cell, neutrophil chemotaxis, and keratinocyte activation and endothelial dysfunction leading to increased atherosclerosis in blood vessels. *IL*, Interleukin; *IFN-γ*, interferon-gamma; *TNF-α*, tumor necrosis factor-alpha. (From Sajja AP, Joshi AA, Teague HL, Dey AK, Mehta NN. Potential immunological links between psoriasis and cardiovascular disease. *Front Immunol*. 2018;9:4.)[78]

rates of major adverse cardiovascular events (MACE) in the absence of lipid-lowering effects. Patients with previous myocardial infarction were randomized to receive canakinumab, a biologic targeting interleukin-1β used in rheumatologic disease, or placebo, and those receiving canakinumab were found to have significantly lower rates of MACE in the absence of changes in LDL. These findings highlight the important contribution of inflammation to cardiovascular disease and suggest this risk can be modified by targeting specific inflammatory pathways.

Other studies have focused on effects of lowering high-sensitivity C-reactive protein (hs-CRP), a marker of systemic inflammation. A primary prevention study, Rosuvastatin to Prevent Vascular Events in Men and Women with Elevated C-Reactive Protein (JUPITER),[12] found that in those without marked hyperlipidemia but elevated hs-CRP, statin therapy reduced MACE by 44% and mortality by 20%.[12] The Evolocumab and Clinical Outcomes in Patients with Cardiovascular disease (FOURIER)[13] and the Cardiovascular Efficacy and Safety of Bococizumab in High-Risk Patients (SPIRE)[14] trials similarly found hs-CRP to be a strong predictor of future MACE despite LDL-C levels as low as 20 to 30 mg/dl while on treatment with both high-intensity statins and PCSK9 (proprotein convertase subtilisin/kexin type 9) inhibitors.

Recently, two large RCTs found colchicine, a medication that attenuates inflammation, effectively reduced risk of MACE in chronic atherosclerosis[15] and lowered risk of ischemic cardiovascular events after myocardial infarction.[16] In response, some physicians have already begun prescribing colchicine to certain high-risk individuals. Though these studies have been done in the general population, they highlight the importance of improving risk stratification and preventive treatments in those with high inflammatory burden, such as patients with chronic inflammatory disease. CCTA is now widely available and can provide anatomical, functional, and dynamic assessment to aid in identifying the vulnerable patient at risk for MACE.[17] Integration of CCTA into clinical care for patients with chronic

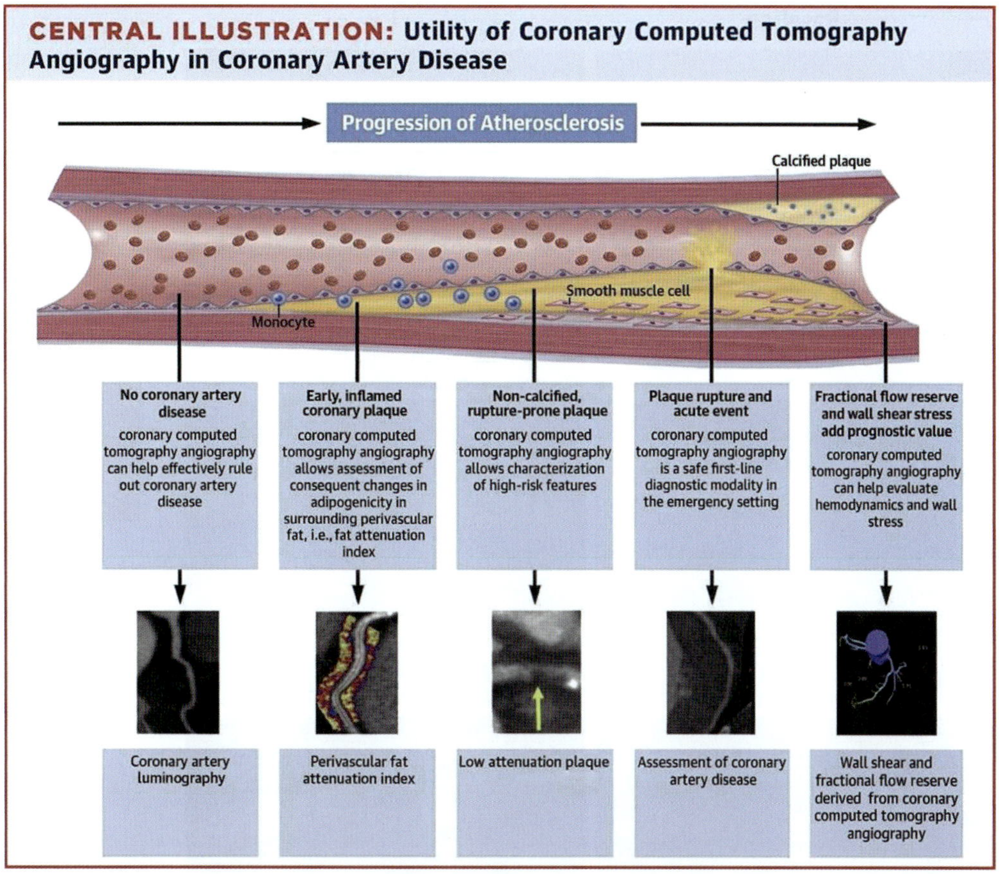

FIG. 17.2 Utility of coronary computed tomography angiography in coronary artery disease. Coronary computed tomography angiography is a powerful clinical tool that can be used to detect and characterize coronary artery disease across various stages from early, subclinical disease to myocardial infarction. (From Abdelrahman KM, Chen MY, Dey AK, et al. Coronary computed tomography angiography from clinical uses to emerging technologies: JACC state-of-the-art review. *J Am Coll Cardiol*. 2020;76:1226–1243.)

inflammatory disease may open new avenues to understand, diagnose, and manage cardiovascular disease.

CURRENT GUIDELINES

It is well known that current risk estimators, including 10-year atherosclerotic cardiovascular disease (ASCVD) and the Framingham Risk Score (FRS), underestimate cardiovascular risk in patients with chronic inflammatory disease.[18] In fact, at the time of MI patients with chronic inflammatory disease have similar ASCVD scores to asymptomatic healthy patients and would not qualify for primary prevention statin therapy based on current guidelines.[19] The American College of Cardiology/American Heart Association (ACC/AHA) 2019 guidelines on primary prevention acknowledge chronic inflammatory diseases as "risk enhancers" for initiating or escalating statin therapy.[20] In those individuals with intermediate risk, where there is clinical uncertainty about statin initiation, further testing to determine presence or extent of subclinical coronary artery disease (CAD) is warranted. Current guidelines recommend using noncontrast coronary artery calcium score (CAC) to document subclinical disease (see Chapter 3, Coronary Artery Calcium Testing: Indications and Patient Management). However, several studies have shown patients with CAC of 0 can have noncalcified plaque, which in some scenarios may represent a higher-risk plaque that is less stable, develops earlier, and is more prone to rupture.[21] For example, in one study conducted in patients with HIV, among those who had CAC of zero, 56% had noncalcified plaque.[22] The ACC/AHA guidelines support these findings by cautioning a CAC of zero may not rule out subclinical noncalcified disease.[20,23]

CAC is a well-established marker of atherosclerotic burden, strongly predicts MACE in the general population, and has been shown to be increased in multiple chronic inflammatory states. However, CAC captures a later stage of atherosclerosis after plaque has already formed. In addition, statin therapy duration increases CAC, making CAC difficult to interpret over time after treatment initiation.[24] CCTA may provide prognostic information over CAC by capturing changes around and in the coronary lumen before overt plaque is recognized (Fig. 17.2). Expanded CCTA-based technologies now also allow CAD characterization in multiple stages of atherosclerosis as well as serial assessment in response to treatment.[17] In patients with chronic inflammatory disease with an accelerated atherosclerotic risk, CCTA may identify potentially intervenable disease before CAC.

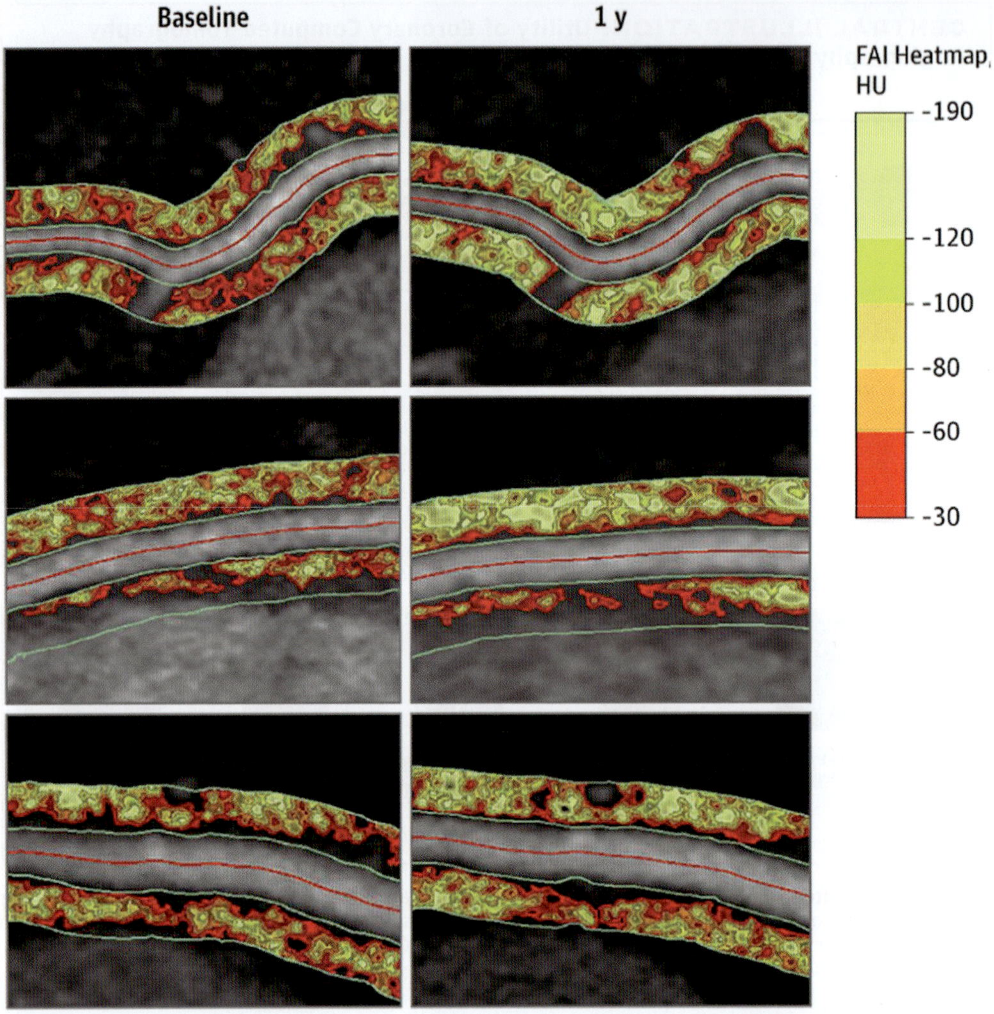

FIG. 17.3 Change in FAI over 1 year after initiation of biologic therapy in patients with psoriasis B. Coronary computed tomography (CT) angiography images of the coronary arteries depicting the perivascular FAI before and after biologic therapy at 1 year of follow-up for patients with excellent response (*top*), moderate response (*middle*), and modest response (*bottom*) to biologic therapy. *FAI*, Perivascular fat attenuation index; *HU*, Hounsfield units. (From Elnabawi YA, Oikonomou EK, Dey AK, et al. Association of biologic therapy with coronary inflammation in patients with psoriasis as assessed by perivascular fat attenuation index. *JAMA Cardiol*. 2019;4:885–891.)

CCTA: FROM EARLY INFLAMMATION TO MYOCARDIAL INJURY

In the past several years, research and clinical applications of CCTA have moved beyond assessing coronary stenosis and instead have focused on comprehensive plaque evaluation.[25,26] Indeed, the presence and extent of nonobstructive disease, compared with no coronary disease, has been associated with a significantly higher risk of 1 year MI and mortality.[27] In addition, CCTA technologies can now identify plaques that are at the highest risk of rupture, assess changes in plaque volume over time, and calculate functional implications of early nonobstructive disease (see Chapter 11, Approaches to Plaque Imaging by CCTA). Several of these technologies have been studied in those with chronic inflammatory disease and are promising techniques for better risk stratifying these populations.

Perivascular Fat Attenuation Index

The perivascular fat attenuation index (FAI) is a novel method for assessing coronary inflammation using CCTA. Inflammation in the coronary arteries drives changes in the composition of surrounding perivascular adipose tissue (PVAT).[28] PVAT is a metabolically active tissue that interacts bidirectionally with the vascular wall and may become dysfunctional in states of chronic inflammation like obesity.[29] Changes in PVAT can be quantified by analyzing three-dimensional gradients of attenuation to calculate the FAI (see Chapter 14, Evaluating Coronary inflammation Using the Fat Attenuation Index). Increased FAI has been associated with cardiac mortality, suggesting early inflammation in the coronary vessels may be a good predictor of MACE.[28] Importantly, FAI can be modified with antiinflammatory treatments in chronic inflammatory states.[30] In psoriasis, one observational study found patients started on systemic biologic therapy had significant reduction in their FAI over 1 year compared with those on topical or light therapy (Fig. 17.3).[30] These findings suggest FAI by CCTA may aid in identifying high-risk patients with chronic inflammation and guide initiation and intensity of treatment. Importantly, response to treatment could also be identified by changes in FAI in just 1 year and allow for personalized risk assessment. Though these findings are promising, larger studies across multiple chronic inflammatory diseases are still needed.

Noncalcified Burden and High-risk Plaque Features

Earlier stages of atherogenesis, prior to calcified plaque formation, include development of noncalcified plaque. Plaques that have noncalcified plaque may be more unstable and are associated with a higher risk of myocardial infarction. RA, SLE, psoriasis, and HIV all have increased prevalence of noncalcified plaque,[31] which may in part explain the increased risk of cardiovascular risk in these diseases. Accordingly, efforts in chronic inflammatory diseases have focused on capturing early atherosclerotic risk, including using the noncalcified burden (NCB) (see Chapter 12, Plaque on CCTA: Lessons from Histology). NCB is derived using quantification of coronary plaque and has been demonstrated to correlate with intravascular ultrasound.[32] In chronic inflammatory diseases, NCB has been used in comparative studies to compare these diseases to general and at-risk populations. For example, we know that patients with psoriasis have a higher NCB.[33] People living with HIV have a two- to threefold increase in NCB compared to those without HIV.[34] NCB can also be used as a surrogate endpoint to understand pathogenesis and progression of atherosclerosis in these diseases. For example, in patients with SLE association of neutrophil subsets with NCB supports the hypothesis that neutrophil subsets contribute to early unstable coronary plaque.[35] Other translational studies using CCTA as an endpoint are discussed in detail later in the chapter.

Importantly, NCB has also been used as an endpoint to assess response to antiinflammatory treatment. In patients with severe psoriasis, NCB quantification before and after 1 year of biologic therapy initiation revealed systemic biologic therapy significantly reduced NCB (Fig. 17.4).[36] Though larger studies are needed, these findings suggest early modulation of inflammation may decrease coronary disease burden in these patients. Studies in other chronic inflammatory diseases are discussed later in the chapter. With the continued development of semiautomatic plaque quantification on CCTA, serial assessment of coronary plaque before and after intervention may ultimately help guide personalized therapy.

Beyond NCB, several high-risk plaque features can be identified on CCTA including low-attenuation plaque (<30 Hounsfield units), positive remodeling index (remodeling index >1.1), napkin-ring sign, and spotty calcifications (see Chapter 11, Approaches to Plaque Imaging by CCTA). Among the various high-risk plaque features, low-attenuation plaque has a strong association with fatal and nonfatal myocardial infarction that is incremental to CAC and the presence of coronary obstruction.[37] The Scottish Computed Tomography of the HEART (SCOT-HEART) study suggests patients with >4% of low-attenuation plaque are five times as likely to have a myocardial infarction. The implications for patients with SLE,[38] RA,[39] psoriasis,[33] and HIV[40]—all cohorts who may have a higher burden of low-attenuation plaque on CCTA compared to the general population—are significant.[38] In patients with RA, initiating biologic disease-modifying medications have been associated with over 70% lower long-term CVD risk in those with low-attenuation plaque at baseline.[41] Identifying presence of these plaques on CCTA could influence clinical decision-making in pursuing more aggressive preventive treatments earlier on.

Lipid-rich Necrotic Core

Lipid-rich necrotic core (LRNC) is the histopathologic correlate of low-attenuation plaque,[42] which can be visualized and quantified using CCTA.[43] Excessive inflammation increases plaque stability by increasing necrosis of foamy lipid laden macrophages that compromise the core.[44] In psoriasis, LRNC was quantified at baseline and at 1 year for participants started on systemic biologic therapy and patients on topical or light therapy.[43] LRNC not only correlated with cardiovascular risk factors including male sex and hypertension, but also significantly decreased over 1 year in patients started on biologic therapy (Fig. 17.5).[43] These findings suggest high-risk plaque could be reversed in the coronary arteries. Out of all chronic inflammatory diseases, LRNC has only been explored in psoriasis patients but could be quantified in other inflammatory diseases with existing CCTA technology.

Fractional Flow Reserve

Beyond anatomical visualization and plaque quantification, FFR by CCTA (FFR_{CT}) now provides functional assessment of the coronaries and has high accuracy of assessing coronary blood flow (*see* Chapter 13, CT-FFR: Current Clinical Evidence and Limitations).[45] Using computational fluid dynamics, FFR_{CT} estimates the coronary blood carrying capacity compared to myocardial tissue demand and is estimated by the coronary artery volume to myocardial mass ratio (V/M). In asymptomatic patients with psoriasis, V/M is reduced. Those with more severe psoriasis have been shown to have lower V/M after adjusting for traditional risk factors. These findings may be explained by endothelial dysfunction in early psoriasis and give insight into how early nonobstructive disease can impair coronary flow.[46] Another study found lower FFR_{CT} in psoriasis was associated with high NCB and those with low FFR_{CT} (≤0.80) had over a 2.5 higher chance of having positive high-sensitivity troponin after adjusting for age, sex, hypertension, hyperlipidemia, waist–hip ratio, lipid therapy, left ventricular hypertrophy, and presence of coronary plaque.[46] These findings suggest chronic inflammation drives early vascular disease and potentially contributes to myocardial injury prior to clinical manifestations. No studies in SLE, RA, or HIV have been done assessing FFR_{CT}; however, one study using PET perfusion found patients with RA had similar impaired coronary flow reserve to those with diabetes.[47] Additional studies in other chronic inflammatory diseases are needed to evaluate coronary microvascular dysfunction. Importantly, a recent study found FFR_{CT} to be significantly more accurate than single-photon emission computerized tomography (SPECT), positron emission tomography (PET), and CCTA in predicting abnormal invasive FFR,[48] supporting the role of combining functional assessment by FFR_{CT} and anatomical assessment by CCTA.

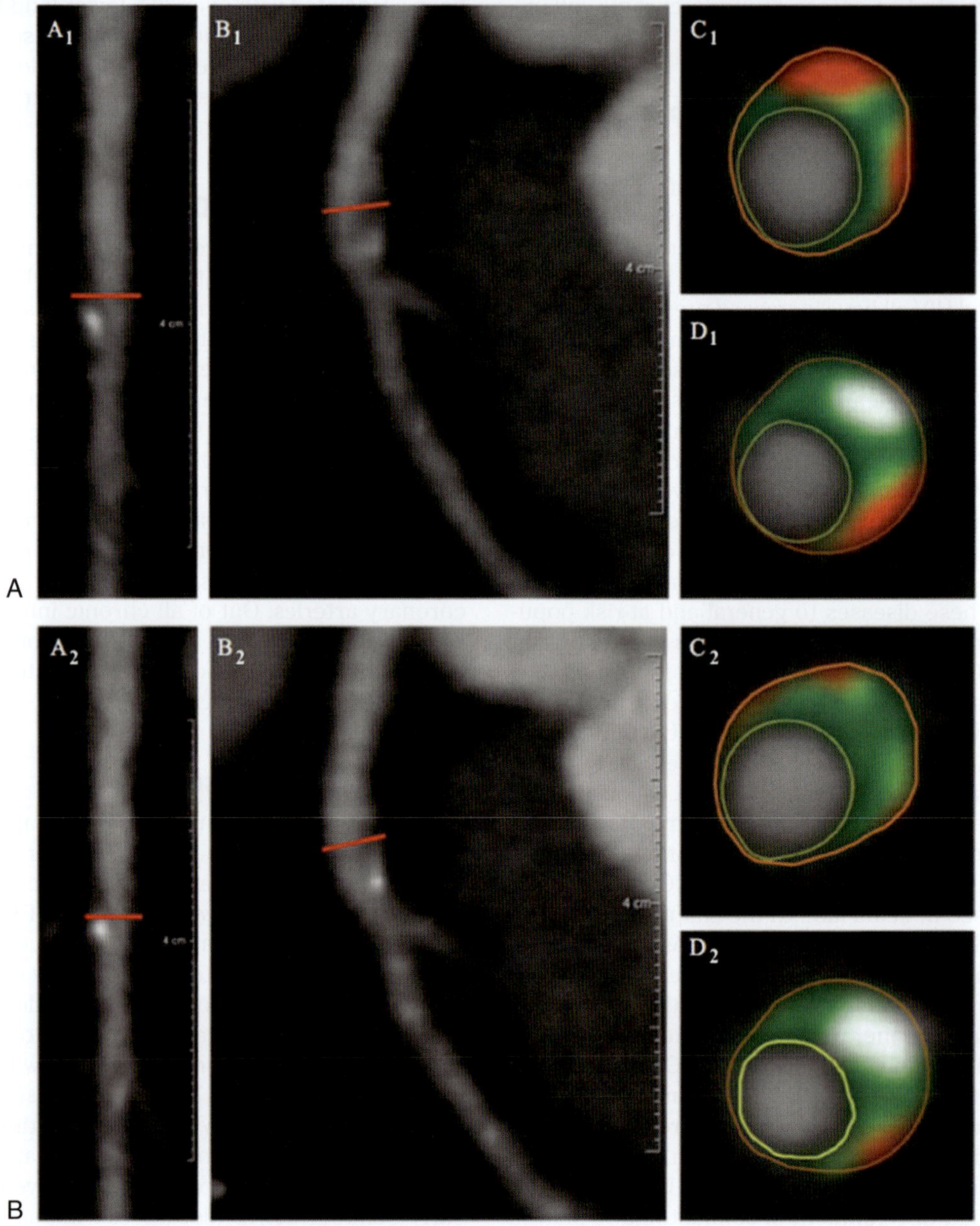

FIG. 17.4 Left anterior descending artery plaque identified before (A) and after (B) biologic therapy. (A) Longitudinal planar and (B) curved planar reformat. (C and D) Representative cross-sectional views with color overlay for plaque subcomponents. Lumen is encircled in *yellow*, vessel wall in *orange* with subcomponents in between, including fibrous (*dark green*), fibro-fatty (*light green*), necrotic (*red*), and dense-calcified (*white*). (B and A) Longitudinal planar and (B) curved planar reformat. (C and D) Representative cross-sectional views with color overlay for plaque subcomponents. Lumen is encircled in *yellow*, vessel wall in *orange* with subcomponents in between, including fibrous (*dark green*), fibro-fatty (*light green*), necrotic (*red*), and dense-calcified (*white*). (From Elnabawi YA, Dey AK, Goyal A, et al. Coronary artery plaque characteristics and treatment with biologic therapy in severe psoriasis: results from a prospective observational study. *Cardiovasc Res*. 2019;115:721–728.)

Wall Shear Stress

Given the heterogenous nature of plaques, it is difficult to determine whether a plaque will progress, resolve, or be stable over time. Disrupted blood flow in arterial branch points is thought to contribute to preferential development of atherosclerotic lesions in these regions. Wall shear stress (WSS) can be used to determine the friction on the vascular endothelium from coronary blood flow. Preclinical studies suggest WSS is atherogenic by promoting inflammation in the artery wall.[49] WSS has traditionally been derived from invasive coronary angiography (the gold standard for assessing WSS) and now can be derived using CCTA, though validation studies are lacking. Importantly, in one small study in patients with stable CAD, higher WSS in the proximal segments of atherosclerotic lesions was significantly better at predicting MI than FFR.[50] Future studies in chronic inflammatory studies using CCTA could assess if differential WSS contributes to early plaque development in these patients.

Beyond the Coronaries: Epicardial Fat

Noncontrast CCTA can be used to quantify epicardial adipose tissue (EAT), a metabolically active tissue between

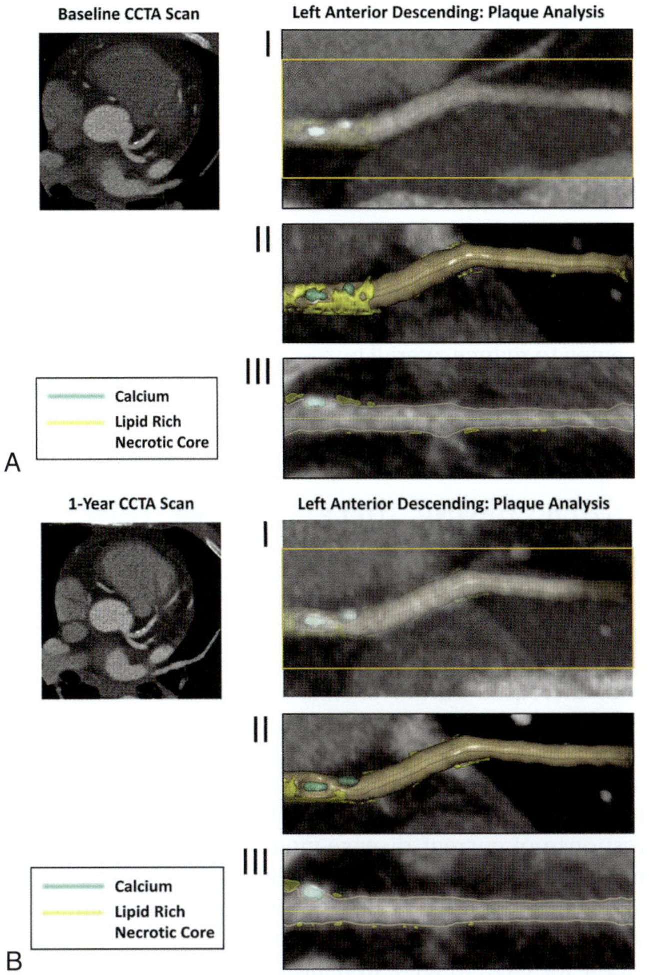

FIG. 17.5 Left anterior descending artery, proximal plaque identified before after 1 year of biologic therapy in a patient with psoriasis. (A), at baseline; (B), at year. I, Coronary artery visualized from coronary computed tomography angiography (CCTA) scan with overlying segmentation of artery and derivation of plaque characteristics (transparent). II, Three-dimensional segmentation of artery in gold with derived plaque characteristics displayed; lipid-rich necrotic core in *yellow* and calcified plaque in *green*. III, Longitudinal planar view through midline of coronary artery with color overlap displaying plaque characteristics. (From Choi H, Uceda DE, Dey AK, et al. Treatment of psoriasis with biologic therapy is associated with improvement of coronary artery plaque lipid-rich necrotic core. *Circ Cardiovasc Imaging*. 2020;13:e011199.)

the myocardium and visceral pericardium using fully automated technology. In healthy states, EAT has antiinflammatory and antifibrotic properties; however, states of metabolic dysfunction like obesity, insulin resistance, and diabetes can cause EAT to become inflammatory.[51] Chronic inflammatory states are associated with a heightened prevalence of obesity, diabetes, and metabolic syndrome. Indeed, SLE, RA, psoriasis, and HIV are associated with EAT accumulation and thickness.[51–53] In RA, EAT volume by CCTA is associated with noncalcified and high-risk plaque, multivessel disease, and multiple inflammatory markers.[52] In HIV, epicardial fat volume by CCTA associates with high-risk plaque beyond cardiovascular risk factors.[53] EAT as an imaging marker would require no further imaging beyond CCTA and may provide prognostic value in predicting CAD in chronic inflammatory diseases.[54]

TRANSLATIONAL STUDIES: LINKING LABORATORY AND CCTA IMAGING BIOMARKERS

Randomized trials in chronic inflammatory diseases studying the effects of antiinflammatory treatment on MACE are difficult, as these diseases have a small sample size and thus small number of events. However, in place of large trials, CCTA-derived imaging biomarkers have been used and can provide information that is directly related with cardiovascular outcomes. In translational studies, NCB has been used as an endpoint to identify blood-based lipid, immune, and inflammatory markers that contribute to inflammation and subclinical atherosclerosis. These studies have furthered our understanding of the complex interplay between inflammation and cardiometabolic disease. NCB has also been serially assessed to determine response to treatment across all inflammatory diseases. Though these studies are promising, they should be followed by randomized controlled trials to increase validity.

Immune Cell Markers

Inflammation triggers increased hematopoiesis from the bone marrow and mobilizes immune cell release from the spleen.[55] This excessive immune activation results in increased number of inflammatory cells in the coronary wall and leads to progression of atherosclerosis. Using CCTA as an endpoint has allowed for mechanistic insights in this process. In patients with SLE, low-density granulocytes but not normal-density granulocytes associate with NCB,[35] suggesting distinct neutrophil subtypes contribute to early vascular disease. In those with psoriasis, neutrophil[56] and monocyte[57] to lymphocyte ratios associate with NCB independent of traditional risk factors, suggesting these markers contribute to residual inflammatory risk.[56,57] Additionally in psoriasis, excessive bone marrow and splenic activation by FDG PET-CT (fluorodeoxyglucose positron emission tomography computed tomography) is related to NCB and LRNC, monocyte subsets, and modulates with initiation of systemic biologic therapy.[58]

Lipoprotein Markers

Chronic inflammatory disorders are associated with increased metabolic disease including dyslipidemia. To better understand how HDL function impacts atherosclerosis severity, reverse cholesterol transport, measured using cholesterol efflux capacity (CEC), was characterized with associations with coronary NCB. In SLE and psoriasis[59] CEC inversely correlates with NCB, whereby those with low HDL function have increased NCB. Deeper characterization of how HDL function may impact ApoB (apolipoprotein B)-LDL pathways in psoriasis demonstrated that oxidized lipids[60] and their receptors[9] associate with both NCB and coronary plaque on CCTA. Additionally, initiation of biologic therapy to treat chronic inflammation in psoriasis reduced levels of oxidized lipid receptors and NCB,[9] opening up future doors to test the impact of modified lipids therapies on inflammatory atherogenesis.

Inflammatory Markers

Although hs-CRP has been widely used to estimate systemic inflammation, other inflammatory markers may be better in those with chronic inflammatory disease. For example, addition of hs-CRP to cardiovascular risk calculators in RA did not significantly improve risk stratification, and hs-CRP may often times be within normal limits in those with chronic inflammatory diseases. An emerging marker assessed by NMR (nuclear magnetic resonance) spectroscopy is glycoprotein acetylation (GlycA), a composite biomarker that integrates protein levels and glycosylation states. GlycA has been associated with MACE in those with normal or low LDL in several large trials in the general population,[61] and GlycA has been widely studied across many chronic inflammatory diseases. Though no studies evaluating levels of GlycA and cardiac events exist in chronic inflammatory diseases, studies using CCTA as an endpoint in RA, SLE, psoriasis, and HIV have found GlycA is significantly associated with NCB.[62]

Myocardial Injury

High-sensitive troponin (hsTn) has been validated in the general population in predicting MACE. hsTn has been correlated with CCTA in multiple chronic inflammatory diseases. In RA, hsTn is a predictor of long-term cardiac events after adjusting for traditional risk factors.[63] In psoriasis, hsTn is associated with NCB at baseline and 1 year.[46] Similar findings are seen in those with HIV.[64] These findings add to a growing body of knowledge that inflammation has physiologic consequences in early vascular inflammation. These findings suggest that hsTn, a myocardial injury marker that is widely available, could add to early risk stratification in chronic inflammatory disease states. However, larger studies are needed to confirm these results.

SEX DIFFERENCES IN CHRONIC INFLAMMATORY DISEASE

In the past decade there has been increased recognition of sex as a biological variable. Cardiovascular disease continues to be the leading cause of mortality in women, and over 45% of women over age 20 years have some form of CVD.[65] Though efforts have been made to reduce sex-based disparities, differences in the treatment of hypertension, diabetes, and dyslipidemia continue to persist.[66] Consideration of sex is especially important in patients with chronic inflammatory disease. For example, according to the Centers of Disease Control (CDC), 9 out of 10 adults with SLE are women and are most likely to develop SLE between the ages of 15 and 44. Women are also three times more likely than men to develop RA, and in 2019 more women were diagnosed with HIV than men. In the general population, young women with acute MI have higher inflammatory levels compared with similar aged men.[67] Increase in plaque severity by CCTA has also been associated with increased mortality in younger women compared to men. [68] In addition, FFR_{CT} may have limitations in women given that women have smaller coronary arteries but lower myocardial mass, leading to a higher V/M ratio compared to men with the same degree of coronary stenosis.[69] Furthermore, nonobstructive disease in women may be more significant. One study found women with nonobstructive left main disease had almost 80% higher risk of MACE than men with nonobstructive left main disease.[70] Finally, early evidence demonstrates that plaque features such as fibrofatty burden may evolve differently over time between men and women with chronic inflammation.[71] Taken together, use of CCTA in women with chronic inflammatory disease may be especially important to prompt more aggressive strategies for prevention and treatment. In addition, careful consideration should be given in reducing traditional risk factors in women to reduce overall burden of cardiovascular disease. For further detail, please see Chapter 5, Sex Differences in Coronary Atherosclerosis.

OTHER CHRONIC INFLAMMATORY STATES

This chapter has focused on CCTA to evaluate cardiovascular risk in patients with SLE, RA, psoriasis, and HIV. However, inflammatory bowel disease (IBD), Sjögren's disease, and systemic sclerosis have all been associated with increased cardiovascular risk. Based on data from other inflammatory diseases, systemic inflammation in these states likely also contributes to CVD. Researchers aiming to study these diseases could consider using CCTA to better characterize atherosclerotic risk and monitor response of current disease-modifying therapies. Though not a chronic inflammatory disease, obesity is also characterized as a chronic low-grade systemic inflammatory state, and increased visceral adipose tissue is a known risk factor for CVD. Indeed, in psoriasis visceral adiposity was shown to increase NCB over time, and the development of visceral adiposity was heavily dependent on systemic inflammation assessed by GlycA.[72] Consideration of these risk factors and evaluating for modifying risk factors defined by the ACC/AHA 2019 guidelines may improve risk stratification in the future.

SERIAL ASSESSMENT USING CCTA

As previously noted, biologic therapy for treatment of psoriasis modulates NCB, LRNC, and FAI. However, several other studies in the past 5 years have assessed plaque response to treatment in chronic inflammatory diseases. In SLE, proportion of time (ranging from 2 to 8 years) on immunosuppressants has been associated with a decrease in noncalcified plaque.[73] Another longitudinal study in RA found disease-modifying therapies resulted in protective calcification of noncalcified lesions and lower likelihood of new plaque formation in patients with early atherosclerosis.[52] In HIV, the effect of antiretroviral therapy (ART) has been mixed. One recent study found use of long-term ART is higher and associated with higher prevalence of coronary disease and high-risk plaque.[74] Another study suggests ARTs may have drug-specific impact on coronary plaque. For example, although abacavir was associated with an increased risk of noncalcified plaque, emtricitabine and tenofovir were associated with a lower risk of plaque.[75] The Pitavastatin to Prevent Cardiovascular Disease in HIV

Infection trial (REPRIEVE) found participants with HIV who received pitavastatin had a lower risk of MACE than those who received a placebo at a follow-up of 5 years.[76] The incidence of MACE was similar in those receiving statin regardless of their screening LDL level, suggesting the antiinflammatory property of statins could benefit those with HIV beyond LDL lowering.

RECOMMENDATIONS IN THE SCOPE OF CURRENT GUIDELINES

Cardiovascular disease is a major cause of mortality in patients with chronic inflammatory disease. These patients are often first seen by primary care physicians, rheumatologists, or infectious disease specialists in the case of patients diagnosed with HIV, and many may never be referred to a cardiologist. Evaluating cardiovascular risk should be included in these initial settings to identify patients at intermediate and high risk for cardiovascular events. Education that classic risk calculators like ASCVD-10 underestimate cardiovascular risk is necessary to ensure intermediate- and high-risk patients are not missed. In those that are high risk, appropriate antiinflammatory treatment including statins and disease-modifying therapy should be started. All physicians should be aware that chronic inflammatory diseases are considered a risk-modifying factor to further classify intermediate-risk patients. Furthermore, all patients should undergo assessment of three Bs in chronic inflammation: **B**lood pressure, **B**ody mass index, and **B**lood measurement of lipids and glucose (Fig. 17.6). Performance of these three by healthcare providers will uncover latent and undiagnosed cardiometabolic diseases early in the course of the disease, permitting appropriate education and treatment measures. Identification of the presence of the metabolic syndrome should also be sought given that the presence of metabolic syndrome in chronic inflammation increased NCB and risk of high-risk plaque.[77]

In the intermediate-risk patient group, further testing for coronary disease should be initiated using CAC or CCTA. When CAC is 0 in a patient with chronic inflammation who is at high risk for CVD (e.g., multiple traditional risk factors or a family history of myocardial infarction), coronary CTA should be obtained. This recommendation reflects the fact that there is a high prevalence of noncalcified disease in those with CAC of 0 in chronic inflammation. On the other hand, the presence of any plaque (on CAC testing or CCTA) should prompt clinicians to intensify pharmacologic and lifestyle therapies. Special consideration should be given to women because despite education on sex differences in cardiology, initiation of appropriate treatment is less likely in women than in men, and women may have increased risk of MACE with nonobstructive disease. Finally, if a plaque is visually identified on CCTA, it may be reasonable in selected cases to repeat CCTA after several years of treatment with disease-modifying therapies in order to guide further interventions.

FUTURE DIRECTIONS

The last 10 years have brought major advancements to CCTA permitting anatomical and functional assessment of obstructive and nonobstructive disease. These technologies will continue to develop and likely be integrated with traditional CCTA techniques in future guidelines. CCTA plaque analysis using a combination of automatic plaque quantification, FFR_{CT}, and WSS will play an increasingly important role in defining an individual's risk for plaque development and MACE. CCTA may also have a future role in evaluating the effects of treatment and tailoring cardiovascular and antiinflammatory therapies. Ultimately, using

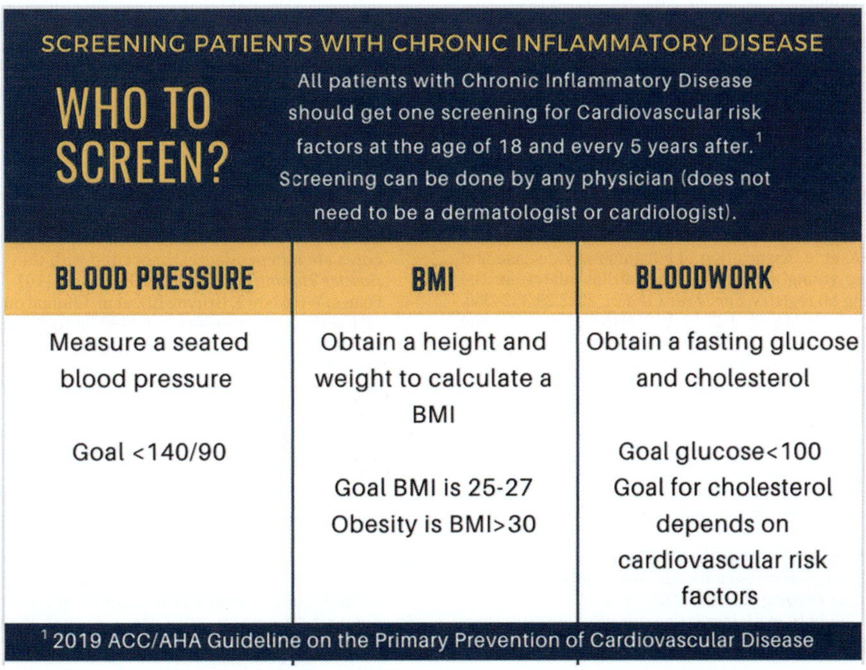

FIG. 17.6 Screening patients with chronic inflammatory disease. Patients with chronic inflammatory disease should undergo screening with the 3Bs: Blood pressure, BMI, and Bloodwork.

CCTA in chronic inflammatory diseases to understand the contribution of inflammation to atherosclerosis may even allow for targeted antiinflammatory therapies for the general population. It is an exciting time in the era of multiple planned clinical trials to assess if targeting inflammatory pathways can improve cardiovascular outcomes. Further education, availability, and adoption of CCTA in clinical cardiology will allow for more precise risk stratification and therapeutic intervention in patients with chronic inflammatory disease.

REFERENCES

1. Conrad N, Verbeke G, Molenberghs G, et al. Autoimmune diseases and cardiovascular risk: a population-based study on 19 autoimmune diseases and 12 cardiovascular diseases in 22 million individuals in the UK. *Lancet.* 2022;400:733–743.
2. England BR, Thiele GM, Anderson DR, Mikuls TR. Increased cardiovascular risk in rheumatoid arthritis: mechanisms and implications. *BMJ.* 2018;361:k1036.
3. Shah ASV, Stelzle D, Lee KK, et al. Global burden of atherosclerotic cardiovascular disease in people living with HIV: Systematic review and meta-analysis. *Circulation.* 2018;138:1100–1112.
4. Alonso A, Barnes AE, Guest JL, Shah A, Shao IY, Marconi V. HIV Infection and incidence of cardiovascular diseases: an analysis of a large healthcare database. *J Am Heart Assoc.* 2019;8:e012241.
5. Gelfand JM, Troxel AB, Lewis JD, et al. The risk of mortality in patients with psoriasis: results from a population-based study. *Arch Dermatol.* 2007;143:1493–1499.
6. Doria A, Iaccarino L, Ghirardello A, et al. Long-term prognosis and causes of death in systemic lupus erythematosus. *Am J Med.* 2006;119:700–706.
7. Soehnlein O, Libby P. Targeting inflammation in atherosclerosis—from experimental insights to the clinic. *Nat Rev Drug Discov.* 2021;20:589–610.
8. Furman D, Campisi J, Verdin E, et al. Chronic inflammation in the etiology of disease across the life span. *Nat Med.* 2019;25:1822–1832.
9. Dey AK, Gaddipati R, Elnabawi YA, et al. Association between soluble lectin-like oxidized low-density lipoprotein receptor-1 and coronary artery disease in psoriasis. *JAMA Dermatol.* 2020;156:151–157.
10. Funderburg NT, Xu D, Playford MP, et al. Treatment of HIV infection with a raltegravir-based regimen increases LDL levels, but improves HDL cholesterol efflux capacity. *Antivir Ther.* 2017;22:71–75.
11. Ridker PM, Everett BM, Thuren T, et al. Antiinflammatory therapy with canakinumab for atherosclerotic disease. *N Engl J Med.* 2017;377:1119–1131.
12. Ridker PM, Danielson E, Fonseca FA, et al. Rosuvastatin to prevent vascular events in men and women with elevated C-reactive protein. *N Engl J Med.* 2008;359:2195–2207.
13. Sabatine MS, Giugliano RP, Keech AC, et al. Evolocumab and clinical outcomes in patients with cardiovascular disease. *N Engl J Med.* 2017;376:1713–1722.
14. Ridker PM, Revkin J, Amarenco P, et al. Cardiovascular efficacy and safety of bococizumab in high-risk patients. *N Engl J Med.* 2017;376:1527–1539.
15. Nidorf SM, Fiolet ATL, Mosterd A, et al. Colchicine in patients with chronic coronary disease. *N Engl J Med.* 2020;383:1838–1847.
16. Tardif JC, Kouz S, Waters DD, et al. Efficacy and safety of low-dose colchicine after myocardial infarction. *N Engl J Med.* 2019;381:2497–2505.
17. Abdelrahman KM, Chen MY, Dey AK, et al. Coronary computed tomography angiography from clinical uses to emerging technologies: JACC state-of-the-art review. *J Am Coll Cardiol.* 2020;76:1226–1243.
18. Lloyd-Jones DM, Braun LT, Ndumele CE, et al. Use of risk assessment tools to guide decision-making in the primary prevention of atherosclerotic cardiovascular disease: A special report from the American Heart Association and American College of Cardiology. *Circulation.* 2019;139:e1162–e1177.
19. Weber B, Biery DW, Singh A, et al. Association of inflammatory disease and long-term outcomes among young adults with myocardial infarction: the Mass general brigham Young-Mi registry. *Eur J Prev Cardiol.* 2022;29:352–359.
20. Arnett DK, Blumenthal RS, Albert MA, et al. 2019 ACC/AHA Guideline on the primary prevention of cardiovascular disease: a report of the American College of Cardiology/American Heart Association task force on clinical practice guidelines. *Circulation.* 2019;140:e596–e646.
21. Joshi NV, Vesey AT, Williams MC, et al. 18F-fluoride positron emission tomography for identification of ruptured and high-risk coronary atherosclerotic plaques: a prospective clinical trial. *Lancet.* 2014;383:705–713.
22. Metkus TS, Brown T, Budoff M, et al. HIV infection is associated with an increased prevalence of coronary noncalcified plaque among participants with a coronary artery calcium score of zero: multicenter AIDS Cohort Study (MACS). *HIV Med.* 2015;16:635–639.
23. Nasir K, Cainzos-Achirica M, Valero-Elizondo J, et al. Coronary atherosclerosis in an asymptomatic U.S. population: miami heart study at baptist health south florida. *JACC Cardiovasc Imaging.* 2022;15:1604–1618.
24. Ngamdu KS, Ghosalkar D, Chung H, et al. Increasing duration of statin therapy is associated with high coronary artery calcium sCORE. *J Am Coll Cardiol.* 2022;79:1245–1245.
25. Hoffmann U, Ferencik M, Udelson JE, et al. Prognostic value of noninvasive cardiovascular testing in patients with stable chest pain: insights from the PROMISE trial (Prospective multicenter imaging study for evaluation of chest pain). *Circulation.* 2017;135:2320–2332.
26. van Rosendael AR, Shaw LJ, Xie JX, et al. Superior risk stratification with coronary computed tomography angiography using a comprehensive atherosclerotic risk score. *JACC Cardiovasc Imaging.* 2019;12:1987–1997.
27. Bittencourt MS, Hulten E, Ghoshhajra B, et al. Prognostic value of nonobstructive and obstructive coronary artery disease detected by coronary computed tomography angiography to identify cardiovascular events. *Circ Cardiovasc Imaging.* 2014;7:282–291.
28. Oikonomou EK, Marwan M, Desai MY, et al. Non-invasive detection of coronary inflammation using computed tomography and prediction of residual cardiovascular risk (the CRISP CT study): a post-hoc analysis of prospective outcome data. *Lancet.* 2018;392:929–939.
29. Kim HW, Shi H, Winkler MA, Lee R, Weintraub NL. Perivascular adipose tissue and vascular perturbation/atherosclerosis. *Arterioscler Thromb Vasc Biol.* 2020;40:2569–2576.
30. Elnabawi YA, Oikonomou EK, Dey AK, et al. Association of biologic therapy with coronary inflammation in patients with psoriasis as assessed by perivascular fat attenuation index. *JAMA Cardiol.* 2019;4:885–891.
31. Patel NH, Dey AK, Sorokin AV, et al. Chronic inflammatory diseases and coronary heart disease: Insights from cardiovascular CT. *J Cardiovasc Comput Tomogr.* 2022;16:7–18.
32. Lin A, Manral N, McElhinney P, et al. Deep learning-enabled coronary CT angiography for plaque and stenosis quantification and cardiac risk prediction: an international multicentre study. *Lancet Digit Health.* 2022;4:e256–e265.
33. Lerman JB, Joshi AA, Chaturvedi A, et al. Coronary plaque characterization in psoriasis reveals high-risk features that improve after treatment in a prospective observational study. *Circulation.* 2017;136:263–276.
34. Boldeanu I, Sadouni M, Mansour S, et al. Prevalence and characterization of subclinical coronary atherosclerotic plaque with CT among individuals with HIV: results from the Canadian HIV and aging cohort study. *Radiology.* 2021;299:571–580.
35. Carlucci PM, Purmalek MM, Dey AK, et al. Neutrophil subsets and their gene signature associate with vascular inflammation and coronary atherosclerosis in lupus. *JCI Insight.* 2018;3:1–15.
36. Elnabawi YA, Dey AK, Goyal A, et al. Coronary artery plaque characteristics and treatment with biologic therapy in severe psoriasis: results from a prospective observational study. *Cardiovasc Res.* 2019;115:721–728.
37. Williams MC, Kwiecinski J, Doris M, et al. Low-attenuation noncalcified plaque on coronary computed tomography angiography predicts myocardial infarction: results from the multicenter scot-heart trial (Scottish computed tomography of the heart). *Circulation.* 2020;141:1452–1462.
38. Stojan G, Li J, Budoff M, Arbab-Zadeh A, Petri MA. High-risk coronary plaque in SLE: low-attenuation non-calcified coronary plaque and positive remodelling index. *Lupus Sci Med.* 2020;7:e000409.
39. Hansen PR, Feineis M, Abdulla J. Rheumatoid arthritis patients have higher prevalence and burden of asymptomatic coronary artery disease assessed by coronary computed tomography: a systematic literature review and meta-analysis. *Eur J Intern Med.* 2019;62:72–79.
40. Soares C, Samara A, Yuyun MF, et al. Coronary artery calcification and plaque characteristics in people living With HIV: a systematic review and meta-analysis. *J Am Heart Assoc.* 2021;10:e019291.
41. Karpouzas GA, Ormseth SR, Hernandez E, Budoff MJ. Biologics may prevent cardiovascular events in rheumatoid arthritis by inhibiting coronary plaque formation and stabilizing high-risk lesions. *Arthritis Rheumatol.* 2020;72:1467–1475.
42. Han D, Torii S, Yahagi K, et al. Quantitative measurement of lipid rich plaque by coronary computed tomography angiography: a correlation of histology in sudden cardiac death. *Atherosclerosis.* 2018;275:426–433.
43. Choi H, Uceda DE, Dey AK, et al. Treatment of psoriasis with biologic therapy is associated with improvement of coronary artery plaque lipid-rich necrotic core. *Circ Cardiovasc Imaging.* 2020;13:e011199.
44. Ota H, Yu W, Underhill HR, et al. Hemorrhage and large lipid-rich necrotic cores are independently associated with thin or ruptured fibrous caps. *Arterioscler Thromb Vasc Biol.* 2009;29:1696–1701.
45. Fearon WF, Nishi T, Bruyne BD, et al. Clinical outcomes and cost-effectiveness of fractional flow reserve–guided percutaneous coronary intervention in patients with stable coronary artery disease. *Circulation.* 2018;137:480–487.
46. Zhou W, Abdelrahman KM, Dey AK, et al. Association among noncalcified coronary burden, fractional flow reserve, and myocardial injury in psoriasis. *J Am Heart Assoc.* 2020;9:e017417.
47. Liao KP, Huang J, He Z, et al. Coronary microvascular dysfunction in rheumatoid arthritis compared to diabetes mellitus and association with all-cause mortality. *Arthritis Care Res (Hoboken).* 2021;73:159–165.
48. Driessen RS, Danad I, Stuijfzand WJ, et al. Comparison of coronary computed tomography angiography, fractional flow reserve, and perfusion imaging for ischemia diagnosis. *J Am Coll Cardiol.* 2019;73:161–173.
49. Samady H, Molony DS, Coskun AU, Varshney AS, De Bruyne B, Stone PH. Risk stratification of coronary plaques using physiologic characteristics by CCTA: focus on shear stress. *J Cardiovasc Comput Tomogr.* 2020;14:386–393.
50. Kumar A, Thompson EW, Lefieux A, et al. High coronary shear stress in patients with coronary artery disease predicts myocardial infarction. *J Am Coll Cardiol.* 2018;72:1926–1935.

51. Packer M. Epicardial adipose tissue may mediate deleterious effects of obesity and inflammation on the myocardium. *J Am Coll Cardiol.* 2018;71:2360–2372.
52. Karpouzas GA, Rezaeian P, Ormseth SR, Hollan I, Budoff MJ. Epicardial adipose tissue volume as a marker of subclinical coronary atherosclerosis in rheumatoid arthritis. *Arthritis Rheumatol.* 2021;73:1412–1420.
53. Sadouni M, Durand M, Boldeanu I, et al. Association of epicardial fat with noncalcified coronary plaque volume and with low attenuation plaque in people with HIV. *AIDS.* 2021;35:1575–1584.
54. West Henry W, Siddique M, Williams Michelle C, et al. Deep-learning for epicardial adipose tissue assessment with computed tomography. *JACC Cardiovasc Imaging.* 2023;16:800–816.
55. Poller WC, Nahrendorf M, Swirski FK. Hematopoiesis and cardiovascular disease. *Circ Res.* 2020;126:1061–1085.
56. Dey AK, Teague HL, Adamstein NH, et al. Association of neutrophil-to-lymphocyte ratio with non-calcified coronary artery burden in psoriasis: findings from an observational cohort study. *J Cardiovasc Comput Tomogr.* 2021;15:372–379.
57. Basyal B, Teague H, Vedantam K, et al. Association between monocyte-lymphocyte ratio and non-calcified coronary burden in psoriasis. *J Am Coll Cardiol.* 2020;75:1937–1937.
58. Patel NH, Osborne MT, Teague H, et al. Heightened splenic and bone marrow uptake of 18F-FDG PET/CT is associated with systemic inflammation and subclinical atherosclerosis by CCTA in psoriasis: an observational study. *Atherosclerosis.* 2021;339:20–26.
59. Purmalek MM, Carlucci PM, Dey AK, et al. Association of lipoprotein subfractions and glycoprotein acetylation with coronary plaque burden in SLE. *Lupus Sci Med.* 2019;6:e000332.
60. Sorokin AV, Remaley AT, Mehta NN. Oxidized lipids and lipoprotein dysfunction in psoriasis. *J Psoriasis Psoriatic Arthritis.* 2020;5:139–146.
61. Otvos JD, Guyton JR, Connelly MA, et al. Relations of GlycA and lipoprotein particle subspecies with cardiovascular events and mortality: a post hoc analysis of the aim-high trial. *J Clin Lipidol.* 2018;12 348-355. e2.
62. Mehta NN, Dey AK, Maddineni R, Kraus WE, Huffman KM. GlycA Measured by NMR spectroscopy is associated with disease activity and cardiovascular disease risk in chronic inflammatory diseases. *Am J Prev Cardiol.* 2020;4:100120.
63. Karpouzas GA, Estis J, Rezaeian P, Todd J, Budoff MJ. High-sensitivity cardiac troponin I is a biomarker for occult coronary plaque burden and cardiovascular events in patients with rheumatoid arthritis. *Rheumatology.* 2018;57:1080–1088.
64. Foster P, Sokoll L, Li J, et al. Circulating levels of cardiac troponin T are associated with coronary noncalcified plaque burden in HIV-infected adults: a pilot study. *Int J STD AIDS.* 2019;30:223–230.
65. Tsao CW, Aday AW, Almarzooq ZI, et al. Heart disease and stroke statistics–2022 update: a report from the American Heart Association. *Circulation.* 2022;145:e153–e639.
66. Peters SAE, Muntner P, Woodward M. Sex differences in the prevalence of, and trends in, cardiovascular risk factors, treatment, and control in the United States, 2001 to 2016. *Circulation.* 2019;139:1025–1035.
67. Lu Y, Zhou S, Dreyer RP, et al. Sex Differences in inflammatory markers and health status among young adults with acute myocardial infarction: results from the VIRGO (Variation in recovery: role of gender on outcomes of young acute myocardial infarction patients) study. *Circ Cardiovasc Qual Outcomes.* 2017;10:e003470.
68. Asif A, Berman DS, Gransar H, et al. SEX differences in prognostic significance of plaque burden and distribution measured by Coronary Computed Tomographic Angiography (CCTA) in younger patients. *J Am Coll Cardiol.* 2022;79:1201–1201.
69. Fairbairn TA, Dobson R, Hurwitz-Koweek L, et al. Sex differences in coronary computed tomography angiography–derived fractional flow reserve: lessons from advance. *JACC Cardiovasc Imaging.* 2020;13:2576–2587.
70. Xie JX, Eshtehardi P, Varghese T, et al. Prognostic significance of nonobstructive left main coronary artery disease in women versus men. *Circ Cardiovasc Imaging.* 2017;10:e006246.
71. Teklu M, Zhou W, Kapoor P, et al. Sex differences in subclinical coronary atherosclerosis in psoriasis by coronary computed tomography angiography. *JACC Cardiovasc Imaging.* 2021;14:2044–2046.
72. Sajja A, Abdelrahman KM, Reddy AS, et al. Chronic inflammation in psoriasis promotes visceral adiposity associated with noncalcified coronary burden over time. *JCI Insight.* 2020;5:1–13.
73. Khan A, Arbab-Zadeh A, Kiani AN, Magder LS, Petri M. Progression of noncalcified and calcified coronary plaque by CT angiography in SLE. *Rheumatol Int.* 2017;37:59–65.
74. Senoner T, Barbieri F, Adukauskaite A, et al. Coronary atherosclerosis characteristics in HIV-infected patients on long-term antiretroviral therapy: insights from coronary computed tomography-angiography. *AIDS.* 2019;33:1853–1862.
75. Kovari H, Calmy A, Doco-Lecompte T, et al. Antiretroviral drugs associated with subclinical coronary artery disease in the swiss human immunodeficiency virus cohort study. *Clin Infect Dis.* 2019;70:884–889.
76. Grinspoon SK, Fitch KV, Zanni MV, et al. Pitavastatin to prevent cardiovascular disease in HIV infection. *N Engl J Med.* 2023;389:687–699.
77. Teklu M, Zhou W, Kapoor P, et al. Metabolic syndrome and its factors are associated with noncalcified coronary burden in psoriasis: an observational cohort study. *J Am Acad Dermatol.* 2021;84:1329–1338.
78. Sajja AP, Joshi AA, Teague HL, Dey AK, Mehta NN. Potential immunological links between psoriasis and cardiovascular disease. *Front Immunol.* 2018;9.

18 Cardiac Computed Tomography in Cardio-oncology

MAROS FERENCIK AND JUAN LOPEZ-MATTEI

KEY POINTS

- Cardio-oncology is an emerging subspecialty of cardiology, which focuses on the care of patients with cancer in the pretreatment period, during active treatment, and in cancer survivors. Cardiovascular computed tomography (CT) has a growing role in cardio-oncology patients.
- Cancer and cardiovascular disease share common risk factors. The assessment of cardiovascular risk and modification of risk factors with lifestyle changes and preventive medications can improve both cardiovascular and cancer outcomes.
- CT can provide accurate risk stratification using coronary artery calcium detection on noncardiac or cardiac CT scans.
- Coronary CT angiography provides reliable assessment for coronary artery disease in cancer patients with suspected cancer therapy–related cardiac dysfunction, vascular toxicities, coronary vasospasm, and presentations with suspected acute coronary syndrome. Subclinical atherosclerosis detected on CT scans provides an opportunity for the implementation of preventive strategies.
- Cardiovascular CT is a complementary imaging technique to echocardiography and cardiac magnetic resonance imaging in cancer patients with radiation-induced heart disease, cardiac masses, valvular abnormalities, and pericardial disease.

Cardio-oncology is an emerging subspecialty of cardiology that focuses on the care of patients with cancer in the pretreatment period, during active treatment, and in cancer survivors (Fig. 18.1). The long-term survival of cancer patients has significantly improved over the past several decades through advances in early detection through imaging and laboratory techniques, pharmacotherapy, radiation therapy, and surgery.[1,2] Sixty-four percent of cancer patients survive 5 years or more.[3] The specialized cardiovascular care of cancer patients and survivors is warranted due to elevated cardiovascular risk in this population. Cancer and cardiovascular disease share common risk factors, and many of the modern cancer therapies can lead to direct cardiovascular damage or increase the future cardiovascular risk, with cardiovascular disease being the leading cause of death in cancer survivors.[4–6]

Cardiac computed tomography (CCT) has become a cornerstone imaging technology in cardiology and its role is supported by major European and American guidelines.[7,8] CCT has a growing role in the population of cancer patients and survivors. Societal guidelines provide recommendations for the care of cardio-oncology patients and the recent expert consensus document summarizes the roles of CCT.[9–20] Guidance documents have been prepared to disseminate the knowledge beyond cardiology and radiology specialists, such as radiation oncologist-specific summary.[21] In this chapter, we will discuss the applications of CCT in cardio-oncology.

CARDIOVASCULAR RISK ASSESSMENT IN CANCER PATIENTS

Symptomatic and asymptomatic cardiovascular disease and cancer often develop in the same period of life and can be seen as a manifestation of aging in many patients. Multiple risk factors (e.g., hypertension, hyperlipidemia, obesity, low physical inactivity, poor diet, diabetes, and smoking) are associated with both cardiovascular disease and cancer.[22–24] The opposite is also true: the absence of subclinical cardiovascular disease (atherosclerosis) as determined by CCT showing a coronary artery calcium (CAC) score of 0 is predicting not only a lower risk of cardiovascular events but also a lower risk of cancer.[25]

Previous studies found that among patients treated for cancer, cardiovascular disease is directly associated with cardiovascular risk factor burden, and cancer patients with concurrent cardiovascular disease have worse cancer outcomes.[26] There are cancer therapies that may cause or accelerate atherosclerosis, such as immune-checkpoint inhibitors, tyrosine kinase inhibitors, antiandrogenic therapies, and radiotherapy.[27–29] Therefore the assessment and detection of cardiovascular risk prior to and during cancer treatment may improve short-term and long-term outcomes. The priority of cardiovascular care of cancer patients is to allow for the delivery of the most efficacious cancer treatment and for the reduction of future adverse cardiovascular events. The accurate cardiovascular risk stratification facilitates the implementation of primary and secondary cardiovascular prevention strategies.[30] It has been shown that preventive cardiovascular measures, including medications and engagement in physical activity, are underutilized in cancer patients.[31] The recent Expert Consensus from the Society of Cardiovascular Computed Tomography emphasizes that "A comprehensive baseline evaluation to screen for, and subsequently optimize any underlying atherosclerotic cardiovascular disease (ASCVD) risk factors is recommended for all patients with cancer and cancer survivors."[20] The Expert Consensus endorses a comprehensive cardiovascular assessment, which includes history, physical examination, basic laboratory evaluation (e.g., lipid panel, hemoglobin A1c), electrocardiogram, and calculation of ASCVD risk using pooled cohort equation or other appropriate online calculators.[20] Preventive measures including the management of elevated lipids, glucose and blood pressure, weight management, and regular physical activity should be discussed and support should be offered to cancer patients.[20]

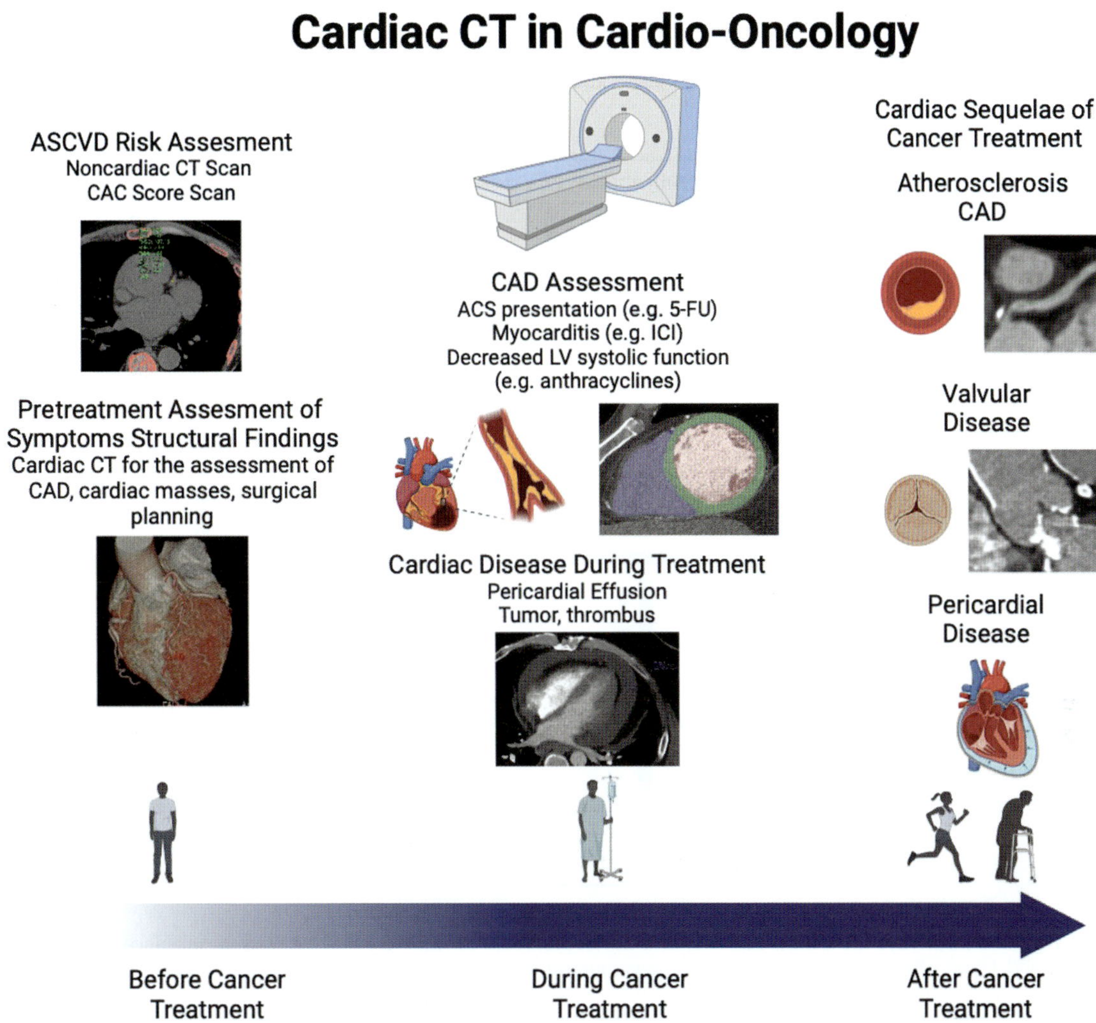

FIG. 18.1 Cardiac Computed Tomography in Cardio-oncology. Cardiac computed tomography has roles in assessing cancer patients before, during, and after treatment. *ACS,* Acute coronary syndrome; *ASCVD,* atherosclerotic cardiovascular disease; *CAC,* coronary artery calcium scoring; *CAD,* coronary artery disease; 5-fluorouracil (5-FU), immune check-point inhibitors (ICI), left ventricle (LV).

CCT can help refine cardiovascular risk assessment by detecting subclinical atherosclerosis. CAC detection and quantification is endorsed by the 2019 American College of Cardiology (ACC)/American Heart Association (AHA) Guideline on the Primary Prevention of CVD in patients at intermediate risk and uncertain risk with regard to preventative therapies.[32] The Expert Consensus from the Society of Cardiovascular Computed Tomography recommends using a similar approach for cancer patients (Fig. 18.2). The subgroups of patients who should be considered for the enhanced cardiovascular risk assessment using CAC include those who have nontraditional risk factors that have known associations with cardiovascular disease (e.g., clonal hematopoiesis of indeterminate potential [CHIP],[33] history of radiation therapy,[27] traditional chemotherapy such as platinum-based therapies and anthracyclines,[28] and certain novel therapies such as tyrosine kinase inhibitors,[34] immune checkpoint inhibitors).[35] In cancer patient populations, the use of preventive therapies (e.g., statins and aspirin) in patients with moderate to severe CAC (CAC score >100 or >75th percentile for age and gender) is endorsed by ACC/AHA, the Society of Cardiovascular Computed Tomography (SCCT), and National Lipid Association (NLA) guidelines.[32,36–39] Although data to support similar approaches in cancer patients are limited, it is reasonable to apply similar recommendations in this specific population. The Expert Consensus from the Society of Cardiovascular Computed Tomography recommends the use of moderate-intensity statin in patients with mild CAC (CAC-DRS 1, Agatston score 1–99) and moderate to high-intensity statin in patients with moderate or severely increased CAC (CAC-DRS 2 and 3, Agatston score ≥100).[20,38]

Diagnosis of patients with cancer presents a special opportunity for the evaluation of the presence of CAC and other extra-coronary calcium and quantification of cardiovascular disease risk. A significant proportion of cardio-oncology patients undergo noncardiac nongated CT (with or without contrast) for cancer screening, cancer diagnosis, staging, treatment planning (e.g., surgery, radiation therapy) or follow-up (Fig. 18.3). The sensitivity for the detection of CAC on noncardiac CT is high,[40] and the evaluation is supported by the Society of Cardiovascular Computed Tomography guidelines.[20,38,41] Although quantification of CAC and calculation of an Agatston score may be feasible on high-quality exams, semiquantitative assessment of CAC (e.g., number of coronary arteries or segments with CAC) or visual assessment (mild, moderate, severe) is a viable alternative for the cardiovascular risk

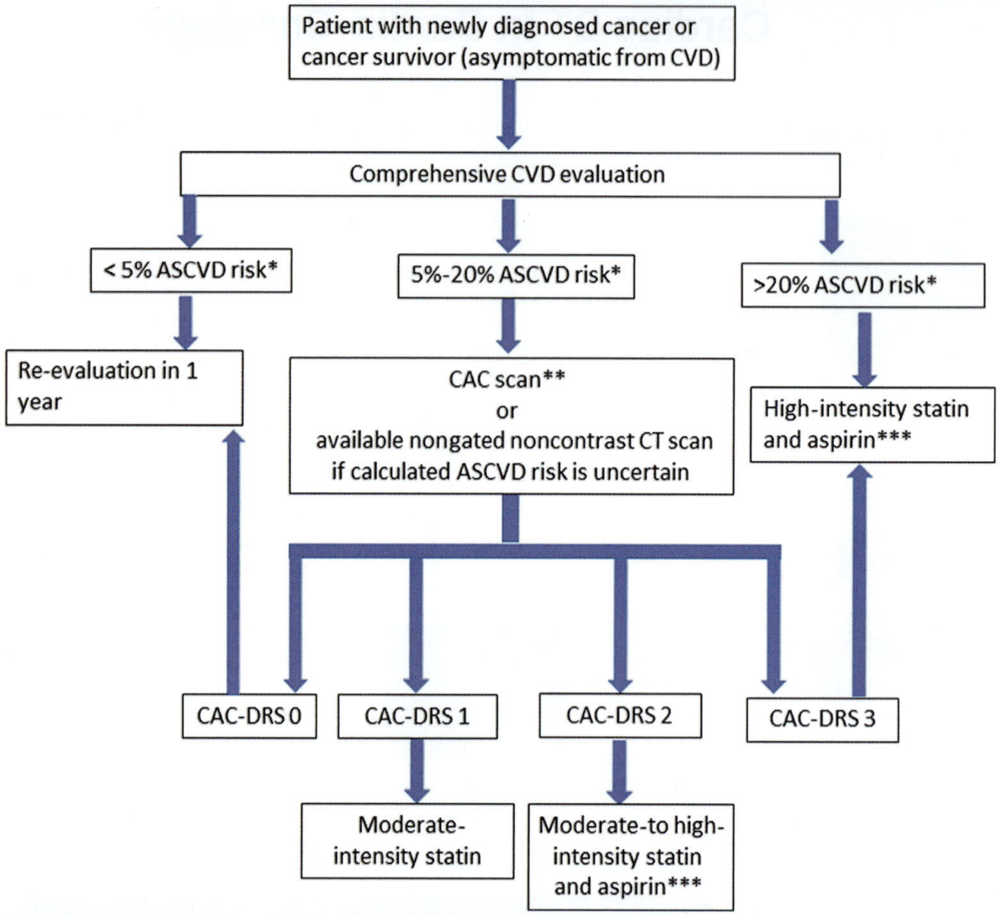

FIG. 18.2 CVD Risk-guided Pathways for Cancer Patients and Survivors. *ASCVD risk score may be used for guidance; however, it has not been validated in a patient population with cancer or those that have been previously treated for cancer. **If available, CAC scan is the preferred method to evaluate CAC quantitatively using the Agatston score in patients with intermediate ASCVD risk. Nongated noncontrast CT scans for cancer imaging may be used for qualitative assessment of CAC-DRS risk categories and should be part of a comprehensive CVD evaluation. ***Caution if thrombocytopenia and evaluate cancer-related bleeding risk before treatment with aspirin. *ASCVD,* Atherosclerotic cardiovascular disease; *CAC,* coronary artery calcium scoring; *CVD,* cardiovascular disease. (Reprinted from Lopez-Mattei J, Yang EH, Baldassarre LA, et al. Cardiac computed tomographic imaging in cardio-oncology: an expert consensus document of the Society of Cardiovascular Computed Tomography (SCCT). Endorsed by the International Cardio-Oncology Society (ICOS). *J Cardiovasc Comput Tomogr*. 2023;17(1):66–83.)

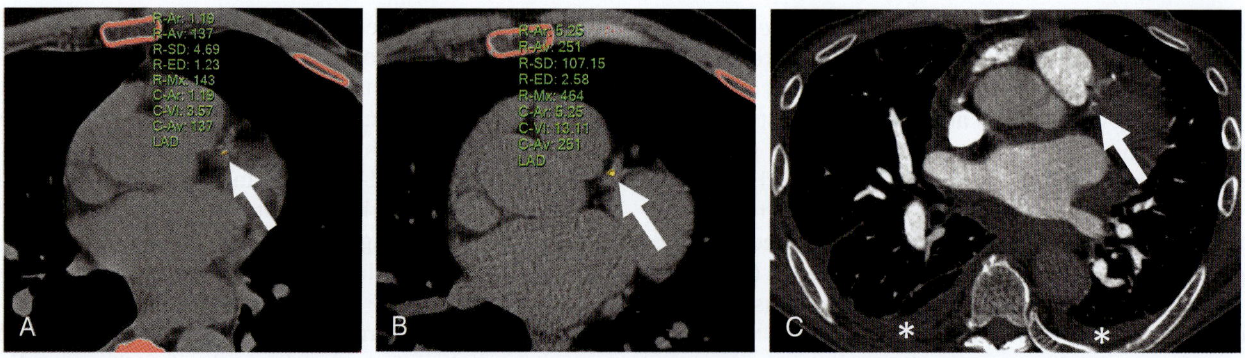

FIG. 18.3 Comparison of Coronary Artery Calcium Detection on Cardiac and Noncardiac Computed Tomography Scans. The detection of a small, calcified plaque in the proximal left anterior ascending coronary artery (*white arrow*) is demonstrated on noncardiac nongated noncontrast chest CT (A). The finding is confirmed on a dedicated cardiac CT scan with electrocardiographic gating obtained with coronary calcium scoring protocol (B). The calcium scoring can be performed on both noncardiac and cardiac scan (*yellow* overlay demonstrating pixels meeting criteria for scoring on Panels A and B). Panel C shows images from a noncardiac nongated contrast-enhanced CT scan obtained 2 years later when the patient was diagnosed with mesothelioma and pleural effusions (*asterisks*). The coronary calcium (Panel C, *arrow*) can be visualized and semiquantitatively assessed on contrast-enhanced scan, but the quantification using calcium scoring is not possible due to the high CT density of the contrast in the lumen.

assessment in cardio-oncology (Fig. 18.3).[41] Semiquantitative assessment (e.g., number of coronary arteries or segments with CAC) has been shown to have prognostic value for future cardiovascular events.[42–44] Preventive therapies can be recommended in patients with moderate or severe CAC (two or more vessels, three or more segments).[42–44] In patients with mild CAC (CAC score 1–99, one vessel, one to two segments), preventive therapies, especially statin therapy, can be considered through the process of shared decision-making, while also incorporating the presence of

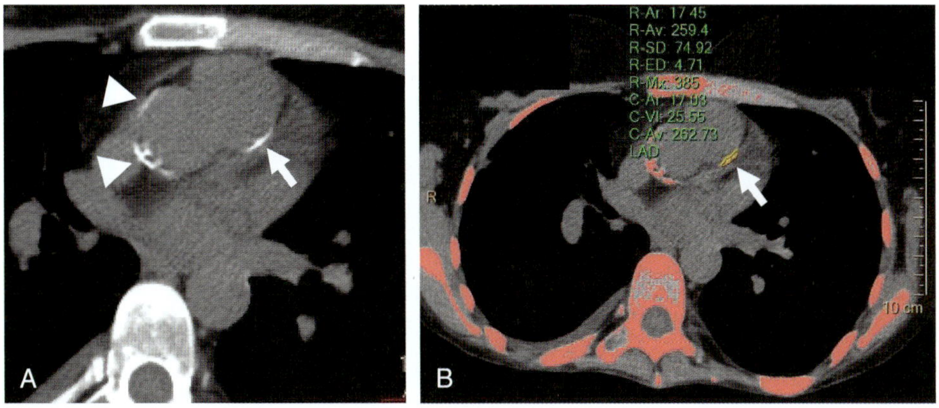

FIG. 18.4 Feasibility of Coronary Artery Calcium Assessment on Noncardiac Computed Tomography Scan Including the Quantification of Coronary Calcium Score. Noncontrast chest CT scan of a 34-year-old woman with a history of acute myeloid leukemia that required treatment with anthracycline (idarubicin) and allogeneic stem cell transplant. Her posttransplant course was complicated by graft-versus-host disease. She was evaluated in cardio-oncology clinic for sinus tachycardia. The review of the noncardiac CT scan revealed moderate calcifications in the left anterior descending coronary artery (Panel A, *arrow*) and moderate calcifications of the wall of the sinuses of Valsalva and the aortic valve (Panel A, *arrowheads*). Although noncardiac CT scans are not optimal for the assessment of coronary artery calcium, prior studies have shown that the quantification of coronary calcium is possible with a fairly good correlation with cardiac CT scans (Panel B, *arrow*). This patient had a coronary calcium (Agatston) score of 102, which represents >99th percentile for her age, sex, and ethnicity. Her other cardiac workup was unremarkable, including a normal transthoracic echocardiogram and normal 14-day EKG monitor. She was diagnosed with inappropriate sinus tachycardia, which can be seen in patients after stem cell transplant and with graft-versus-host disease. Preventive therapies with aspirin and statin were commenced due to increased cardiovascular risk.

other underlying cardiovascular disease risk factors (Fig. 18.2).[37] Discussion of initiation of aspirin and statins should include input from oncologists to avoid drug-drug interactions and increased bleeding complications in those at risk. The disclosure of the presence of CAC to the patient is associated with increased adherence to preventive therapies, including heart-healthy, regular exercise, and weight reduction.[45]

The evaluation of cardiovascular risk with the additional value of CAC detection is even more important in cancer survivors. As mentioned earlier, cancer survivors who develop clinical cardiovascular disease have a much higher total mortality rate and they are disproportionately affected by coronary artery disease (CAD). Clinical manifestations of CAD are responsible for approximately three-quarters of all cardiovascular mortality in cancer survivors.[26,46] Therefore the detection and quantitative or semiquantitative assessment of CAC on follow-up CT scans should be also recommended (Fig. 18.4). The initialization of preventive therapies (e.g., aspirin, statin) should be recommended to patients with moderate or severe CAC.

The sensitivity and accuracy of nongated chest CT scans for CAC evaluation have limitations due to lower spatial resolution and the presence of motion artifacts. Therefore a formal noncontrast CAC scan with electrocardiographic (ECG) gating should be considered for the quantification of CAC when there is clinical uncertainty (see Chapter 3, Coronary Artery Calcium Testing: Indications and Patient Management).

CARDIAC CT IMAGING IN THE EVALUATION OF CANCER THERAPY–RELATED CARDIAC DYSFUNCTION (CARDIOTOXICITY)

The evaluation of patients with a decrease in left ventricular systolic function is one of the most common clinical problems in cardio-oncology practice. Cardiac dysfunction can be seen in patients undergoing traditional chemotherapy and targeted or immune-based therapies. The decrease in the left ventricular function is typically detected on a routine follow-up transthoracic echocardiography or when the patients develop clinical symptoms suggestive of heart failure. Cardiac magnetic resonance imaging (CMR) is used in a subset of patients who need a more accurate assessment of left ventricular function or additional characterization of cardiomyopathy. CCT has limited value in the evaluation of left ventricular function (Fig. 18.5). Its role lies as part of the workup to identify the etiology of reduction in systolic function especially when coupled with rise of cardiac biomarkers where obstructive CAD needs to be excluded in the context of possible cardiotoxicity. The most common causes of cardiovascular toxicities and the role of CCT in their evaluation are summarized in Table 18.1.

Coronary CT angiography (CTA) is a well-established noninvasive anatomic test with a high negative predictive value (approaching 99%) for the exclusion of obstructive CAD[47–52] (see Chapter 7, Diagnostic Accuracy of CCTA). Therefore coronary CTA is an ideal technique for the exclusion of obstructive CAD as the possible etiology of left ventricular systolic dysfunction in patients undergoing cancer treatment and who have suspected cancer therapy–related cardiac dysfunction (Fig. 18.6). The detection of CAD is important as coronary revascularization may lead to improvement of left ventricular function, thus enabling effective cancer treatments. Coronary CTA (CCTA) may be the preferred test over stress testing with imaging in patients with no prior history of CAD and abnormal wall motion, which may decrease the specificity of stress testing with imaging. Furthermore, several cancer treatments have been implicated in the development of cardiac ischemia, coronary events, coronary vasospasm (Fig. 18.7), or cardiac inflammation/myocarditis[18] and in select cases coronary CTA prior to the planned treatment can provide

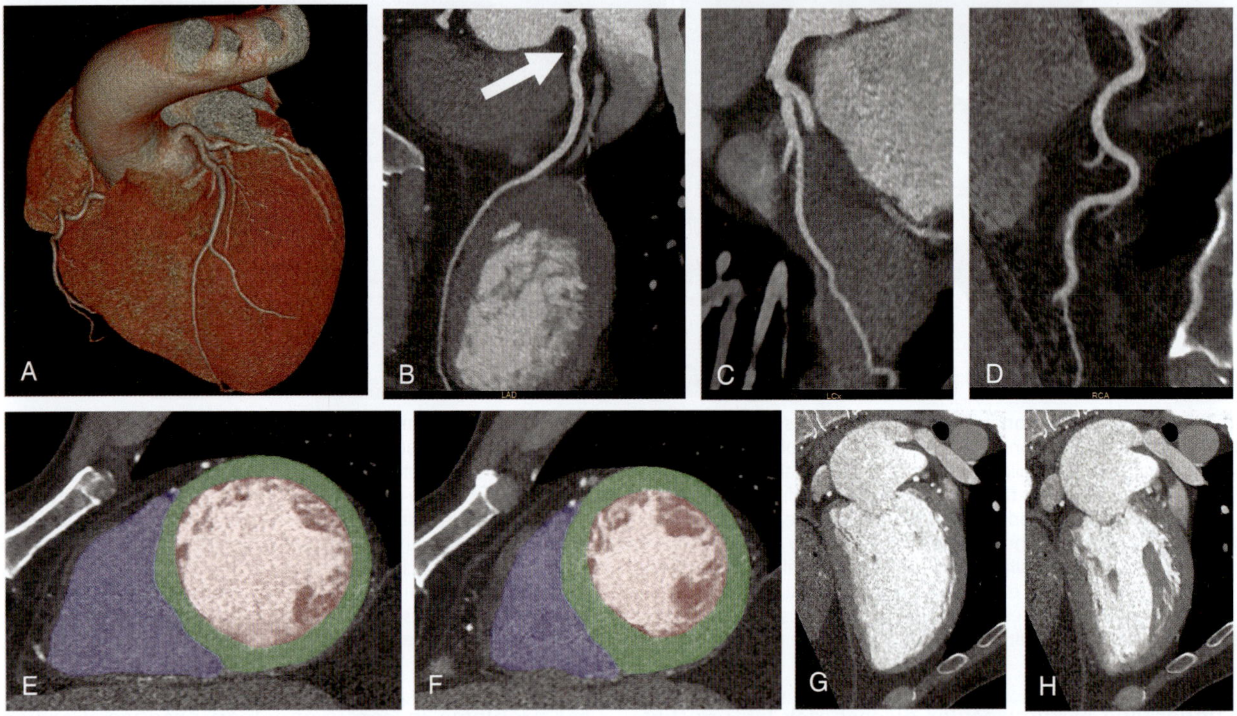

FIG. 18.5 Feasibility of Combined Coronary Artery and Left Ventricular Function Assessment With Cardiac Computed Tomography. A 66-year-old man with a history of prostate cancer on antiandrogen therapy developed signs and symptoms of congestive heart failure. He was found to have atrial fibrillation on ECG and decreased left ventricular systolic function on transthoracic echocardiogram. Coronary CT angiography (CCTA) was obtained with retrospective ECG gating to exclude obstructive coronary artery disease. CCTA of diagnostic quality was obtained despite a heart rate of 85 beats per minute and atrial fibrillation (Panel A, 3D volume reformatted image). There was a small amount of partially calcified plaque in the proximal LAD (*white arrow*) with minimal (<25%) luminal stenosis (Panel B, curved multiplanar reformatted image). There was no obvious coronary atherosclerosis or stenosis in the left circumflex (Panel C) and right (Panel D) coronary artery. The segmentation of the left ventricular cavity (*red*), left ventricular myocardium (*green*), and right ventricular cavity was performed in end diastole (Panel E) and end systole (Panel F). The two-chamber view of the left ventricle is depicted in end diastole (Panel G) and end systole (Panel H). The automatic segmentation was performed on the cardiac workstation, and the left ventricular (30%) and right ventricular (39%) ejection fraction was calculated. The findings were similar to the assessment from transthoracic echocardiography.

risk stratification prior to the cancer treatment and optimization of medical therapies.

CCTA also plays a role in patients with acute chest pain and suspected acute coronary syndrome (ACS).[8,53] It has a growing role in the evaluation of these patients, especially in the setting of low- to moderate-risk ACS (e.g., transient ECG abnormalities, mildly elevated troponin, wall motion abnormalities with no other significant findings; Fig. 18.8).[54–56] The advantage of CCTA is its ability to detect obstructive CAD and, if present, permit timely initiation of treatment according to the current ACC/AHA guidelines.[8] Cancer therapy–related thrombocytopenia and anemia places cancer patients at increased risk of procedural complications (e.g., bleeding) from invasive procedures such as invasive coronary angiography. The Society for Cardiovascular Angiography and Interventions (SCAI) guidelines addressed this issue and provided a recommendation that CCTA could be a preferred method for the evaluation of cancer patients.[13] CCTA has growing role in the evaluation of suspected type 2 myocardial infarction.[57,58] CCTA has a unique noninvasive capability to detect nonobstructive atherosclerosis and characterize coronary atherosclerosis.[59–62] Medical therapies can be initiated based on the results of coronary CTA and lead to improved outcomes if this allows for the continuation of cancer treatments.

CARDIAC CT IN THE EVALUATION OF THE EFFECTS OF RADIATION THERAPY

Chest radiation therapy (RT) is an essential component of the treatment for some of the malignancies involving the thoracic region. Although modern RT methods have significantly reduced the radiation dose to the heart and vascular structure, there is still a risk of radiation damage to those structures, which may lead to an increased risk of the development and progression of CAD, valvular and pericardial disease, and subsequent cardiovascular mortality.[27,63–66] CAD from the RT is an important competing cause of death in cancer survivors who underwent RT.[27,63,67–69]

CCT may play a role in pretreatment risk stratification and pos-treatment evaluation for RT-induced CAD. The assessment of CAC, which can be detected on RT planning and cancer staging CT scans may be used to assess for the presence of coronary atherosclerosis prior to RT to establish baseline cardiovascular risk. CAC detected on pretreatment CT scans is associated with an increased risk of acute coronary events after RT, even after correcting for radiation dose to the heart.[70] As described in the section on cardiovascular risk assessment, the detection of CAC should lead to the implementation of preventive measures for those at increased cardiovascular risk, including the

TABLE 18.1 The Most Common Types of Cancer Treatment–related Cardiac Dysfunction and the Role of Cardiac Computed Tomography

ONCOLOGIC THERAPY TYPE	COMMON CARDIOVASCULAR SIDE EFFECTS	POSSIBLE ROLES OF CARDIOVASCULAR CT
Anthracyclines (doxorubicin, daunorubicin, idarubicin, mitoxantrone)	Cardiomyopathy (toxicity increases in a cumulative, dose-dependent fashion) Myopericarditis Arrhythmia Pericardial effusion	• CCTA to rule out obstructive CAD as the etiology of decreased left ventricular systolic function/ cardiomyopathy • CCTA to rule out obstructive CAD in patients with troponin elevation, when an alternative diagnosis for myocardial injury other than coronary thrombosis is more likely • CAC assessment on noncardiac CT scans for baseline risk assessment
HER2/neu Receptor Inhibitors (transtuzumab, pertuzumab)	Cardiomyopathy	• CCTA to rule out obstructive CAD as the etiology of decreased left ventricular systolic function/ cardiomyopathy • CCTA to rule out obstructive CAD in patients with troponin elevation, when an alternative diagnosis for myocardial injury other than coronary thrombosis is more likely • CAC assessment on noncardiac CT scans for baseline risk assessment
Alkylating Agents (cyclophosphamide)	Hemorrhagic myopericarditis	• Cardiac CT to evaluate pericardial effusion (HU measurements for characterization of the effusion if clinically relevant) • CCTA to rule out obstructive CAD in patients with troponin elevation, when an alternative diagnosis for myocardial injury other than coronary thrombosis is more likely (e.g., myopericarditis) • CAC assessment on noncardiac CT scans for baseline risk assessment
Fluoropyrimidines (5-fluorouracil, capecitabine)	Anginal chest pain (incidence up to 18%) Coronary vasospasm Myocardial infarction	• CCTA to rule out obstructive CAD in patients presenting with symptoms of chest pain suspected to be coronary vasospasm to exclude other concomitant processes that could account for an acute coronary event. • Coronary CTA to evaluate coronary atherosclerosis prior to therapy • CAC assessment on noncardiac CT scans for baseline risk assessment
Taxanes (paclitaxel, docetaxel)	Myocardial ischemia Coronary vasospasm Cardiomyopathy Arrhythmias	• CCTA to rule out obstructive CAD as the etiology of decreased left ventricular systolic function/ cardiomyopathy • CCTA to rule out obstructive CAD in patients with troponin elevation, when an alternative diagnosis for myocardial injury other than coronary thrombosis is more likely • CAC assessment on noncardiac CT scans for baseline risk assessment
Vascular Endothelial Growth Factor Inhibitors (bevacizumab, sunitinib, sorafenib, pazopanib	Arterial hypertension Acute thromboembolic events, including ACS	• CCTA to rule out ACS in patients with acute presentation • CCTA to rule out obstructive CAD in patients with troponin elevation, when an alternative diagnosis for myocardial injury other than coronary thrombosis is more likely
Immune Checkpoint Inhibitors (pembrolizumab, nivolumab, ipilimumab, atezolizumab)	Myocarditis Increased risk of coronary atherosclerosis	• CCTA to rule out obstructive CAD when myocarditis is suspected (e.g., elevated troponin) • CCTA to evaluate coronary atherosclerosis prior to therapy • CAC assessment on noncardiac CT scans
CAR-T Therapy	Cytokine release syndrome Elevated troponin Cardiomyopathy Arrhythmias	• CCTA to rule out obstructive CAD in patients with troponin elevation, when an alternative diagnosis for myocardial injury other than coronary thrombosis is more likely • CCTA to rule out obstructive CAD as the etiology of decreased left ventricular systolic function/ cardiomyopathy
Hematopoietic Stem Cell Transplantation	Population with an increased prevalence of CV risk factors	• CAC assessment on noncardiac CT scans or CAC scan for baseline risk assessment • CCTA to rule out obstructive CAD in patients with symptoms suggestive of obstructive CAD

ACS, Acute coronary syndrome; *CAC*, coronary artery calcium scoring; *CAD*, coronary artery disease; *CAR-T*, chimeric antigen receptor therapy; *CCTA*, coronary computed tomography angiography; *CT*, computed tomography; *HU*, Hounsfield units.

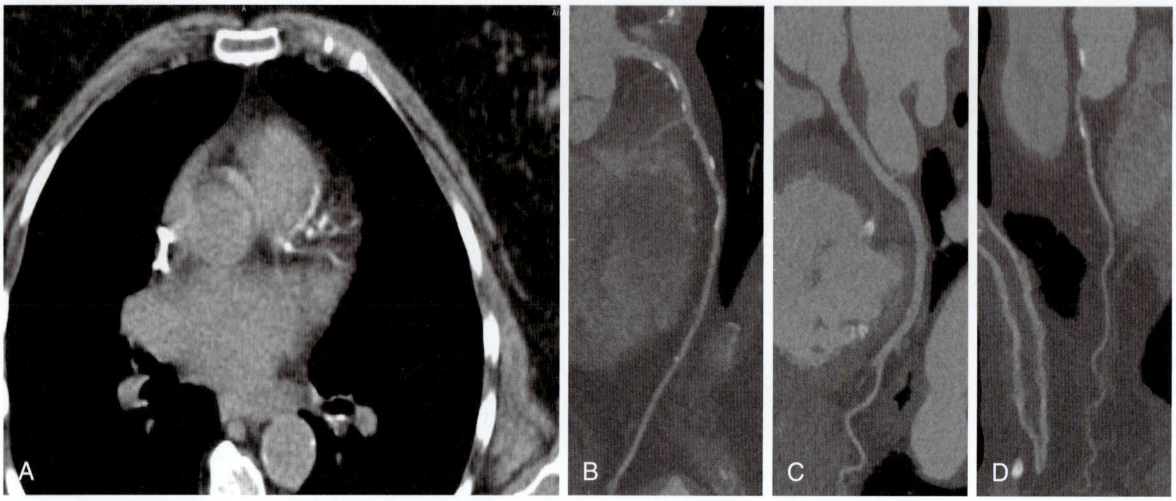

FIG. 18.6 Coronary Computed Tomography Angiography Evaluation in a Patient With New Onset Left Ventricular Dysfunction After Anthracycline Therapy. A 66-year-old woman with large B-cell lymphoma who underwent six cycles of chemotherapy (total dose of doxorubicin 300 mg/m²) and developed a new left ventricular systolic dysfunction (left ventricular ejection fraction of 35%). A noncontrast nongated CT exam showed moderate coronary calcifications (Panel A). She underwent a coronary CT angiography (CCTA) to assess for the presence of obstructive coronary artery disease and exclusion of ischemic cardiomyopathy due to the presence of cardiovascular risk factors and a strong family history of coronary artery disease. Panel B represents the curved multiplanar reformatted reconstruction of the left anterior descending coronary artery, Panel C represents the dominant left circumflex coronary artery, and Panel D a small right coronary artery. All vessels demonstrated mild stenosis (<50%) with calcified and noncalcified plaque. Cardiomyopathy was attributed to anthracycline exposure and the patient was started on statin in addition to guideline-directed medical therapies for heart failure.

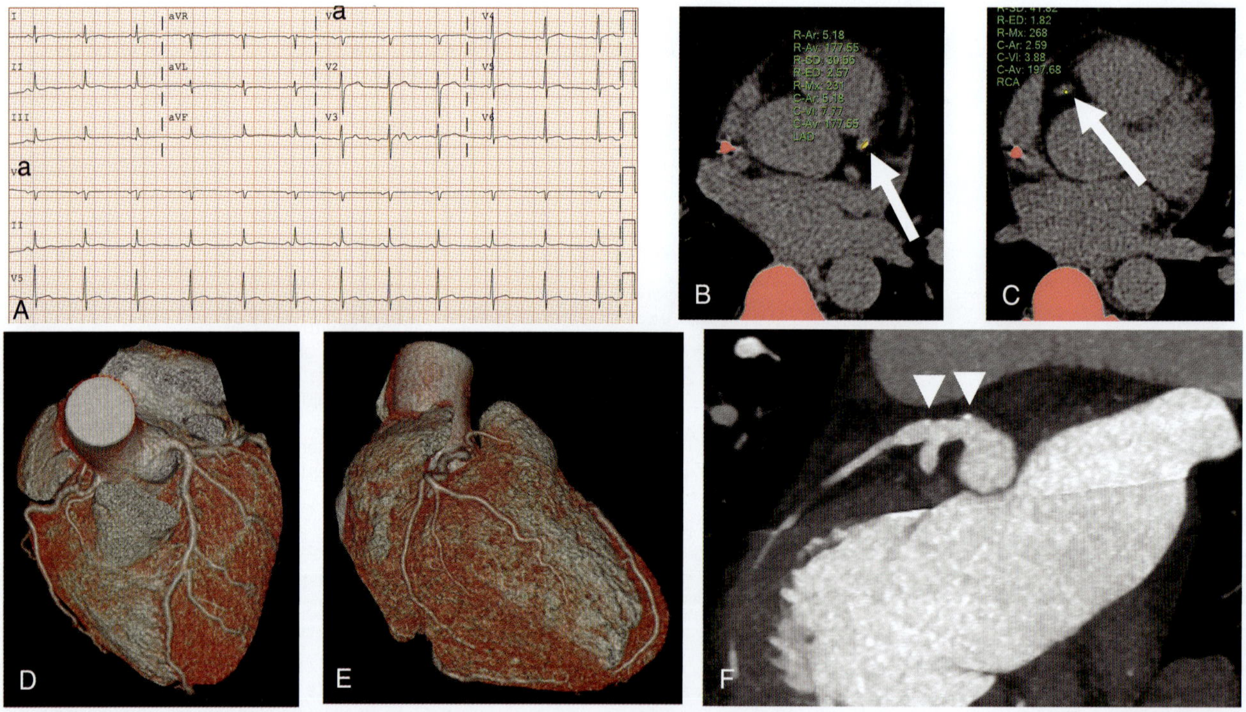

FIG. 18.7 Coronary Computed Tomography Angiography Evaluation in a Patient with Suspected Coronary Vasospasm During Fluoropyrimidine Therapy. A 47-year-old man with a history of essential hypertension and rectal cancer who was treated with radiation therapy and chemotherapy including capecitabine and then 5-fluorouracil. He developed resting chest pain while taking capecitabine and with 5-fluorouracil infusions. He had evidence of borderline ST segment elevations (Panel A) and normal cardiac troponin. We performed coronary CT angiography (CCTA) to evaluate for the presence of coronary artery disease. Noncontrast ECG-gated scan demonstrated coronary calcium in the left main, left anterior descending (*white arrow*, Panel B), and right coronary artery (*white arrow*, Panel C) with a coronary calcium (Agatston) score of 23 (83rd percentile for age, sex, and ethnicity). CCTA did not show any significant stenosis (3D reformatted images in Panels D and E). There was a small amount of calcified and noncalcified plaque in the distal left main and proximal left anterior descending coronary artery (*arrowheads*, multiplanar image in Panel F). The patient was treated with isosorbide mononitrate, amlodipine, and L-arginine. He was able to complete his chemotherapy regimen with the improvement of chest pain symptoms. He was also started on atorvastatin and aspirin.

start of preventive medications and risk factor modification.[40] The development of new CAC after RT is another important sign of increased cardiovascular risk and should trigger aggressive cardiovascular risk modification.[71,72]

CCTA may be a useful tool to evaluate for the presence of coronary artery disease after RT.[71,73] Smaller studies in asymptomatic survivors of Hodgkin's lymphoma who were treated with chest radiation have found that CCTA

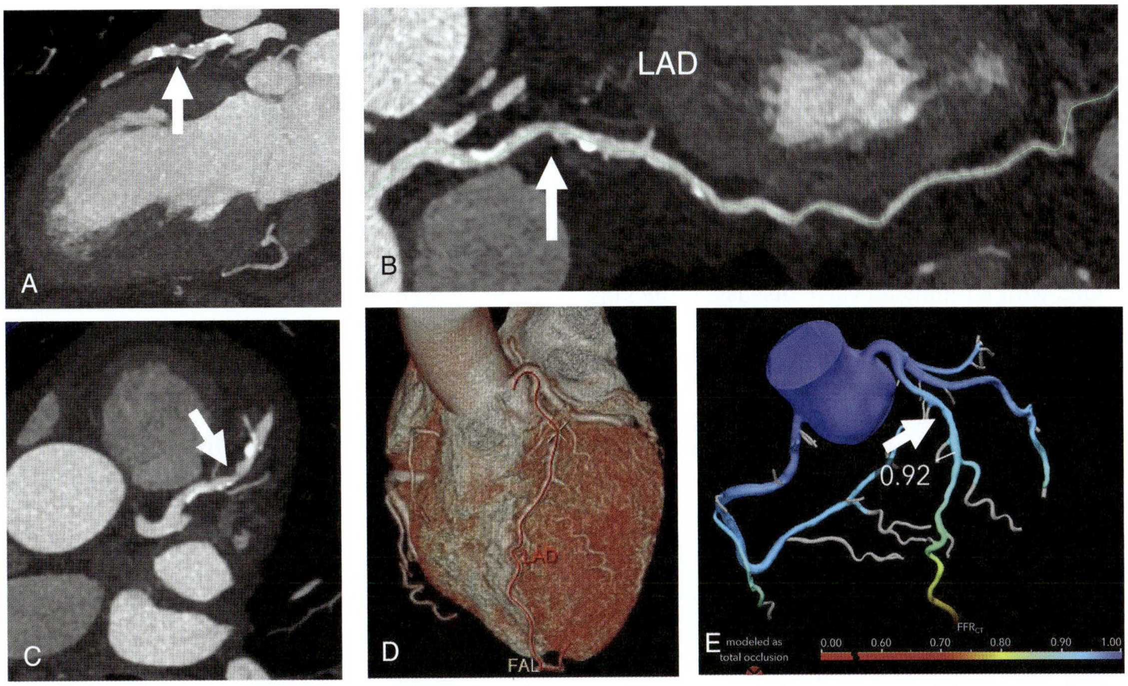

FIG. 18.8 Coronary Computed Tomography Angiography Evaluation of Complications of Immune Checkpoint Inhibitor Therapy. A 77-year-old man was treated for metastatic melanoma. He was initially treated with surgery followed by nivolumab and pembrolizumab. He had an episode of loss of consciousness/syncope while working on his farm that per the report required cardiovascular resuscitation although no arrhythmia was recorded. The initial workup did not reveal any ischemic ECG changes, and high-sensitivity cardiac troponin showed mild elevation. He underwent a transthoracic echocardiogram that showed normal cardiac function. The E14-day EKG monitor did not reveal any significant arrhythmia. Cardiac magnetic resonance showed normal cardiac function and no evidence of myocarditis, which can complicate the therapy with immune checkpoint inhibitors. Coronary CT angiography (CCTA) was obtained to rule out obstructive coronary artery disease. CTA demonstrated a large amount of calcified and noncalcified plaque in the left anterior descending coronary artery. There was mild to moderate (~50%) stenosis in the mid-left anterior descending (LAD) seen in two perpendicular views on the maximum intensity projection images (Panels A and B, *arrow*) and also on the curved multiplanar reformatted image (Panel C, *arrow*). The three-dimensional volume reformatted image is shown in Panel D. The hemodynamic significance of the mid-LAD stenosis was evaluated by noninvasive CT-based fractional flow reserve (FFR CT). FFR CT value distal to the stenosis (Panel **E**, *arrow*) was 0.92, suggesting that the stenosis was not hemodynamically significant (abnormal value is <0.80). The patient was eventually diagnosed with seizures in the setting of a brain metastasis.

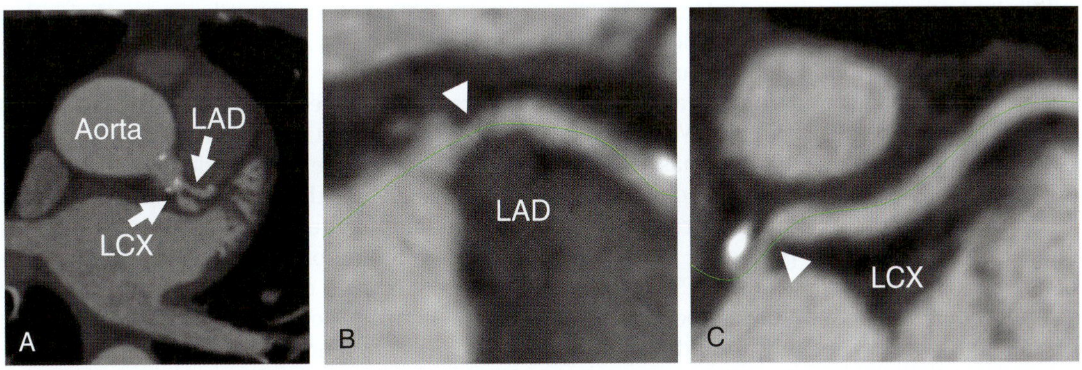

FIG. 18.9 Radiation Therapy-induced Coronary Artery Disease. A 70-year-old woman treated with radiation therapy for left-sided breast cancer 29 years ago presented with chest pain, elevated cardiac troponin, and mildly decreased left ventricular systolic function. Coronary CT angiography (CCTA) demonstrated calcified plaque in the distal left main coronary artery and severe ostial stenosis of the left anterior descending (LAD) and left circumflex (LCX) coronary artery (Panel A, maximum intensity projection image of the left main coronary artery bifurcation; Panel B, curved multiplanar reformatted image of the ostial LAD stenosis, *arrowhead*; Panel C, curved multiplanar reformatted image of the ostial LCX stenosis, *arrowhead*). The patients underwent coronary artery bypass surgery.

can reliably detect CAD.[71,73–75] Prior guidelines have recommended noninvasive stress testing for CAD detection 5 to 10 years after RT in asymptomatic high-risk patients, followed by reassessment every 5 years.[76–79] CCTA is an alternative test for patients who have suspected symptomatic or asymptomatic CAD (Fig. 18.9).[47–52] The strength of CCTA is its ability to rule in or rule out obstructive CAD and detect nonobstructive CAD. The latter information can be used for the decision to start preventive therapies (e.g., statins and aspirin).

RT-induced valvular heart disease develops in a subgroup of patients who received chest radiation therapy 10 to 20 years after the exposure. The reported prevalence of RT-induced valvular disease has varied widely across studies with the range of 2% to 37% for patients treated for Hodgkin's lymphoma and 0.5% to 4.2% for patients treated for breast cancer.[80] The imaging of patients with suspected RT-induced valvular disease should detect anatomical valve abnormalities, valve dysfunction, and left ventricular function. Transthoracic echocardiography provides a comprehensive evaluation of patients with prior radiation exposure. In a selected subgroup of patients, CMR imaging can complement echocardiography for the detailed assessment of valvular function and left ventricular characterization. CCT has a supplementary role in the assessment of patients with RT-induced valve disease, especially for detailed assessment of valvular calcification. CCT plays a critical role in preprocedural planning of transcatheter valvular interventions (transcatheter aortic, mitral, and tricuspid valve replacement) in patients with prior RT. Preinterventional CCT imaging is considered the gold standard for the anatomic assessment of aortic, mitral, and tricuspid valve interventions.[81–86]

CCT IN THE EVALUATION OF CARDIAC MASSES AND TUMORS

Tumors of the heart can be primary cardiac or secondary tumors (i.e., metastases). The primary tumors are rare. Among primary cardiac tumors, only 5% to 6% of them are malignant, most commonly sarcomas, lymphomas, and mesotheliomas.[87] Cardiac metastases are up to 40 times more common than primary cardiac tumors.[88] The diagnosis, localization, and characterization of cardiac tumors requires often multimodality cardiac imaging (Table 18.2).[89] Transthoracic echocardiography is widely available and is typically used as the first imaging test. It provides high temporal resolution and allows the evaluation of tissue characteristics. Transesophageal echocardiography can be used when there are limited acoustic windows and image quality is limited in transthoracic imaging. Echocardiography is ideal for the evaluation of small mobile masses and masses on the heart valves and provides additional evaluation of valvular function with color Doppler imaging. CMR imaging is used for further characterization of cardiac masses. The strength of CMR is its ability for detailed tissue characterization and multiplanar evaluation of cardiac structures as well as parametric tissue mapping, perfusion, presence, and pattern of late gadolinium enhancement. CCT can play an important role in the identification of the location of a cardiac tumor, including its relationship to and potential involvement of surrounding cardiac structures, especially the coronary arteries (see also Chapter 21, Cardiac Masses). The imaging protocols for the assessment of cardiac masses may include noncontrast imaging, first-pass imaging during CTA acquisition, and delayed imaging. The strengths of CCT include the high spatial resolution with isotropic voxel size. Multiplanar reformatted images in any imaging plane and three-dimensional imaging are optimal for the demonstration of spatial relationships between the tumor and other cardiac structures both for the diagnosis and surgical planning. CCT may also help differentiate intra-cavitary tumor from thrombus[90] and benign from malignant cardiac tumors in some instances with the addition of fluorodeoxyglucose positron emission tomography (FDG-PET).[91,92] CCT is the optimal technique for the imaging of calcified masses such as mitral annular calcification, which can be challenging on echocardiography and CMR (Fig. 18.10). CCT can also characterize adipose structures such as lipoma and lipomatous hypertrophy of the interatrial septum. Additionally, CCTA can be simultaneously obtained for a noninvasive exclusion of significant obstructive CAD before surgery and for planning to assess the proximity of the mass to coronary arteries. This can provide a less invasive, low-risk assessment for a patient with a low pretest probability of CAD, as patients—particularly with left-sided masses—may be at risk for embolic events with invasive coronary angiography.

CCT IN THE EVALUATION OF PERICARDIAL DISEASE

The pathologic changes of the pericardium in cancer patients include the changes after RT and the effect of anticancer drugs. The inflammation of the pericardium can occur acutely after therapeutic RT. This can lead to acute pericarditis and pericardial effusion. More often chronic changes with fibrotic changes and calcification are observed years after RT. This can lead to clinical presentation with pericardial constriction.[93] Several classes of chemotherapeutic agents have been associated with pericardial disease including anthracyclines, alkylating agents (e.g., cyclophosphamide), cytarabine, and tyrosine kinase inhibitors.[94–96] The clinical presentations include acute pericarditis and chronic changes leading to fibrosis and rarely to pericardial constriction. The direct tumor invasion into the pericardium from the surrounding structures (e.g., lung cancer, breast cancer) or direct involvement of the pericardium from primary pericardial tumors, or more often metastases can result in pericardial inflammation and effusion (Fig. 18.11). The pericardial effusion often accumulates gradually and tends to be hemorrhagic.

Transthoracic echocardiography is the first-line modality for the evaluation of pericardial disease. Echocardiography can provide reliable detection and quantification of the effusion. Furthermore, the hemodynamic evaluation for the tamponade and constriction can be obtained with the combination of two-dimensional imaging and Doppler. CMR is used as a complementary imaging tool for the assessment of pericardiac effusion and constriction. CMR can assess for ventricular interdependence, pericardial adhesions, and late-gadolinium enhancement of the pericardium (which is present in active inflammation or fibrosis) and to evaluate for myopericarditis. CCT has a more limited role but may identify the presence of acute pericarditis with the presence of the iodinated contrast enhancement of the pericardium on the first-pass imaging. On CCT, the pericardium in the setting of acute or chronic pericarditis will appear thickened (>4 mm) and may demonstrate the presence of a pericardial effusion.[93,97] Characteristics of the pericardial effusion on CCT may be obtained by measuring the CT attenuation of the fluid using Hounsfield units (HU)[98]:

- Transudative effusion (similar CT attenuation to water, <10 HU)
- Exudative effusion with high protein content (>10 HU)

TABLE 18.2 Imaging Characteristics of Cardiac Masses on Multimodality Imaging

CARDIAC MASSES	ECHOCARDIOGRAPHY	CARDIAC MAGNETIC RESONANCE IMAGING	CARDIAC COMPUTED TOMOGRAPHY	MORPHOLOGIC CHARACTERISTICS OF THE MASS
Benign Tumors				
Cardiac myxoma	Hyperechoic	T1: hypo/isointense; T2: hyperintense; LGE: peripheral, vascular pedicle, heterogeneous	Hypodense; calcifications; high iodine concentration on delayed-enhancement images	Irregular borders; pedunculated and usually arises from the interatrial septum, near the fossa ovalis; intracavitary, left atrium (75%), right atrium (20%), ventricles (5%)
Lipoma	Hyperechoic	T1/T2: hyperintense; fat saturation: hypointense	Hypodense; fat attenuation	Smooth, broad base; interatrial septum, intramural, intracavitary
Papillary fibroelastoma	Heterogeneous	T1/T2: hyperintense, homogeneous; LGE: high, homogeneous delayed	Hypodense	Frond, pedicle; valvular, small size; developed "head" or with elongated strand-like projections
Rhabdomyoma	Hyperechoic	T1: isointense; T2: iso/ hyperintense; T2: iso/ hyperintense	Hypodense	Smooth, broad base; intramural
Fibroma	Hyperechoic	T1: isointense; T2: hypointense; LGE: hyperenhancement	Hypodense; punctate calcification enhancement	Smooth, broad base; intramural
Hemangioma	Enhancement with echo-contrast	T1: isointense, heterogeneous; T2: hyperintense; first-pass: high-contrast intensity	Hypodense; heterogenous; calcifications intense enhancement	Intracavitary
Malignant Tumors				
Sarcomas	Isoechoic to hyperechoic	T1: iso (rhabdo-, undifferentiated)/ heterogeneous (angio); T2: heterogeneous (angio)/ hyperintense (rhabdo-, undifferentiated); LGE: heterogeneous (angio-), homogeneous (rhabdo-)	Isodense	Lobular; broad base: left atrium (undifferentiated, osteo-, fibro-, leiomyosarcoma, right atrium (angiosarcoma)
Lymphomas	Homogeneous echogenicity, thickened wall	T1: isointense, homogeneous; T2: isointense; LGE: variable	Hypo/isodense	Lobular; right atrium, right ventricle, mediastinum
Metastases	Isoechoic to hyperechoic	T1: hypo/isointense; T2: iso/ hyperintense; LGE: heterogeneous, strong	Isodense; ± calcifications	Mulitple locations, pericardial effusion
Thrombus				
Thrombus	Hyperechoic	T1: homogenous, high (low if chronic); T2: iso/high (low if chronic); fat saturation: isointense; first-pass perfusion and LGE: hypointense at long inversion times	Low-attenuation, nonenhancing; crescentic shape (chronic)	Left atrial appendage, apical thrombus with severe left ventricular dysfunction, associated with indwelling catheters
Paracardial Lesions				
Pericardial cyst	Echolucent	Low intensity on T1-weighted and high intensity on T2-weighted images, no post-contrast-enhancement	Thin-walled, sharply defined, oval homogeneous, attenuation is slightly higher than water, no post-contrast-enhancement	Smooth and regular limits adjoining the cardiac border, often in right cardiophrenic angle
Tumor-like				
Lipomatous hypertrophy of interatrial septum	Hyperechoic	T1/T2: hyperintense; fat saturation: hypointense	Low CT attenuation, nonenhancing on contrast images	Smooth, well-marginated expansion of the interatrial septum >1.5 cm in transverse diameter; dumbbell shaped
Caseous calcification of mitral annulus	Echolucent center and the more echogenic periphery	T1/T2 hypointense, SSFP hypointense, no first-pass perfusion, enhanced border and nonenhanced core	Calcific rim with high CT attenuation and central homogeneous liquefied calcium with lower CT attenuation	Round, ovoid shape, typically located in the posterior mitral annulus

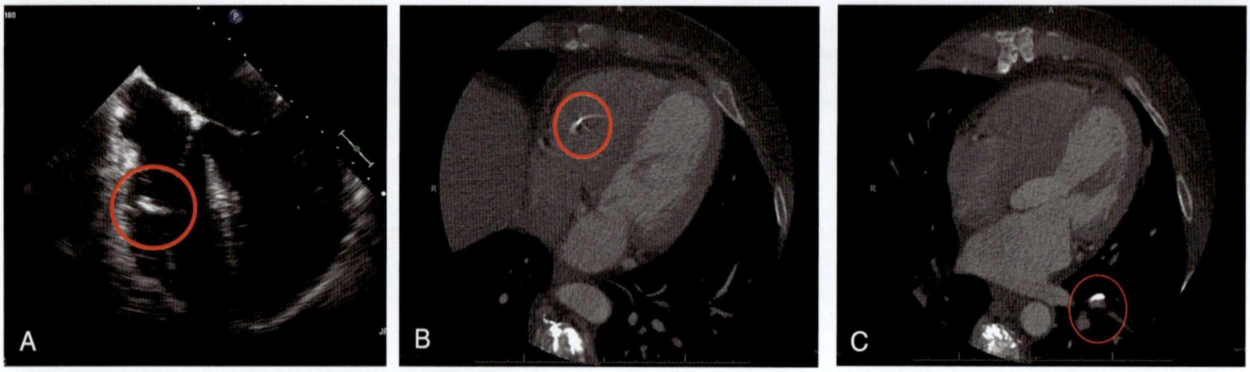

FIG. 18.10 Cardiac Mass Assessment With Cardiac Computed Tomography. An 83-year-old man with multiple myeloma was referred for a transesophageal echocardiogram evaluation due to an ill-defined echogenicity in the right ventricle (*red circle* in Panel A) seen originally on routine transthoracic echocardiogram. Cardiac CT was ordered for a detailed assessment. A high CT density was noted in the right ventricle (*red circle* in Panel B) as well as in a pulmonary branch (*red circle* in Panel C). This was consistent with embolized bone cement from an interventional radiology procedure that the patient underwent 2 weeks before the echocardiogram.

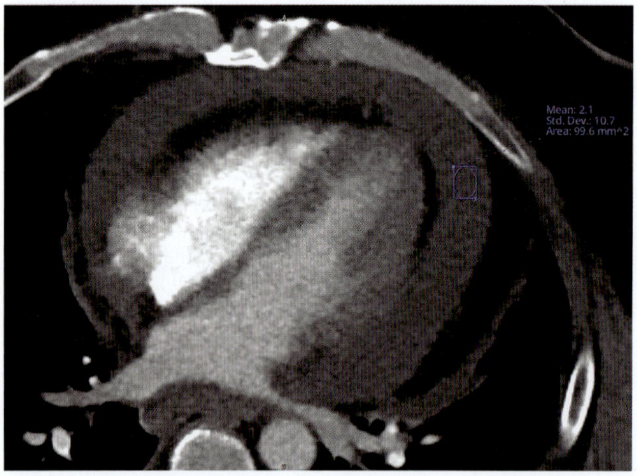

FIG. 18.11 Computed Tomography Evaluation of Pericardial Effusion. A 46-year-old man with a viral illness and prior history of melanoma with clinical presentation of cough and shortness of breath underwent contrast-enhanced computed tomography to rule out pulmonary embolism. A large circumferential pericardial effusion was seen with a mean CT density of +2 Hounsfield units (HU) consistent. Transthoracic echocardiogram showed findings suggestive of increased intra-pericardial pressures. The patient underwent pericardiocentesis with the improvement of his symptoms. The analysis of pericardial fluid was negative for the presence of malignant cells. No cardiac masses were seen in cardiac imaging studies and the patient was treated for presumed viral pericarditis.

- Purulent, malignant, or myxedematous exudative effusion (20–60 HU)
- Hemorrhagic effusion (>60 HU)

Although CCT cannot provide hemodynamic assessment for constriction, the presence of significantly thickened pericardium and advanced diffuse pericardial calcifications support the diagnosis of constrictive pericarditis.[98]

CONCLUSIONS

In the growing field of cardio-oncology, CCT has diverse applications in the clinical care of cancer patients and survivors (Fig. 18.1). The assessment for the presence of CAC on nongated chest CT obtained routinely for cancer patients provides a unique opportunity for the optimization of cardiovascular risk prediction and modification of risk factors. Preventive treatments are especially important, as cardiovascular mortality is the most common cause of death in long-term cancer survivors. CCTA is uniquely positioned to provide an assessment of CAD in patients undergoing cancer treatments due to its noninvasive nature and high negative predictive value. Many cardiovascular toxicities from cancer therapies can be differentiated from ACS by using CCT. CCT is a complementary technique to echocardiography and CMR in the evaluation of pericardial disease, RT-induced heart disease, and cardiac masses.

Disclosures: Maros Ferencik Grants NIH, AHA, Consulting Siemens Healthineers, Elucid, HeartFlow, Stock options Elucid

Funding: None

REFERENCES

1. Ahn SG, Lee HM, Lee SA. Long-term survival analysis of korean breast cancer patients at a single center: improving outcome over time. *Yonsei Med J.* 2014;55(5):1187–1195. doi:10.3349/ymj.2014.55.5.1187.
2. DeSantis CE, Lin CC, Mariotto AB, et al. Cancer treatment and survivorship statistics, 2014. *CA Cancer J Clin.* 2014;64(4):252–271. doi:10.3322/caac.21235.
3. Groarke JD, Nguyen PL, Nohria A, Ferrari R, Cheng S, Moslehi J. Cardiovascular complications of radiation therapy for thoracic malignancies: the role for non-invasive imaging for detection of cardiovascular disease. *Eur Heart J.* 2014;35(10):612–623. doi:10.1093/eurheartj/eht114.
4. Mertens AC, Liu Q, Neglia JP, et al. Cause-specific late mortality among 5-year survivors of childhood cancer: the childhood cancer survivor study. *J Natl Cancer Inst.* 2008;100(19):1368–1379. doi:10.1093/jnci/djn310.
5. Bradshaw PT, Stevens J, Khankari N, Teitelbaum SL, Neugut AI, Gammon MD. Cardiovascular disease mortality among breast cancer survivors. *Epidemiology.* 2016;27(1):6–13. doi:10.1097/EDE.0000000000000394.
6. Armstrong GT, Chen Y, Yasui Y, et al. Reduction in late mortality among 5-year survivors of childhood cancer. *N Engl J Med.* 2016;374(9):833–842. doi:10.1056/NEJMoa1510795.
7. Knuuti J, Wijns W, Saraste A, et al. 2019 ESC Guidelines for the diagnosis and management of chronic coronary syndromes. *Eur Heart J;.* 2020:407–477.
8. Writing Committee M, Gulati M, Levy PD, et al. 2021 AHA/ACC/ASE/CHEST/SAEM/SCCT/SCMR Guideline for the evaluation and diagnosis of chest pain: a report of the American College of Cardiology/American Heart Association joint committee on clinical practice guidelines. *J Am Coll Cardiol;.* 2021:e187–e285.
9. Armenian SH, Lacchetti C, Barac A, et al. Prevention and monitoring of cardiac dysfunction in survivors of adult cancers: American society of clinical oncology clinical practice guideline. *J Clin Oncol.* 2017;35(8):893–911. doi:10.1200/JCO.2016.70.5400.
10. Campia U, Moslehi JJ, Amiri-Kordestani L, et al. Cardio-oncology: vascular and metabolic perspectives: a scientific statement from the American Heart Association. *Circulation.* 2019;139(13):e579–e602. doi:10.1161/CIR.0000000000000641.
11. Curigliano G, Lenihan D, Fradley M, et al. Management of cardiac disease in cancer patients throughout oncological treatment: ESMO consensus recommendations. *Ann Oncol.* 2020;31(2):171–190. doi:10.1016/j.annonc.2019.10.023.
12. Gilchrist SC, Barac A, Ades PA, et al. Cardio-oncology rehabilitation to manage cardiovascular outcomes in cancer patients and survivors: a

scientific statement from the American Heart Association. *Circulation*. 2019;139(21):e997–e1012. doi:10.1161/CIR.0000000000000679.

13. Iliescu CA, Grines CL, Herrmann J, et al. SCAI Expert consensus statement: evaluation, management, and special considerations of cardio-oncology patients in the cardiac catheterization laboratory (endorsed by the cardiological society of india, and sociedad Latino Americana de Cardiologia Intervencionista). *Catheter Cardiovasc Interv*. 2016;87(5):E202–E223. doi:10.1002/ccd.26379.
14. Lancellotti P, Suter TM, Lopez-Fernandez T, et al. Cardio-oncology services: rationale, organization, and implementation. *Eur Heart J*. 2019;40(22):1756–1763. doi:10.1093/eurheartj/ehy453.
15. Lyon AR, Dent S, Stanway S, et al. Baseline cardiovascular risk assessment in cancer patients scheduled to receive cardiotoxic cancer therapies: a position statement and new risk assessment tools from the Cardio-Oncology study group of the heart failure association of the European Society of Cardiology in collaboration with the International Cardio-Oncology Society. *Eur J Heart Fail*. 2020;22(11):1945–1960. doi:10.1002/ejhf.1920.
16. Plana JC, Galderisi M, Barac A, et al. Expert consensus for multimodality imaging evaluation of adult patients during and after cancer therapy: a report from the American Society of Echocardiography and the European Association of cardiovascular imaging. *J Am Soc Echocardiogr*. 2014;27(9):911–939. doi:10.1016/j.echo.2014.07.012.
17. Virani SA, Dent S, Brezden-Masley C, et al. Canadian cardiovascular society guidelines for evaluation and management of cardiovascular complications of cancer therapy. *Can J Cardiol*. 2016;32(7):831–841. doi:10.1016/j.cjca.2016.02.078.
18. Zamorano JL, Lancellotti P, Rodriguez Munoz D, et al. 2016 ESC Position paper on cancer treatments and cardiovascular toxicity developed under the auspices of the ESC committee for practice guidelines: the task force for cancer treatments and cardiovascular toxicity of the European Society of Cardiology (ESC). *Eur Heart J*. 2016;37(36):2768–2801. doi:10.1093/eurheartj/ehw211.
19. Lyon AR, Lopez-Fernandez T, Couch LS, et al. 2022 ESC Guidelines on cardio-oncology developed in collaboration with the European Hematology Association (EHA), the European Society for Therapeutic Radiology and Oncology (ESTRO) and the International Cardio-Oncology Society (IC-OS). *Eur Heart J Cardiovasc Imaging*. 2022;23(10):e333–e465. doi:10.1093/ehjci/jeac106.
20. Lopez-Mattei J, Yang EH, Baldassarre LA, et al. Cardiac computed tomographic imaging in cardio-oncology: an expert consensus document of the Society of Cardiovascular Computed Tomography (SCCT). Endorsed by the International Cardio-Oncology Society (ICOS). *J Cardiovasc Comput Tomogr*. 2023;17(1):66–83. doi:10.1016/j.jcct.2022.09.002.
21. Wright JL, Amini A, Bergom C, Milgrom SA. Summary of cardiac computed tomographic imaging in cardio-oncology: an expert consensus document of the society of cardiovascular computed tomography. *Pract Radiat Oncol*. 2023;13(6):488–495. doi:10.1016/j.prro.2023.08.008.
22. Eyre H, Kahn R, Robertson RM, et al. Preventing cancer, cardiovascular disease, and diabetes. *Circulation*. 2004;109(25):3244–3255. doi:10.1161/01.Cir.0000133321.00456.00.
23. Calle EE, Rodriguez C, Walker-Thurmond K, Thun MJ. Overweight, obesity, and mortality from cancer in a prospectively studied cohort of U.S. adults. *N Engl J Med*. 2003;348(17):1625–1638. doi:10.1056/NEJMoa021423.
24. Whelton SP, Al Rifai M, Dardari Z, et al. Coronary artery calcium and the competing long-term risk of cardiovascular vs. cancer mortality: the CAC consortium. *Eur Heart J Cardiovasc Imaging*. 2019;20(4):389–395. doi:10.1093/ehjci/jey176.
25. Handy CE, Desai CS, Dardari ZA, et al. The association of coronary artery calcium with noncardiovascular disease: the multi-ethnic study of atherosclerosis. *JACC Cardiovasc Imaging*. 2016;9(5):568–576. doi:10.1016/j.jcmg.2015.09.020.
26. Armenian SH, Xu L, Ky B, et al. Cardiovascular disease among survivors of adult-onset cancer: a community-based retrospective cohort study. *J Clin Oncol*. 2016;34(10):1122–1130. doi:10.1200/JCO.2015.64.0409.
27. Darby SC, Ewertz M, McGale P, et al. Risk of ischemic heart disease in women after radiotherapy for breast cancer. *N Engl J Med*. 2013;368(11):987–998. doi:10.1056/NEJMoa1209825.
28. Hassan SA, Palaskas N, Kim P, et al. Chemotherapeutic agents and the risk of ischemia and arterial thrombosis. *Curr Atheroscler Rep*. 2018;20(2):10. doi:10.1007/s11883-018-0702-5.
29. Suero-Abreu GA, Zanni MV, Neilan TG. Atherosclerosis with immune checkpoint inhibitor therapy: evidence, diagnosis, and management: JACC: cardio-oncology state-of-the-art review. *JACC Cardio Oncol*. 2022;4(5):598–615. doi:10.1016/j.jaccao.2022.11.011.
30. Marvel FA, Whelton SP, Blumenthal RS. A cardio-oncology cardiovascular prevention framework. *JACC Cardio Oncol*. 2019;1(2):252–255. doi:10.1016/j.jaccao.2019.11.012.
31. Sayed A, Munir M, Addison D, et al. The underutilization of preventive cardiovascular measures in patients with cancer. An analysis of the behavioural risk factor surveillance system, 2011–2022. *Eur J Prev Cardiol*. 2023. doi:10.1093/eurjpc/zwad146.
32. Arnett DK, Blumenthal RS, Albert MA, et al. 2019 ACC/AHA Guideline on the primary prevention of cardiovascular disease: a report of the American College of Cardiology/American Heart Association task force on clinical practice guidelines. *Circulation*. 2019;140(11):e596–e646. doi:10.1161/CIR.0000000000000678.
33. Jaiswal S, Natarajan P, Silver AJ, et al. Clonal hematopoiesis and risk of atherosclerotic cardiovascular disease. *N Engl J Med*. 2017;377(2):111–121. doi:10.1056/NEJMoa1701719.
34. Seijkens TTP, Lutgens E. Cardiovascular oncology: exploring the effects of targeted cancer therapies on atherosclerosis. *Curr Opin Lipidol*. 2018;29(5):381–388. doi:10.1097/MOL.0000000000000538.
35. Drobni ZD, Alvi RM, Taron J, et al. Association between immune checkpoint inhibitors with cardiovascular events and atherosclerotic plaque. *Circulation*. 2020;142(24):2299–2311. doi:10.1161/CIRCULATIONAHA.120.049981.
36. Cainzos-Achirica M, Miedema MD, McEvoy JW, et al. Coronary artery calcium for personalized allocation of aspirin in primary prevention of cardiovascular disease in 2019: the MESA study (Multi-ethnic study of atherosclerosis). *Circulation*. 2020;141(19):1541–1553. doi:10.1161/CIRCULATIONAHA.119.045010.
37. Mitchell JD, Fergestrom N, Gage BF, et al. Impact of statins on cardiovascular outcomes following coronary artery calcium scoring. *J Am Coll Cardiol*. 2018;72(25):3233–3242. doi:10.1016/j.jacc.2018.09.051.
38. Hecht HS, Blaha MJ, Kazerooni EA, et al. CAC-DRS: coronary artery calcium data and reporting system. An expert consensus document of the Society of Cardiovascular Computed Tomography (SCCT). *J Cardiovasc Comput Tomogr*. 2018;12(3):185–191. doi:10.1016/j.jcct.2018.03.008.
39. Orringer CE, Blaha MJ, Blankstein R, et al. The National Lipid Association scientific statement on coronary artery calcium scoring to guide preventive strategies for ASCVD risk reduction. *J Clin Lipidol*. 2021;15(1):33–60. doi:10.1016/j.jacl.2020.12.005.
40. Gernaat SA, Isgum I, de Vos BD, et al. Automatic coronary artery calcium scoring on radiotherapy planning CT scans of breast cancer patients: reproducibility and association with traditional cardiovascular risk factors. *PLoS One*. 2016;11(12):e0167925. doi:10.1371/journal.pone.0167925.
41. Hecht HS, Cronin P, Blaha MJ, et al. 2016 SCCT/STR Guidelines for coronary artery calcium scoring of noncontrast noncardiac chest CT scans: a report of the society of cardiovascular computed tomography and society of thoracic radiology. *J Cardiovasc Comput Tomogr*. 2017;11(1):74–84. doi:10.1016/j.jcct.2016.11.003.
42. Blaha MJ, Budoff MJ, Tota-Maharaj R, et al. Improving the CAC score by addition of regional measures of calcium distribution: multi-ethnic study of atherosclerosis. *JACC Cardiovasc Imaging*. 2016;9(12):1407–1416. doi:10.1016/j.jcmg.2016.03.001.
43. Dzaye O, Dudum R, Mirbolouk M, et al. Validation of the Coronary Artery Calcium Data and Reporting System (CAC-DRS): dual importance of CAC score and CAC distribution from the Coronary Artery Calcium (CAC) consortium. *J Cardiovasc Comput Tomogr*. 2020;14(1):12–17. doi:10.1016/j.jcct.2019.03.011.
44. Ferencik M, Pencina KM, Liu T, et al. Coronary artery calcium distribution is an independent predictor of incident major coronary heart disease events: results from the framingham heart study. *Circ Cardiovasc Imaging*. 2017;10(10). doi:10.1161/CIRCIMAGING.117.006592.
45. Mamudu HM, Paul TK, Veeranki SP, Budoff M. The effects of coronary artery calcium screening on behavioral modification, risk perception, and medication adherence among asymptomatic adults: a systematic review. *Atherosclerosis*. 2014;236(2):338–350. doi:10.1016/j.atherosclerosis.2014.07.022.
46. Sturgeon KM, Deng L, Bluethmann SM, et al. A population-based study of cardiovascular disease mortality risk in US cancer patients. *Eur Heart J*. 2019;40(48):3889–3897. doi:10.1093/eurheartj/ehz766.
47. Budoff MJ, Dowe D, Jollis JG, et al. Diagnostic performance of 64-multidetector row coronary computed tomographic angiography for evaluation of coronary artery stenosis in individuals without known coronary artery disease: results from the prospective multicenter ACCURACY (Assessment by Coronary Computed Tomographic Angiography of Individuals Undergoing Invasive Coronary Angiography) trial. *J Am Coll Cardiol*. 2008;52(21):1724–1732. doi:10.1016/j.jacc.2008.07.031.
48. Danad I, Raijmakers PG, Driessen RS, et al. Comparison of coronary CT angiography, SPECT, PET, and hybrid imaging for diagnosis of ischemic heart disease determined by fractional flow reserve. *JAMA Cardiol*. 2017;2(10):1100–1107. doi:10.1001/jamacardio.2017.2471.
49. Knuuti J, Ballo H, Juarez-Orozco LE, et al. The performance of non-invasive tests to rule-in and rule-out significant coronary artery stenosis in patients with stable angina: a meta-analysis focused on post-test disease probability. *Eur Heart J*. 2018;39(35):3322–3330. doi:10.1093/eurheartj/ehy267.
50. Meijboom WB, Meijs MF, Schuijf JD, et al. Diagnostic accuracy of 64-slice computed tomography coronary angiography: a prospective, multicenter, multivendor study. *J Am Coll Cardiol*. 2008;52(25):2135–2144. doi:10.1016/j.jacc.2008.08.058.
51. Miller JM, Rochitte CE, Dewey M, et al. Diagnostic performance of coronary angiography by 64-row CT. *N Engl J Med*. 2008;359(22):2324–2336. doi:10.1056/NEJMoa0806576.
52. Schuetz GM, Schlattmann P, Dewey M. Use of 3x2 tables with an intention to diagnose approach to assess clinical performance of diagnostic tests: meta-analytical evaluation of coronary CT angiography studies. *BMJ*. 2012;345:e6717. doi:10.1136/bmj.e6717.
53. Collet JP, Thiele H, Barbato E, et al. 2020 ESC Guidelines for the management of acute coronary syndromes in patients presenting without persistent ST-segment elevation. *Eur Heart J*. 2021;42(14):1289–1367. doi:10.1093/eurheartj/ehaa575.
54. Kumar V, Weerakoon S, Dey AK, et al. The evolving role of coronary CT angiography in acute coronary syndromes. *J Cardiovasc Comput Tomogr*. 2021;15(5):384–393. doi:10.1016/j.jcct.2021.02.002.

55. Lee KK, Bularga A, O'Brien R, et al. Troponin-guided coronary computed tomographic angiography after exclusion of myocardial infarction. *J Am Coll Cardiol.* 2021;78(14):1407–1417. doi:10.1016/j.jacc.2021.07.055.
56. Linde JJ, Kelbæk H, Hansen TF, et al. Coronary CT angiography in patients with non-ST-segment elevation acute coronary syndrome. *J Am Coll Cardiol.* 2020;75(5):453–463. doi:10.1016/j.jacc.2019.12.012.
57. McCarthy CP, Murphy SP, Amponsah DK, et al. Coronary computed tomographic angiography with fractional flow reserve in patients with type 2 myocardial infarction. *J Am Coll Cardiol.* 2023. doi:10.1016/j.jacc.2023.08.020.
58. Meah MN, Bularga A, Tzolos E, et al. Distinguishing type 1 from type 2 myocardial infarction by using CT coronary angiography. *Radiology.* 2022;4(5):e220081. doi:10.1148/ryct.220081.
59. Abdelrahman KM, Chen MY, Dey AK, et al. Coronary computed tomography angiography from clinical uses to emerging technologies: JACC state-of-the-art review. *J Am Coll Cardiol.* 2020;76(10):1226–1243. doi:10.1016/j.jacc.2020.06.076.
60. Achenbach S, Moselewski F, Ropers D, et al. Detection of calcified and noncalcified coronary atherosclerotic plaque by contrast-enhanced, submillimeter multidetector spiral computed tomography: a segment-based comparison with intravascular ultrasound. *Circulation.* 2004;109(1):14–17. doi:10.1161/01.CIR.0000111517.69230.0F.
61. Ahmadi A, Argulian E, Leipsic J, Newby DE, Narula J. From subclinical atherosclerosis to plaque progression and acute coronary events: JACC state-of-the-art review. *J Am Coll Cardiol.* 2019;74(12):1608–1617. doi:10.1016/j.jacc.2019.08.012 doi:papers3://publication/doi/.
62. Arbab-Zadeh A, Fuster V. From detecting the vulnerable plaque to managing the vulnerable patient: JACC state-of-the-art review. *J Am Coll Cardiol.* 2019;74(12):1582–1593. doi:10.1016/j.jacc.2019.07.062.
63. van Nimwegen FA, Schaapveld M, Cutter DJ, et al. Radiation dose-response relationship for risk of coronary heart disease in survivors of Hodgkin lymphoma. *J Clin Oncol.* 2016;34(3):235–243. doi:10.1200/JCO.2015.63.4444.
64. Carr ZA, Land CE, Kleinerman RA, et al. Coronary heart disease after radiotherapy for peptic ulcer disease. *Int J Radiat Oncol Biol Phys.* 2005;61(3):842–850. doi:10.1016/j.ijrobp.2004.07.708.
65. Dess RT, Sun Y, Matuszak MM, et al. Cardiac events after radiation therapy: combined analysis of prospective multicenter trials for locally advanced non-small-cell lung cancer. *J Clin Oncol.* 2017;35(13):1395–1402. doi:10.1200/JCO.2016.71.6142.
66. Wang K, Eblan MJ, Deal AM, et al. Cardiac toxicity after radiotherapy for Stage III non-small-cell lung cancer: pooled analysis of dose-escalation trials delivering 70 to 90 Gy. *J Clin Oncol.* 2017;35(13):1387–1394. doi:10.1200/JCO.2016.70.0229.
67. Aleman BM, van den Belt-Dusebout AW, De Bruin ML, et al. Late cardiotoxicity after treatment for Hodgkin lymphoma. *Blood.* 2007;109(5):1878–1886. doi:10.1182/blood-2006-07-034405.
68. Clarke M, Collins R, Darby S, et al. Effects of radiotherapy and of differences in the extent of surgery for early breast cancer on local recurrence and 15-year survival: an overview of the randomised trials. *Lancet.* 2005;366(9503):2087–2106. doi:10.1016/S0140-6736(05)67887-7.
69. van Nimwegen FA, Schaapveld M, Janus CP, et al. Cardiovascular disease after Hodgkin lymphoma treatment: 40-year disease risk. *JAMA Intern Med.* 2015;175(6):1007–1017. doi:10.1001/jamainternmed.2015.1180.
70. Roos CTG, van den Bogaard VAB, Greuter MJW, et al. Is the coronary artery calcium score associated with acute coronary events in breast cancer patients treated with radiotherapy? *Radiother Oncol.* 2018;126(1):170–176. doi:10.1016/j.radonc.2017.10.009.
71. Rademaker J, Schoder H, Ariaratnam NS, et al. Coronary artery disease after radiation therapy for Hodgkin's lymphoma: coronary CT angiography findings and calcium scores in nine asymptomatic patients. *Am J Roentgenol.* 2008;191(1):32–37. doi:10.2214/AJR.07.3112.
72. Andersen R, Wethal T, Gunther A, et al. Relation of coronary artery calcium score to premature coronary artery disease in survivors >15 years of Hodgkin's lymphoma. *Am J Cardiol.* 2010;105(2):149–152. doi:10.1016/j.amjcard.2009.09.005.
73. Kupeli S, Hazirolan T, Varan A, et al. Evaluation of coronary artery disease by computed tomography angiography in patients treated for childhood Hodgkin's lymphoma. *J Clin Oncol.* 2010;28(6):1025–1030. doi:10.1200/JCO.2009.25.2627.
74. Daniels LA, Krol AD, de Graaf MA, et al. Screening for coronary artery disease after mediastinal irradiation in Hodgkin lymphoma survivors: phase II study of indication and acceptancedagger. *Ann Oncol.* 2014;25(6):1198–1203. doi:10.1093/annonc/mdu130.
75. Girinsky T, M'Kacher R, Lessard N, et al. Prospective coronary heart disease screening in asymptomatic Hodgkin lymphoma patients using coronary computed tomography angiography: results and risk factor analysis. *Int J Radiat Oncol Biol Phys.* 2014;89(1):59–66. doi:10.1016/j.ijrobp.2014.01.021.
76. Desai MY, Windecker S, Lancellotti P, et al. Prevention, diagnosis, and management of radiation-associated cardiac disease: JACC scientific expert panel. *J Am Coll Cardiol.* 2019;74(7):905–927. doi:10.1016/j.jacc.2019.07.006.
77. Lancellotti P, Nkomo VT, Badano LP, et al. Expert consensus for multi-modality imaging evaluation of cardiovascular complications of radiotherapy in adults: a report from the European Association of cardiovascular imaging and the American Society of Echocardiography. *J Am Soc Echocardiogr.* 2013;26(9):1013–1032. doi:10.1016/j.echo.2013.07.005.
78. Kirkham AA, Virani SA, Campbell KL. The utility of cardiac stress testing for detection of cardiovascular disease in breast cancer survivors: a systematic review. *Int J Womens Health.* 2015;7:127–140. doi:10.2147/IJWH.S68745.
79. Heidenreich PA, Schnittger I, Strauss HW, et al. Screening for coronary artery disease after mediastinal irradiation for Hodgkin's disease. *J Clin Oncol.* 2007;25(1):43–49. doi:10.1200/JCO.2006.07.0805.
80. Gujral DM, Lloyd G, Bhattacharyya S. Radiation-induced valvular heart disease. *Heart.* 2016;102(4):269–276. doi:10.1136/heartjnl-2015-308765.
81. Blanke P, Dvir D, Cheung A, et al. A simplified D-shaped model of the mitral annulus to facilitate CT-based sizing before transcatheter mitral valve implantation. *J Cardiovasc Comput Tomogr.* 2014;8(6):459–467. doi:10.1016/j.jcct.2014.09.009.
82. Banks T, Razeghi O, Ntalas I, et al. Automated quantification of mitral valve geometry on multi-slice computed tomography in patients with dilated cardiomyopathy—implications for transcatheter mitral valve replacement. *J Cardiovasc Comput Tomogr.* 2018;12(4):329–337. doi:10.1016/j.jcct.2018.04.003.
83. Agricola E, Asmarats L, Maisano F, et al. Imaging for tricuspid valve repair and replacement. *JACC Cardiovasc Imaging.* 2021;14(1):61–111. doi:10.1016/j.jcmg.2020.01.031.
84. Gheorghe LL, Mobasseri S, Agricola E, et al. Imaging for native mitral valve surgical and transcatheter interventions. *JACC Cardiovasc Imaging.* 2021;14(1):112–127. doi:10.1016/j.jcmg.2020.11.021.
85. Little SH, Bapat V, Blanke P, Guerrero M, Rajagopal V, Siegel R. Imaging guidance for transcatheter mitral valve intervention on prosthetic valves, rings, and annular calcification. *JACC Cardiovasc Imaging.* 2021;14(1):22–40. doi:10.1016/j.jcmg.2019.10.027.
86. Pulerwitz TC, Khalique OK, Leb J, et al. Optimizing cardiac CT protocols for comprehensive acquisition prior to percutaneous MV and TV repair/replacement. *JACC Cardiovasc Imaging.* 2020;13(3):836–850. doi:10.1016/j.jcmg.2019.01.041.
87. Cresti A, Chiavarelli M, Glauber M, et al. Incidence rate of primary cardiac tumors: a 14-year population study. *J Cardiovasc Med (Hagerstown).* 2016;17(1):37–43. doi:10.2459/JCM.0000000000000059.
88. Butany J, Nair V, Naseemuddin A, Nair GM, Catton C, Yau T. Cardiac tumours: diagnosis and management. *Lancet Oncol.* 2005;6(4):219–228. doi:10.1016/S1470-2045(05)70093-0.
89. Tyebally S, Chen D, Bhattacharyya S, et al. Cardiac tumors: JACC cardio-oncology state-of-the-art review. *JACC CardioOncol.* 2020;2(2):293–311. doi:10.1016/j.jaccao.2020.05.009.
90. Bittencourt MS, Achenbach S, Marwan M, et al. Left ventricular thrombus attenuation characterization in cardiac computed tomography angiography. *J Cardiovasc Comput Tomogr.* 2012;6(2):121–126. doi:10.1016/j.jcct.2011.12.006.
91. D'Angelo EC, Paolisso P, Vitale G, et al. Diagnostic accuracy of cardiac computed tomography and 18-F fluorodeoxyglucose positron emission tomography in cardiac masses. *JACC Cardiovasc Imaging.* 2020;13(11):2400–2411. doi:10.1016/j.jcmg.2020.03.021.
92. Lopez-Mattei JC, Lu Y. Multimodality imaging in cardiac masses: to standardize recommendations, the time is now!. *JACC Cardiovasc Imaging.* 2020;13(11):2412–2414. doi:10.1016/j.jcmg.2020.04.009.
93. Chetrit M, Xu B, Kwon DH, et al. Imaging-guided therapies for pericardial diseases. *JACC Cardiovasc Imaging.* 2020;13(6):1422–1437. doi:10.1016/j.jcmg.2019.08.027.
94. Chang HM, Moudgil R, Scarabelli T, Okwuosa TM, Yeh ETH. Cardiovascular complications of cancer therapy: best practices in diagnosis, prevention, and management: Part 1. *J Am Coll Cardiol.* 2017;70(20):2536–2551. doi:10.1016/j.jacc.2017.09.1096.
95. Chang HM, Okwuosa TM, Scarabelli T, Moudgil R, Yeh ETH. Cardiovascular complications of cancer therapy: best practices in diagnosis, prevention, and management: Part 2. *J Am Coll Cardiol.* 2017;70(20):2552–2565. doi:10.1016/j.jacc.2017.09.1095.
96. Klein AL, Abbara S, Agler DA, et al. American Society of Echocardiography clinical recommendations for multimodality cardiovascular imaging of patients with pericardial disease: endorsed by the society for cardiovascular magnetic resonance and society of cardiovascular computed tomography. *J Am Soc Echocardiogr.* 2013;26(9). doi:10.1016/j.echo.2013.06.023 965-1012 e15.
97. Munden RF, Carter BW, Chiles C, et al. Managing incidental findings on thoracic CT: mediastinal and cardiovascular findings. a white paper of the ACR incidental findings committee. *J Am Coll Radiol.* 2018;15(8):1087–1096. doi:10.1016/j.jacr.2018.04.029.
98. Wang ZJ, Reddy GP, Gotway MB, Yeh BM, Hetts SW, Higgins CB. CT and MR imaging of pericardial disease. *Radiographics.* 2003;23 Spec No:S167-80. doi:10.1148/rg.23si035504.

19 Cardiac Computed Tomography for Transcatheter Aortic Valve Replacement

ABDUL RAHMAN IHDAYHID, PHILIPP BLANKE, AND JONATHON A. LEIPSIC

KEY POINTS

- Cardiac CT has played an essential role in translating the use of TAVR into routine practice by providing clinicians with an accurate and reproducible means to guide procedural planning and optimize results.
- Pre-TAVR Cardiac CT is used to identify aortic valve morphology, size TAVR devices, define optimal interventional projection angle, and predict complications and guide procedural strategy.
- Post-TAVR Cardiac CT is increasingly utilized for assessment of mechanisms of valve degeneration such as leaflet thrombus and risk stratifying future procedures such as repeat coronary angiography or valve intervention.

INTRODUCTION

Degenerative aortic stenosis (AS) is characterized by progressive calcification of the aortic valve and annulus, which ultimately restricts leaflet mobility and promotes valve obstruction. AS is the leading cause of valvular heart disease–related mortality, affecting approximately 12% individuals above the age of 75, and with an aging population its prevalence is expected to double in the next 20 years.[1,2] Symptomatic severe AS confers a poor prognosis with mortality approaching 50% at 2 years and is inevitably fatal without valve replacement.[3] Minimally invasive, percutaneous transcatheter aortic valve replacement (TAVR) is increasingly utilized as a safe and effective alternative to traditional surgical treatment.[3,4] Since the first TAVR was implanted in 2002, there has been increasing randomized control trial data supporting its effectiveness as either superior or noninferior to conventional surgical aortic valve replacement (SAVR).[3–7]

Cardiac CT has played an essential role in translating the use of TAVR into routine practice by providing clinicians with a noninvasive, accurate, and reproducible means to guide procedural planning and optimize results. ECG-gated CT acquisition of the heart provides a three-dimensional, patient-specific delineation of the aortic anatomy which is used to (1) assess annular and aortic root dimensions, (2) identify high-risk features for procedural complications, (3) guide procedural strategy, and (4) provide insight on important clinical scenarios following TAVR such as feasibility of coronary access and repeat valve intervention.

TAVR PREPROCEDURAL PLANNING

Anatomic Definitions

Knowledge of the aortic root and valve anatomy is fundamental for accurate sizing of the TAVR prosthesis, optimizing procedural strategy and minimizing complications. The aortic root consists of the valvular leaflets, fibrous interleaflet triangles, coronary ostia, sinuses of Valsalva, and the sinotubular junction. The aortic root extends from the basal attachment of the aortic valve leaflets within the left ventricle, also known as the aortic annulus to the level of the sinotubular junction, which is identified by the sinus ridge and superior attachment of the valvular leaflets[8] (Fig. 19.1).

Valve Morphology

Characterization of the valve morphology (tricuspid, bicuspid, quadri-cuspid) is an important step in the preprocedural assessment for TAVR. The majority of clinical trials demonstrating the safety and efficacy of TAVR have been performed in patients with tricuspid aortic valves, which represents the most common morphology. Bicuspid aortic valves (BAV) are the most frequent congenital heart disease, occurring in 1% to 2% of the population, and are associated with higher rates and early onset of AS, aortic insufficiency, and aorta/aortic root dilation compared to patients with tricuspid valve morphology.[9–12] BAV stenosis accounts for around 10% of patients being treated with TAVR, and with expanding indications into younger cohorts, this is expected to increase in the future.[13] BAV stenosis represents a more complex and challenging anatomy to treat with TAVR. The aortic dimensions of BAV are typically larger than tricuspid valves, increasing the likelihood of annular dimensions being outside the range of conventional transcatheter heart valve (THV) devices. Furthermore, BAV are more heavily and eccentrically calcified and, in the presence of a calcified raphe, can prevent optimal expansion of the THV and increase the risk of procedural complications.[14–16] Early TAVR studies in patients with bicuspid anatomy demonstrated lower device success, higher paravalvular regurgitation (PVR), and increased in-hospital mortality compared with tricuspid

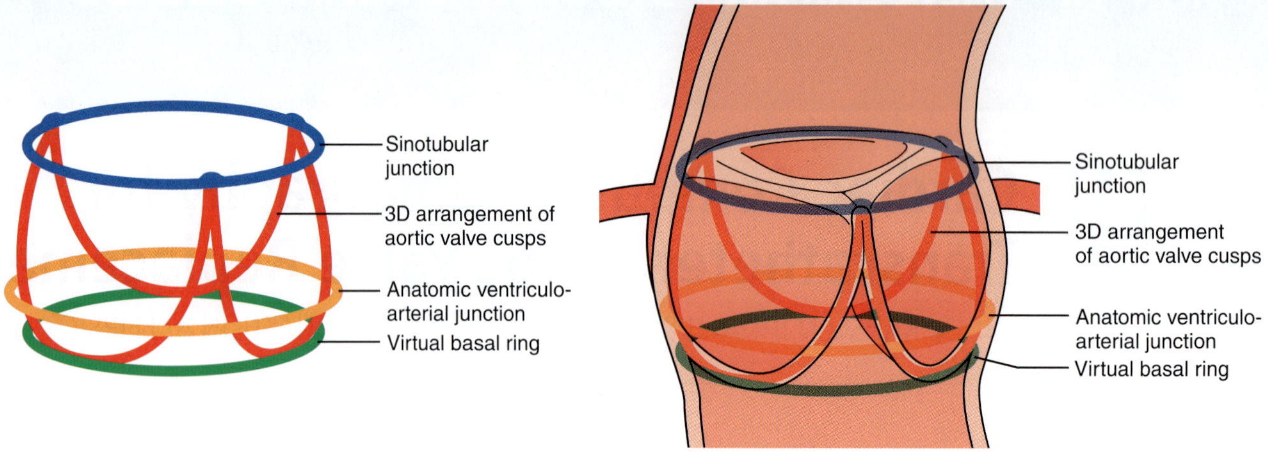

FIG. 19.1 **Anatomy of Aortic Root and Annulus.** Aortic annulus is defined by virtual ring formed from the basal hinge points of the valve cusps.

valve morphology.[17,18] Subsequent improvements in THV technology by means of smaller delivery systems and improved outer sealing skirts, in addition to a greater utilization of CT-guided procedural planning, has seen a significant improvement in short-term clinical outcomes for TAVR in BAV disease.[19–22] Overall, both randomized control trials and long-term follow-up is needed to better define the anatomic features of BAV most suitable for TAVR and its impact on valve durability and clinical outcomes compared with SAVR.

CT provides a more accurate and reproducible method for defining the presence and subtype of BAV morphology compared with echocardiography.[23,24] Several BAV classifications exist, with the Seivers classification based on the number and location of raphe most commonly used in the surgical literature.[25] Procedural success and long-term outcomes in TAVR are more dependent on the overall calcific burden and the presence of raphe; therefore a TAVI-centered classification system has been created that categorizes the bicuspid aortic valve morphology based on whether there is (1) two or three commissures and (2) the presence or absence of a raphe. This classification divides bicuspid anatomy into three types: (1) tricommissural, or also known as "functional/acquired"; (2) bicommissural with raphe (equivalent to Sievers Type 1); and (3) bicommissural without raphe (equivalent to Sievers Type 0).[26] In addition to valve morphology, the raphe location and length should be assessed including the extent of raphe and leaflet calcification in a qualitative manner (mild, moderate, severe). The presence on CT of significant raphe and/or leaflet calcification is independently associated with all-cause mortality including more frequent procedural complications such as aortic root injury and moderate-to-severe PVR.[27] Finally, the aortic root and ascending aorta should also be assessed due to the association of BAV with aortic dilatation, aneurysms, and coarctation.[12]

Aortic Stenosis Severity

The assessment of AS severity is routinely performed using echocardiography, and severe AS is defined by an aortic valve area (AVA) <1 cm^2, peak aortic jet velocity >4 m/s, and mean gradient >40 mmHg.[28] In most cases, these parameters are concordant and the severity of AS is clear. In some scenarios, there is discordance between the AVA and mean gradient, such that the calculated AVA is in the severe range, but the mean gradient suggests mild or moderate disease, signifying a diagnostic dilemma on the underlying severity of AS. This scenario is also referred to as "low-flow low-gradient" (LFLG) AS and is indicative of a low-flow hemodynamic state secondary to reduced indexed left ventricular (LV) stroke volume ($\leq$35 mL/m^2).[28] The main subtypes of LFLG AS include (1) classical LFLG AS where low stroke volume is secondary to reduced LV ejection fraction and (2) paradoxical LFLG AS in which, despite a preserved LV function, a low stroke volume is observed secondary to small-cavity concentric LV hypertrophy with increased arterial afterload. Recognition of these conditions is important as LFLG AS carries a worse prognosis and higher mortality compared with traditional high-gradient AS and patients obtain prognostic benefit from valve replacement.[29,30] Calcium scoring of the aortic valve has emerged as a useful arbitrator in diagnosing severe AS in LFLG scenarios.[31] Aortic valve calcification is quantified using the same acquisition protocol used for a coronary artery calcium scoring. A noncontrast ECG-gated cardiac CT scan is acquired in diastole at 120 to 140 kV.[31] Quantification is performed on the axial images including both valve leaflet and annular calcification while taking care to exclude nonvalvular calcification in the left ventricular outflow tract (LVOT), aortic sinus, coronary arteries, and mitral annulus. Although using Multi-planar reconstruction (MPR) to create an "en-face" view of the valve can improve differentiation of valvular and nonvalvular calcification, quantification is not recommended in this view given concerns it underestimates aortic valve calcification.[31] Sex-specific thresholds have been defined to identify severe AS with high diagnostic accuracy and ability to predict adverse outcomes.[32,33] A CT aortic valve calcium score (CT-AVC) of >1300 in women (sensitivity 86%, specificity 89%) and >2000 in men (sensitivity 89%, specificity 80%) is considered severe, and the use of CT-AVC has been endorsed by European guidelines for the management of patients with aortic stenosis.[28,31]

Annular Sizing

Accurate identification and measurement of the aortic annulus is an essential step in appropriate sizing of THV and

Measurements | **Multiplanar Reformats**

Aortic Annulus Dimensions

Segment using cubic spline tool
Measure area, perimeter, diameter

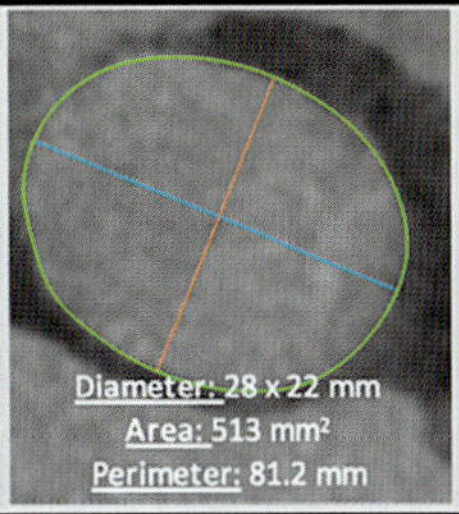

Coronary Heights

Measured with a caliper tool perpendicularly from annular plane to lower edge of coronary artery ostium

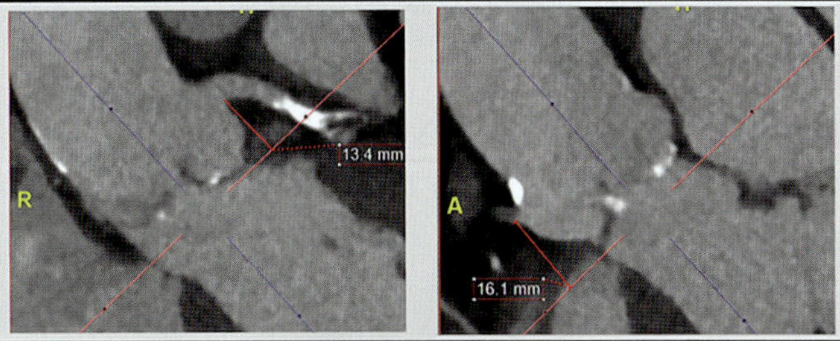

Sinus of Valsalva

Measured in parallel with annular plane and at widest dimensions
Three cusp to commissure distance taken with average of three.

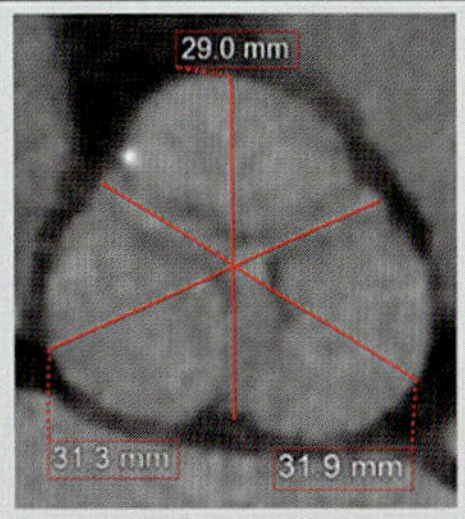

Sinotubular Junction

Height: Caliper tool used to measure perpendicular from annular plane to STJ

Diameter: Aligned with STJ which is typically not parallel to annular plane.

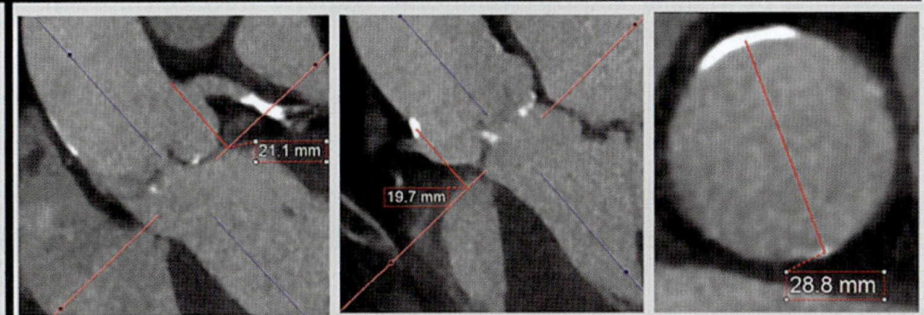

Aortic Angulation

Measured as angle between horizontal plane and plane of the aortic annulus

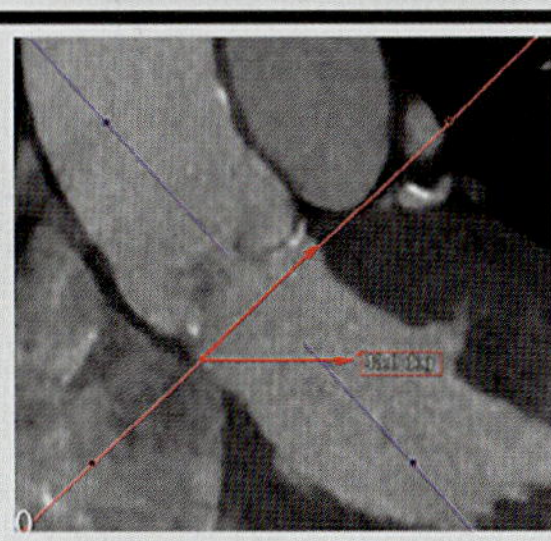

FIG. 19.2 Routine CT Measurements for Transcatheter Aortic Valve Replacement. *STJ,* Sinotubular junction.

optimizing outcomes. Using commercially available software packages, the basal attachment points of the three aortic valve cusps can be routinely identified to delineate the virtual plane known as the aortic annulus.[34] Annular measurements should be performed on ECG-gated multiphasic cardiac CT to determine the annular area, perimeter, and diameter (Fig. 19.2). The aortic annulus undergoes dynamic change in its dimensions throughout the cardiac cycle with a larger annular area and perimeter in systole compared to diastole. Therefore, to minimize the risk of THV undersizing, the recommendation is to use the multiphasic reconstructions to identify the phase with the largest dimensions, which is typically in systole.[35] A caveat is that in some patients with a prominent basal septum, annular dimensions can be largest in diastole.[34]

Identification and quantification of calcification in the aortic annulus, valve cusps, and LVOT, also known as "landing zone calcification," is an essential consideration in sizing strategies of THV. Annular and LVOT calcification is graded qualitatively on the basis of its anatomic distribution and degree of protrusion. Calcification in the LVOT is most commonly found below the noncoronary and left

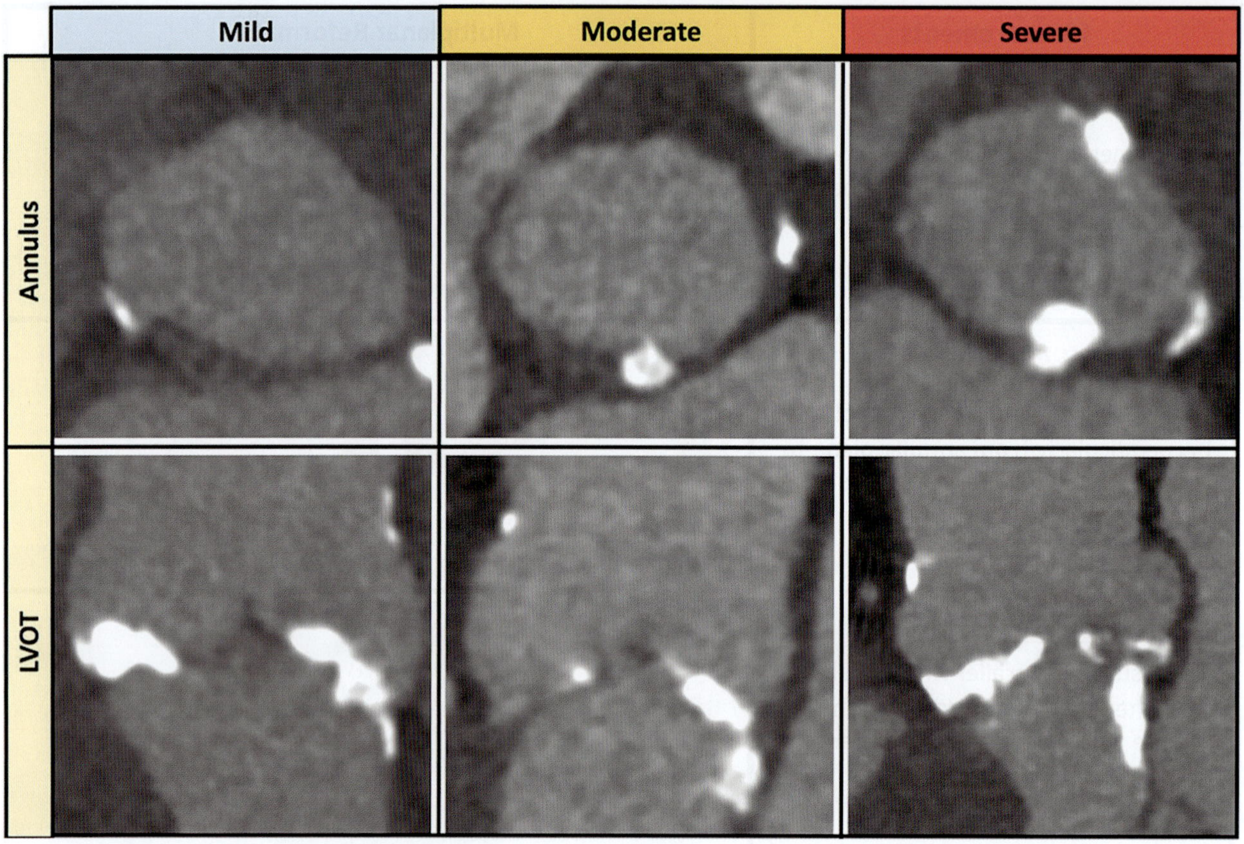

FIG. 19.3 **Grading of Annular and Left Ventricular Outflow Tract Calcification. Mild:** Single, adherent, non-protruding focus of calcification. **Moderate:** Two or more nodules of calcification or single nodule with limited protrusion into annulus/LVOT. **Severe:** Single or multiple nodules of calcification protruding into annular lumen and/or extending into the LVOT. *LVOT,* Left ventricular outflow tract.

coronary cusp along the intervalvular fibrosa.[34] The presence of severe LVOT or annular calcification is associated with increased risk of PVR, annular rupture, and conduction disturbance requiring permanent pacemaker (PPM) insertion.[36]

The annular area is typically used to guide sizing strategies for balloon-expandable valves and perimeter for self-expanding valves. The presence and extent of annular/LVOT calcification, underlying conduction disturbance, and patient characteristics are other factors that also influence THV device selection and sizing (Fig. 19.3). Although not routinely reported, the degree of THV oversizing in relation to the annulus can be useful to provide a quantitative metric to guide THV sizing.[37] The optimal oversizing thresholds are specific to each device and change with improvements in THV technology. For example, initial recommendations for balloon-expandable devices were to oversize annular area by >10% to minimize the risk of significant PVR. However, improvements in the sealing-skirt associated with THV devices and operator technique have led to a significant reduction in PVR and the ability to achieve optimal results with even nominal degrees of oversizing.[37–39]

In patients with BAV anatomy, there has been some debate regarding the optimal measurement technique to guide THV sizing. Several studies have observed that in BAV, THV anchoring can occur above the annulus with underexpansion greatest at the valve orifice rather than the annulus.[40,41] Therefore it has been suggested that supra-annular sizing may be more suitable for BAV. A major limitation to supra-annular measurements has been the lack of standardization and limited reproducibility compared with annular sizing.[42,43] The clinical translation of cardiac CT to guide TAVR has largely been driven by its accuracy and reproducibility, and therefore annular sizing in BAV remains the most reliable and recommended approach.

Optimal Projection Angle

During valve implantation, the position of the THV prior to deployment is guided by the 2D images projected from conventional angiography. Identifying the plane of the aortic annulus during the procedure is essential to ensure appropriate THV deployment depth to minimize risk of complications such as PVR, conduction disturbance, and valve embolization. Pre-TAVR cardiac CT can provide the optimal C-arm angulations for a perpendicular view of all three cusps in a line, thereby minimizing the need for repeat predeployment aortic root angiograms and reducing contrast usage, procedural time, and radiation exposure[44,45] (Fig. 19.4). The standard three-cusp view serves balloon-expandable THV well as they position more naturally in the center and perpendicular to the aortic annulus. In contrast, with self-expanding devices, the delivery catheter is typically positioned toward the outer curve of the aortic root and expands from the noncoronary cusp

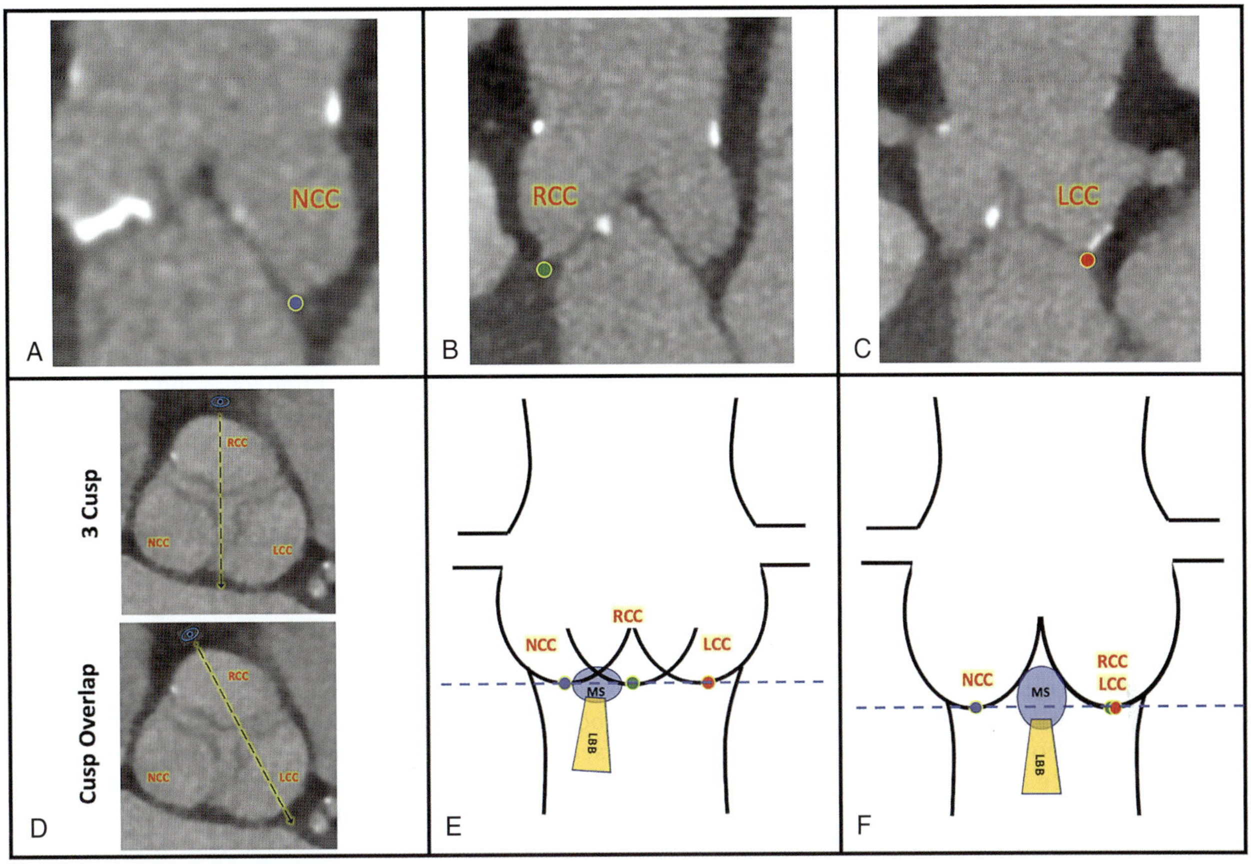

FIG. 19.4 Three-Cusp and Cusp-Overlap Optimal Projection Angle. (A–C): The annular plane is defined by a parallel line along the nadir of all three cusps. (D) Projection of three-cusp and cusp-overlap. (E) Classical three-cusp coplanar view with the RCC centered in the middle. The membranous septum lies caudal to the NCC and RCC commissure with the LBB in close vicinity. (F) Cusp-overlap view with NCC on the left and RCC and LCC overlapped on the right and membranous septum arising caudal and in-between. Cusp-overlap view elongates the LVOT, reducing foreshortening of the NCC and allows for more precise evaluation of NCC depth and location of the membranous septum, therefore facilitating high THV deployment and lower PPM rate. *LBB*, Left bundle branch; *LCC*, left coronary cusp; *LVOT*, left ventricular outflow tract; *NCC*, noncoronary cusp; *MS*, membranous septum; *PPM*, permanent pacemaker; *RCC*, right coronary cusp; *THV*, transcatheter heart valve.

toward the left coronary cusp. This often results in a parallax or misalignment of the delivery system with the annulus, making an estimation of implant depth unclear and likely contributing to an increase risk of new permanent PPM insertion. To address this limitation, the cusp overlap technique has been developed to improve the deployment of self-expanding THV.[46] The technique is based on using CT to determine a coplanar angle that overlaps the right and left coronary cusps, thus isolating the noncoronary cusp and reducing parallax of the THV in relation to the annular plane. The optimal angle is often in a right anterior oblique (RAO) and caudal orientation, which visually elongates the LVOT, providing the operator with better visualization of the noncoronary cusp hinge point that allows for a more precise THV implantation depth[46] (Fig. 19.4). Overall, the technique has allowed higher implants of self-expanding THV and has contributed to a reduced risk of PPM.[47,48]

PREDICTING COMPLICATIONS

Annular Rupture

Annular rupture is among the most serious complications of TAVR. The definition is broad and includes injury along the aortic root complex, which includes the LVOT, sinuses, and sinotubular junction. The reported incidence is between 0.5% to 1.0% but is likely higher due to contained ruptures without clinical manifestations.[49,50] Uncontained ruptures are associated with very high in-hospital mortality exceeding 75%.[49–52] Pre-TAVR CT plays an important role in assessing the risk of annular rupture that includes moderate to severe subannular calcification, particularly the presence of protruding calcification and within the upper part of the LVOT (within 2 mm below annular).[34,51] Calcification below the noncoronary cusp also confers a higher risk as THV expansion along the rigid intervalvular fibrosa transmits counterbearing forces toward the free-muscular portion of the LVOT that is below the left coronary cusp and is more susceptible to rupture.[53] Procedural risk factors include THV oversizing >20% and use of balloon-expandable valves,[51,54] although aggressive postdilatation of self-expanding devices in the presence of subannular calcification, can also induce injury. It is important to also recognize that "annular injury" can occur above the annulus and involve the sinotubular junction. The height of sinotubular junction (ST) from the annulus and its mean diameter should be measured on CT and compared with the expected THV height and size (Fig. 19.2). THV that are anticipated to interact with a narrow and calcified STJ can cause annular injury, presenting as an aortic dissection or coronary artery occlusion. Overall, the identification of risk factors for annular rupture on pre-TAVR CT can influence device selection (i.e., self-expanding THV), sizing (smaller THV with less oversizing), and procedural technique (higher implant to avoid LVOT calcium, lower implant to avoid narrow STJ, and cautious post-dilatation).

Coronary Obstruction

Coronary artery occlusion is a relatively rare complication that occurs in <1% of TAVR for native aortic valve stenosis and is associated with a 30-day mortality between 40% and 50%.[55,56] Anatomic risk factors can be readily identified on pre-TAVR CT and include a coronary height of <12 mm measured perpendicular to the annular plane and a mean sinus of Valsalva (SoV) diameter of <30 mm.[55] The combination of low coronary heights and small sinuses contributes to several potential mechanisms of coronary obstruction: (1) in the majority of cases it occurs due to displacement of bulky calcified leaflets over a coronary ostium; (2) coronary embolization or valve debris or thrombus; (3) inadvertent alignment of a THV commissural post in front of coronary ostium preventing coronary flow; and (4) THV sealing skirt directly overlying the coronary ostium, particularly in high implants. The presence of a low coronary height <12 mm in addition to a small SoV measuring <30 mm is found in approximately 1 in 10 patients,[57] and given the incidence of coronary obstruction is considerably less, it highlights the need to interpret these anatomic risk factors in the overall context of a patient's anatomy, risk profile, and procedural strategy.

Conduction Disturbance

Despite significant advances in procedural safety, new conduction disturbance requiring PPM implantation remains a frequent and important consequence of TAVR. New-onset persistent left bundle branch block (LBBB) occurs in approximately 23%, and according to a recent metaanalysis, the overall rate of PPM implantation with new-generation THV ranges between 2.3% and 36.1%.[58] The highest risk is observed in supra-annular self-expanding devices (15% to 27%) compared with balloon expandable (4 to 24%) and in those with underlying right bundle branch block (RBBB).[58] Conduction disturbance following TAVR has clinical implications, with a new-onset LBBB or PPM insertion associated with increased all-cause mortality and reduced functional status.[59,60] The mechanism underlying the development of conduction disturbance relates to the close proximity of the aortic annulus with the His bundle, which passes through the membranous septum (Fig. 19.4). Therefore, the deeper the THV implant or shorter the membranous septal length, the increased likelihood the THV frame will impinge on the bundle of His, leading to conduction disturbance. The membranous septal length (MSL) can be measured on pre-TAVR CT as the longest point between the annulus and muscular septum. An MSL <8 mm predicts conduction disturbance as does the presence of LVOT calcification beneath the left coronary cusp.[61,62] Early studies have demonstrated that measurement of MSL to guide depth of self-expanding THV implant reduced the rate of new PPM insertion from 10% to 3%.[47] However, given the increasing adoption of the cusp-overlap technique, similar improvements in the PPM rate have been observed by employing routine high implantation of self-expanding THV,[63,64] therefore potentially negating the widespread use of MSL measurements in clinical practice.

POST-TAVR CT

Echocardiography is the imaging modality routinely used to assess heart valve function following TAVR.[65] ECG-gated post-TAVR cardiac CT allows for precise imaging of the THV geometry, implant position, and leaflets.[34] The use of post-TAVR cardiac CT is an evolving area, and although there is no clear consensus on its routine use in practice, emerging evidence provides a strong rationale for identifying complications, assessing mechanisms of valve degeneration, and risk-stratification of future procedures such as repeat coronary angiography or valve intervention. The post-TAVR CT is typically acquired across the entire cardiac cycle to allow for multiphasic reconstruction and assessment of both anatomy and function. In patients without residual severe valve stenosis, image quality can be optimized with beta blockers to reduce the heart rate and nitroglycerin to improve the visualization of the coronary arteries.

Leaflet Thrombus

Leaflet thrombus (LT) of bioprosthetic aortic valves is characterized by hypoattenuated leaflet thickening (HALT) and reduced leaflet motion (RLM) noted on multiphasic post-TAVR cardiac CT. HALT is identified as a meniscal leaflet thickening that is greater at the base and extends toward the center of the leaflet[34] (Fig. 19.5). The burden of HALT is quantified on CT based on the number of leaflets involved (1, 2, or 3) and severity graded using a 4-tier ordinal scale: none, ≤25%, 26% to 50%, 51% to 75%, and >75%.[34] Clinical valve thrombosis is rare, affecting <1% following TAVR, and can present as symptomatic bioprosthetic valve stenosis, heart failure, or thromboembolism.[66] Subclinical LT is more common, affecting 10% to 15% following TAVR and manifests most commonly without clinical or hemodynamic sequalae or in asymptomatic patients with elevated transvalvular gradients on echocardiography.[67] Recent evidence from serial post-TAVR CT highlights the natural history and dynamic nature of HALT with a significant proportion of patients demonstrating resolution of HALT at 1 year (42–54%) and others developing HALT after initially showing no evidence at 30 days (21–35%).[68,69]

The pathophysiology of LT involves an interplay between the THV, the native aortic root, corresponding flow dynamics, and patient systemic factors. Unlike SAVR where the native valve leaflets are removed, TAVR results in a new neo-sinus located between the THV leaflets and a combination of the displaced native leaflets and THV frame (Fig. 19.6). In vitro hemodynamic studies have demonstrated that the neosinus is susceptible to regions of blood stasis and contributes to thrombus formation.[70] The frame geometry and its relationship to the surrounding

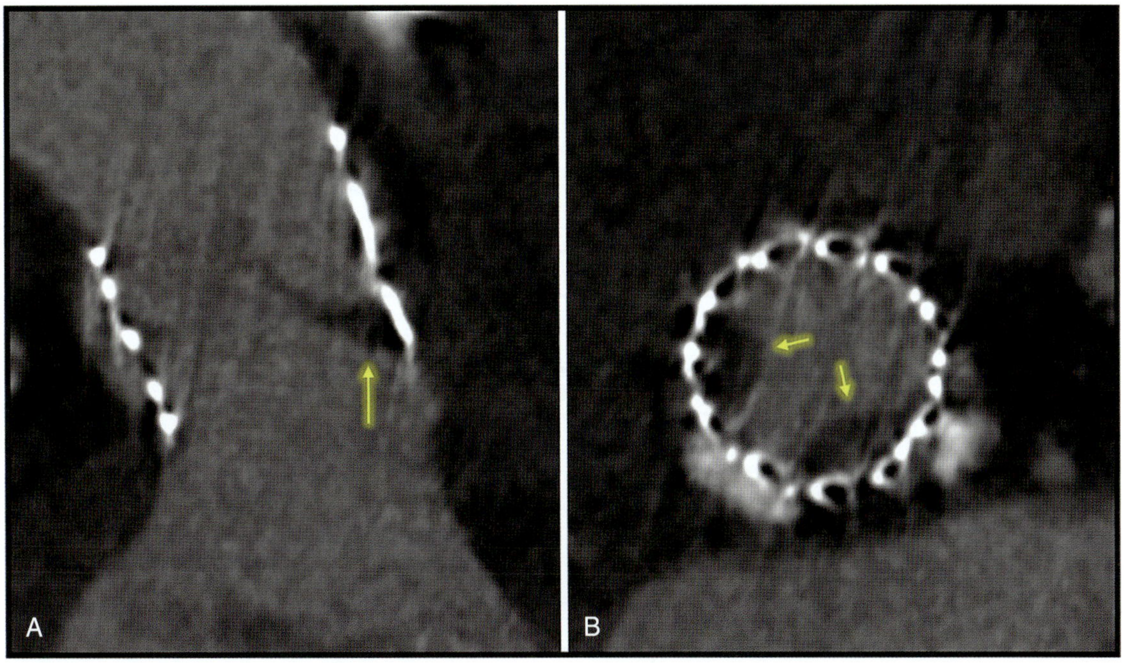

FIG. 19.5 **Example of leaflet thrombus.** (A and B) Example of leaflet thrombus characterized by hypoattenuated leaflet thickening evident on long- and short-axis reconstruction (*yellow arrows*). Long-axis image (A) highlights typical meniscal hypoattenuation and leaflet thickening.

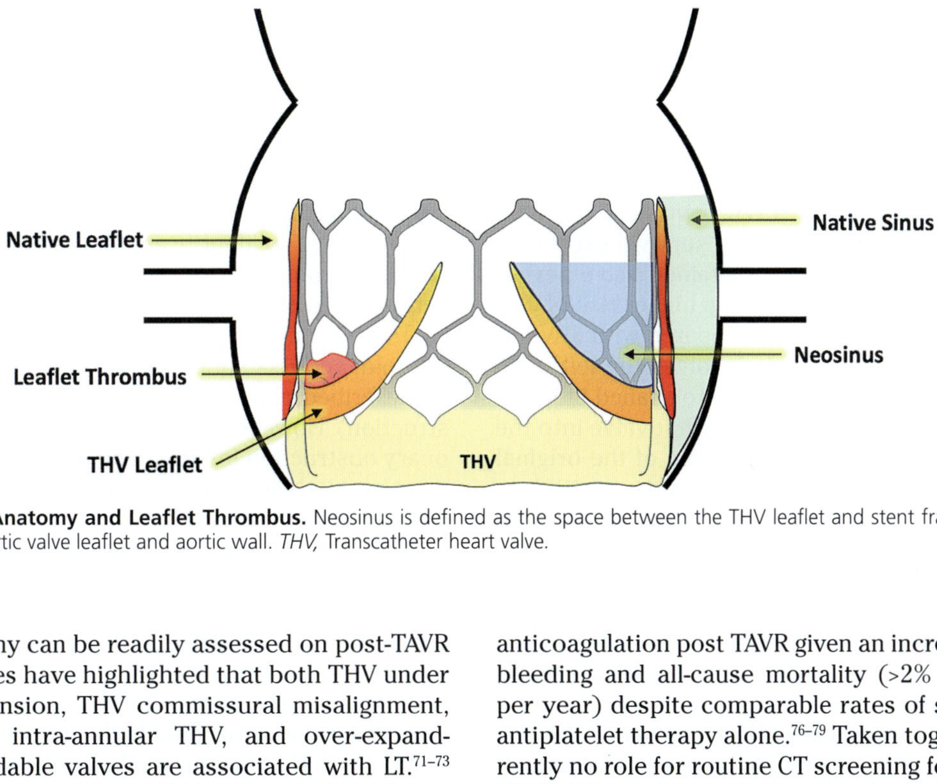

FIG. 19.6 **Neosinus Anatomy and Leaflet Thrombus.** Neosinus is defined as the space between the THV leaflet and stent frame. Native sinus exists between the native aortic valve leaflet and aortic wall. *THV,* Transcatheter heart valve.

aortic root anatomy can be readily assessed on post-TAVR CT. Recent analyses have highlighted that both THV under or eccentric expansion, THV commissural misalignment, deeper implants, intra-annular THV, and over-expanded balloon-expandable valves are associated with LT.[71–73] These risk factors contribute to LT by altering the relative size of the neo-sinus and its associated flow dynamics in addition to impacting leaflet kinematics and shear stress, which together promote thrombogenesis.[73] The clinical impact of subclinical LT remains uncertain and an area of ongoing investigation, although concerns from observational data point toward an increased risk of stroke, valve degeneration, and all-cause mortality.[74,75] Anticoagulation is effective for both prevention and treatment of subclinical LT; however, randomized trials caution against routine anticoagulation post TAVR given an increased risk of major bleeding and all-cause mortality (>2% absolute increase per year) despite comparable rates of stroke as those on antiplatelet therapy alone.[76–79] Taken together, there is currently no role for routine CT screening for HALT, with post-TAVR CT imaging in this setting focused in patients with elevated or rising THV gradients on echocardiography or those with acute thromboembolism (Fig. 19.7).

Valve-in-Valve

Bioprosthetic transcatheter and surgical valve leaflets consist of animal tissue that can degenerate and develop restenosis over time, requiring repeat valve replacement. Valve-in-valve (ViV) TAVR, predominately for failed surgical

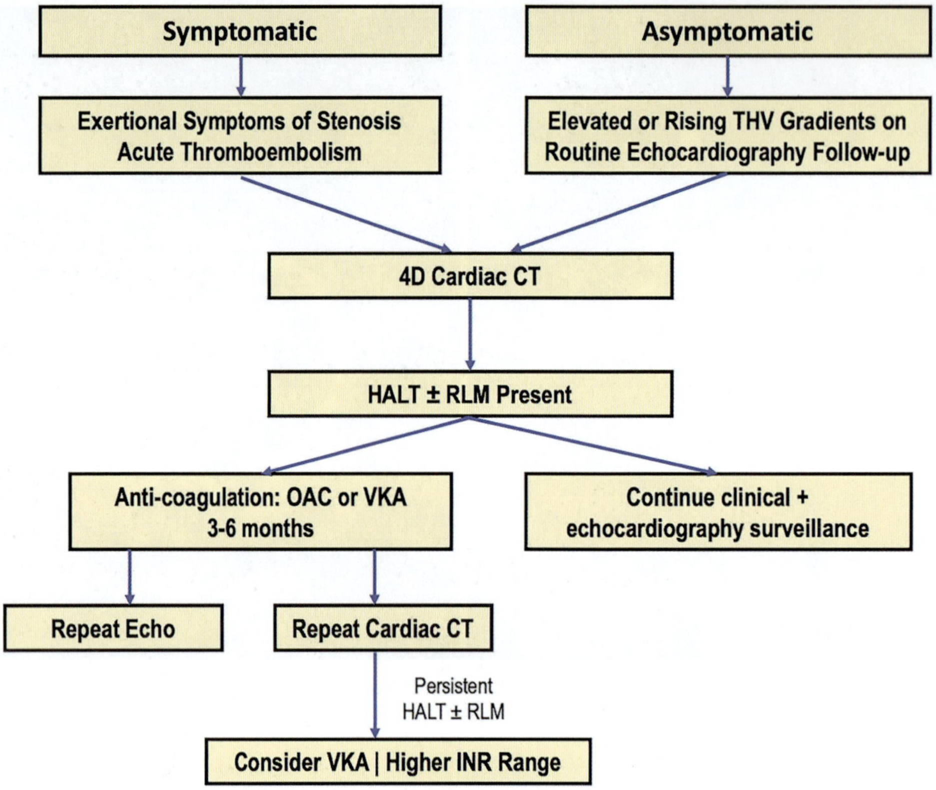

FIG. 19.7 Clinical Approach to Leaflet Thrombus. *HALT,* Hypoattenuated leaflet thickening; *INR*, International Normalized Ratio; *OAC,* oral anticoagulant; *RLM,* reduced leaflet mobility/motion; *THV,* Transcatheter heart valve; *VKA*, vitamin K antagonist.

bioprosthesis, has emerged as a safe and effective alternative to SAVR and accounts for close to 5% of all TAVR procedures.[80] Registry data of ViV TAVR have demonstrated high rates of technical success, 1-year survival exceeding 80%, improved quality of life, and sustained valve performance up to 5 years.[81,82] ViV TAVR has a higher risk of coronary obstruction at 2.3% to 3.5% compared with TAVR in native valves and most commonly involves the left main coronary artery.[57,83] Implanting a THV into a failed bioprosthetic valve displaces the leaflets of the first valve into the open position, therefore sealing the frame of the original valve and creating a covered stent graft in the aortic root (Fig. 19.8). There is risk of direct coronary obstruction when the displaced leaflets are in close proximity of the coronary ostium in patients with a narrow SoV. Indirect coronary obstruction can also occur when the displaced leaflets are in close proximity or direct contact with the STJ, thereby sequestering the SoV and preventing blood flow into the coronaries.

Preprocedural CT plays a key role in evaluating the risk of coronary obstruction. The risk of coronary obstruction is evaluated by using MPR to first depict the degenerated bioprosthesis as an en-face view (Fig. 19.9). A virtual ring of the same diameter as the planned THV is then positioned in the center of the original valve and positioned at the level of the coronary ostium. The distance between the virtual ring and coronary ostium is then measured and defined as the virtual THV to coronary distance (VTC).[34] A VTC of <4 mm has been validated as an accurate measure to identify high risk of coronary obstruction.[57] When the surgical valve posts or displaced valve leaflets are in close proximity to the STJ or projected to extend above the coronary ostium, a similar virtual THV distance with the neighboring aortic sinus (VTS) and STJ (VTSTJ) should be performed to identify anatomies at risk of coronary obstruction from sinus sequestration. Implantation of a THV within a stentless surgical valve is biomechanically similar as TAVR in native stenosis due to the absence of a rigid scaffold, and risk should be assessed in the same manner as described above (see above section on Coronary Obstruction). However, it should be noted that the risk of coronary obstruction for stentless ViV carries the highest risk due to underlying small and distorted root anatomies with low coronary heights.[34,83]

As the indications for TAVR expand to younger patients with lower surgical risk, THV degeneration is anticipated to become an important issue with patients requiring repeat TAVR (THV-in-THV) as their anticipated life expectancy exceeds the lifespan of their initial THV. The experience with THV-in-THV is less than in surgical bioprosthesis, though early registry data highlight promising procedural outcomes and 1-year survival compared with ViV.[84,85] There are some differences in the assessment of coronary obstruction for THV-in-THV (Fig. 19.10). First, the second THV is assumed to be the same size as the initial THV; therefore a virtual ring is not utilized. Second, the height at which the displaced leaflets are pinned in the open position, also known as the "leaflet plane" or "neoskirt height," often does not extend to the top of the frame and differs between THVs. Bench testing has provided important pictorial insight into the respective leaflet planes of commonly used THV, which is essential for performing the VTC, VTS/VTSTJ

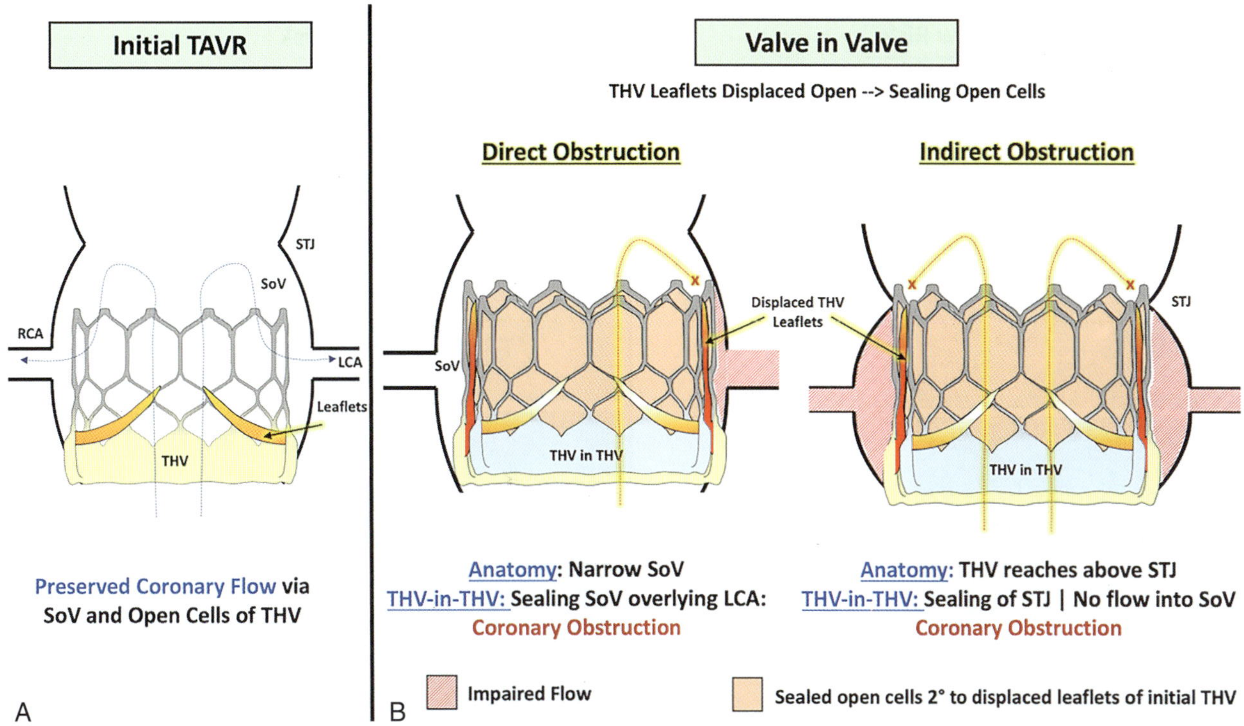

FIG. 19.8 Valve-in-Valve Intervention: Mechanisms of Coronary Obstruction. (A) Schematic illustration of preserved coronary blood flow following TAVR. (B) Direct coronary obstruction and indirect mechanisms of coronary obstruction in setting of THV in THV deployment. *LCA,* Left coronary artery; *RCA,* right coronary artery; *SoV,* sinus of Valsalva; *STJ,* sinotubular junction; *TAVR,* transcatheter aortic valve replacement; *THV,* transcatheter heart valve.

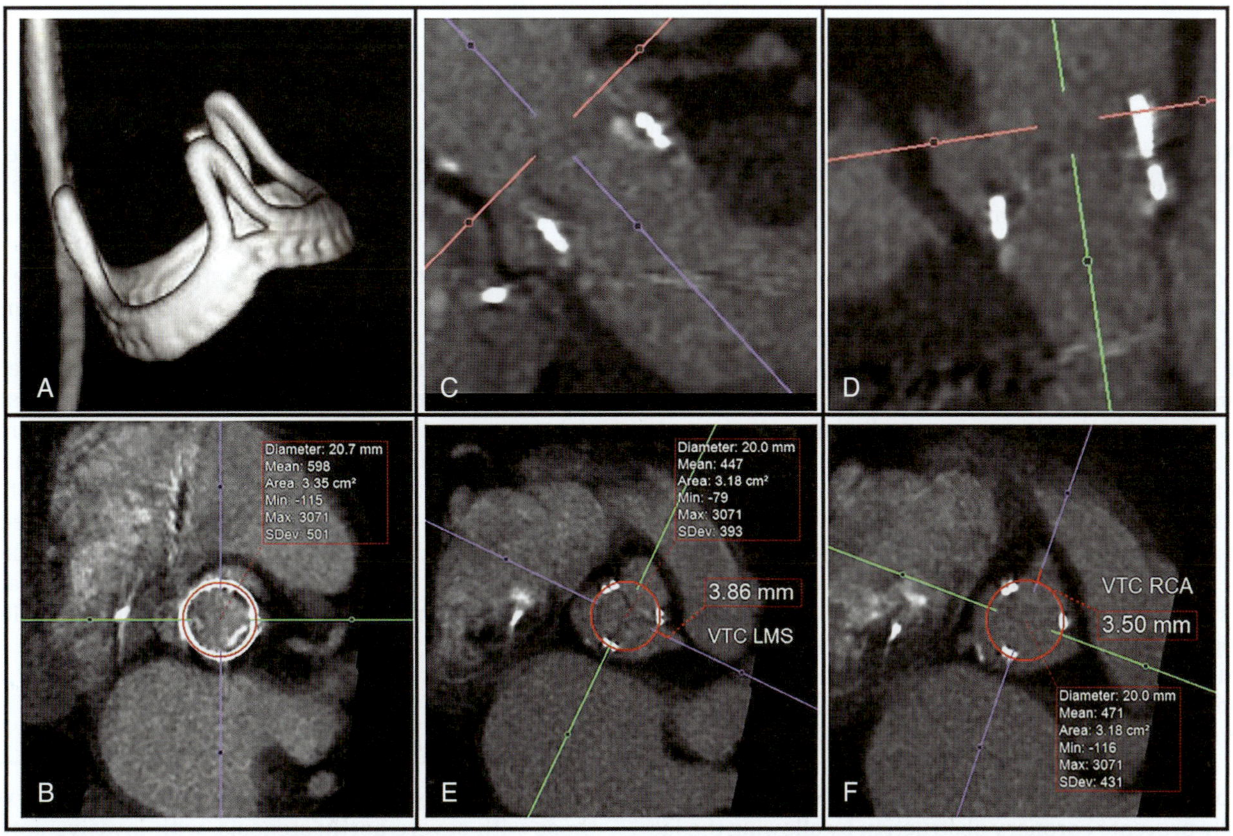

FIG. 19.9 Preprocedural Risk Assessment of Coronary Obstruction Using Cardiac CT in Patients Undergoing THV in Bioprosthetic Surgical Heart Valve. (A) Volume-rendered reconstruction of PERIMOUNT bioprosthetic surgical heart valve. (B) Internal dimensions of valve consistent with 20-mm device. (C, E) Bioprosthetic valve posts extend to upper aspect of LCA and RCA ostium, rendering patient at potential risk of coronary obstruction. (D, F) Based on valve type and size, a 20-mm virtual THV is simulated within the surgical valve. Virtual THV to coronary (VTC) distance of the LCA and RCA is small (<4 mm) and highlights increased risk of coronary obstruction for valve-in-valve TAVR. *LCA,* Left coronary artery; *RCA,* right coronary artery; *TAVR,* transcatheter aortic valve replacement; *THV,* transcatheter heart valve.

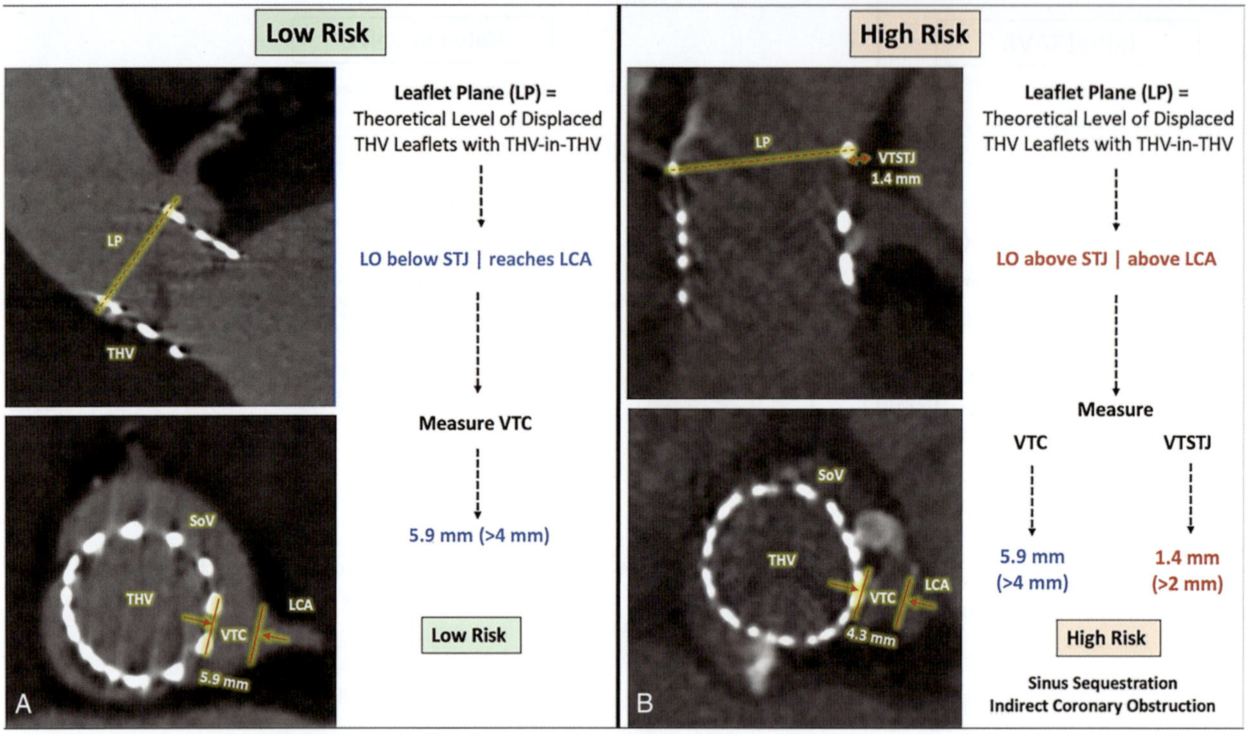

FIG. 19.10 Preprocedural Risk Assessment of Coronary Obstruction Using Cardiac CT in Patients Undergoing THV-in-THV. Leaflet plane (LP) represents the theoretic level of displaced leaflets in setting of THV in THV. (A) Post-TAVR CT of balloon-expandable THV with the LP reaching the LCA but not the STJ. Virtual distance between the THV frame and coronary ostium (VTC) measures 5.9 mm, which represents a low-risk coronary obstruction for future THV in THV. (B) Post-TAVR CT demonstrates LP of original THV extending above the LCA and STJ. VTC is normal at 5.9 mm; however, virtual THV distance to STJ (VTSTJ) is small at 1.9 mm, representing a high-risk coronary obstruction by means of sinus sequestration. *LCA,* Left coronary artery; *LP,* leaflet plane; *STJ,* sinotubular junction; *TAVR,* transcatheter aortic valve replacement; *THV,* transcatheter heart valve.

measurements.[86] The mechanisms of coronary obstruction are similar to ViV; however, given the higher frame heights and the supra-annular nature of some THV designs, the displaced leaflets of the original THV often extend above the coronary ostium, making indirect coronary obstruction by means of sinus sequestration a greater concern. Using a conservative threshold VTSTJ/VTS of <2.0 mm, repeat THV with a supra-annular self-expanding THV has a potential risk of coronary obstruction in 46% compared with 2% using an intra-annular balloon-expandable device.[87] Further work is needed to the refine appropriate thresholds and risk-assessment algorithms for predicting coronary obstruction. In particular, using an isolated anatomic measure of risk (i.e., VTC) does not take into account the complete 3D relationship of the THV with the native anatomy and its impact on coronary blood flow, highlighting opportunities for CT-guided computational modeling to refine risk assessment in the future.[88]

Procedural techniques to mitigate the risk of coronary obstruction includes "snorkel stenting" from the coronary ostium into the aorta, or using an emerging transcatheter electro-surgery technique to perform intentional laceration of the at-risk bioprosthetic or native aortic leaflet immediately before TAVR, also known as BASILICA.[89] BASILICA potentially prevents coronary obstruction by allowing the lacerated leaflet to splay to the side following TAVR, thereby maintaining coronary flow. CT provides important information on the feasibility of BASILICA and procedural guidance by means of optimal C-arm angulation for leaflet laceration. Cardiac CT can (1) assess the pattern of calcification on the target leaflet, with heavy calcification at the nadir a potential obstacle to successful laceration using radiofrequency energy[89]; and (2) using short-axis images, assess the commissural alignment of the original bioprosthetic valve or alignment of the target leaflet with the coronary ostium (Fig. 19.11). If the commissural post lies in front of the coronary ostium or the ostium is eccentric to the midline of the leaflet, then leaflet laceration may not adequately improve coronary flow to prevent obstruction.[90] CT analysis of native aortic valves has highlighted that although the left coronary artery often arises from the midline of the cusp, the right coronary is frequently offset toward the noncoronary commissure.[90] Therefore deployment techniques that aim to align the THV with the native commissure may still not adequately optimize patients for repeat TAVR procedures. This understanding provides an opportunity to use cardiac CT to refine future THV deployment techniques that also consider "coronary alignment" to ensure adequate lifetime management of patients with AS.

CORONARY ARTERY DISEASE

Coronary artery disease (CAD) is frequently observed in those with severe aortic stenosis, with invasive coronary angiography (ICA) prior to TAVR routine practice to identify the presence and severity of disease.[91] Despite the uncertainty regarding the indication and prognostic value of revascularisation in this cohort, an invasive procedure to identify CAD remains a key aspect of the workup prior

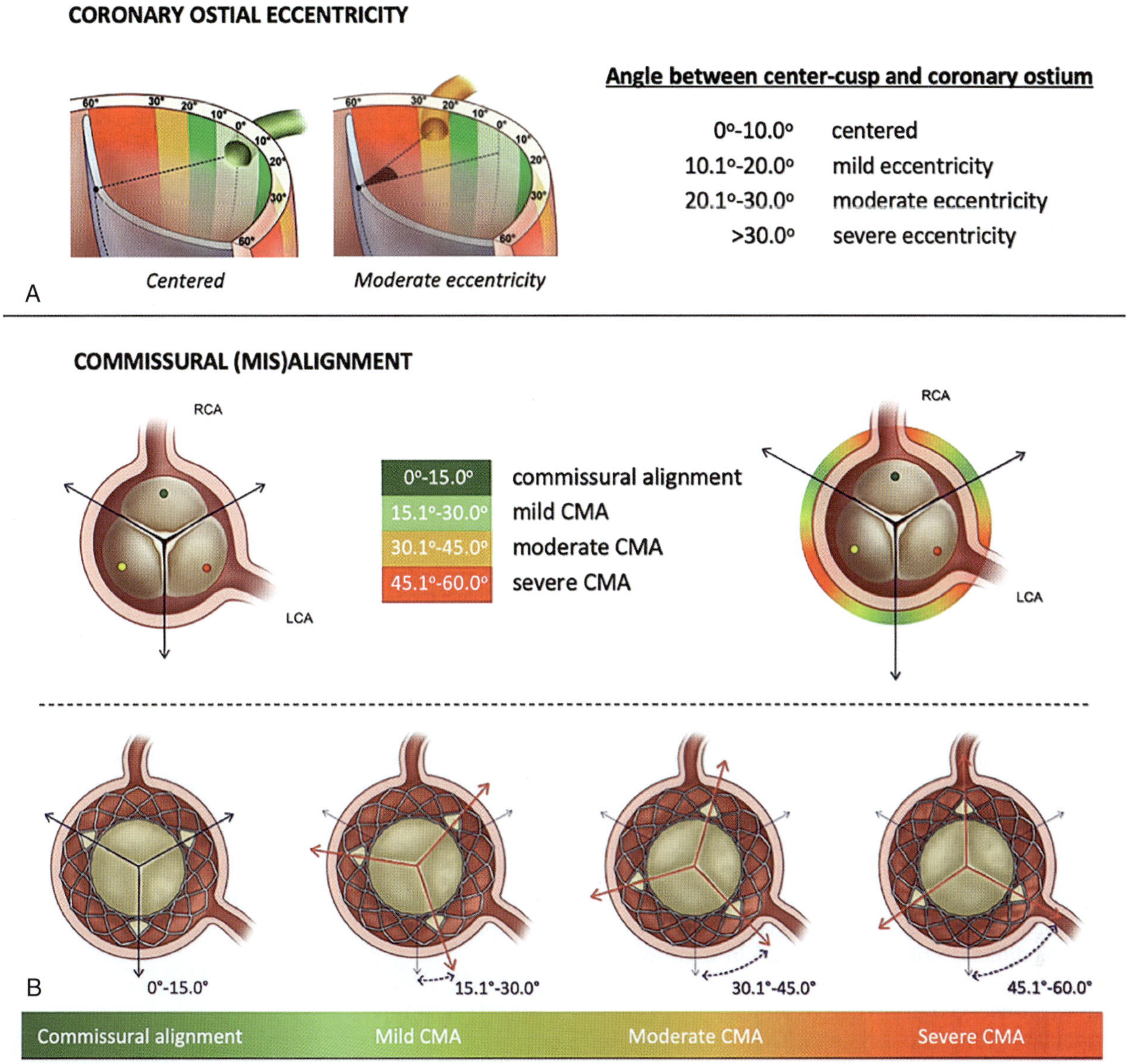

FIG. 19.11 Definition of Coronary Eccentricity and Commissural Alignment. Definitions of (A) coronary ostial eccentricity and (B) commissural (mis) alignment. *CMA,* Commissural alignment; *LCA,* left coronary artery; *LCC,* left coronary cusp; *NCC,* noncoronary cusp; *RCA,* right coronary artery; *RCC,* right coronary cusp; *TAVR,* transcatheter aortic valve replacement. (Adapted from Tang GHL, Amat-Santos IJ, De Backer O, et al. Rationale, definitions, techniques, and outcomes of commissural alignment in TAVR: from the Align-TAVR consortium. *JACC Cardiovasc Interv*. 2022;15(15):1497–1518.)

to TAVR. Coronary CT angiography (CCTA) is increasingly utilized as a first-line noninvasive modality to identify the presence of coronary artery disease in patients with stable angina.[92] Although cardiac CT is integral for preprocedural planning of TAVR, the widespread adoption of reporting CAD from the pre-TAVR CT has been limited due to the frequently observed high calcific plaque burden and the reluctance to optimize image quality with nitroglycerin and beta blockers[34] negatively impacting specificity and overall accuracy.[93] Preliminary studies have observed a high negative predictive value, and therefore CTCA use has been commonly limited to excluding significant disease in the left main and proximal coronary arteries.[93] With the shift in risk profile of TAVR to younger patients and the potential challenges of future coronary access, a more complete CAD evaluation is needed. It is likey that use of photon-counting CT (PCCT; see Chapters 2 and 7 for further detail) will further expand the capabilites of assessing for obstructive CAD among individual referred for pre-TAVR evaluation. A small pilot study highlighted the potential safety of using nitroglycerin to optimize CTCA in stable patients with severe AS and also demonstrated the accuracy of CT-derived fractional flow reserve (CT-FFR).[94] The ability to accurately leverage the coronary information captured from the pre-TAVR CT warrants further investigation and heralds an opportunity to provide a comprehensive "one-stop" noninvasive evaluation and risk stratification of patients being considered for TAVR.

As TAVR is now indicated in younger patients with longer life expectancies, there is an increased likelihood that they may have progression of their CAD that requires post-TAVR invasive coronary angiography (ICA) and percutaneous coronary intervention (PCI). Due to the anatomic relationship of the coronary ostia with the THV frame, commissures, and

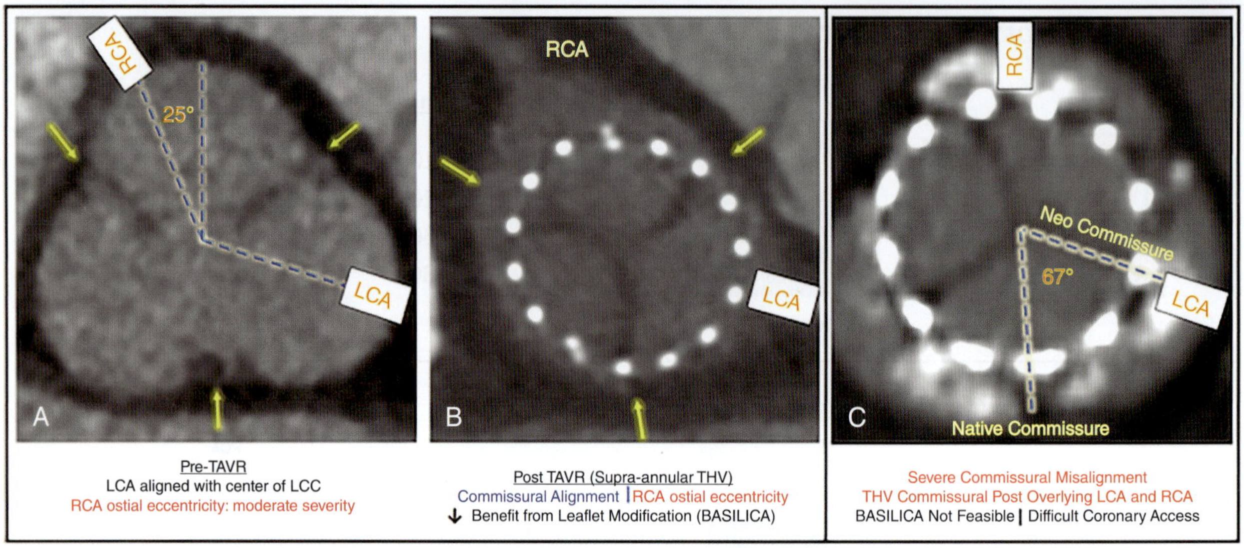

FIG. 19.12 Example of Coronary Eccentricity and Commissural Alignment. (A) Example of tricuspid aortic valve with moderate eccentricity of RCA in relation to midline of RCC and an LCA aligned with LCC. (B) Post-TAVR CT demonstrates the self-expanding THV neo-commissures are aligned with the native commissures (*yellow arrows*). In the event the patient needs THV-in-THV, the eccentricity of the RCA in relation to the midline of THV leaflet may reduce the efficacy of intentional leaflet laceration (BASILICA). (C) Balloon-expandable THV with severe commissural misalignment resulting in THV commissural post overlying both LCA and RCA and therefore anticipated difficulty for future coronary access during invasive coronary angiography. *LCA,* Left coronary artery; *LCC,* left coronary sinus; *RCA,* right coronary artery; *TAVR,* transcatheter aortic valve replacement; *THV,* transcatheter heart valve.

sealing skirt, coronary access may be challenging or prohibitive. This appears more problematic for self-expanding supra-annular THV compared with shorter-frame intra-annular devices.[95,96] The former have a taller frame design that extends above the coronaries, smaller stent cells, a higher leaflet position, and an asymmetric sealing skirt that can contribute to difficult coronary access. A recent multicenter registry in patients presenting with ST-elevation myocardial infarction (STEMI) following TAVR emphasized the clinical implications of difficult coronary access.[97] In a cohort of 118 patients, longer door-to-balloon times and a higher PCI failure rate was observed likely due to an inability or difficulty in cannulating the coronary ostia. This contributed to a significantly higher mortality (42%) compared to STEMI patients without TAVR (25%).[97]

Analysis of post-TAVR CT has provided insight into factors that potentially facilitate or preclude future coronary access (Fig. 19.12). A THV commissure in the proximity or overlapping the coronary ostium creates a physical barrier that can render coronary access after TAVR challenging or not feasible. Using MPR to define a short-axis view of the post-TAVR CT in diastole, the angle between the THV commissure and both the native commissure and coronary ostium can be defined. A THV commissure landing within 0 to 20 degrees of the coronary ostium is defined as severe coronary overlap and a >45 degree offset from the native commissure defines severe commissural misalignment[98] (Fig. 19.11). Other contributing factors include the coronary ostium lying below the sealing skirt or the distance between the THV frame and aortic sinus/STJ being <2 mm.[87,99,100] Overall, CT-identified risk factors for unfavorable coronary access appear to be more common in supra-annular self-expanding THV compared with intra-annular balloon-expandable devices (22.7% vs. 11.3% for LMCA; 21.2% vs. 8.1% for RCA).[87] Routine post-TAVR CT to evaluate the feasibility of coronary access is currently not recommended; however, knowledge of these factors has (1) informed new deployment techniques to optimize THV commissural alignment leading to increased rates of successful coronary access with self-expanding devices[101]; (2) increased awareness that aiming for a high THV deployment to minimize risk of conduction disturbance can come at a trade-off of difficult coronary access in the future; and (3) highlighted the even greater challenges of coronary access in setting of THV-in-THV, particularly for supra-annular devices.[102]

FUTURE DIRECTIONS—COMPUTER SIMULATION

Cardiac CT has been crucial to translating TAVR into clinical practice by providing clinicians with a noninvasive, accurate, and reproducible means to size the aortic anatomy, select the appropriate device, and guide procedural strategy.[34] However, with the indications of TAVR shifting to younger patients, there is a need for CTA to evolve and meet the new demands that come with treating patients with longer life expectancy. The patient journey with AS does not end following TAVR. The use of TAVR in younger patients has highlighted new issues of utmost importance such as long-term valve durability, feasibility of repeat TAVR, and minimizing the prognostic impact of procedural complications. Current assessment methods with cardiac CT focus on static quantitative and qualitative anatomic measurements derived from CT. Although assessment of annular size and degree of calcification from static cardiac CT provides some insight into the risk of developing complications such as PVR or annular injury, it does not take into account the mechanical interaction of the THV with the native anatomy, and therefore a full appreciation of potential outcomes and complications.

An underutilized strength of cardiac CT is its ability to generate an accurate, three-dimensional, and patient-specific model of the cardiac geometry. Advances in image processing and biomedical engineering provide an opportunity to transform a standard cardiac CT into a model that simulates the mechanical interaction of the THV deployment on the patient-specific native anatomy to predict clinical outcomes. Patient-specific virtual THV implantation is based on the principles of finite element modeling with different material properties defined for the THV device and surrounding tissue such as the aortic wall, leaflets, and calcium nodules.[103] Early studies of virtual THV implantation have shown promise at predicting deformation of the aortic anatomy and displacement of calcium nodules.[104] The technique has also been accurate at predicting PVR and by modeling the level and force of THV contact against the membranous septum and at predicting the need for subsequent PPM.[105,106] The field is still in its infancy and requires further validation across the spectrum of THV devices, as well as prospective evaluation of its impact at enhancing preprocedural decision-making and optimizing TAVR outcomes.

REFERENCES

1. Osnabrugge RL, Mylotte D, Head SJ, et al. Aortic stenosis in the elderly: disease prevalence and number of candidates for transcatheter aortic valve replacement: a meta-analysis and modeling study. *J Am Coll Cardiol.* 2013;62(11):1002–1012.
2. Nkomo VT, Gardin JM, Skelton TN, Gottdiener JS, Scott CG, Enriquez-Sarano M. Burden of valvular heart diseases: a population-based study. *Lancet.* 2006;368(9540):1005–1011.
3. Leon MB, Smith CR, Mack M, et al. Transcatheter aortic-valve implantation for aortic stenosis in patients who cannot undergo surgery. *N Engl J Med.* 2010;363(17):1597–1607.
4. Mack MJ, Leon MB, Thourani VH, et al. Transcatheter aortic-valve replacement with a balloon-expandable valve in low-risk patients. *N Engl J Med.* 2019;380(18):1695–1705.
5. Popma JJ, Deeb GM, Yakubov SJ, et al. Transcatheter aortic-valve replacement with a self-expanding valve in low-risk patients. *N Engl J Med.* 2019;380(18):1706–1715.
6. Smith CR, Leon MB, Mack MJ, et al. Transcatheter versus surgical aortic-valve replacement in high-risk patients. *N Engl J Med.* 2011;364(23):2187–2198.
7. Leon MB, Smith CR, Mack MJ, et al. Transcatheter or surgical aortic-valve replacement in intermediate-risk patients. *N Engl J Med.* 2016;374(17):1609–1620.
8. Piazza N, de Jaegere P, Schultz C, Becker AE, Serruys PW, Anderson RH. Anatomy of the aortic valvar complex and its implications for transcatheter implantation of the aortic valve. *Circ Cardiovasc Interv.* 2008;1(1):74–81.
9. Siu SC, Silversides CK. Bicuspid aortic valve disease. *J Am Coll Cardiol.* 2010;55(25):2789–2800.
10. Yutzey KE, Demer LL, Body SC, et al. Calcific aortic valve disease: a consensus summary from the alliance of investigators on calcific aortic valve disease. *Arterioscler Thromb Vasc Biol.* 2014;34(11):2387–2393.
11. Michelena HI, Desjardins VA, Avierinos JF, et al. Natural history of asymptomatic patients with normally functioning or minimally dysfunctional bicuspid aortic valve in the community. *Circulation.* 2008;117(21):2776–2784.
12. Verma S, Siu SC. Aortic dilatation in patients with bicuspid aortic valve. *N Engl J Med.* 2014;370(20):1920–1929.
13. Kim WK, Liebetrau C, Fischer-Rasokat U, et al. Challenges of recognizing bicuspid aortic valve in elderly patients undergoing TAVR. *Int J Cardiovasc Imaging.* 2020;36(2):251–256.
14. Philip F, Faza NN, Schoenhagen P, et al. Aortic annulus and root characteristics in severe aortic stenosis due to bicuspid aortic valve and tricuspid aortic valves: implications for transcatheter aortic valve therapies. *Catheter Cardiovasc Interv.* 2015;86(2):E88–E98.
15. van Rosendael PJ, Kamperidis V, Kong WK, et al. Comparison of quantity of calcific deposits by multidetector computed tomography in the aortic valve and coronary arteries. *Am J Cardiol.* 2016;118(10):1533–1538.
16. Tchetche D, de Biase C, van Gils L, et al. Bicuspid aortic valve anatomy and relationship with devices: the Bavard multicenter registry. *Circ Cardiovasc Interv.* 2019;12(1):e007107.
17. Mylotte D, Lefevre T, Sondergaard L, et al. Transcatheter aortic valve replacement in bicuspid aortic valve disease. *J Am Coll Cardiol.* 2014;64(22):2330–2339.
18. Yoon SH, Bleiziffer S, De Backer O, et al. Outcomes in transcatheter aortic valve replacement for bicuspid versus tricuspid aortic valve stenosis. *J Am Coll Cardiol.* 2017;69(21):2579–2589.
19. Makkar RR, Yoon SH, Leon MB, et al. Association between transcatheter aortic valve replacement for bicuspid vs tricuspid aortic stenosis and mortality or stroke. *JAMA.* 2019;321(22):2193–2202.
20. Forrest JK, Kaple RK, Ramlawi B, et al. Transcatheter aortic valve replacement in bicuspid versus tricuspid aortic valves from the STS/ACC TVT registry. *JACC Cardiovasc Interv.* 2020;13(15):1749–1759.
21. Halim SA, Edwards FH, Dai D, et al. Outcomes of transcatheter aortic valve replacement in patients with bicuspid aortic valve disease: a report from the society of thoracic surgeons/American College of Cardiology transcatheter valve therapy registry. *Circulation.* 2020;141(13):1071–1079.
22. Waksman R, Craig PE, Torguson R, et al. Transcatheter aortic valve replacement in low-risk patients with symptomatic severe bicuspid aortic valve stenosis. *JACC Cardiovasc Interv.* 2020;13(9):1019–1027.
23. Tanaka R, Yoshioka K, Niinuma H, Ohsawa S, Okabayashi H, Ehara S. Diagnostic value of cardiac CT in the evaluation of bicuspid aortic stenosis: comparison with echocardiography and operative findings. *Am J Roentgenol.* 2010;195(4):895–899.
24. Hayashida K, Bouvier E, Lefevre T, et al. Transcatheter aortic valve implantation for patients with severe bicuspid aortic valve stenosis. *Circ Cardiovasc Interv.* 2013;6(3):284–291.
25. Sievers HH, Schmidtke C. A classification system for the bicuspid aortic valve from 304 surgical specimens. *J Thorac Cardiovasc Surg.* 2007;133(5):1226–1233.
26. Jilaihawi H, Chen M, Webb J, et al. A bicuspid aortic valve imaging classification for the TAVR Era. *JACC Cardiovasc Imaging.* 2016;9(10):1145–1158.
27. Yoon SH, Kim WK, Dhoble A, et al. Bicuspid aortic valve morphology and outcomes after transcatheter aortic valve replacement. *J Am Coll Cardiol.* 2020;76(9):1018–1030.
28. Vahanian A, Beyersdorf F, Praz F, et al. 2021 ESC/EACTS Guidelines for the management of valvular heart disease: developed by the task force for the management of valvular heart disease of the European Society of Cardiology (ESC) and the European Association for Cardio-Thoracic Surgery (EACTS). *Rev Esp Cardiol (Engl Ed).* 2022;75(6):524.
29. Maes F, Lerakis S, Barbosa Ribeiro H, et al. Outcomes from transcatheter aortic valve replacement in patients with low-flow, low-gradient aortic stenosis and left ventricular ejection fraction less than 30%: a substudy from the Topas-Tavi registry. *JAMA Cardiol.* 2019;4(1):64–70.
30. Fischer-Rasokat U, Renker M, Liebetrau C, et al. 1-Year Survival after TAVR of patients with low-flow, low-gradient and high-gradient aortic valve stenosis in matched study populations. *JACC Cardiovasc Interv.* 2019;12(8):752–763.
31. Pawade T, Sheth T, Guzzetti E, Dweck MR, Clavel MA. Why and how to measure aortic valve calcification in patients with aortic stenosis. *JACC Cardiovasc Imaging.* 2019;12(9):1835–1848.
32. Clavel MA, Messika-Zeitoun D, Pibarot P, et al. The complex nature of discordant severe calcified aortic valve disease grading: new insights from combined Doppler echocardiographic and computed tomographic study. *J Am Coll Cardiol.* 2013;62(24):2329–2338.
33. Clavel MA, Pibarot P, Messika-Zeitoun D, et al. Impact of aortic valve calcification, as measured by MDCT, on survival in patients with aortic stenosis: results of an international registry study. *J Am Coll Cardiol.* 2014;64(12):1202–1213.
34. Blanke P, Weir-McCall JR, Achenbach S, et al. Computed tomography imaging in the context of Transcatheter Aortic Valve Implantation (TAVI)/Transcatheter Aortic Valve Replacement (TAVR): an expert consensus document of the society of cardiovascular computed tomography. *JACC Cardiovasc Imaging.* 2019;12(1):1–24.
35. Murphy DT, Blanke P, Alaamri S, et al. Dynamism of the aortic annulus: effect of diastolic versus systolic CT annular measurements on device selection in transcatheter aortic valve replacement (TAVR). *J Cardiovasc Comput Tomogr.* 2016;10(1):37–43.
36. Blanke P, Willson AB, Webb JG, et al. Oversizing in transcatheter aortic valve replacement, a commonly used term but a poorly understood one: dependency on definition and geometrical measurements. *J Cardiovasc Comput Tomogr.* 2014;8(1):67–76.
37. Blanke P, Pibarot P, Hahn R, et al. Computed tomography-based oversizing degrees and incidence of paravalvular regurgitation of a new generation transcatheter heart valve. *JACC Cardiovasc Interv.* 2017;10(8):810–820.
38. Ihdayhid AR, Leipsic J, Hahn RT, et al. Impact of annular oversizing on paravalvular regurgitation and valve hemodynamics: new insights from PARTNER 3. *JACC Cardiovasc Interv.* 2021;14(19):2158–2169.
39. Tang GHL, Hooda A, Chuang MA, et al. Outcomes of SAPIEN 3 ultra TAVR in extremely undersized versus equivalent nominally sized anatomies. *JACC Cardiovasc Interv.* 2022;15(4):463–466.
40. Xiong TY, Feng Y, Li YJ, et al. Supra-annular sizing for transcatheter aortic valve replacement candidates with bicuspid aortic valve. *JACC Cardiovasc Interv.* 2018;11(17):1789–1790.
41. Xiong TY, Li YJ, Feng Y, et al. Understanding the interaction between transcatheter aortic valve prostheses and supra-annular structures from post-implant stent geometry. *JACC Cardiovasc Interv.* 2019;12(12):1164–1171.
42. Kim WK, Renker M, Rolf A, et al. Annular versus supra-annular sizing for TAVI in bicuspid aortic valve stenosis. *EuroIntervention.* 2019;15(3):e231–e238.
43. Weir-McCall JR, Attinger-Toller A, Blanke P, et al. Annular versus supra-annular sizing for transcatheter aortic valve replacement in bicuspid aortic valve disease. *J Cardiovasc Comput Tomogr.* 2020;14(5):407–413.
44. Samim M, Stella PR, Agostoni P, et al. Automated 3D analysis of pre-procedural MDCT to predict annulus plane angulation and C-arm positioning: benefit on procedural outcome in patients referred for TAVR. *JACC Cardiovasc Imaging.* 2013;6(2):238–248.

45. Hell MM, Biburger L, Marwan M, et al. Prediction of fluoroscopic angulations for transcatheter aortic valve implantation by CT angiography: influence on procedural parameters. *Eur Heart J Cardiovasc Imaging.* 2017;18(8):906–914.
46. Tang GHL, Zaid S, Michev I, et al. "Cusp-Overlap" view simplifies fluoroscopy-guided implantation of self-expanding valve in transcatheter aortic valve replacement. *JACC Cardiovasc Interv.* 2018;11(16):1663–1665.
47. Jilaihawi H, Zhao Z, Du R, et al. Minimizing permanent pacemaker following repositionable self-expanding transcatheter aortic valve replacement. *JACC Cardiovasc Interv.* 2019;12(18):1796–1807.
48. Pascual I, Hernandez-Vaquero D, Alperi A, et al. Permanent pacemaker reduction using cusp-overlapping projection in TAVR: a propensity score analysis. *JACC Cardiovasc Interv.* 2022;15(2):150–161.
49. Arsalan M, Kim WK, Van Linden A, et al. Predictors and outcome of conversion to cardiac surgery during transcatheter aortic valve implantation. *Eur J Cardiothorac Surg.* 2018;54(2):267–272.
50. Pineda AM, Harrison JK, Kleiman NS, et al. Incidence and outcomes of surgical bailout during TAVR: insights from the STS/ACC TVT registry. *JACC Cardiovasc Interv.* 2019;12(18):1751–1764.
51. Barbanti M, Yang TH, Rodes Cabau J, et al. Anatomical and procedural features associated with aortic root rupture during balloon-expandable transcatheter aortic valve replacement. *Circulation.* 2013;128(3):244–253.
52. Barbanti M, Buccheri S, Rodes-Cabau J, et al. Transcatheter aortic valve replacement with new-generation devices: a systematic review and meta-analysis. *Int J Cardiol.* 2017;245:83–89.
53. Girdauskas E, Owais T, Fey B, et al. Subannular perforation of left ventricular outflow tract associated with transcatheter valve implantation: pathophysiological background and clinical implications. *Eur J Cardiothorac Surg.* 2017;51(1):91–96.
54. Hansson NC, Norgaard BL, Barbanti M, et al. The impact of calcium volume and distribution in aortic root injury related to balloon-expandable transcatheter aortic valve replacement. *J Cardiovasc Comput Tomogr.* 2015;9(5):382–392.
55. Ribeiro HB, Webb JG, Makkar RR, et al. Predictive factors, management, and clinical outcomes of coronary obstruction following transcatheter aortic valve implantation: insights from a large multicenter registry. *J Am Coll Cardiol.* 2013;62(17):1552–1662.
56. Ribeiro HB, Nombela-Franco L, Urena M, et al. Coronary obstruction following transcatheter aortic valve implantation: a systematic review. *JACC Cardiovasc Interv.* 2013;6(5):452–461.
57. Ribeiro HB, Rodes-Cabau J, Blanke P, et al. Incidence, predictors, and clinical outcomes of coronary obstruction following transcatheter aortic valve replacement for degenerative bioprosthetic surgical valves: insights from the VIVID registry. *Eur Heart J.* 2018;39(8):687–695.
58. Faroux L, Chen S, Muntane-Carol G, et al. Clinical impact of conduction disturbances in transcatheter aortic valve replacement recipients: a systematic review and meta-analysis. *Eur Heart J.* 2020;41(29):2771–2781.
59. Chamandi C, Barbanti M, Munoz-Garcia A, et al. Long-term outcomes in patients with new-onset persistent left bundle branch block following TAVR. *JACC Cardiovasc Interv.* 2019;12(12):1175–1184.
60. Jorgensen TH, De Backer O, Gerds TA, Bieliauskas G, Svendsen JH, Sondergaard L. Mortality and heart failure hospitalization in patients with conduction abnormalities after transcatheter aortic valve replacement. *JACC Cardiovasc Interv.* 2019;12(1):52–61.
61. Fujita B, Kutting M, Seiffert M, et al. Calcium distribution patterns of the aortic valve as a risk factor for the need of permanent pacemaker implantation after transcatheter aortic valve implantation. *Eur Heart J Cardiovasc Imaging.* 2016;17(12):1385–1393.
62. Hamdan A, Guetta V, Klempfner R, et al. Inverse relationship between membranous septal length and the risk of atrioventricular block in patients undergoing transcatheter aortic valve implantation. *JACC Cardiovasc Interv.* 2015;8(9):1218–1228.
63. Mendiz OA, Noc M, Fava CM, et al. Impact of cusp-overlap view for TAVR with self-expandable valves on 30-day conduction disturbances. *J Interv Cardiol.* 2021;2021:9991528.
64. Pisaniello AD, Makki HBE, Jahangeer S, Daniels MJ, Hasan R, Fraser DGW. Low rates of permanent pacing are observed following self-expanding transcatheter aortic valve replacement using an annular plane projection for deployment. *Circ Cardiovasc Interv.* 2021;14(1):e009258.
65. Kappetein AP, Head SJ, Genereux P, et al. Updated standardized endpoint definitions for transcatheter aortic valve implantation: the Valve Academic Research Consortium-2 consensus document. *J Am Coll Cardiol.* 2012;60(15):1438–1454.
66. Van Mieghem NM, Unverdorben M, Hengstenberg C, et al. Edoxaban versus Vitamin K antagonist for atrial fibrillation after TAVR. *N Engl J Med.* 2021;385(23):2150–2160.
67. Chakravarty T, Sondergaard L, Friedman J, et al. Subclinical leaflet thrombosis in surgical and transcatheter bioprosthetic aortic valves: an observational study. *Lancet.* 2017;389(10087):2383–2392.
68. Makkar RR, Blanke P, Leipsic J, et al. Subclinical leaflet thrombosis in transcatheter and surgical bioprosthetic valves: partner 3 cardiac computed tomography substudy. *J Am Coll Cardiol.* 2020;75(24):3003–3015.
69. Blanke P, Leipsic JA, Popma JJ, et al. Bioprosthetic aortic valve leaflet thickening in the evolut low risk sub-study. *J Am Coll Cardiol.* 2020;75(19):2430–2442.
70. Trusty PM, Sadri V, ID Madukauwa-David, et al. Neosinus flow stasis correlates with thrombus volume post-TAVR: a patient-specific in vitro study. *JACC Cardiovasc Interv.* 2019;12(13):1288–1290.
71. Hatoum H, Dollery J, Lilly SM, Crestanello JA, Dasi LP. Implantation depth and rotational orientation effect on valve-in-valve hemodynamics and sinus flow. *Ann Thorac Surg.* 2018;106(1):70–78.
72. Madukauwa-David ID, Sadri V, Kamioka N, et al. Transcatheter aortic valve deployment influences neo-sinus thrombosis risk: an in vitro flow study. *Catheter Cardiovasc Interv.* 2020;95(5):1009–1016.
73. Rashid HN, Michail M, Ihdayhid AR, et al. Prosthesis geometrical predictors of leaflet thrombosis following transcatheter aortic valve replacement with intra-annular prostheses. *Heart Lung Circ.* 2022;31(5):678–684.
74. Fukui M, Bapat VN, Garcia S, et al. Deformation of transcatheter aortic valve prostheses: implications for hypoattenuating leaflet thickening and clinical outcomes. *Circulation.* 2022;146(6):480–493.
75. Garcia S, Fukui M, Dworak MW, et al. Clinical impact of hypoattenuating leaflet thickening after transcatheter aortic valve replacement. *Circ Cardiovasc Interv.* 2022;15(3):e011480.
76. Dangas GD, Tijssen JGP, Wohrle J, et al. A controlled trial of rivaroxaban after transcatheter aortic-valve replacement. *N Engl J Med.* 2020;382(2):120–129.
77. De Backer O, Dangas GD, Jilaihawi H, et al. Reduced leaflet motion after transcatheter aortic-valve replacement. *N Engl J Med.* 2020;382(2):130–139.
78. Collet JP, Van Belle E, Thiele H, et al. Apixaban vs. standard of care after transcatheter aortic valve implantation: the ATLANTIS trial. *Eur Heart J.* 2022;43(29):2783–2797.
79. Andreotti F, Massetti M, Ten Berg J. Defining optimal antithrombotic therapy post-TAVI: the contribution of ATLANTIS. *Eur Heart J.* 2022;43(29):2798–2800.
80. Vemulapalli S, Carroll JD, Mack MJ, et al. Procedural volume and outcomes for transcatheter aortic-valve replacement. *N Engl J Med.* 2019;380(26):2541–2550.
81. Webb JG, Murdoch DJ, Alu MC, et al. 3-Year outcomes after valve-in-valve transcatheter aortic valve replacement for degenerated bioprostheses: the Partner 2 registry. *J Am Coll Cardiol.* 2019;73(21):2647–2655.
82. Hahn RT, Webb J, Pibarot P, et al. 5-Year follow-up from the partner 2 aortic valve-in-valve registry for degenerated aortic surgical bioprostheses. *JACC Cardiovasc Interv.* 2022;15(7):698–708.
83. Dvir D, Webb J, Brecker S, et al. Transcatheter aortic valve replacement for degenerative bioprosthetic surgical valves: results from the global valve-in-valve registry. *Circulation.* 2012;126(19):2335–2344.
84. Landes U, Webb JG, De Backer O, et al. Repeat transcatheter aortic valve replacement for transcatheter prosthesis dysfunction. *J Am Coll Cardiol.* 2020;75(16):1882–1893.
85. Landes U, Sathananthan J, Witberg G, et al. Transcatheter replacement of transcatheter versus surgically implanted aortic valve bioprostheses. *J Am Coll Cardiol.* 2021;77(1):1–14.
86. Akodad M, Sellers S, Gulsin GS, et al. Leaflet and neoskirt height in transcatheter heart valves: implications for repeat procedures and coronary access. *JACC Cardiovasc Interv.* 2021;14(20):2298–2300.
87. Ochiai T, Oakley L, Sekhon N, et al. Risk of coronary obstruction due to sinus sequestration in redo transcatheter aortic valve replacement. *JACC Cardiovasc Interv.* 2020;13(22):2617–2627.
88. Heitkemper M, Hatoum H, Azimian A, et al. Modeling risk of coronary obstruction during transcatheter aortic valve replacement. *J Thorac Cardiovasc Surg.* 2020;159(3) 829–838. e3.
89. Khan JM, Greenbaum AB, Babaliaros VC, et al. The BASILICA trial: prospective multicenter investigation of intentional leaflet laceration to prevent TAVR coronary obstruction. *JACC Cardiovasc Interv.* 2019;12(13):1240–1252.
90. Komatsu I, Leipsic J, Webb JG, et al. Coronary ostial eccentricity in severe aortic stenosis: guidance for BASILICA transcatheter leaflet laceration. *J Cardiovasc Comput Tomogr.* 2020;14(6):516–519.
91. Faroux L, Guimaraes L, Wintzer-Wehekind J, et al. Coronary artery disease and transcatheter aortic valve replacement: JACC state-of-the-art review. *J Am Coll Cardiol.* 2019;74(3):362–372.
92. Writing Committee M, Gulati M, Levy PD, et al. 2021 AHA/ACC/ASE/CHEST/SAEM/SCCT/SCMR Guideline for the evaluation and diagnosis of chest pain: a report of the American College of Cardiology/American Heart Association joint committee on clinical practice guidelines. *J Am Coll Cardiol.* 2021;78(22):e187–e285.
93. Gatti M, Gallone G, Poggi V, et al. Diagnostic accuracy of coronary computed tomography angiography for the evaluation of obstructive coronary artery disease in patients referred for transcatheter aortic valve implantation: a systematic review and meta-analysis. *Eur Radiol.* 2022;32(8):5189–5200.
94. Michail M, Ihdayhid AR, Comella A, et al. Feasibility and validity of computed tomography-derived fractional flow reserve in patients with severe aortic stenosis: the CAST-FFR study. *Circ Cardiovasc Interv.* 2021;14(1):e009586.
95. Nai Fovino L, Scotti A, Massussi M, et al. Incidence and feasibility of coronary access after transcatheter aortic valve replacement. *Catheter Cardiovasc Interv.* 2020;96(5):E535–E541.
96. Barbanti M, Costa G, Picci A, et al. Coronary cannulation after transcatheter aortic valve replacement: the RE-ACCESS study. *JACC Cardiovasc Interv.* 2020;13(21):2542–2555.
97. Faroux L, Lhermusier T, Vincent F, et al. ST-segment elevation myocardial infarction following transcatheter aortic valve replacement. *J Am Coll Cardiol.* 2021;77(17):2187–2199.
98. Tang GHL, Amat-Santos IJ, De Backer O, et al. Rationale, definitions, techniques, and outcomes of commissural alignment in TAVR: from the ALIGN-TAVR consortium. *JACC Cardiovasc Interv.* 2022;15(15):1497–1518.
99. Rogers T, Greenspun BC, Weissman G, et al. Feasibility of coronary access and aortic valve reintervention in low-risk TAVR patients. *JACC Cardiovasc Interv.* 2020;13(6):726–735.

100. Abdelghani M, Landt M, Traboulsi H, Becker B, Richardt G. Coronary access after TAVR with a self-expanding bioprosthesis: insights from computed tomography. *JACC Cardiovasc Interv*. 2020;13(6):709–722.
101. Tarantini G, Nai Fovino L, Scotti A, et al. Coronary access after transcatheter aortic valve replacement with commissural alignment: the align-access study. *Circ Cardiovasc Interv*. 2022;15(2):e011045.
102. De Backer O, Landes U, Fuchs A, et al. Coronary access after TAVR-in-TAVR as evaluated by multidetector computed tomography. *JACC Cardiovasc Interv*. 2020;13(21):2528–2538.
103. de Jaegere P, Rocatello G, Prendergast BD, de Backer O, Van Mieghem NM, Rajani R. Patient-specific computer simulation for transcatheter cardiac interventions: what a clinician needs to know. *Heart*. 2019;105(Suppl 2):s21–s27.
104. Schultz C, Rodriguez-Olivares R, Bosmans J, et al. Patient-specific image-based computer simulation for theprediction of valve morphology and calcium displacement after TAVI with the medtronic CoreValve and the Edwards Sapien valve. *EuroIntervention*. 2016;11(9):1044–1052.
105. de Jaegere P, De Santis G, Rodriguez-Olivares R, et al. Patient-specific computer modeling to predict aortic regurgitation after transcatheter aortic valve replacement. *JACC Cardiovasc Interv*. 2016;9(5):508–512.
106. Rocatello G, El Faquir N, De Santis G, et al. Patient-specific computer simulation to elucidate the role of contact pressure in the development of new conduction abnormalities after catheter-based implantation of a self-expanding aortic valve. *Circ Cardiovasc Interv*. 2018;11(2):e005344.

20 Use of Cardiac Computed Tomography in Structural Heart Disease Interventions

JOAO CAVALCANTE AND DAVIDE MARGONATO

CARDIAC COMPUTED TOMOGRAPHY FOR TRANSCATHETER MITRAL VALVE INTERVENTIONS

Introduction

The considerable efficacy and safety of transcatheter valve therapies over the last decade offer many patients improved quality and quantity of life. This immense progress and growth are due not only to safer devices and increased operators' expertise, but also through the major improvements and systematic integration of advanced imaging techniques into direct patient care. This is particularly true for multidetector computed tomography (MDCT), whose contribution in the context of multimodality imaging is nowadays pervasive for preprocedural planning and follow-up of patients with valvular heart disease being considered for transcatheter interventions.[1] Following the success of transcatheter aortic valve implantation (TAVI), there is now great interest in new transcatheter technologies, specifically designed for repair and replacement of atrioventricular valves. However, their anatomy and pathophysiology are significantly more complex than the aortic valve, leading to an important need for appropriate multimodality imaging evaluation with standardized definition of imaging selection criteria for different devices. In the context of mitral valve (MV) disease, echocardiography can help identify when if mitral regurgitation (MR) or mitral stenosis (MS) are amenable to percutaneous therapy, especially for the large number of patients with contraindications for surgery or for those who are at high operative risk.[2] Subsequently, MDCT can provide information for a more comprehensive systematic evaluation of MV pathology and for the feasibility of transcatheter treatment.

Transcatheter mitral valve replacement (TMVR) has been approved by the U.S. Food and Drug Administration for the treatment of high-risk patients with failed bioprosthetic valves (valve-in-valve [ViV] TMVR) and of prior MV annuloplasty repair (valve-in-ring [ViR] TMVR) with the use of a balloon-expandable transcatheter aortic valve device (Edwards SAPIEN 3, Edwards Lifesciences, Irvine, CA). Multimodality imaging including echocardiography and MDCT are crucial for selecting appropriate TMVR candidates and procedural planning. MDCT is useful to assess suitability of patients for TMVR, device selection, and procedural planning and evaluate potential complications such as left ventricular outflow tract obstruction (LVOTO). In patients not suitable for transcatheter repair, in the presence of sufficient mitral annular calcification (MAC), the option for TMVR valve-in-MAC (ViMAC) has also been performed under research registries,[3] either with specific native TMVR devices or with SAPIEN 3.

Data Acquisition

The MDCT acquisition protocol for TMVR planning may differ according to several factors: particularly, the type of scanner, iodine contrast concentration, renal function of the patient, and body habitus. Each institution should customize its acquisition protocol accordingly.[4] In our center, we mainly use the third-generation MDCT dual-source Somatom Force scanner (Siemens Healthineers), which offers excellent temporal resolution (66 msec). This allows for harmonious imaging even in patients with irregular rhythm or high heart rate, and premedication for heart rate control is usually not necessary. Although dual-source scanners provide the best temporal resolution, volumetric MDCT scanners are recommended as they offer whole heart coverage in a single heartbeat, although with worse temporal resolution.

The acquisition protocol starts with a single contrast bolus injection (iodine concentration of 350 mg/mL and a total volume of 60–120 cc) at a flow rate of 4 to 7 mL/s[4], followed by a 60-mL saline chaser. The cardiac scan acquisition is triggered using a bolus tracking method, with the region of interest (ROI) placed at the descending aorta at the carina level. An attenuation threshold is set based on the selected kilovolt peak (80–120 kVp, depending on the patient's body mass index), typically around 120 Hounsfield units (HU). A retrospective electrocardiogram (ECG) gated scan is performed, covering the full cardiac cycle without dose modulation to allow for both systolic and diastolic measurements. Functional images are reconstructed with isotropic voxels of 1.0 mm at every 5% of the R-R interval (0–95%). In cases with highly irregular heart rate, manual ECG editing and absolute reconstruction (at every 50 msec) based on the duration of the shortest R-R interval are performed to reduce motion artifacts.

Obtaining high-quality functional images is crucial for the pre-TMVR MDCT assessment. Although a 64-detector-row single-source MDCT scanner is the minimum requirement for TMVR, it can present challenges and issues due to inadequate temporal resolution with potential significant blurring in the presence of faster heart rates or arrhythmias, in addition to longer acquisition and breath-holding times. These factors increase the risk of misregistration and motion artifacts, especially in symptomatic patients with arrhythmias or faster heart rates. The insufficient temporal resolution can further exacerbate these imaging artifacts, making TMVR planning difficult, particularly in the presence of MAC, high-density prosthetic materials, or cardiac arrhythmias.

Data Analysis

MITRAL VALVE LEAFLETS

The anterior MV leaflet is roughly semicircular, with the base attached to the anterior MV annulus that extends to the mitral-aortic fibrous intervalvular fibrosa. Despite the absence of true anatomic carvings, the anterior leaflet has been historically divided in three scallops due to surgical purposes: the lateral (A1), the central (A2), and the medial (A3). The posterior MV leaflet is shorter and typically presents as a quadrangular shape. Although its morphology can vary, the posterior leaflet is usually divided by two carvings in three scallops: the lateral (P1), the central (P2, usually the larger), and the medial (P3). The leaflets are separated by two deep incisures named commissures (anterolateral and posteromedial) and present on their ventricular surfaces the attachment of the chordae tendinae through which they are connected to the papillary muscles.

These anatomic characteristics are easily identifiable via MDCT and seen in both reconstructed short-axis and long-axis views. Although echocardiography is considered the primary imaging modality to assess the MV apparatus, different leaflet measurements can also be precisely obtained from MDCT, including leaflet length, area, tenting height, and coaptation angle[5]; moreover, MDCT can distinguish between leaflet fibrosis and leaflet calcification, an important aspect that echocardiography often may not distinguish due to ultrasound beam absorption properties. MDCT can also exclude direct insertion of the papillary muscles on the leaflets, another parameter that should be ruled out before TMVR.

In the context of TMVR, the MV annulus may serve as a point of anchoring for TMVR devices, whereas the anterior leaflet may contribute to left ventricular outflow tract obstruction (LVOTO) after implantation of some TMVR devices (see specific paragraph on neo-LVOT).

Lastly, although transesophageal echocardiography—particularly with the use of 3D imaging—has considerably improved our visualization and understanding of the mechanism and severity of MR, functional CTA with high temporal resolution and adequate leaflet rendering can also provide an exquisite evaluation (Fig. 20.1).

MITRAL VALVE ANNULUS

The MV annulus is a nonplanar structure with an ellipsoidal shape and two diameters: the major or inter-commissural and the minor or septal-lateral. From a functional perspective, it is divided in an anteromedial and a posterolateral parts. The anteromedial is delimited by the right and left fibrous trigone. It is noteworthy that the trigones are

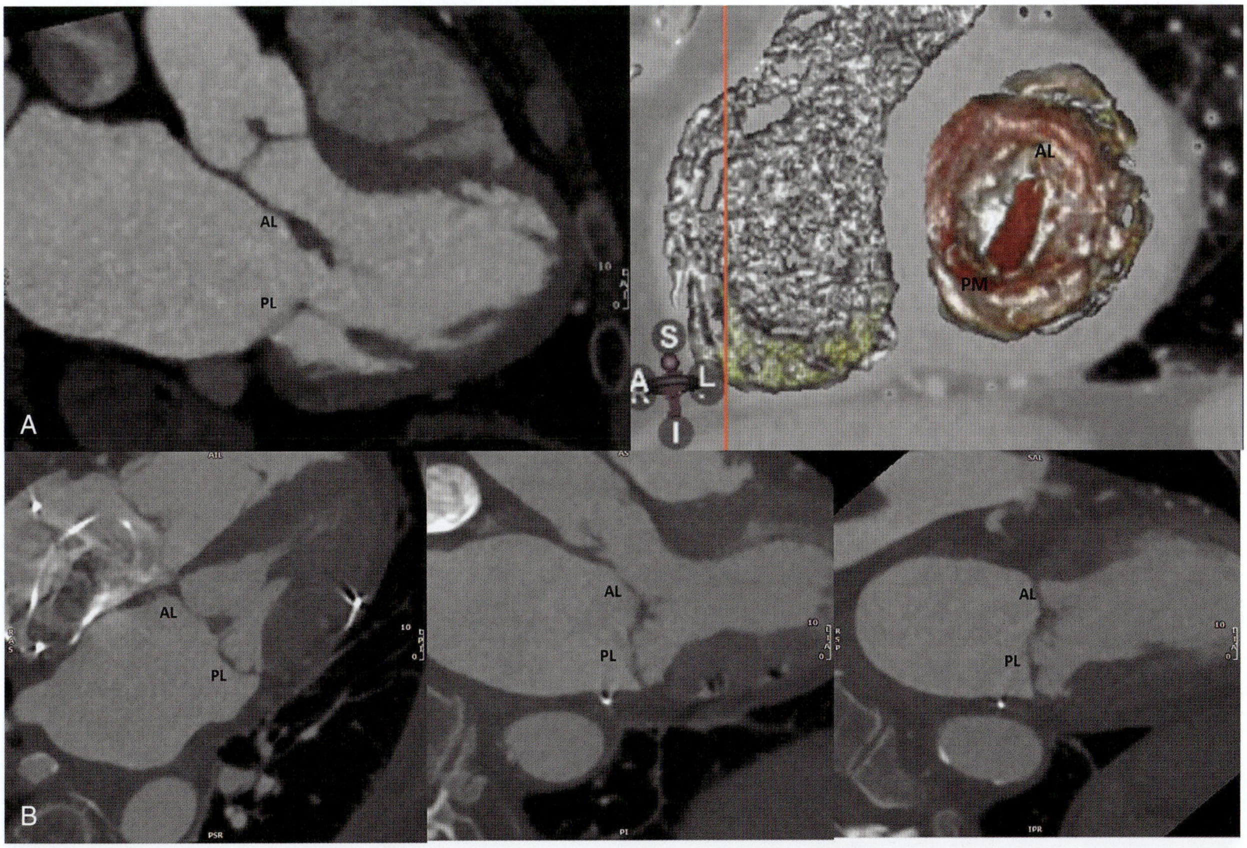

FIG. 20.1 Different MR etiologies identified by MDCT. In Panel A, a patient with rheumatic disease: on the left, the typical rheumatic thickening of the distal edge of the anterior leaflet in three-chambers view, on the right the "fish-mouth" appearance of the MV seen from the LV due to bicommissural fusion in a 3D rendering model. In Panel B, a prolapse of the central portion (P2) of the posterior leaflet is shown in four-, three-, and two-chamber views, respectively. *AL*, Anterior leaflet; *AL (right upper image)*, anterolateral commissure; *PL*, posterior leaflet; *PM*, posteromedial commissure.

connected by a fibrous tissue continuity formed by the anterior MV leaflet and the left interleaflet triangle: the presence of this robust fibrous structure, named the mitral-aortic continuity, justifies the rigidity of this portion of the annulus, which is highly resistant to deformation. The posterolateral part of the annulus is made of fibrous tissue interspersed with regions of muscular fibers. These anatomical conformations explain two important concepts.[6] First, the sphincteric role of the muscular fibers in this part of the annulus may reduce its area by up to 25% in systole. Second, the absence of a true fibrous structure makes this posterolateral part amenable to progressive dilatation.

Sizing the annulus is a crucial step to choose the most appropriate transcatheter MV prosthesis (Fig. 20.2). Due to its dynamic nature, MDCT data acquisition should cover the entire cardiac cycle, optimally without dose modulation. For TMVR screening and planning, the annulus can be considered not only in its classical saddle nonplanar shape, but even in a "D-shape" form obtained by connecting the two trigones with a straight line: its segmentation is then performed using dedicated software with the semi-automated creation of multiplanar reformat images and a user-defined interpolated cubic spline in order to measure its diameters, perimeter, and area both in systole and in diastole.[4]

Given the high closing forces of the mitral valve, and to avoid complications such as paravalvular leak or device embolization, some degree of oversizing in these above

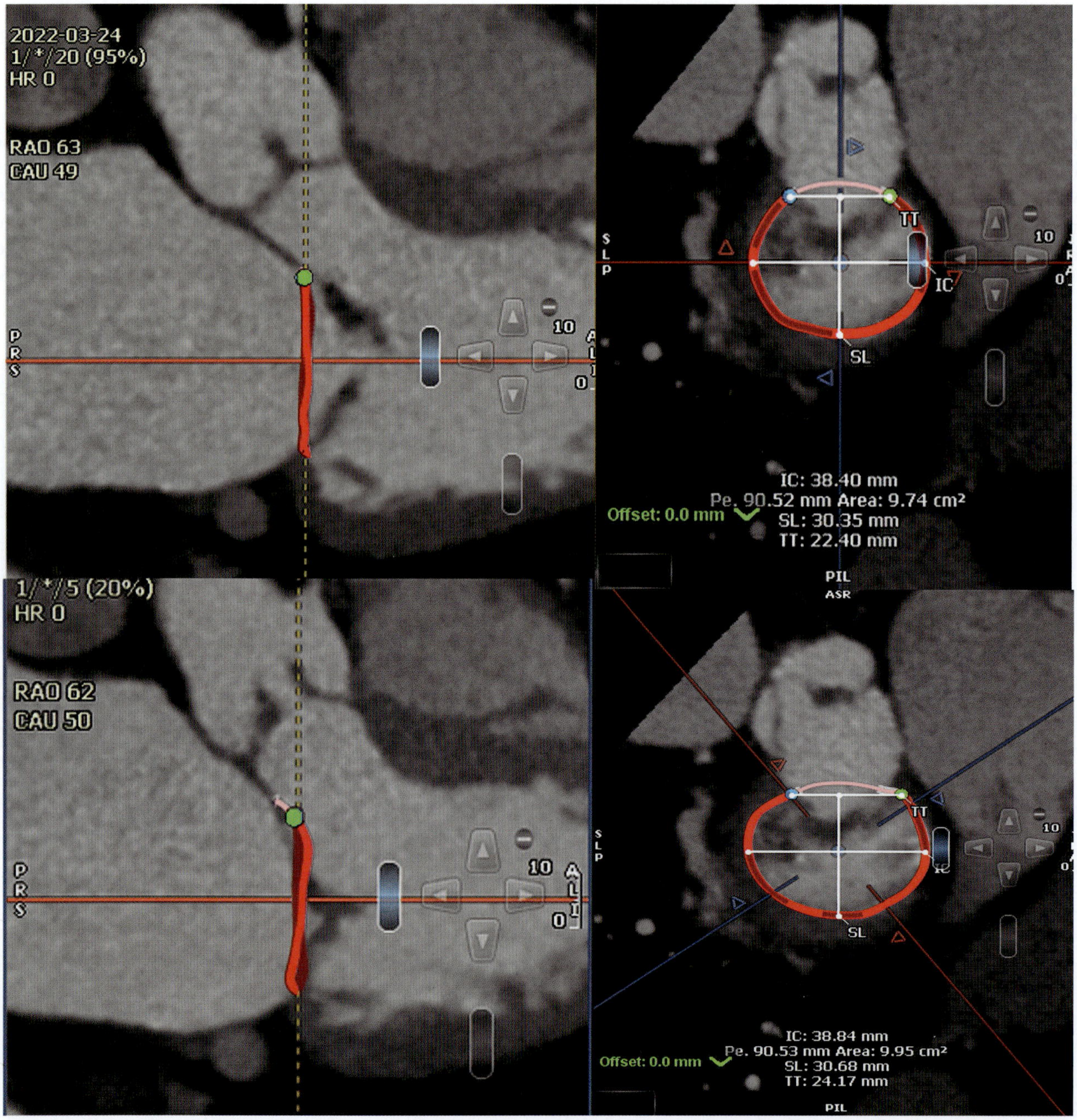

FIG. 20.2 Mitral valve annulus analysis by cardiac computed tomography. For transcatheter mitral valve replacement planning, the mitral annulus segmentation is performed using dedicated software with the semi-automated measurement of inter-commissural (IC), septo-lateral (SL), trigone-to-trigone (TT) distances, and MV perimeter (PE) and area, both in systole (*upper panel*) and in diastole (*lower panel*).

mentioned parameters is needed when planning a suitable TMVR strategy through MDCT evaluation, and the presence and extension of MAC has to be assessed. Moreover, to prevent problem with anchoring in degenerative myxomatous disease, the presence of mitral-annular disjunction must be excluded, as the excessive mitral annular motion and relative protrusion of the basal ventricular myocardium can potentially interfere with prosthesis cages.[7] On the contrary, in functional MR, tethering of the posterior leaflet causes the formation of an inward deflection of the basal myocardium at the annular level (so-called "myocardial shelf"), representing the true anchoring zone of prosthesis designed to engage the myocardium: the absence of this myocardial shelf must be reported as it might prevent adequate sealing in the landing zone.

CALCULATION OF THE NEO-LVOT AREA

The native LVOT is an anatomic space located proximal to the aortic valve plane and bordered anteriorly by the basal segment of the interventricular septum and posteriorly by the mitral-aortic continuity, which in MDCT appears as a relatively thicker tissue that extends from the aortic annulus into the LVOT. A neo-LVOT is created when an implanted TMVR prosthesis extends the circumferential anatomy of the native LVOT deeper into the left ventricle. Specifically, the posterior border of the neo-LVOT becomes the anterior circumference of the prosthesis along with the native anterior MV leaflet. The neo-LVOT usually appears as a crescent-shaped structure in cross-section imaging, due to the circular outer surface of the prosthesis. Of note, this anatomic description applies for neo-LVOT definition after TMVR ViV as well.

Evaluation of the neo-LVOT area ideally requires a dedicated postprocessing software, although standard MPR assessment can be done with difficulties with the creation of the neo-LVOT blood flow centerline and orthogonal alignment with that path.[8] The dynamism of the MV annulus can vary according to the underlying MV pathology. For example, in case of organic MV disease due to MV prolapse, the annulus may be largest in mid-end systole,[9] whereas in functional/secondary MR from dilated cardiomyopathy it is largest in early diastole.[10] For complete annuloplasty ring or bioprosthesis, end-diastole sizing is not needed, as the failed surgical device dimensions will not change throughout cardiac cycle. Subsequently, sizing for TMVR ViV or ViR using a balloon expandable aortic device (Sapien 3, Edwards Lifesciences, CA) requires greater degree of oversizing than in the aortic position and is typically guided by the true internal diameter of the surgical prosthesis for ViV, or the inner area for ViR. Use of the Mitral ViV mobile app (https://apps.apple.com/us/app/valve-in-valve-mitral/id703369667), allows for comprehensive evaluation and procedural guidance for the best-fitting prosthesis size. Sizing for native TMVR-specific devices is beyond the scope of this book chapter, especially given their unique design and different mechanisms of fixation, which require dedicated assessment of not only the mitral annulus but other anatomical parameters. In addition, iterations of TMVR-specific devices make this a dynamic field, and analysis for suitability remains mostly done by imaging core labs. As such, the remainder of this book chapter will focus on the current FDA-approved treatment for a balloon-expandable aortic transcatheter prosthesis for high-risk surgical patients—ViV and ViR TMVR. TMVR in MAC is off label.

The cardiac cycle phase used for neoLVOT area measurement for ViV or ViR TMVR should be the end systolic identified as the last phase when the aortic valve is fully open, typically around 30% of the cardiac cycle, and with less blurring/motion artifact of the mitral device of interest. After segmenting in this phase, a virtual model of the chosen mitral device type and size must be inserted in the optimal position, with the depth adjusted so the external skirt of the SAPIEN 3 valve contacts the entire landing zone (typically 25–30% atrial and 75–70% ventricular). Attention should be paid to the aortic annulus/mitral annulus angle given to potential canting of the failed surgical devices. Lastly, a blood flow centerline along the predicted residual open pathway connecting the aortic root and the left-ventricular cavity is drawn.[11] Scrolling along this 3D pathway in cross-section view, the smallest visible neo-LVOT area can be identified and measured (Fig. 20.3).

There are several issues that renders the evaluation of neo-LVOT area of pivotal importance at the moment of MDCT TMVR planning:

- LVOTO can be a dramatic complication of TMVR leading to periprocedural hemodynamic failure, and independently predicts 30 days and long-term mortality in this scenario.[3,12,13] This complication is not so rare, as its incidence can range from 2.2% to 39.7%, according to TMVR type (ViV, ViR, ViMAC).[3] Besides, chronic LVOTO, by increasing LV afterload, can lead to maladaptive remodeling of the LV, indirectly worsening long-term prognosis. Therefore preprocedural identification of patients at high LVOTO risk is mandatory, and preventing the risk of LVOTO is the key to improve outcomes.[14]
- Uncertainties persist in the context of neo-LVOT measurement. First, the upper limit for significant risk for LVOTO according to neo-LVOT projected area is unclear. A reduction of 35% in LVOT area has been shown to generate exponential increases in LVOT pressure gradients, and the commonly used risk threshold of 2 cm2, mainly derived from past studies on obstructive hypertrophic cardiomyopathy, is still debated.[11] Second, because substantial cardiac output has already occurred by 30% of cardiac phase, a borderline end systolic neo-LVOT may be a finding of small concern, if this is way larger in earlier phases of the cycle. Eventually, late systolic neo-LVOT area is not the sole determinant of post TMVR LVOTO risk, as many other anatomical predictors of fixed or dynamic LVOTO are involved. These predictors are mostly derived from the surgical arena and may include the length of the anterior MV leaflet that is displaced toward the LVOT by the MV prosthesis implanted in the fully-open native MV, a hypertrophic basal interventricular septum (usually >14 mm), particularly in the context of a small hyperdynamic LV, and an acute mitral-aortic angle (<120 degrees).[15]
- Pre-TMVR interventional strategies can be used to reduce the risk of LVOTO, and the best options must be carefully tailored to each patient, even according to MDCT findings. Preprocedural alcohol septal ablation has been proposed for patients with asymmetric

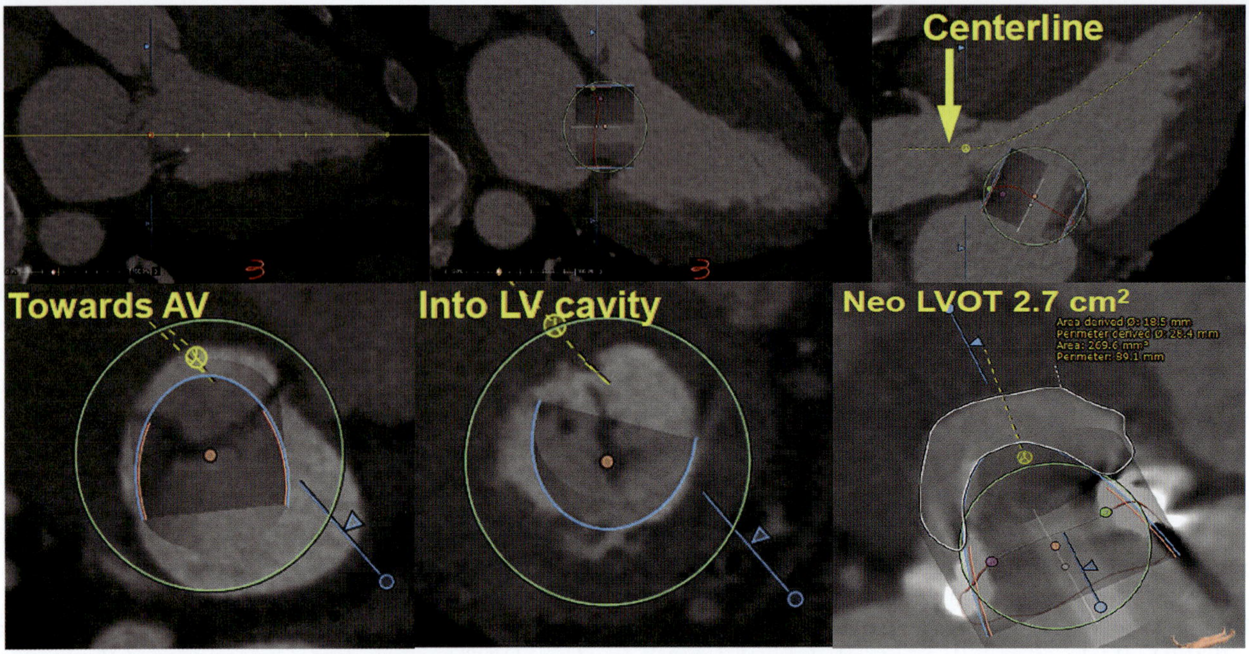

FIG. 20.3 How to model neo-LVOT. First, segment mitral annulus at late systole (typically 30% of cardiac cycle). Insert the virtual prosthesis model into optimal annular position and draw centerline for the neo-LVOT. Measure neo-LVOT area at the narrowest point through neo-LVOT centerline axis. In this figure, an example of a low-risk anatomy for outflow tract obstruction after TMVR is shown. *LVOT*, Left ventricular outflow tract; *TMVR*, transcatheter mitral valve replacement.

hypertrophy of the basal septum; however, this technique carries a risk iatrogenic conduction disorder that is nonneglectable in such a high-risk population.[11] LAMPOON technique has been developed to percutaneously split the anterior MV leaflet and prevent iatrogenic LVOT obstruction in high-risk cases, with successful, although limited, results[16]: the blood will flow through the open cells of the TMVR, limited mainly by its external skirt (the so called skirt neo-LVOT).

TRANSEPTAL PUNCTURE AND FLUOROSCOPIC ANGLES

The access site for TMVR has moved from initially transapical to now transseptal. A successful puncture is crucial to obtain a coaxial trajectory to the MV plane and increase the possibility for a safe and successful TMVR procedure.

Puncture site for TMVR is usually performed in the postero-inferior part of the fossa ovalis, but a mid-posterior puncture also provides adequate working height in the left atrium and a coaxial plane to the failed MV device.

Defining the fluoroscopic angles for optimal device deployment and anchoring is also an important role of preprocedural MDCT. The two main coplanar fluoroscopic projections used for navigation and deployment are the septal-lateral and the trigone-to-trigone, based on the above-mentioned MV annular measurements, which are orthogonal to the MV plane. A compromise view between these two views is usually provided due to C-arm angulation constraints to achieve perfect reproduction of these planes.[17] This information is essential to guide the procedure in nonradiopaque degenerated bioprosthetic valves, particularly for patients receiving ViV TMVR.

VALVE-IN-VALVE, VALVE-IN-RING, AND VALVE-IN-MAC

Preprocedural evaluation should primarily exclude other causes of high transvalvular gradients, in particular the presence of thrombosis, acute endocarditis, or patient-prosthesis mismatch, which should be treated with either medical therapy or a surgical approach.[18]

Then, the next step is to identify the size and type of the degenerated bioprosthetic heart valve (BHV), and MDCT is the most accurate imaging modality to confirm its diameters (Fig. 20.4).

Although the patient's medical records typically provide reliable information on the type and size of the BHV, there are instances where this information may be incorrect, incomplete, or missing. As a result, precise details regarding the BHV type and size may not be available during MDCT image analysis and workup for assessing the risk of post-procedural LVOTO.

To ensure accurate identification and confirmation of the size and type of the BHV, we recommend utilizing 3D maximal intensity projections (MIP) to verify the key anatomic features of the BHV and measure it from center to center.[19] It is important to emphasize that for ViV procedure the relevant measurement is represented by the smallest internal dimension (true ID), as the new valve will be inserted inside the old one. Yet the labeled dimensions for BHV may include the external diameter, as the dimensions could vary depending on the manufacturer[19]; further assistance with this is available via a free online application tool.[20] By examining the 3D projections, one can confirm the characteristics of the BHV and align them with the information provided by the ViV app. For mitral ViV, the desired oversizing should be larger than the average 10% for aortic ViV because of superior stress on the valve and more powerful closing forces; however, excessive oversizing must be avoided as it can cause abnormal leaflet mobility, higher gradient, and ViV deformation.[21] In addition to the previously described evaluation for neoLVOT, it is noteworthy that the risk of LVOTO may depend on intrinsic characteristics of the degenerated

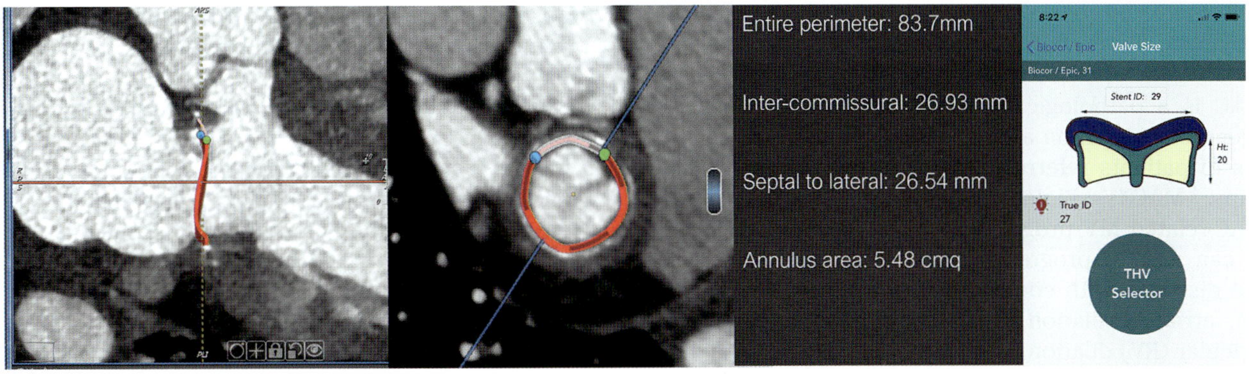

FIG. 20.4 Preprocedural planning by cardiac computed tomography for valve-in-valve procedure. On the left and central panels, internal diameters of the bioprosthesis are measured; radiographic appearance should match the expected appearance. The complementary role of cardiac computed tomography and of the Valve in Valve app (*right panel*) are pivotal to identify valve type and size.

BHV, particularly whether BHV leaflet extend all the way to the end of prosthesis stent frame (bovine pericardial BHV versus porcine leaflets, which, although shorter, result in smaller true ID). In addition, BHV canting towards the interventricular septum and shallower the angle between the aortic and mitral annulus device (typically <120 degrees) might increase the risk of LVOTO.

TMVR for ViR has a higher rate of complications, with a 5% to 8% reported incidence of LVOTO, 12% incidence of second valve intervention, and 18.4% incidence of postprocedural paravalvular leak.[3,14,22] The procedure is not technically easy to perform, as these data suggest. The first and foremost point to address is that properties of each ring is unique, and hence not all rings are ideal for ViR. The ideal ring should provide both adequate anchoring and circularity, be radiopaque, and have a proper size in the range of the currently available TAVI devices: in general, this is translated into a semirigid complete annulus ring being the most ideal, as opposed to an incomplete band (Fig. 20.5). Rigid rings do not allow for full expansion and circularity of the new valve; instead, the valve deforms itself to fit the oval shape of the ring, and this may lead to valve dysfunction and paravalvular leaks.[22]

MDCT is the most important preprocedural imaging technique for ViV as it provides intercommissural distance and internal annular area in order to choose the most appropriate SAPIEN3 size according to sizing charts.[5,19] Again, aggressive oversizing (>20%) is suggested in this setting to prevent leaks and atrial embolization of the valve. Compared to native TMVR ViV, some consideration must be underlined in this peculiar scenario:

- When evaluating the neo-LVOT area, it must be taken into account that the native anterior MV leaflet is preserved, increasing the risk of dynamic or fixed LVOTO; moreover, interestingly, if the native anterior leaflet is longer than the height of the SAPIEN 3 (approximately >22 mm), it has been reported that the displaced anterior MV leaflet can interfere with new TMVR THV functioning and cause intraprosthetic regurgitation.[23]
- An angle between the centerline of the MV and the LV apex should be measured in MDCT (the so called "Emory angle"): if this angle is >15 degrees, there is an increased

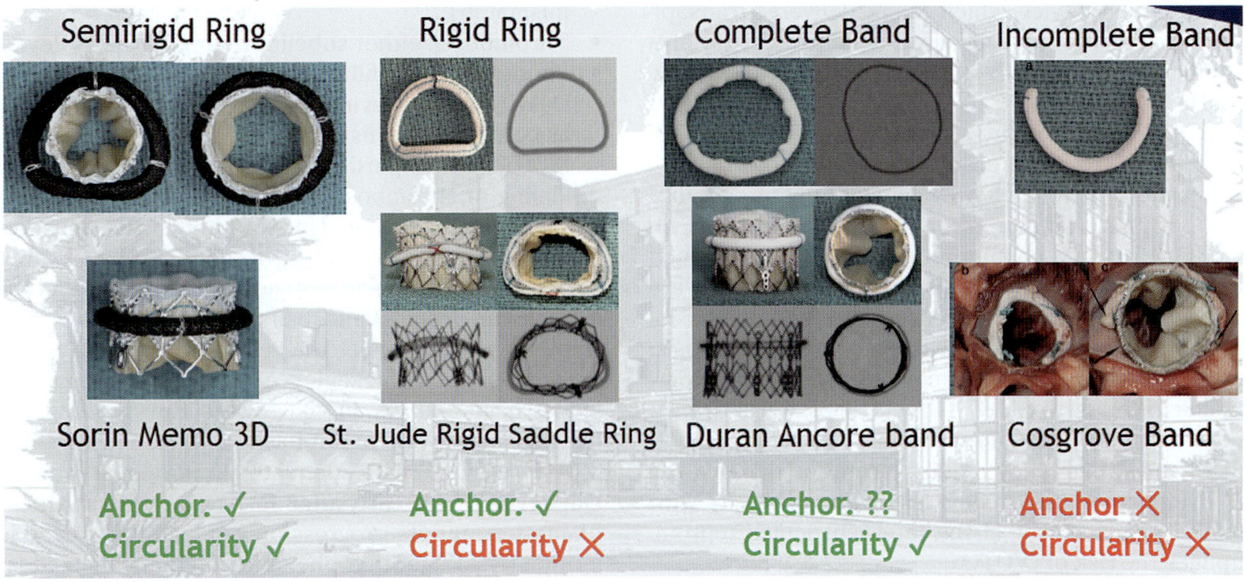

FIG. 20.5 Different types of surgical rings. Feasibility of Valve-in Ring can be foreseen according to the characteristics of each ring. (Courtesy Dr. Vinayak Bapat.)

risk of reduced coaxiality at the moment of prosthesis deployment, increasing the risk of prosthesis dysfunction and/or paravalvular leak.

MAC is a pathological process with a prevalence in the general population around 25%, increasing up to two-thirds of patients referred for transcatheter aortic valve therapy.[24] MAC is a biologically active process whose rate of MAC-related MV progression is not well understood.[25] MAC can lead to progressive MV dysfunction—typically mixed disease—with consequences such as left atrial dilation, atrial fibrillation, pulmonary hypertension, right ventricular (RV) dilation/dysfunction, etc.[26]

TMVR for MAC is a technically challenging procedure, with a reported incidence of valve embolization, residual relevant MR, and LVOTO of approximately 7%, 13%, and 40%, respectively.[11] This adds up to the fact the MAC is independently associated with all-cause mortality, acute myocardial infarction, stroke, and atrial fibrillation[24]: therefore MAC probably represents a marker of a very advanced stage of clinical deterioration for patients with valvular heart disease. Currently, there is no FDA label approval for balloon-expandable Sapien 3 use in high-risk MAC patients, and data from MITRAL II trial (NCT04408430) will help in better understanding of whether this could be a valuable approach. In parallel, several reports of adequate procedural outcomes using TMVR-specific devices in MAC patients provide the possibility for treatment with more predictable procedural results. Recently, the transapical fully retrievable and repositionable MV prosthesis Tendyne (Abbott Structural Heart, Menlo Park, CA) has been tested for compassionate use in 20 patients with MR and severe MAC, showing encouraging acute outcomes, mid-term durability, and clinical improvement[27]; the same device is under investigation for use in symptomatic patients with MR (with or without MAC) through a dedicated registry arm of the SUMMIT trial (NCT03433274). Another proposed device proposed to target MAC is the Intrepid valve (Medtronic, Dublin, Ireland), presenting a dual-structure design consisting of a circular inner stent that hosts a trileaflet bovine pericardial valve and a congenial outer fixation stent; this device, which can be delivered transapically or transeptally, is specifically tested in a registry arm for patients with MAC in the APOLLO (NCT03242642) pivotal trials.

When performing preprocedural MDCT for TMVR ViMAC (Fig. 20.6), specific precautions are as follows:

- The reasons for the high prevalence of postprocedural LVOTO in this scenario are multifactorial. It has been proposed that MV coaptation point might be pushed anteriorly by MAC itself[28]; also, as these patients are typically older and with increased afterload due to comorbidities such as hypertension or aortic stenosis. Furthermore, some patients may have small and hyperdynamic or hypertrophied left ventricles, a well-known risk factor for LVOTO. The anterior MV leaflet is present, and when >22 mm, may require laceration. RV dilation and dysfunction also creates less filling of the LV with leftward displacement of the interventricular septum, amplifies the risk of LVOTO.
- The compliance of the new valve within the MAC and its achievable deformation is rarely predictable. In the absence of specific prediction model, neo-LVOT-obtained values must be cautiously interpreted, and higher cutoff may be needed.
- Recently, a very detailed scoring system has been proposed by Guerrero and colleagues[29] aimed at grading MAC by computed tomography in order to predict anchoring and embolization risk. This MAC score presents four anatomic variables summed in a score that increases along with calcific lesion complexity: calcium thickness (<5 mm, 5–9.9 mm, >10 mm), calcium distribution (<180 degrees, 180–270 degrees, >270 degrees), trigone involvement (none, one, both), and leaflet involvement (none, anterior leaflet, both). This MAC scoring classification has resulted in a better systematic evaluation of MAC distribution and extension, providing important considerations for patient selection. Patients with a score ≤6 had high risk for device migration or embolization compared with patients with MAC scores of 7 or greater (60% versu s 9.7%, $P < .001$). Equally important as having a higher MAC score for anchoring is providing adequate oversizing and ventricular flaring of the THV stent frame to avoid embolization.

POST-TMVR IMAGING EVALUATION

Routine post TMVR follow-up, from predischarge to long-term reevaluations, is based on transthoracic echocardiography (TTE) evaluation of prosthesis function. The aims are to assess peak gradient through the neo-LVOT, transprosthetic gradients, any intra- or paravalvular regurgitation, valve migration, and acute changes in biventricular systolic function and pulmonary artery pressures. In case of red flags for bioprosthetic valve dysfunction (BVD), MDCT analysis should be considered. BVD can be classified as follows[18]:

- Structural Valve Deterioration, any intrinsic permanent change to the prosthetic valve (such as leaflet fibrosis or calcification)
- Nonstructural Valve Dysfunction, any abnormality not intrinsic to the prosthetic valve resulting in valve dysfunction (such as paravalvular leak, patient prosthesis mismatch)
- Thrombosis, either subclinical or clinically relevant
- Endocarditis, fulfilling at least one between positive Duke Criteria or evidence of abscess, pus, or vegetation as confirmed by histological studies or on autopsy

MDCT can be particularly useful if intrinsic leaflet remodeling or thrombosis is suspected. Calcification is the common final pathway of bioprosthetic valve degeneration and can be easily detected with noncontrast CT, although sometimes it can be challenging to differentiate valve leaflet calcium from stent struts related metallic artifact.[30] Hypo-attenuated leaflet thickening (HALT) is a meniscoid crescent-shaped thickening of the leaflet, starting at the leaflet base and expanding toward the free edge. It can be visualized with multiphasic gated contrast-enhanced MDCT (Fig. 20.7) with adequate temporal resolution. HALT can develop very early after aortic or mitral prosthesis implantation, and its progression can lead to reduced leaflet motion (RLM), another phenomenon that can be identified by MDCT; we suggest diagnosing RLM only in the presence of HALT, as due to MDCT limited temporal resolution, RLM

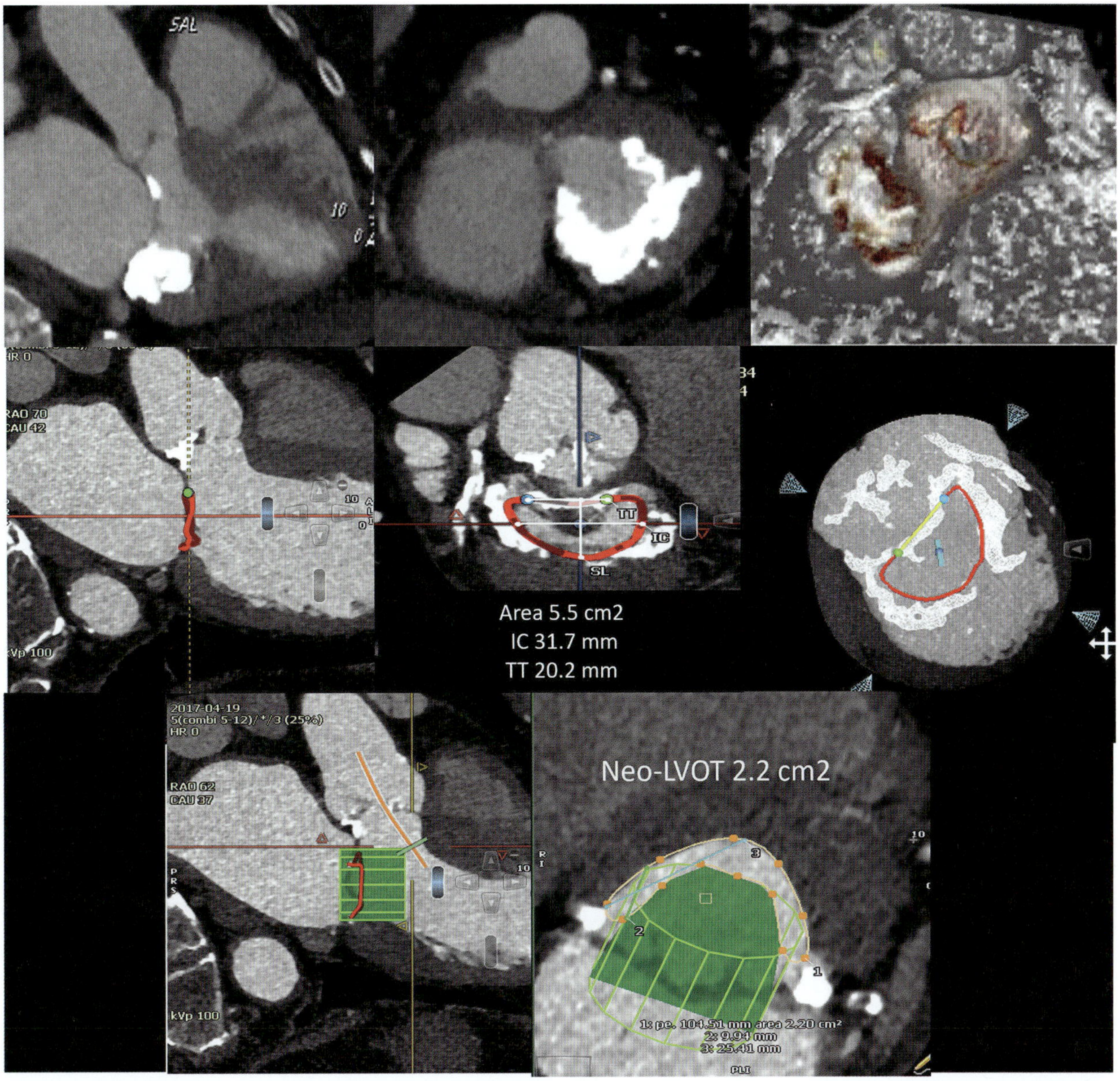

FIG. 20.6 A case of severe MAC. In the upper panels, the circumferential distribution and thickness of calcium and leaflet/trigone involvement can be evaluated, both in 2D as well as in 3D (*upper right panel*) images. Annular and neo-LVOT measurements are performed in the central and lower panels to plan ViMAC. *LVOT*, Left ventricular outflow tract; *MAC*, mitral annular calcification; *ViMAC*, valve-in-MAC.

in the absence of HALT may be a false-positive finding due to image artifact. Interestingly, a recent study,[31] unique in its design, has described detailed histomorphometric findings from a series of explanted transcatheter valve prosthesis, showing that there is a time-dependent degeneration of the prosthesis, starting from the very hours after implantation, consisting of thrombus formation, endothelial hyperplasia, fibrosis, and calcifications. Of note, thrombus was noted in all patients on both the atrial and ventricular size of the prosthesis and regardless of concomitant antithrombotic therapy. Although not specifically evaluated for MV prosthesis, these findings, if confirmed on larger populations, suggest a potential for early postprocedural MDCT assessment of prosthesis in patients at risk of prosthesis thrombosis/failure. This idea has been recently underlined by another small but pioneer study[32] on early post TMVR MDCT evaluation, demonstrating that prosthesis early deformation is common after TMVR and may be affected by excessive oversizing and a shallower implant depth. Furthermore, there is a higher incidence of HALT in patients with a higher degree of deformation and an INR <2.5 (Fig. 20.8).

CARDIAC COMPUTED TOMOGRAPHY FOR TRANSCATHETER TRICUSPID VALVE INTERVENTIONS

Introduction

The independent prognostic role of tricuspid regurgitation (TR), regardless of its etiology or RV function, has been demonstrated through several studies.[33–35] Patients suffering from severe TR often have high surgical risk given their

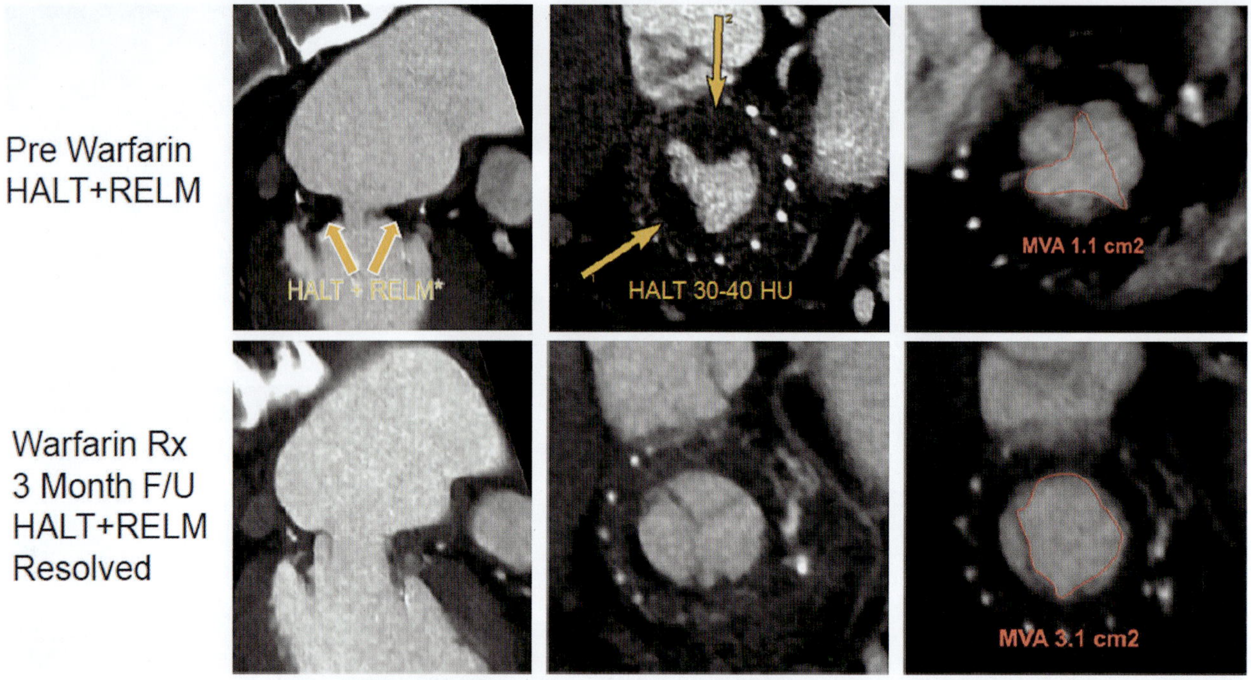

FIG. 20.7 Hypo-attenuated leaflet thickening (HALT). An example of HALT's typical appearance on cardiac computed tomography is in the upper panel. In the lower panel, resolution of HALT due to antithrombotic therapy leading to a significant improvement of leaflet excursion and therefore an increase in mitral valve area (MVA) is shown.

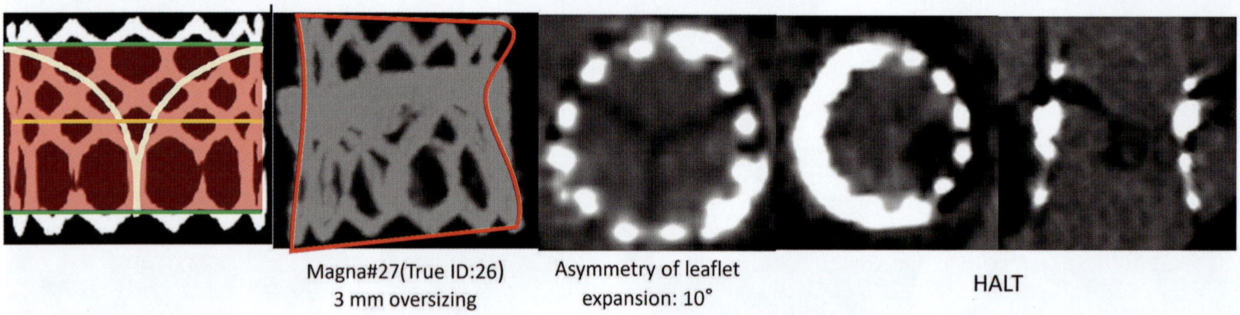

FIG. 20.8 An example of valve deformation and hypo-attenuated leaflet thickening (HALT) in a patient with mitral ViV evaluated with MDCT. First panel on the left represent the three levels where expansion area and eccentricity are measured: leaflet inflow (*upper green line*), narrowest level (*yellow line*), and leaflet outflow (*lower green line*). *MDCT*, Multidetector computed tomography; *ViV*, valve-in-valve. (Courtesy Dr. Miho Fukui.)

age, prior surgical intervention, and cardiac and noncardiac comorbidities. Therefore surgical consideration is not frequently entertained, and such patients are often treated with medical treatment.[36] However, in recent years, different transcatheter tricuspid valve replacement (TTVR) devices—some borrowed directly from MV design whereas others have been specifically developed for TTVR—have reshaped the therapeutical approach to TR. For some of them, feasibility and efficacy have been shown in early feasibility or pivotal studies, albeit with short follow-up time.[37–39]

TTE and TEE (Transesophageal Echocardiography) are the first-line imaging techniques. The triscuspid valve (TV) has a complex three-dimensional (3D) structure, and it is challenging to visualize all three leaflets in a single two-dimensional plane because of the variability of imaging planes from different transducer angles: therefore 3D imaging is crucial for a complete evaluation of the TV.

Indeed, transcatheter treatment of these patients present several challenges, due to the peculiar characteristics of the TV apparatus and of the right heart chambers. In particular, the large dimension of the nonplanar tricuspid annulus (TA) lacks annular calcifications as its anchoring system and is a fragile tissue. Moreover, navigation beyond the TV plane may be demanding due to RV trabeculae and muscular bands and the chordae tendinae. Lastly, the proximity of the tricuspid annulus to other cardiac structures, such as the atrioventricular node or the right coronary artery, and the possibility of a transvalvular lead, may require further caution when planning interventional treatment of severe TR patients.

Therefore multimodality imaging has a fundamental role in the etiological classification, evaluation of procedural feasibility, preprocedural planning, and intraprocedural monitoring of transcatheter therapies for TR.

The complementary role of MDCT is now an integral part of preprocedural evaluation for transcatheter TV intervention, both repair and replacement (TTVR), as a comprehensive assessment of the right heart can be provided[40]: TA annulus segmentation and its distance from surrounding structures, leaflet morphology, RV volumes and global contractile function, and the relationship between the TV and the caval system.

CT Data Acquisition for TTVR

Patients with TR often have atrial arrhythmias, difficulty in breath-holding, chronic kidney disease, and intracardiac leads, making data acquisition a challenging process. Similar to the MV, we need appropriate images throughout the entire cardiac cycle, so an ECG-gated sequential acquisition covering the whole cardiac cycle, without dose modulation and using the smallest available collimation, is the standard for high-quality imaging reconstruction.[40,41] In case of regular rhythm, the entire cardiac cycle by 5% phases is reconstructed; in the presence of atrial arrhythmias, absolute millisecond reconstruction is preferred at 50 msec intervals.

The major challenge is posed by the mixing of noncontrast and contrast blood in the right atrium: to avoid this, a mildly diluted biphasic contrast injection is suggested (80%/20% up to 50%/50% blend of contrast/ saline at 4.5 mL/s, followed by a 60-mL saline chaser at 4.5 mL/s). A long injection time (at least 20 seconds) provides more time for the right atrium (RA) to be uniformly enhanced before imaging begins. If enhancement of the RV only is needed, a bolus tracking technique with the ROI at the level of the pulmonary trunk is used to obtain a homogeneous right heart opacification, possibly greater than 300 HU without streak artifacts in the superior vena cava (SVC) or mixing artifacts in the right atrium. For biventricular enhancement, the Hounsfield units trigger can be use a lower threshold at the level of the descending thoracic aorta or of the left atrium.[40,41] Following cardiac scan, a 90-second delayed venous scan of the chest/abdomen/pelvis to map out the access to the RA and to the TV is often obtained to ascertain venous access size and ensure an appropriate trajectory for TTVR replacement devices; here. Of note, systolic contrast reflux in the inferior vena cava can support the diagnosis of severe TR. A standard medium smooth kernel with 1-mm slices to improve leaflets visualization is suggested.

Data Analysis

LEAFLET ANATOMY AND TETHERING

Whereas for routine TTVR assessment the leaflet anatomy and morphology is not a determinant factor, understanding the mechanism of TR and the implications for other potential edge-to-edge repair requires evaluation of the TV leaflets.

The TV is the most caudal heart valve and the one with the largest orifice. The most common valve morphology is made of three leaflets, the anterior (AL), posterior (PL), and septal (SL): AL is the largest and presents a quadrangular shape and the greatest excursion; PL is the smallest with a triangular shape; and SL presents a semicircular shape.[42] Both the AL and PL arise from the corresponding RV free wall and are dependent on a large anterior papillary muscle with a single head that incorporates the moderator band. The SL originate directly from the annulus above the membranous septum, is connected to the interventricular septum via chordal attachment to the septal papillary muscle or directly to the septum, and it is apically inserted compared to the septal insertion of the anterior MV leaflet.[43] The classical three-leaflet morphology, however, is not the only one, and multiple anatomical variants have been previously reported by pathological and surgical studies.[44,45] A recent study[46] has proposed a novel systematic classification for TV leaflet morphology to provide a common nomenclature based on four morphological types identified at TEE: type I, the classical with 3 leaflets, was present only in 54% out of 579 patients; conversely, 46% presented either 2 leaflets (type II), 4 leaflets with 2 anterior (type IIIA), 4 leaflets with 2 posterior (type IIIB), 4 leaflets with 2 septal (type IIIC) or, eventually, >4 leaflets (type IV).

In the presence of appropriate right heart enhancement, an optimal visualization of the tricuspid leaflets with MDCT is possible, given the high spatial and particularly the temporal resolution of dual-source MDCT scanners that allows identifying very fine anatomic details such as the septal atrioventricular junction, the chordae tendineae direct or indirect attachment, or the arrangement of the papillary muscles.[40,47]

Therefore the identification of the number of the leaflets and of their appearance (to suspect fibrotic or calcific remodelling) and the presence of cleft/indentations may provide an idea concerning the complexity of the anatomy of the TV, directly affecting patient management if a decision between TV repair or replacement has not been made yet.

Furthermore, leaflet tethering should be assessed, as this is an important predictive parameter for residual TR after surgical annuloplasty and to predict transcatheter TV repair futility.[36] This can be done with a reconstructed RV four-chamber view, measuring the distance between annular plane and coaptation point between the anterior/ posterior and septal leaflets; tenting angle and area can also be obtained in this view as well[40] (Fig. 20.9).

By reconstructing (with double-oblique multiplanar views) a mid-systolic (30–40%) coronal image at the level of leaflet tips, the coaptation gap dimension and location can be measured, as this is another important parameter if edge-to-edge repair is considered.[37]

In addition, quantification of TR can be obtained with MDCT by measuring the anatomical regurgitant orifice area[48] (Fig. 20.10). Although yet to be validated as a predictive parameter for transcatheter procedural success by further studies, this novel anatomic measurement is the morphological correspondent of the 3D vena contracta measured by echocardiography, which correlates with TR severity, and may be particularly useful when echocardiographic images are suboptimal. This parameter has adequate reproducibility and can be obtained from an en face plane of the TV aligned at the leaflet's free edge by measuring the narrowest mid-systolic area of the regurgitant orifice. MDCT can provide data on the optimal fluoroscopic projection and trajectory simulation for preprocedural TTVR planning (Fig. 20.11).

ANNULAR REMODELING AND IMPLICATIONS FOR TTVR

The TA is the largest annulus of the heart, a complex interconnected 3D structure 20% larger and less symmetric

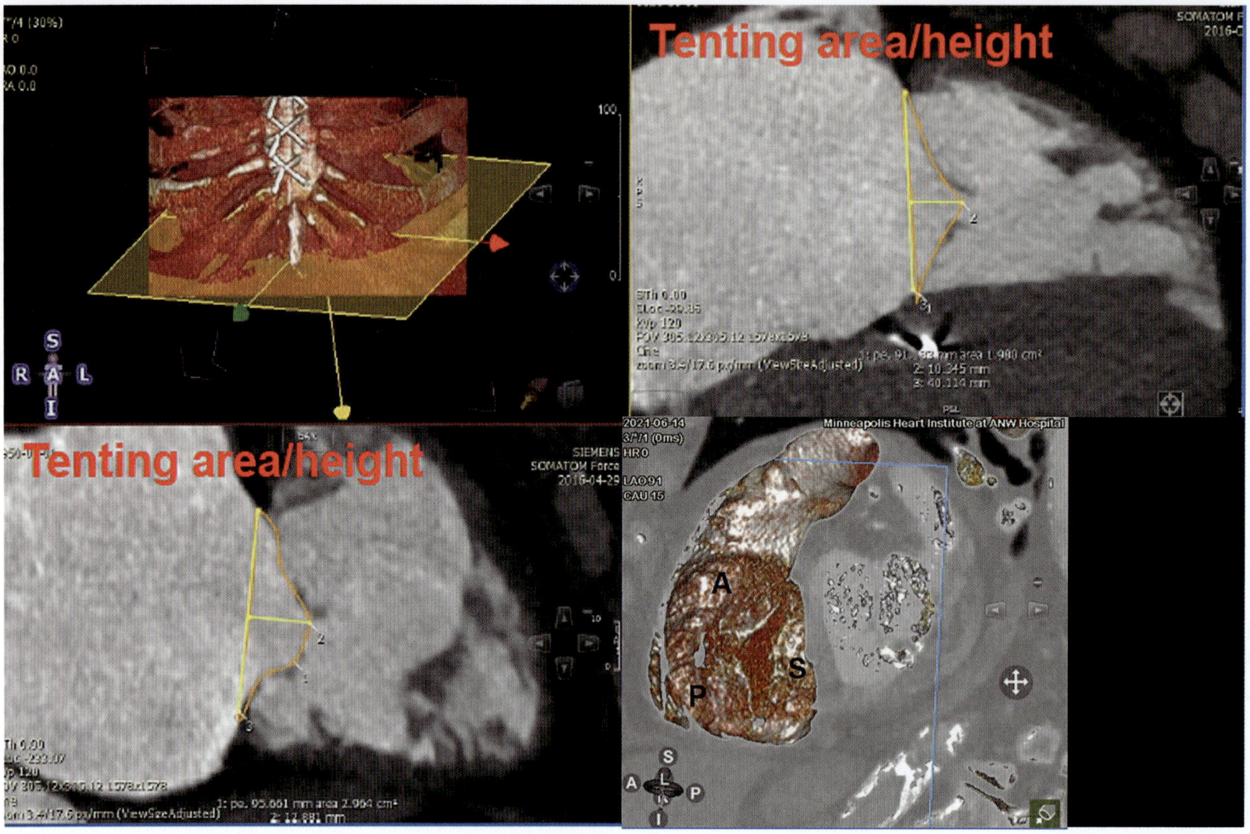

FIG. 20.9 Assessment of tricuspid valve anatomy. Tenting parameters, crucial to decide between repair or replacement of the tricuspid valve, are easily evaluated through MDCT. In the right-lower panel, en face–rendered reconstruction of the tricuspid valve leaflets allows evaluation of the tricuspid morphology (in this case, the most common three-leaflet morphology). *MDCT*, Multidetector computed tomography.

than the mitral annulus.[42] Although in normal subjects it is a nonplanar oval shape, with its posterolateral part being more apical, in patients with functional TR it tends to dilate in an anteroposterior direction, partly acquiring a more circular and planar shape. Dilation occurs mainly in this direction because its SL portion is relatively still due to its fixed position close to the fibrous trigones.[49] Compared to the mitral annuus, the TA is more prone to progressive elongation or dilatation because it is almost exclusively composed of fibro-adipose tissue, and its only true fibrous part is where the leaflets are attached to the central fibrous body: therefore it lacks a real continuous fibrous structure.

The TA is highly dynamic during the cardiac cycle, reducing its area up to 30% during systole, whereas its shape remains more constant. This is due to the contraction of the surrounding myocardium. In fact, at the hinge of the leaflets, muscular fibers from the RA may overlap the leaflet for up to 2 mm, as the AL and PL are inserted directly on the ventricular myocardium. Thus vigorous sphincteric contraction and relaxation of the annulus are direct consequences of the adjoining RA and RV walls.[49] The other main motion of the TA follows the longitudinal contraction of the RV, which displaces the TA during systole, whereas the RV apex remains fixed due to its connections with the diaphragm.

Transcatheter annuloplasty devices target annular dilation as the major pathophysiological mechanism in functional atrial TR. The goal is to reshape the TA, either by a transfemoral ring or suture-based approach, by applying tension to obtain a controlled reduction of both the major and minor TA diameters.[43] Such devices require preprocedural MDCT to assess TA diameters, perimeter and area throughout the cardiac cycle for device size selection, and for anatomic landmarks to identify the ideal positioning of anchors (Fig. 20.12). The major concern when planning annuloplasty procedure with MDCT is the anatomic relationship with the right coronary artery (RCA). The RCA runs in the right atrioventricular groove, separated by the TA only for few millimeters. Often, the closest spot is with the postero-septal segment of the TV, which on average is 5.5 mm from the RCA, whereas the longest distance is from the anterior part, approximately 7 mm.[42,50] Nonetheless, it is important to keep in mind that the RCA anatomic course is highly variable. This anatomical relation is of major concern and has to be systematically evaluated during both preprocedural MDCT and intraprocedural TEE monitoring, in order to avoid RCA spasm or injury.

One of the limitations for current TTVR devices that were directly brought from the mitral space has to do with their smaller profile, relative to a much larger TA area that needs to be covered. Therefore there is a substantial number of patients who screen-fail, and a need for more dedicated TTVR devices with a larger size, as currently being evaluated in clinical trials. Preliminary early-feasibility studies have shown increased procedural safety, albeit the concerns for venous bleeding, higher pacemaker rates (in part due to oversizing), and prosthesis durability remain issues that will need to be systematically evaluated. For these reasons, although TR elimination might not be as

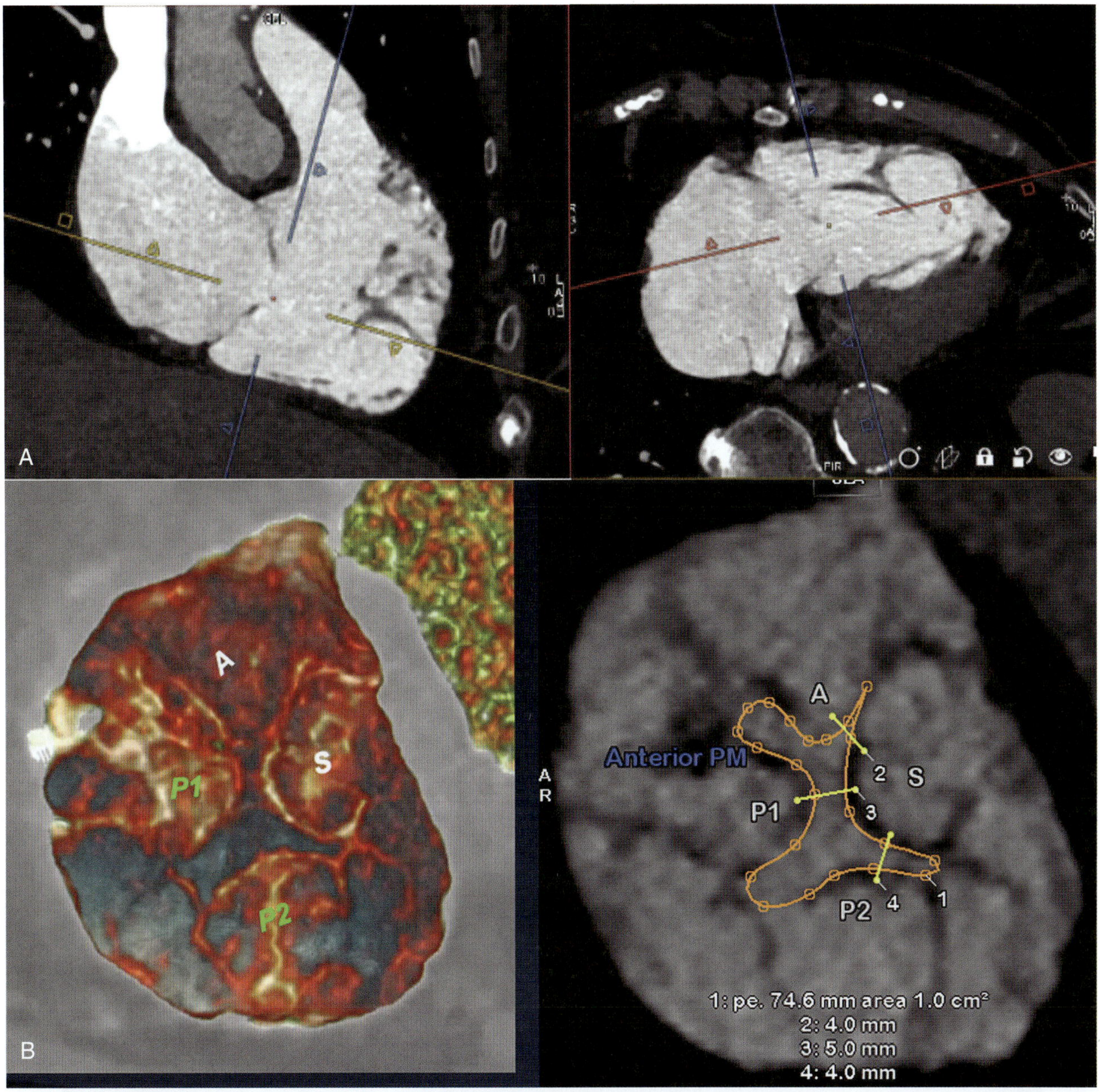

FIG. 20.10 Anatomical regurgitant orifice area and coaptation gap measurement. In mid-end systole (30–40%), the reference plane is aligned at the leaflet tips in the long-axis views (*upper panels*). Once the smallest orifice (*lower left panel*) is identified, the anatomical regurgitant orifice area and the coaptation gap/s can be measured (*lower right panel*). Note the quadricuspid morphology of the tricuspid valve in this example, which has two posterior leaflets. *A*, Anterior leaflet; *P1*, first posterior leaflet; *P2*, second posterior leaflet; *S*, septal leaflet.

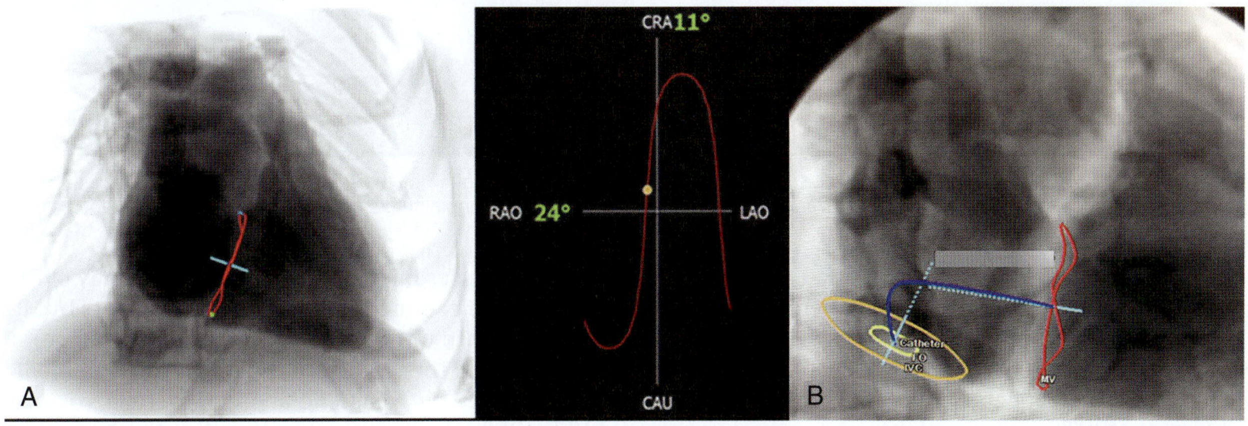

FIG. 20.11 Panel A, preprocedural prediction of the fluoroscoping angle using MDCT. In Panel B, the trajectory of the catheter from the inferior vena cava plane coaxial to the tricuspid valve plane is simulated (the mark "MV" at the level of the tricuspid annulus is automatically reported from the software). *MDCT*, Multidetector computed tomography.

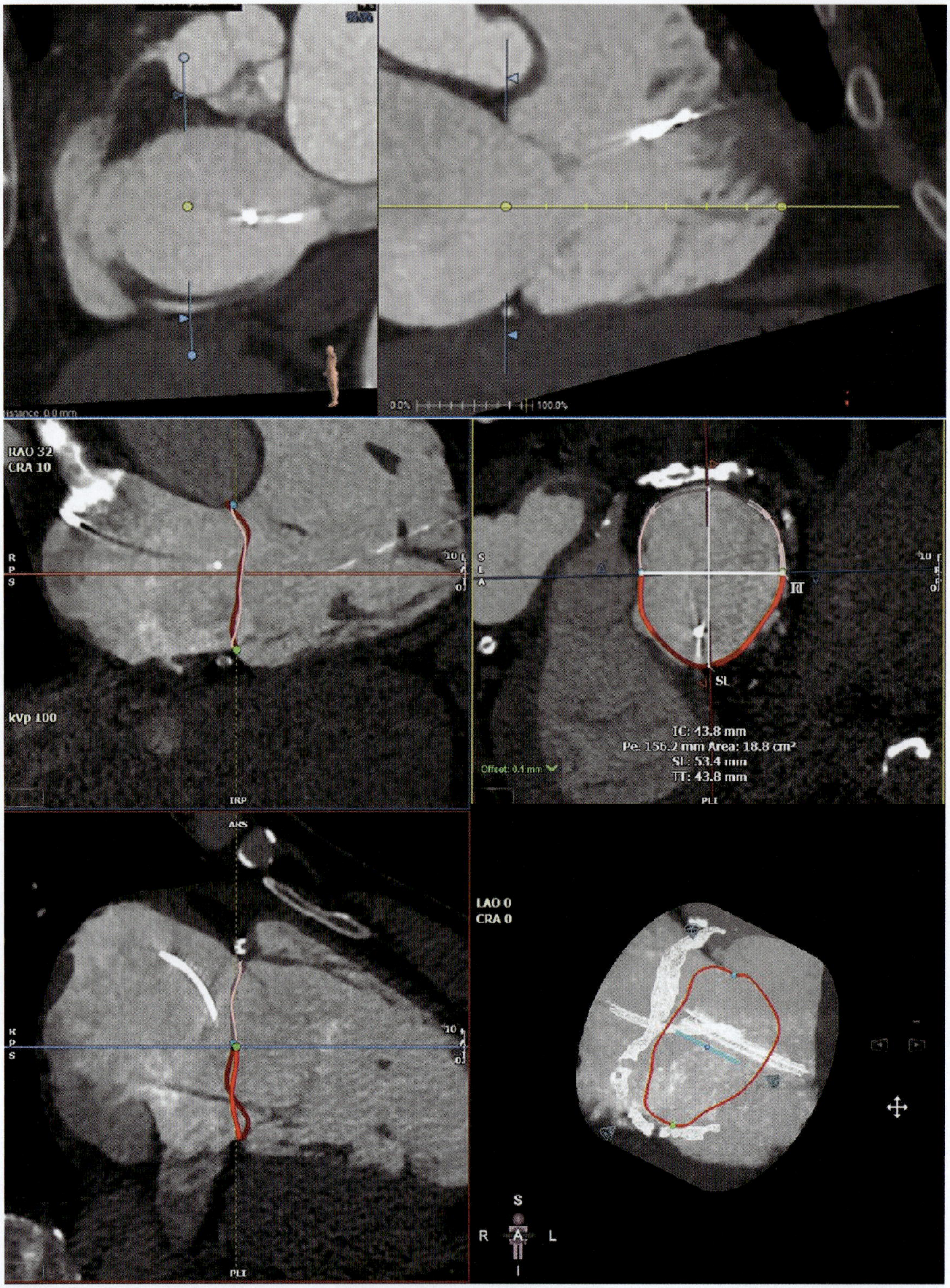

FIG. 20.12 Tricuspid valve annulus analysis by cardiac computed tomography. The segmentation of the tricuspid valve annulus is based on the same technique as for mitral valve, in order to evaluate annular area, perimeter, and major and minor diameters both in systole and in diastole.

effective as edge-to-edge repair is for TTVR, the incredible safety profile is attractive to some frail patients.

RIGHT VENTRICLE EVALUATION BY MDCT

To further improve patients selection for transcatheter TV treatment, MDCT can be useful for a comprehensive assessment of the RV. With the use of dedicated postprocessing software, right-sided chambers volumetric and functional assessment is feasible, and accuracy of RV volumetric and ejection fraction (EF) measurements by MDCT is comparable to CMR (Cardiac Magnetic Resonance), which is considered the gold standard for EF measurement.[51] Accordingly, RV end-diastolic and end-systolic volumes and RVEF (Right Ventricular Ejection Fraction) can be measured, similarly to CMR, using the disk summation method on a contiguous stack of short-axis image reconstructed

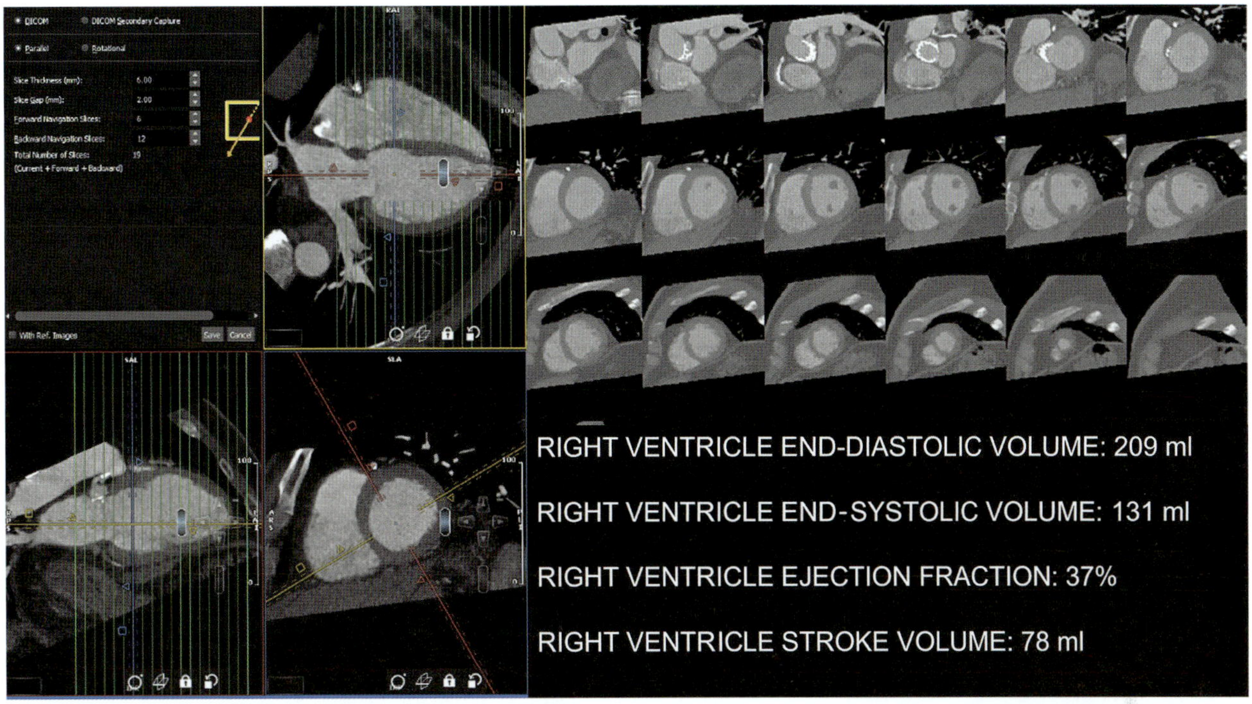

FIG. 20.13 Right ventricle assessment using cardiac computed tomography reconstructions in the short axis. Through the disk-summation method, functional and volumetric measurements are obtained.

with 6-mm slice thickness with 4-mm interslice gap, and the prognostic role of this CT-derived measurement has recently been confirmed[52] (Fig. 20.13).

Specific patterns of RV remodeling can help identify a RV cardiomyopathy or confirm the underline mechanism of TR. For example, recently atrial functional (AFTR) TR has been recognized as a distinct TR subtype with its own peculiar anatomic and clinical characteristics. The leading mechanism of AFTR is an enlargement of both the TA and the RV basal diameter (RV conical shape) with normal leaflet length, reduced systolic annular coverage in the absence of significant valve tethering.[36] MDCT allows an accurate evaluation of these specific morphologic abnormalities affecting the TV apparatus in AFTR by precisely measuring annular dimension and coaptation gap/s (see section on Annular Remodeling) and by confirming the typical RV conical remodeling pattern (RV end-diastolic basal dimension >> mid dimension).[43] Moreover, although prognostic data have not been reported, MDCT can add insights into the RV-to-pulmonary artery coupling by dividing the RV stroke volume by the RV end-systolic volume or by integrating its functional values to invasive or echo-derived pulmonary artery pressures.[53] At last, with the use of dedicated postprocessing software, an analysis of specific RV contraction patterns (longitudinal, circumferential, and radial[54]) can be obtained in order to add insights into RV global function beyond EF and therefore have implications when treating patients with TTVR. In fact, the required annular oversizing might compromise RV contractility that might be already impaired despite pseudo-normal RVEF due to severe TR regurgitant volume.

CIED (CARDIAC IMPLANTABLE ELECTRONIC DEVICE)-RELATED TR

The prevalence CIED-related TR is still a matter of debate, with an initial reported frequency of TR following lead implantation ranging from 7% up to 45%.[55] These conflicting reports are not surprising, as many past studies were based on 2D TTE evaluation of the TV, which presents severe limitations for the assessment of the TV apparatus for the identification of leads crossing the annulus and for the specific mechanism leading to lead-induced TR. However, due to increased recognition regarding the etiology and importance of CIED-related TR, this entity now has its own dedicated diagnosis and management.[55,56] In particular, in the absence of a clear causative relationship between CIED and TR, the proposed term is "lead-associated TR," as the evolution of TR is dependent on the typical risk factors.[55] If, through multimodality imaging, a causative relationship between CIED and TR is established, the term suggested is "lead-related TR": TR worsens by at least 1 grade after CIED implantation in about 20% of patients, and here the presence of the lead clearly accelerates TR progression.[36,55] In the context of lead-related TR, two mechanisms may be observed: CIED impingement is characterized by normal diastolic excursion of the TV leaflet with separation from the lead but permanent lead-leaflet contact in systole with reduced systolic leaflet excursion; CIED adhesion is diagnosed when leaflet and lead move together throughout the cardiac cycle with reduced systolic leaflet excursion.[55,57] Whether the number and type of leads (implantable cardioverter defibrillator [ICD] versus pacing) crossing the TV annulus, the position of the leads within the RV, or the degree of right ventricular pacing are correlated to a more severe presentation of TR remains unclear. MDCT plays an important complementary role to define the CIED TR mechanism (Fig. 20.14). If transvenous lead extraction is considered, useful information such as vascular access routes, exclusion of lead fibrosis/significant ingrowth of the subvalvular apparatus in proximity of the lead, and vein stenoses may be identified in order predict lead

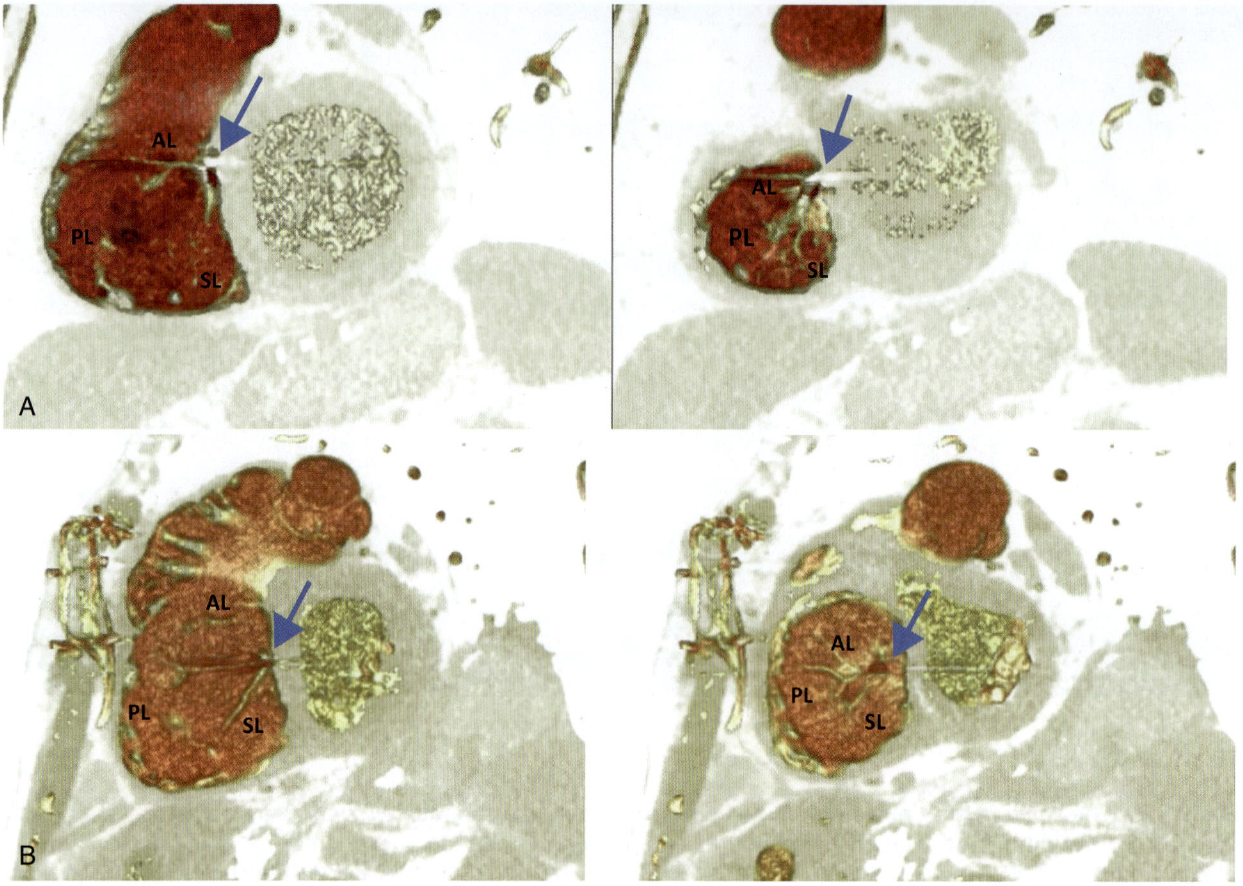

FIG. 20.14 Determining the anatomic and functional relationship between the transvalvular lead and tricuspid valve leaflets. In Panel A, the lead is in the anteroseptal commissure, being just a bystander that does not seem to affect leaflet coaptation. In Panel B, an example of lead-associated tricuspid regurgitation in the presence of septal leaflet impingement due to a fixed adherent lead. For both panels, on the left is the diastolic frame, on the right, the systolic frame. *AL*, Anterior leaflet; *PL*, posterior leaflet; *SL*, septal leaflet.

extraction feasibility or potential complications.[58] Moreover, a detailed dynamic analysis of lead-leaflet interaction is useful to address the relationship between the TV apparatus and the lead in order to determine if the lead is a just a bystander or if there is lead adhesion/impingement. This information, along with evaluation of leaflet-tethering parameters and TA dimensions, might improve TR intervention planning by determining the landing zone for implantable transcatheter valves and anticipating the need for lead jailing. Lastly, the evaluation of TV-lead/leaflet relationship can be demanding as CIED leads can cause blooming artifacts along with the cardiac motion, therefore requiring great right-sided contrast opacification with no dose modulation, optimal scanner temporal resolution, and often absolute millisecond reconstruction.

There are several issues from an electrophysiology perspective that will need further attention by imaging and medical community. For example, the longer-term implications of jailing of CIED leads, in particular ICD leads, as well as the leadless pacemakers or coronary sinus leads, which have been used in cases of post-TTVR, need to be better understood. These considerations would be important if this therapy is to be approved and expanded beyond inoperable patients.

Importance of Inferior Vena Cava-Tricuspid Annulus Relationship

The relationship between the inferior vena cava (IVC) and the TA represent a major challenge for transcatheter TV treatment. In fact, the short distance between the IVC orifice and the TV annulus with unfavorable angulation may result in a complete lack of stabilization and difficult coaxiality. This relationship has serious implications for both TTVR and heterotopic caval valve devices.

As for TTVR, the delivery systems vary in size from 28 Fr to 42 Fr, and venous access must be measured to assess the sheath/femoral vein ratio. Measurement of the IVC dimension is therefore crucial, in addition to its relationship to the TA to ensure adequate navigation of the delivery system.[40,41] As previously reported, in this context preprocedural MDCT simulation of delivery system trajectory can predict complication or intraprocedural steering difficulties according to each patient's anatomy and increase the chances of a successful landing and anchoring of the prosthesis to avoid paravalvular regurgitation or device migration.

Caval heterotopic devices are conceived with the aim to mitigate the effect of TR for patients ineligible for TV repair and for TTVR due to anatomic and/or functional reasons,

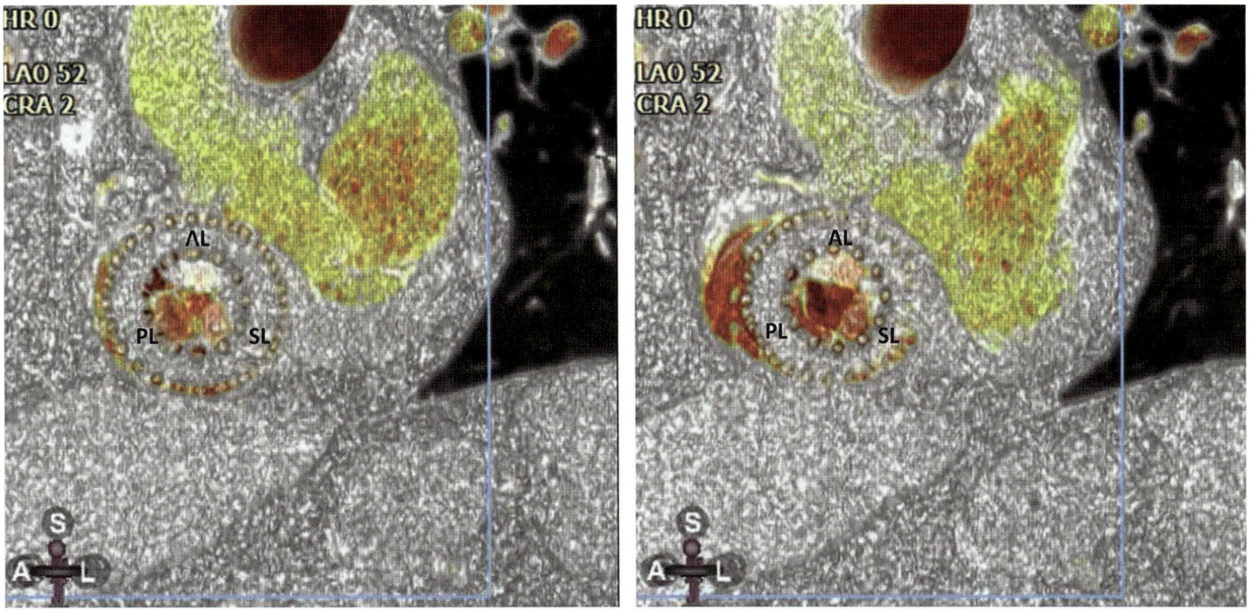

FIG. 20.15 Hypo-attenuated leaflet thickening of a tricuspid valve bioprosthesis causing restricted leaflet motion. 3D endoluminal systolic (*left panel*) and diastolic (*right panel*) views clearly demonstrate severe restriction of the excursion of both the anterior and septal leaflets, but only mild restriction of the posterior leaflet. *AL*, Anterior leaflet; *PL*, posterior leaflet; *SL*, septal leaflet.

providing a palliative relief for congestive heart failure symptoms and potentially a better management of diuretic therapy. The intervention, accordingly, does not address TR itself but the regurgitation of blood into the caval veins. In this procedure, a stented valve is implanted in either the IVC or both superior and inferior cavae veins to reduce the reflux from the RA.[59]

Dimensions of the SVC and IVC are measured with MDCT at the transition level with the right atrium and with the first hepatic vein in mid-systole. The distance between these two transitions planes is then measured to ensure for optimal valve positioning to avoid hepatic vein obstruction.

Post TTVR Imaging Evaluation

Follow-up after transcatheter TV intervention is essentially based on TTE and, for clinical research protocols, MDCT evaluation is required. In case of TTVR, data regarding HALT prevalence and association with clinical outcomes, at the present time, have not been reported, but our experience indicates that it is something we need to better understand. Therefore it is conceivable that as the number of patients treated with these novel devices increases, this complication could have a nonneglectable prevalence due to the slower-flow/lower-pressure status of the right heart compared with left chambers and to the average larger size of TTVR devices[39] (Fig. 20.15). Data[60] from an international registry of 306 patients who had undergone transcatheter TV ViV, performed with a Melody valve in 138 patients (45%) or a Sapien valve in 168 (55%), reported an incidence of prosthesis-related outcomes (endocarditis, thrombosis, or significant dysfunction) at 3 years of 8%. Of note, thrombosis occurred in three patients in the short term, in two patients within 2 months, and in three patients after 6 months; as the authors reported, prosthesis thrombosis was not investigated systematically with CT to detect subtle or minor cases, and therefore the real incidence could be higher. Eventually, MDCT evaluation, by including RV volumetric and functional measurements pre- and post-TTVR, could identify and address the presence of RV afterload mismatch, a potential short- and long-term complication due to the sudden increase of RV end-systolic volume following severe TR treatment.[61]

REFERENCES

1. Prendergast BD, Baumgartner H, Delgado V, et al. Transcatheter heart valve interventions: where are we? Where are we going? *Eur Heart J.* 2019;40(5):422–440. doi:10.1093/eurheartj/ehy668.
2. Iung B, Vahanian A. Epidemiology of valvular heart disease in the adult. *Nat Rev Cardiol.* 2011;8(3):162–172. doi:10.1038/nrcardio.2010.202.
3. Yoon SH, Whisenant BK, Bleiziffer S, et al. Outcomes of transcatheter mitral valve replacement for degenerated bioprostheses, failed annuloplasty rings, and mitral annular calcification. *Eur Heart J.* 2019;40(5):441–451. doi:10.1093/eurheartj/ehy590.
4. Hashimoto G, Lopes BBC, Sato H, et al. Computed tomography planning for transcatheter mitral valve replacement. *Struct Heart.* 2022;6(1):100012. doi:10.1016/j.shj.2022.100012.
5. Patel KP, Vandermolen S, Herrey AS, et al. Cardiac computed tomography: application in valvular heart disease. *Front Cardiovasc Med.* 2022;9:849540. doi:10.3389/fcvm.2022.849540.
6. Faletra F. *Echocardiography in Mitral Valve Disease*. 2013th ed. Springer.
7. Dejgaard LA, Skjølsvik ET, Lie ØH, et al. The mitral annulus disjunction arrhythmic syndrome. *J Am Coll Cardiol.* 2018;72(14):1600–1609. doi:10.1016/j.jacc.2018.07.070.
8. Weir-McCall JR, Blanke P, Naoum C, Delgado V, Bax JJ, Leipsic J. Mitral valve imaging with CT: relationship with transcatheter mitral valve interventions. *Radiology.* 2018;288(3):638–655. doi:10.1148/radiol.2018172758.
9. Rizvi A, Marcus RP, Guo Y, et al. Dynamic computed tomographic assessment of the mitral annulus in patients with and without mitral prolapse. *J Cardiovasc Comput Tomogr.* 2020;14(6):502–509. doi:10.1016/j.jcct.2020.02.005.
10. Banks T, Razeghi O, Ntalas I, et al. Automated quantification of mitral valve geometry on multi-slice computed tomography in patients with dilated cardiomyopathy—implications for transcatheter mitral valve replacement. *J Cardiovasc Comput Tomogr.* 2018;12(4):329–337. doi:10.1016/j.jcct.2018.04.003.
11. Reid A, Ben Zekry S, Turaga M, et al. Neo-LVOT and transcatheter mitral valve replacement: expert recommendations. *JACC Cardiovasc Imaging.* 2021;14(4):854–866. doi:10.1016/j.jcmg.2020.09.027.
12. Guerrero M, Urena M, Himbert D, et al. 1-Year outcomes of transcatheter mitral valve replacement in patients with severe mitral annular calcification. *J Am Coll Cardiol.* 2018;71(17):1841–1853. doi:10.1016/j.jacc.2018.02.054.
13. Descoutures F, Himbert D, Maisano F, et al. Transcatheter valve-in-ring implantation after failure of surgical mitral repair. *Eur J Cardiothorac Surg.* 2013;44(1):e8–15. doi:10.1093/ejcts/ezt155.

14. Maisano F, Taramasso M. Mitral valve-in-valve, valve-in-ring, and valve-in-MAC: the good, the bad, and the Ugly. *Eur Heart J.* 2019;40(5):452–455. doi:10.1093/eurheartj/ehy725.
15. Alfieri O, Lapenna E. Systolic anterior motion after mitral valve repair: where do we stand in 2015? *Eur J Cardiothorac Surg.* 2015;48(3):344–346. doi:10.1093/ejcts/ezv230.
16. Khan JM, Babaliaros VC, Greenbaum AB, et al. Anterior leaflet laceration to prevent ventricular outflow tract obstruction during transcatheter mitral valve replacement. *J Am Coll Cardiol.* 2019;73(20):2521–2534. doi:10.1016/j.jacc.2019.02.076. Erratum in: *J Am Coll Cardiol.* 2019;74(4):595.
17. Blanke P, Dvir D, Naoum C, et al. Prediction of fluoroscopic angulation and coronary sinus location by CT in the context of transcatheter mitral valve implantation. *J Cardiovasc Comput Tomogr.* 2015;9(3):183–192. doi:10.1016/j.jcct.2015.02.007.
18. Pibarot P, Herrmann HC, Wu C, et al. Standardized definitions for bioprosthetic valve dysfunction following aortic or mitral valve replacement: JACC state-of-the-art review. *J Am Coll Cardiol.* 2022;80(5):545–561. doi:10.1016/j.jacc.2022.06.002.
19. Tzimas G, Haugan D, Akodad M, et al. Computed tomography reference dimensions for identification of stented surgical mitral bioprostheses valve size. *J Cardiovasc Comput Tomogr.* 2022;16(6):517–523. doi:10.1016/j.jcct.2022.07.001.
20. Bapat VN, Attia R, Thomas M. Effect of valve design on the stent internal diameter of a bioprosthetic valve: a concept of true internal diameter and its implications for the valve-in-valve procedure. *JACC Cardiovasc Interv.* 2014;7(2):115–127. doi:10.1016/j.jcin.2013.10.012.
21. Bapat V. Valve-in-valve apps: why and how they were developed and how to use them. *EuroIntervention.* 2014;10(Suppl U):U44–U51. doi:10.4244/EIJV10SUA7.
22. Guerrero M, Vemulapalli S, Xiang Q, et al. Thirty-day outcomes of transcatheter mitral valve replacement for degenerated mitral bioprostheses (Valve-in-Valve), failed surgical rings (Valve-in-Ring), and native valve with severe mitral annular calcification (Valve-in-Mitral Annular Calcification) in the United States: data from the society of Thoracic Surgeons/American College of Cardiology/Transcatheter valve therapy registry. *Circ Cardiovasc Interv.* 2020;13(3):e008425. doi:10.1161/CIRCINTERVENTIONS.119.008425.
23. Babaliaros VC, Lederman RJ, Gleason PT, et al. The art of SAPIEN 3 transcatheter mitral valve replacement in valve-in-ring and valve-in-mitral-annular-calcification procedures. *JACC Cardiovasc Interv.* 2021;14(20):2195–2214. doi:10.1016/j.jcin.2021.08.044.
24. Guerrero ME, Grayburn P, Smith 2nd RL, et al. Diagnosis, classification, and management strategies for mitral annular calcification: a heart valve collaboratory position statement. *JACC Cardiovasc Interv.* 2023;16(18):2195–2210. doi:10.1016/j.jcin.2023.06.044. PMID: 37758378.
25. Massera D, Trivieri MG, Andrews JPM, et al. Disease activity in mitral annular calcification. *Circ Cardiovasc Imaging.* 2019;12(2):e008513. doi:10.1161/CIRCIMAGING.118.008513.
26. Churchill TW, Yucel E, Deferm S, Levine RA, Hung J, Bertrand PB. Mitral valve dysfunction in patients with annular calcification: JACC review topic of the week. *J Am Coll Cardiol.* 2022;80(7):739–751. doi:10.1016/j.jacc.2022.05.032.
27. Gössl M, Thourani V, Babaliaros V, et al. Early outcomes of transcatheter mitral valve replacement with the Tendyne system in severe mitral annular calcification. *EuroIntervention.* 2022;17(18):1523–1531. doi:10.4244/EIJ-D-21-00745.
28. Yoshida N, Miyoshi T, Ninomaru T, et al. Left ventricular outflow tract obstruction caused by massive mitral annular calcification in a patient with hypertensive heart disease. *J Cardiol Cases.* 2015;12(3):87–90. doi:10.1016/j.jccase.2015.05.008.
29. Guerrero M, Wang DD, Pursnani A, et al. A cardiac computed tomography-based score to categorize mitral annular calcification severity and predict valve embolization. *JACC Cardiovasc Imaging.* 2020;13(9):1945–1957. doi:10.1016/j.jcmg.2020.03.013.
30. Mahjoub H, Mathieu P, Larose E, et al. Determinants of aortic bioprosthetic valve calcification assessed by multidetector CT. *Heart.* 2015;101(6):472–477. doi:10.1136/heartjnl-2014-306445.
31. Sellers SL, Turner CT, Sathananthan J, et al. Transcatheter aortic heart valves: histological analysis providing insight to leaflet thickening and structural valve degeneration. *JACC Cardiovasc Imaging.* 2019;12(1):135–145. doi:10.1016/j.jcmg.2018.06.028.
32. Fukui M, Okada A, Burns MR, et al. Deformation of transcatheter heart valves with mitral valve-in-valve. *EuroIntervention.* 2023;19(11):e937–e947. doi:10.4244/EIJ-D-23-00614.
33. Topilsky Y, Nkomo VT, Vatury O, et al. Clinical outcome of isolated tricuspid regurgitation. *JACC Cardiovasc Imaging.* 2014;7(12):1185–1194. doi:10.1016/j.jcmg.2014.07.018.
34. Benfari G, Antoine C, Miller WL, et al. Excess mortality associated with functional tricuspid regurgitation complicating heart failure with reduced ejection fraction. *Circulation.* 2019;140(3):196–206. doi:10.1161/CIRCULATIONAHA.118.038946.
35. Zhan Y, Debs D, Khan MA, et al. Natural history of functional tricuspid regurgitation quantified by cardiovascular magnetic resonance. *J Am Coll Cardiol.* 2020;76(11):1291–1301. doi:10.1016/j.jacc.2020.07.036.
36. Margonato D, Ancona F, Ingallina G, et al. Tricuspid regurgitation in left ventricular systolic dysfunction: marker or target? *Front Cardiovasc Med.* 2021;8:702589. doi:10.3389/fcvm.2021.702589.
37. Sorajja P, Whisenant B, Hamid N, et al. Transcatheter repair for patients with tricuspid regurgitation. *N Engl J Med.* 2023;388(20):1833–1842. doi:10.1056/NEJMoa2300525.
38. Kodali S, Hahn RT, Makkar R, et al. Transfemoral tricuspid valve replacement and one-year outcomes: the TRISCEND study. *Eur Heart J.* 2023;44(46):4862–4873. doi:10.1093/eurheartj/ehad667.
39. Oliveira DC, Oliveira CGC. The forgotten, not studied or not valorized tricuspid valve: the transcatheter revolution is coming. *Cardiol Res.* 2019;10(4):199–206. doi:10.14740/cr874.
40. Lopes BBC, Hashimoto G, Bapat VN, Sorajja P, Scherer MD, Cavalcante JL. Cardiac computed tomography and magnetic resonance imaging of the tricuspid valve: preprocedural planning and postprocedural follow-up. *Interv Cardiol Clin.* 2022;11(1):27–40. doi:10.1016/j.iccl.2021.09.004.
41. Pulerwitz TC, Khalique OK, Leb J, et al. Optimizing cardiac CT protocols for comprehensive acquisition prior to percutaneous MV and TV repair/replacement. *JACC Cardiovasc Imaging.* 2020;13(3):836–850. doi:10.1016/j.jcmg.2019.01.041.
42. Ancona F, Stella S, Taramasso M, et al. Multimodality imaging of the tricuspid valve with implication for percutaneous repair approaches. *Heart.* 2017;103(14):1073–1081. doi:10.1136/heartjnl-2016-310939.
43. Hahn RT, Badano LP, Bartko PE, et al. Tricuspid regurgitation: recent advances in understanding pathophysiology, severity grading and outcome. *Eur Heart J Cardiovasc Imaging.* 2022;23(7):913–929. doi:10.1093/ehjci/jeac009. Erratum in: Eur Heart J Cardiovasc Imaging. 2022.
44. Hołda MK, Zhingre Sanchez JD, Bateman MG, Iaizzo PA. Right atrioventricular valve leaflet morphology redefined: implications for transcatheter repair procedures. *JACC Cardiovasc Interv.* 2019;12(2):169–178. doi:10.1016/j.jcin.2018.09.029.
45. Kocak A, Govsa F, Aktas EO, Boydak B, Yavuz IC. Structure of the human tricuspid valve leaflets and its chordae tendineae in unexpected death. A forensic autopsy study of 400 cases. *Saudi Med J.* 2004;25(8):1051–1059.
46. Hahn RT, Weckbach LT, Noack T, et al. Proposal for a standard echocardiographic tricuspid valve nomenclature. *JACC Cardiovasc Imaging.* 2021;14(7):1299–1305. doi:10.1016/j.jcmg.2021.01.012.
47. Hell MM, Emrich T, Kreidel F, et al. Computed tomography imaging needs for novel transcatheter tricuspid valve repair and replacement therapies. *Eur Heart J Cardiovasc Imaging.* 2021;22(6):601–610. doi:10.1093/ehjci/jeaa308.
48. Lopes BBC, Sorajja P, Hashimoto G, et al. Tricuspid anatomic regurgitant orifice area by functional DSCT: a novel parameter of tricuspid regurgitation severity. *JACC Cardiovasc Imaging.* 2021;14(8):1669–1672. doi:10.1016/j.jcmg.2021.02.002.
49. Faletra FF, Leo LA, Paiocchi VL, et al. Imaging-based tricuspid valve anatomy by computed tomography, magnetic resonance imaging, two and three-dimensional echocardiography: correlation with anatomic specimen. *Eur Heart J Cardiovasc Imaging.* 2019;20(1):1–13. doi:10.1093/ehjci/jey136.
50. van Rosendael PJ, Kamperidis V, Kong WK, et al. Computed tomography for planning transcatheter tricuspid valve therapy. *Eur Heart J.* 2017;38(9):665–674. doi:10.1093/eurheartj/ehw499.
51. Maffei E, Messalli G, Martini C, et al. Left and right ventricle assessment with Cardiac CT: validation study vs. cardiac MR. *Eur Radiol.* 2012;22(5):1041–1049. doi:10.1007/s00330-011-2345-6.
52. Fukui M, Sorajja P, Hashimoto G, et al. Right ventricular dysfunction by computed tomography associates with outcomes in severe aortic stenosis patients undergoing transcatheter aortic valve replacement. *J Cardiovasc Comput Tomogr.* 2022;16(2):158–165. doi:10.1016/j.jcct.2021.11.005.
53. He Q, Lin Y, Zhu Y, et al. Clinical usefulness of right ventricle-pulmonary artery coupling in cardiovascular disease. *J Clin Med.* 2023;12(7):2526. doi:10.3390/jcm12072526.
54. Kresoja KP, Rommel KP, Lücke C, et al. Right ventricular contraction patterns in patients undergoing transcatheter tricuspid valve repair for severe tricuspid regurgitation. *JACC Cardiovasc Interv.* 2021;14(14):1551–1561. doi:10.1016/j.jcin.2021.05.005.
55. Andreas M, Burri H, Praz F, et al. Tricuspid valve disease and cardiac implantable electronic devices. *Eur Heart J.* 2023;45(5):346–365.
56. Praz F, Muraru D, Kreidel F, et al. Transcatheter treatment for tricuspid valve disease. *EuroIntervention.* 2021;17(10):791–808. doi:10.4244/EIJ-D-21-00695.
57. Mediratta A, Addetia K, Yamat M, et al. 3D Echocardiographic location of implantable device leads and mechanism of associated tricuspid regurgitation. *JACC Cardiovasc Imaging.* 2014;7(4):337–347. doi:10.1016/j.jcmg.2013.11.007.
58. Svennberg E, Jacobs K, McVeigh E, Pretorius V. Birgersdotter-Green U. Computed tomography-guided risk assessment in percutaneous lead extraction. *JACC Clin Electrophysiol.* 2019;5(12):1439–1446. doi:10.1016/j.jacep.2019.09.007.
59. Lauten A, Figulla HR, Unbehaun A, et al. Interventional treatment of severe tricuspid regurgitation: early clinical experience in a multicenter, observational, first-in-man study. *Circ Cardiovasc Interv.* 2018;11(2):e006061. doi:10.1161/CIRCINTERVENTIONS.117.006061.
60. McElhinney DB, Aboulhosn JA, Dvir D, et al. Mid-term valve-related outcomes after transcatheter tricuspid valve-in-valve or valve-in-ring replacement. *J Am Coll Cardiol.* 2019;73(2):148–157. doi:10.1016/j.jacc.2018.10.051.
61. Demir OM, Regazzoli D, Mangieri A, et al. Transcatheter tricuspid valve replacement: principles and design. *Front Cardiovasc Med.* 2018;5:129. doi:10.3389/fcvm.2018.00129.

21 Cardiac Masses

AYAZ AGHAYEV, SUMIT GUPTA, AND MICHAEL L. STEIGNER

KEY POINTS

- Advanced imaging is an essential step in diagnosing cardiac masses, particularly in differentiating between benign and malignant neoplasms.
- When further imaging is required following echocardiography, cardiac magnetic resonance imaging (CMR) and cardiac computed tomography (CCT) can provide more detailed tissue characterization. When the differential diagnosis is a malignant neoplasm, F-fluorodeoxyglucose positron emission tomography/computed tomography can be performed to differentiate primary from secondary/metastatic tumors.
- Although certain cardiac masses have specific imaging features, they can mimic each other. Therefore clinical context, mass location, and imaging features should be considered during the assessment.

INTRODUCTION

Cardiac masses are rare entities with an estimated prevalence of 0.02% to 2.3% at autopsy and 0.15% on imaging series. However, they can be associated with high morbidity and mortality.[1,2] Various cardiac masses can be encountered, including nonneoplastic and neoplastic (primary or secondary/metastasis) masses (Table 21.1). Nonneoplastic masses, particularly thrombi, are the most frequent cardiac masses, followed by cardiac metastases.[3,4] The diagnosis and management of cardiac masses can be challenging due to the difficulty of obtaining a tissue biopsy. Moreover, unlike other body parts, masses in the heart, even benign masses, require proper diagnosis and subsequent surgical or medical treatment, given the associated hemodynamic and arrhythmic complications. Therefore imaging plays a vital role in characterizing masses, assessing complications associated with masses, surgical planning, and surveillance.

This chapter aims to discuss the diagnostic approach, available imaging modalities, and imaging features of cardiac masses, emphasizing cardiac computed tomography (CCT).

DIAGNOSTIC APPROACH TO CARDIAC MASSES

The diagnostic approach can vary because patients may be symptomatic or completely asymptomatic, with a mass being incidentally detected on imaging. Symptoms can be systemic, such as embolic, paraneoplastic, or constitutional (fever, weight loss, and fatigue) symptoms, or local, such as chest pain, dyspnea, syncope due to mass effect on cardiac structures, including valves, or arrhythmia.[4] Whether the cardiac mass was incidentally detected or detected due to symptoms, the following parameters should be considered as a part of the diagnostic algorithm:

1. **Clinical context**: Clinical context can provide critical information to narrow down the diagnosis. For example, the probability of a new cardiac mass being a melanoma metastasis is exceptionally high in patients with a history of metastatic disease such as melanoma. Similarly, in patients with recent myocardial infarctions and new left ventricular mass on echocardiography, the mass could be diagnosed as a thrombus without any requirement for advanced imaging. Furthermore, diagnosing a valvular mass in a patient with bacteremia (i.e., vegetation) might be completely different from that in an asymptomatic patient (i.e., papillary fibroelastoma).
2. **Mass Location:** In symptomatic or asymptomatic patients, the mass location within the heart or in the vicinity of the pericardium can help with the differential diagnosis. Fig. 21.1 shows the typical sites of the common masses. For example, a mass within a chamber or attached to a central line is most likely a thrombus, and a mass in the cardiac groove is likely paraganglioma.[5]
3. **Multimodality imaging features:** Imaging features can guide imagers to diagnose or provide differential diagnoses of the masses. Multimodality imaging is essential for the diagnosis of cardiac masses. In symptomatic patients, echocardiography is usually the first-line imaging modality and can be integrated with other modalities, including CCT, cardiac magnetic resonance imaging (CMR), or positron emission tomography/computed tomography (PET/CT). Similarly, these advanced imaging modalities can also assess incidentally discovered cardiac masses on echocardiography or chest CT. Currently, CMR is the preferred imaging modality to characterize cardiac masses. However, every imaging modality has its advantages and disadvantages. For example, CT has a superb spatial resolution compared to other imaging modalities, MRI has an excellent tissue resolution, and PET/CT with different tracers can provide details about the metabolic activity of the masses. The following section provides a detailed description of each modality.

IMAGING OF CARDIAC MASSES

CCT

In the last decade, electrocardiogram-gated CCT has become an increasingly used imaging modality when other modalities are limited or contraindicated.[6] Additionally, CCT can be combined with other imaging modalities, such

TABLE 21.1 Common Non-neoplastic and Neoplastic Cardiac Masses

NONNEOPLASTIC	NEOPLASTIC PRIMARY		NEOPLASTIC SECONDARY
	BENIGN	MALIGNANT	Metastases
Thrombus/ vegetations	Myxoma	Lymphoma	
Lipomatous hypertrophy	Lipoma	Sarcomas • Angiosarcoma • Undifferentiated • Rhabdomyosarcoma • Osteosarcoma • Liposarcoma	
Crista terminalis	Papillary fibroelastoma		
Coumadin ridge	Fibroma		
	Hemangioma		
	Pericardial cyst		
	Paraganglioma		

as PET.[7] CCT is the fastest imaging modality that offers a 3D volumetric dataset with a high spatial/temporal resolution and multiplanar reconstruction capability.[8] Therefore there is a potential benefit in using CCT in the diagnosis/ management of small masses or vegetation.[9] Furthermore, CCT can provide reasonable but limited tissue characterization, mainly when obtained in multiple contrast phases, including the noncontrast, arterial, and delayed phases. Fatty or calcified masses can easily be differentiated based on tissue density on noncontrast CCT. The arterial phase images can delineate masses from the coronary arteries (aneurysms/pseudoaneurysms) or hypervascular masses. Furthermore, the perfusion pattern on postcontrast images can help distinguish between enhancing and nonenhancing solid masses. Dual-energy option in CT may help characterize the enhancement pattern of various masses. Additionally, CCT can be performed dynamically to assess the relationship of the masses with adjacent structures, including valves, myocardium, coronary arteries, and pulmonary or systemic veins.

Considering all the above-mentioned options, the scan protocol of CCT should be tailored based on the clinical question. For the majority of masses, three-phase contrast imaging is required: (1) precontrast imaging (ECG-gated noncontrast), (2) arterial phase (bolus tracking or time bolus techniques after injecting iodine-based contrast agents), and (3) delayed phase (40–60 s after contrast injection). If the mass is known, its location plays a crucial role in the scan planning. Based on the mass location, image acquisition can be categorized as follows: (1) left-sided, (2) right-sided, or (3) epicardial/pericardial masses. For valvular masses, contrast timing should be adjusted based on the valve. Additionally, data acquisition for valvular masses should be obtained throughout the cardiac cycle in either a prospective or retrospective nature. The valvular and intracavitary masses can be demonstrated as filling defects in the arterial phase. If there is any enhancing component, it can be better seen on delayed images. For epicardial masses, particularly coronary artery aneurysm/pseudoaneurysm, proper coronary computed tomography angiography (CCTA) should be obtained. On rare occasions where the mass location is unknown, the timing of the arterial phase should be adjusted to opacify all four chambers (see Chapter 1, Image Acquisition Protocols for Different Types of Cardiac CT).

Other Imaging Modalities

Echocardiography. Echocardiography, a first-line imaging modality in a patient with a suspected cardiac mass, can determine the presence or absence and location of the mass. In specific clinical scenarios, echocardiography alone can

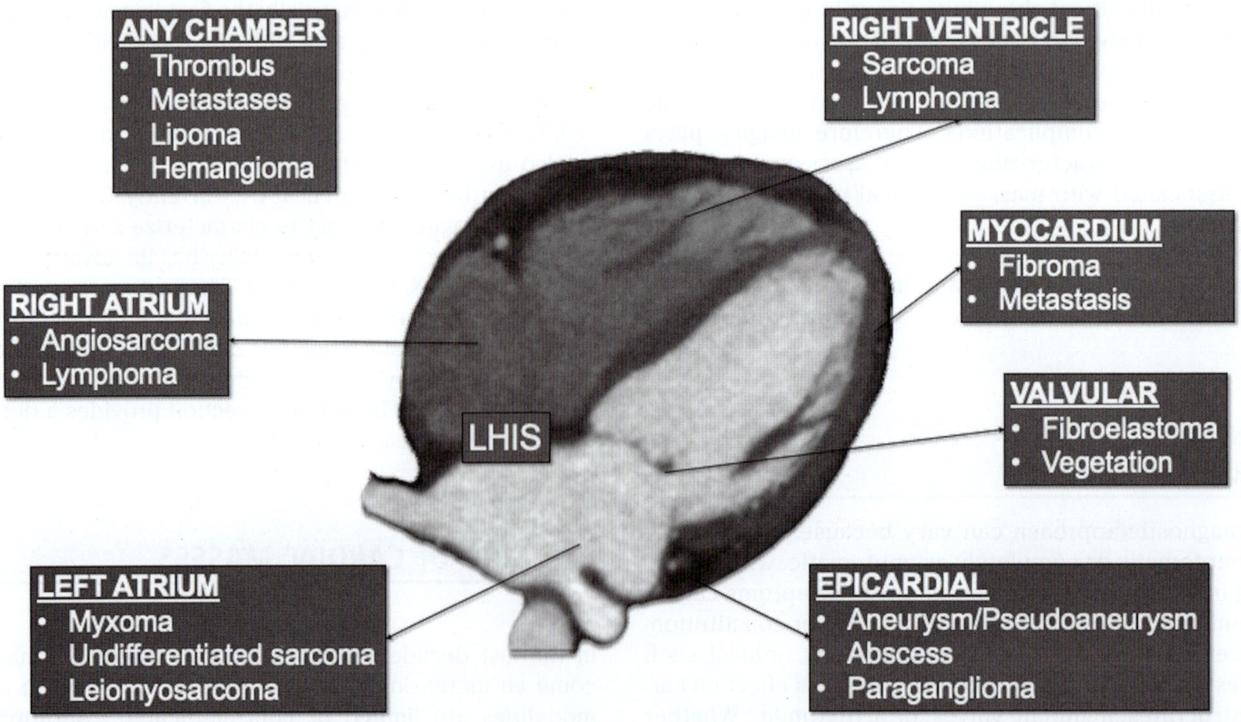

FIG. 21.1 Typical locations for common nonneoplastic and neoplastic cardiac masses. *LHIS*, Lipomatous hypertrophy of the interatrial septum.

be sufficient for diagnosing the masses or guiding the clinician on how to proceed with advanced imaging. Echocardiography is an excellent tool for detecting highly mobile, small cardiac masses (<1 cm) due to its high temporal resolution. Additionally, it is an ideal tool for assessing hemodynamically significant obstructions caused by cardiac masses. The potential limitations of echocardiography have been overcome with advanced echocardiography techniques, including transesophageal echocardiography (TEE), real-time three-dimensional echocardiography, and the use of ultrasound-enhancing agents (UEAs). TEE offers an even higher spatial and temporal resolution to localize highly mobile masses and assess hemodynamic complications. Furthermore, UEAs can be used to evaluate perfusion patterns of cardiac masses. Generally, the main limitations of echocardiography are its poor acoustic window, particularly in large patients, and the lack of tissue characterization.

CMR. CMR is considered the most useful imaging modality for cardiac masses detected on echocardiography or CT due to its ability to characterize the tissue.[10] CMR uses a magnetic field and radiofrequency. Therefore it is free from radiation exposure. CMR starts with assessing the location, morphology, and mobility of the masses. A CMR mass protocol will often start with a stack of balanced steady-state-free precession or spoiled gradient echo (GRE) in at least two planes. Next, tissue characterization using double inversion recovery (DIR) fast spin-echo (FSE) T1- or T2-weighted (T1-w or T2-w) sequences are obtained, which can also be acquired with fat suppression and require additional pre-pulse (triple inversion recovery) to assess fatty components of the mass. Enhancement features on postcontrast sequences for tissue characterization include first-pass perfusion (FPP), postcontrast DIR FSE T1-w, late gadolinium enhancement (LGE) with phase-sensitive inversion recovery (PSIR), and free-breathing/respiratory/electrocardiogram-gated contrast-enhanced magnetic resonance angiography (MRA). Injection of 0.05 to 0.1 mmol/kg of gadolinium-based contrast agent is required during the FPP sequence, and images should be obtained in multiple planes. After 7 to 10 min of contrast injection, an LGE sequence with PSIR should be obtained. Besides regular LGE sequences with an inversion time (TI) of ~300 ms, a long TI (>500 ms) can be acquired for adequate recovery of the signal of the enhancing components of the mass.[11]

PET/CT. PET/CT, particularly with F-fluorodeoxyglucose (FDG) tracer, is a routinely used imaging modality in patients with cancer. However, its role is not well established in cardiac masses. Studies have shown that FDG-PET/CT can be used in selected cases.[12–15] PET/CT can be performed as a routine oncology study with a skull base to mid-thigh coverage, and dedicated ECG-gated cardiac PET can be acquired if desired. FDG is the most common tracer for an evaluation of cardiac masses or infections. However, for specific indications, for example, neuroendocrine tumors (cardiac paraganglioma), newer tracers such as Gallium-68 DOTATATE can be used.[16] A high-fat, low-carbohydrate diet should be prescribed to suppress normal myocardial FDG uptake if the cardiac mass is known based on other imaging modalities.

NONNEOPLASTIC CARDIAC MASSES

Thrombus and Vegetation

Thrombus is the most common cardiac mass.[3] Patients with a hypercoagulable state, ischemic cardiomyopathy (with focal wall motion abnormality), atrial fibrillation, malignancy, or a catheter extending into the chambers are at a high risk of developing a thrombus. Typically, thrombi appear as mobile, lobular, or linear/layering intracavitary masses. Furthermore, they can occur anywhere in the heart. For example, they can occur in the left ventricle, particularly in areas with a hypokinetic, akinetic, or aneurysmal wall, and in the left atrial appendage and the right ventricle or atrium as an isolated or extension of a thrombus from the inferior vena cava (IVC) or superior vena cava (SVC). Thrombi can often be detected on echocardiography or chest CT, and a diagnosis can be made based on the clinical context/location. Based on the location and relationship with the cardiac structures, CCT can easily diagnose thrombus (Fig. 21.2). For example, a mass in the left

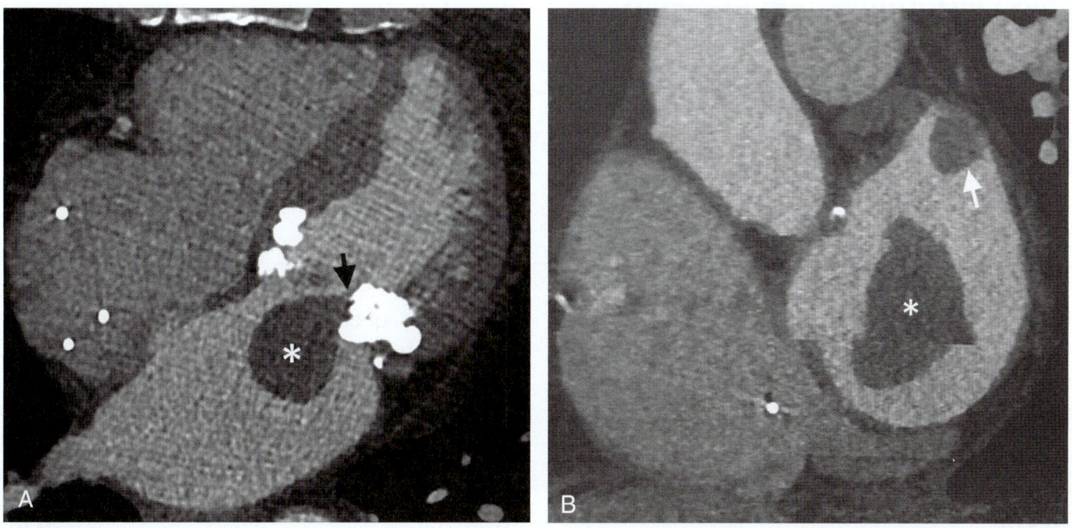

FIG. 21.2 A 82-year-old male with severe mitral valve stenosis and mitral annulus calcifications presented for valvular assessment. Echocardiography revealed a large mass in the left atrium (not shown). Four-chamber (A) and short-axis (B) cardiac CT images of the heart revealed a large mass (*asterisk*) attached to the mitral valve calcification (*black arrow*); additional mass in the upper wall of the left atrium, extending from the left atrial appendage (*white arrow*).

atrial appendage is almost always a thrombus but requires delayed phase acquisition at 60 s to exclude stasis-related artifacts. In certain clinical scenarios, they may require additional imaging, most of the time with CMR, for tissue characterization. The signal characteristics of the thrombi on CMR are not helpful. They can present as hyperintense or hypointense on T1-w and T2-w images based on the age of the thrombi.[10] The most important imaging feature of the thrombus is that it is not enhanced on postcontrast sequences, including FPP or LGE. Additionally, long TI (~600 ms) LGE sequences can confirm the diagnosis of thrombus.[17] Thrombi do not demonstrate any FDG uptake on PET/CT images.

Regarding vegetation, any injury along the endothelium in the heart leads to platelet-fibrin nidus/thrombus formation. When the nidus or thrombus is infected due to bacteremia, it results in infective endocarditis (IE) and produces a vegetation with a mass-like appearance, particularly along the valves.[18] Transthoracic echocardiography (TTE) or TEE should be the first imaging modality when there is a clinical concern for IE. TEE is particularly sensitive for the detection of valvular lesions. However, acoustic shadowing can limit proper evaluation of the leaflet when there is a large amount of calcification or prosthetic valve, and CCT can help assess the leaflets for thrombus/vegetation.[19] Although the role of CMR is not well established in diagnosing vegetations, it usually shows signal characteristics similar to thrombus in large vegetations. FDG-PET/CT has been performed for diagnosing IE, particularly in prosthetic valve infections or paravalvular abscesses.[20] However, vegetations are often photopenic with no FDG uptake and could result in a false negative on PET when performed without correlative studies such as CTA or echocardiography due to the fact that they are small and avascular lesions.[21] Mural endocarditis is a rare subset of endocarditis when the vegetation involves the nonvalvular structures, such as papillary muscle or endocardium.[22] It can mimic benign masses such as myxoma due to its location. Therefore clinical context is important in the differential diagnosis.

Mitral Annulus Calcification (MAC)/Caseous MAC (CMAC)

MAC is a chronic degenerative process of the fibrous component of the mitral valve, commonly the posterior mitral annulus.[23] It can be encountered incidentally by echocardiography. However, CT is the ideal modality to delineate the border of calcification and show calcification in the myocardium. CMR can demonstrate peripheral enhancement in MAC with central hypointensity due to calcification. CMAC is a rare MAC variant, which has been shown to have higher cardioembolic events than regular MAC (Fig. 21.3). In CMAC, degeneration or liquefaction of the central calcified component results in hypodense areas on CCT, which in rare cases can fistulize with the cardiac chambers.[24]

Lipomatous Hypertrophy of the Interatrial Septum (LHIS)

LHIS is an accumulation of adipocytes in the atrial septum that results in the thickening, hypertrophy, and mass-like appearance of the septum. Contrary to the true intracardiac lipoma, it does not have a discrete capsule.[25] It occurs in older and obese patients and is incidentally detected on imaging.[26] Due to its fat content, it follows the same signal characteristics as fat in all imaging modalities, that is, echogenic mass in the echo and fat density/hypodense on CT. An important imaging feature is that LHIS spares the fossa ovalis. Furthermore, LHIS can demonstrate FDG uptake. Therefore it is important not to confuse it with a metastatic focus in patients with known cancer. Fig. 21.4 shows the imaging features of LHIS in all available imaging modalities.

Mass Mimicking Anatomic Structures

Normal anatomic structures or bands in the heart can mimic masses. The most problematic of these structures are the coumadin ridge and crista terminalis. Coumadin ridge or left lateral ridge appears because the left atrial wall folds between the left superior vein and left atrial appendage.[27] It can appear as a prominent pedunculated nodular mass in the LA wall and mimic a thrombus on echocardiography. On CCT or CMR images, it can follow tissue characteristics of the atrial wall, and the location should be sufficient to diagnose this entity. However, in rare cases, benign or malignant cardiac neoplasms can develop along the coumadin ridge. Therefore a prominent and nodular coumadin ridge may warrant advanced imaging for additional tissue characterization.

Crista terminalis c-shaped muscular structure in the right atrial wall extends between the SVC and IVC orifice. It is an embryological remnant tissue from the septum spurium.[27] It may appear as a linear structure in most patients. However, a prominent crista terminalis has been reported on echocardiography up to 15 mm in width, which can mimic a mass.[28] Therefore CCT or CMR can help differentiate normal crista terminalis from a mass, particularly a thrombus, in patients with indwelling right heart catheters. Additionally, the imaging features on CCT or CMR, including the location of the structure, smooth, well-defined contours, and similar density or signal intensity as that of the inner wall of the right atrium, can help identify crista terminalis (Fig. 21.5). Crista terminalis can be prominent in patients with LHIS due to fatty deposits.

BENIGN CARDIAC NEOPLASMS

Myxoma

Myxoma is the most common benign cardiac neoplasm, accounting for ~50% of all benign cardiac tumors. Approximately 75% of cardiac myxomas are located in the left atrium attached to the fossa ovalis. Histologically, cardiac myxoma contains scattered tumor cells (spindle cells) and fibrotic tissue within a mucopolysaccharide-rich-myxoid stroma. It is usually an echogenic, mobile mass with a thin stalk on echocardiography. Myxomas typically appear as a filling defect on CCT, attached to the atrial wall with a small neck (Fig. 21.6). Enhancement patterns may vary on CMR based on the myxoid stroma and tumor cell component ratio. It is usually hyperintense on T2-w images and isointense on T1-w images.

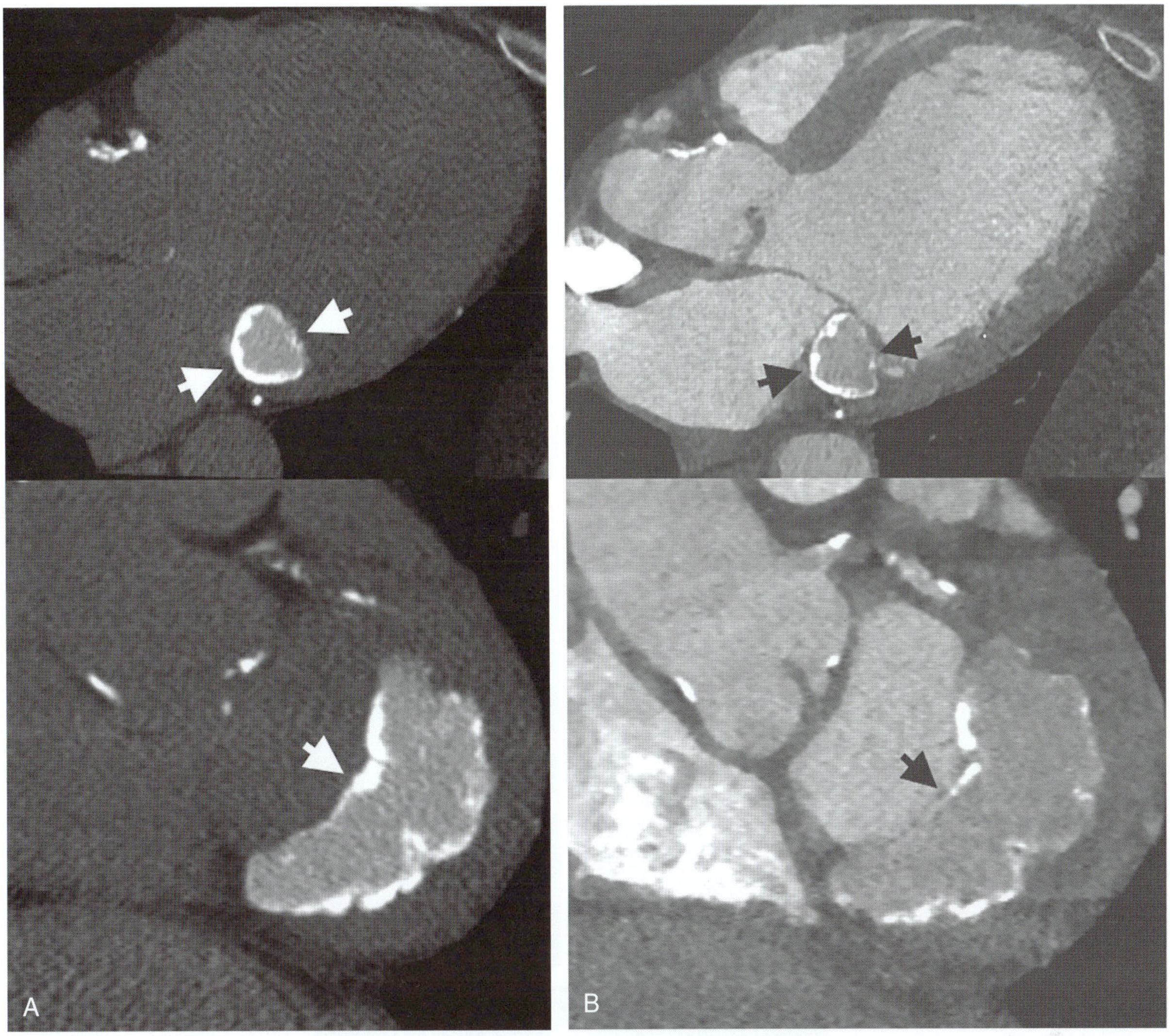

FIG. 21.3 A 77-year-old male presented with multifocal acute ischemic infarcts, and echocardiography revealed a mass in the mitral annulus. Noncontrast (A) and postcontrast (B) three-chamber and short-axis cardiac CT images demonstrate a large crescentic shape mass (*arrows*). In the mitral annulus with a relatively hypodense central component compared to the periphery of the mass, which is a classic imaging feature for caseous mitral annulus calcification (CMAC).

The tumoral (spindle cells) and fibrotic components demonstrate enhancement on perfusion and LGE images. However, myxoid stroma does not show any enhancement.[29] Cardiac myxomas do not demonstrate FDG uptake.

Lipoma

Lipoma is the second most common primary tumor of the heart, occurring sporadically at all ages. They can arise either from the subendocardium or subepicardium and can have a mass effect when they grow larger.[30] Regardless of their location, they are well-circumscribed tumors that contain mature adipocytes. Like LHIS, lipomas demonstrate fat features on imaging modalities and can be easily diagnosed on CCT or CMR. They do not show any perfusion on postcontrast images. However, it is important to acknowledge that LGE images are not fat suppressed. Therefore hyperintense mass on LGE images does not indicate enhancement.

Papillary Fibroelastoma

Papillary fibroelastoma is a small (<1.5 cm) cardiac tumor almost always located at the free edges of the heart valves. It is located on the downstream side of the leaflet (the aortic site of the aorta and ventricular aspect of the mitral valve).[4] Although patients with papillary fibroelastoma are asymptomatic, it can be detected on echocardiography as a part of the workup for embolism. Papillary fibroelastoma can be detected with state-of-the-art CCT (scanners with high temporal resolution capability) (Fig. 21.7). However, tissue characterization is difficult. Similarly, it appeared as a highly mobile small mass that is connected to the valve via a stalk on CMR. Additionally, considering the fibrohialinous stroma, LGE images can depict gadolinium retention if it is possible to capture the mass. However, first-past perfusion images are often not helpful due to the small size of these lesions. PET/CT plays no role in the workup due to its size and mobility.

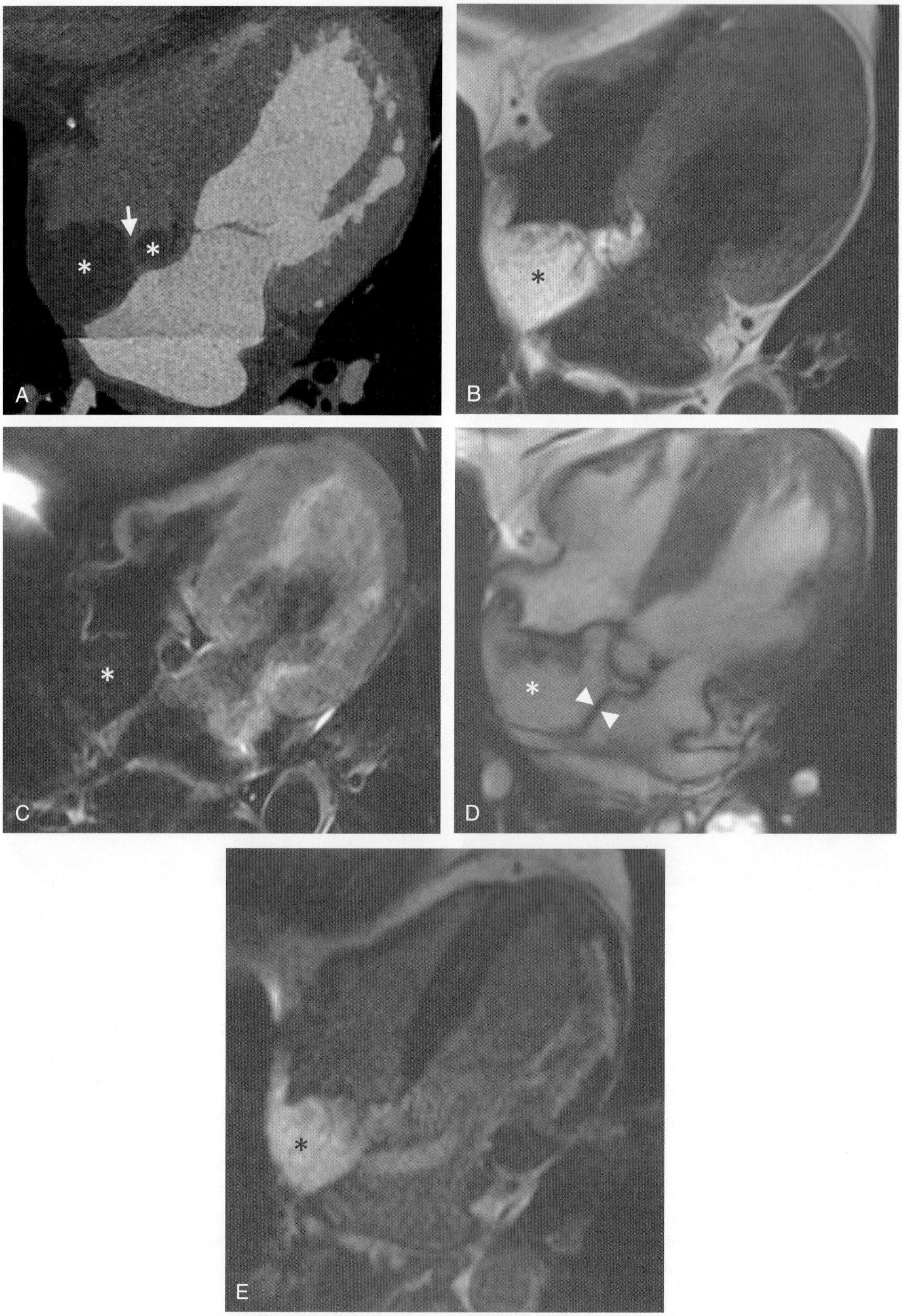

FIG. 21.4 A 74-year-old female presented with new onset of dyspnea and reduced 34% EF on TTE. The patient underwent CCT for coronary artery assessment. In addition to severe coronary artery disease, a large mass was detected in the interatrial septum (A), which has a fat density (*asterisk*) and spared fossa ovalis (*arrow*). CCT imaging features were consistent with LHIS, which was confirmed on CMR—(B) precontrast T1-weighted image shows a hyperintense mass in the interatrial septum (*asterisk*), which demonstrates complete suppression on precontrast T2-weighted fat-suppressed image (*asterisk*) (C). Balanced steady-state free precession (bSSFP) image (D) shows a hyperintense mass (*asterisk*) with a dark rim (*arrowheads*) around the mass, which is known as a "chemical-shift artifact." The mass is hyperintense (*asterisk*) on LGE image (E), which can be confusing; however, LGE images inherently are not fat suppressed. *CCT*, Cardiac CT; *CMR*, cardiac magnetic resonance imaging; *LGE*, late gadolinium enhancement; *LHIS*, lipomatous hypertrophy of the interatrial septum; *TTE*, transthoracic echocardiography.

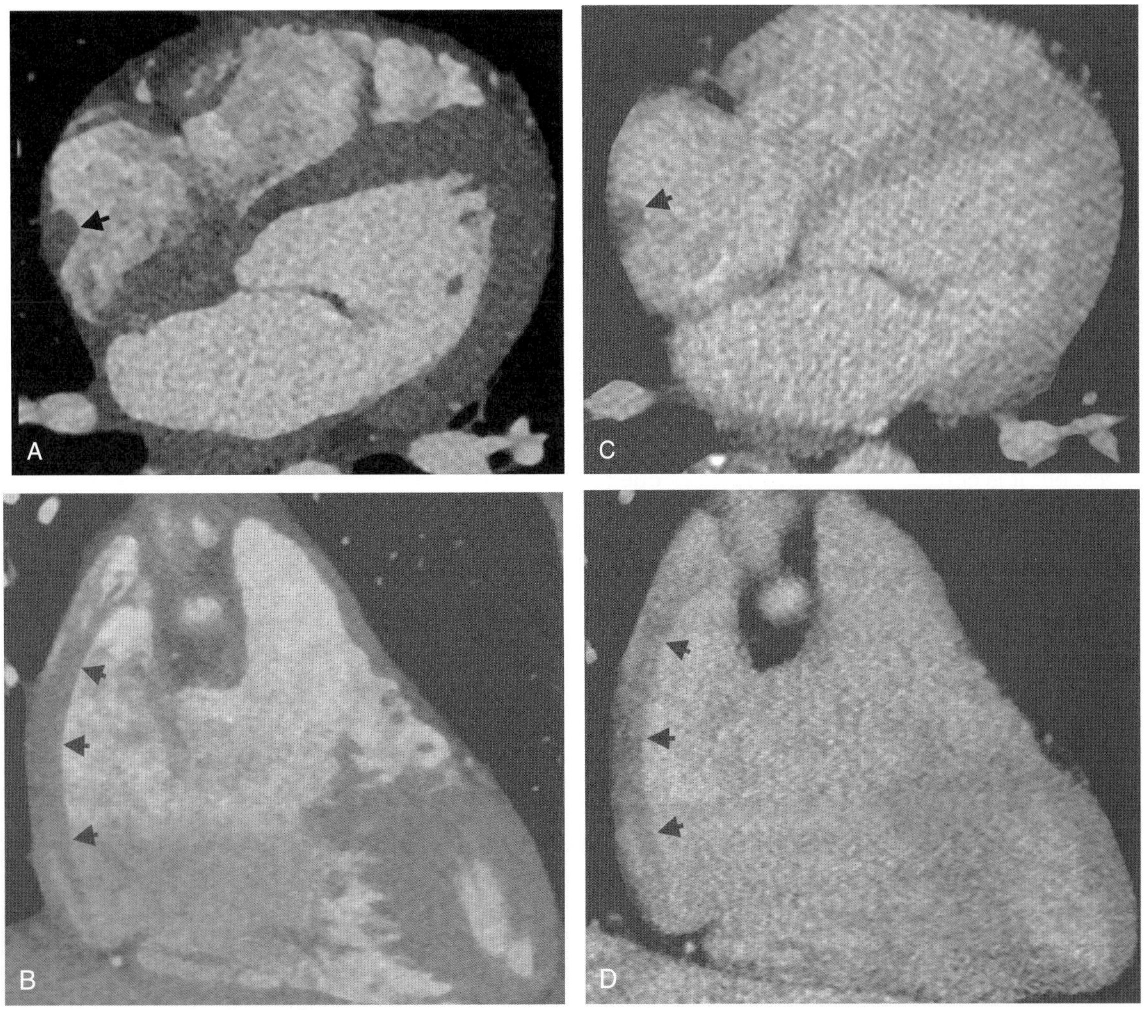

FIG. 21.5 A 47-year-old male presented with atrial fibrillation. Echocardiography revealed a mass in the right atrial wall. Four-chamber-view arterial phase cardiac CT (CCT) image (A, B) revealed an oblong hypodense lesion along the right atrial wall (*arrows*), which is not enhanced on delayed phase CCT image (C, D) and is consistent with prominent crista terminalis.

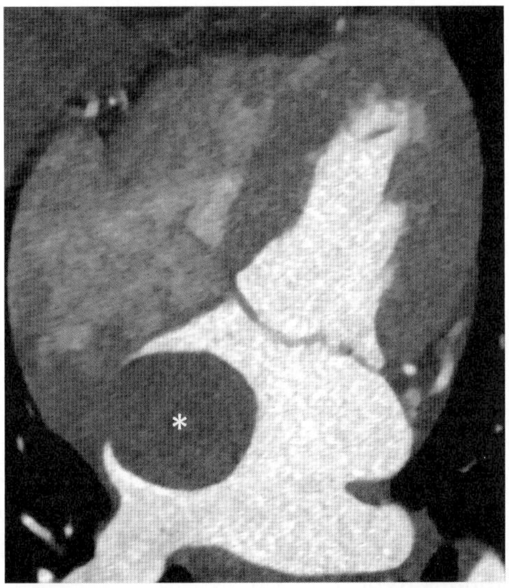

FIG. 21.6 A 63-year-old female presented with chest pain and a large mass detected in the chest CT (not shown). Four-chamber view cardiac CT image of the heart demonstrates a large mass in the left atrium (*asterisk*) attached to the interatrial septum. The mass was successfully resected, and pathology confirmed the diagnosis.

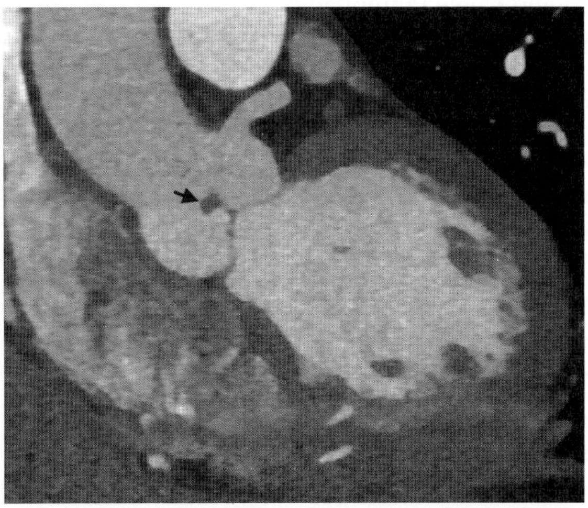

FIG. 21.7 A 59-year-old female incidentally found to have a mass in the aortic valve echocardiography (not shown). The patient underwent cardiac CT (CCT) to evaluate coronary arteries for presurgical assessment, which revealed no coronary artery disease. Multiplanar reformatted (MPR) CCT image shows a 5 mm mass (*arrow*) in the noncoronary cusp of the aortic valve, consistent with papillary fibroelastoma, which was confirmed on pathology.

Fibroma

Fibroma is a common primary cardiac tumor that can affect children and adults. Patients can present with heart failure due to the mass effect or sudden cardiac death due to arrhythmia. Fibroma is associated with certain syndromes, such as Gorlin syndrome and familial adenomatous polyposis. It usually appears to be a large, solid mass within the myocardium and contains fibroblast, collagen, and frequently with foci of calcifications.[31] These tumors appear on echocardiography as isoechoic nodular or discrete masses in the wall of the left ventricle. CCT shows a soft tissue-attenuated mass with foci of calcifications. These tumors tend to demonstrate fibrotic tissue characteristics on CMR due to fibroblasts, including isointense on T1-w images and hypointense on T2-w images. The mass is not enhanced on FPP images, but it is enhanced on LGE sequences due to gadolinium retention.[32] The LGE pattern is a characteristic of fibroma.[33] On FDG-PET/CT, fibroma can demonstrate moderate FDG uptake and rarely can mimic malignant neoplasm due to intense FDG uptake[12,34] (Fig. 21.8).

Cardiac/Pericardial Cyst

Pericardial cyst is a rare congenital anomaly located along the pericardium. It is usually located at the anterior right cardiophrenic angle. However, it can arise from anywhere along the pericardial line. Classic imaging features on CCT are fluid-attenuation mass along the right atrium with no mass effect on the adjacent structures. It shows homogeneous T2 hyperintensity on CMR with no enhancement on postcontrast images.

Hemangioma

Cardiac hemangioma is a rare benign tumor with diverse clinical presentations based on location, size, and growth rate. Decreased exercise tolerance is considered the most common reported symptom.[35] In rare cases, particularly pericardial hemangiomas, cardiac hemangiomas can bleed and cause tamponade and, thus, sudden death. Although diagnosing cardiac hemangiomas can be difficult on imaging, certain imaging findings can help with differential diagnosis. For example, CCT and CMR postcontrast images demonstrate peripheral nodular enhancement in early phases, and more enhancement on delayed images are classic findings in cardiac hemangioma.[36] Precontrast images are nonspecific, including hypodense mass on CCT, isointense on T1-w, and hyperintense on T2-w images.[33]

Paraganglioma

Paraganglioma is a rare neuroendocrine neoplasm derived from the mediastinal sympathetic ganglia. They are usually located along the epicardium and cardiac grooves, commonly in the aortopulmonary, atrioventricular, and interatrial grooves.[5] Catecholamine-related symptoms, including palpitation, tremors, and hypertension, are their common presentations. Most paragangliomas are benign entities. However, some of these tumors have malignant potential. According to the World Health Organization, "malignancy" is defined by the presence of distant metastasis, not local invasion.[37] Cardiac paragangliomas demonstrate nonspecific, heterogeneous echotexture on echocardiography. CCT shows avidly enhanced mass in the cardiac grooves with the large-feeding vessels from the coronaries to the mass. CMR features are markedly hyperintense on T2-w images and isointense to myocardium on T1-w images.[10] They are highly vascular masses demonstrating avid enhancement during the FPP and heterogeneously hyperintense signal characteristics on LGE images. PET/CT imaging with a conventional FDG tracer shows intense uptake in the mass and potential metastatic foci. Additionally, alternative tracers, such as Gallium-68 DOTATATE, can help diagnose somatostatin receptor-positive paragangliomas with high sensitivity and specificity[38] (Fig. 21.9).

MALIGNANT CARDIAC NEOPLASMS

Metastasis

Cardiac metastases are 20 to 40 times more common than primary cardiac tumors.[1] They present in 10% to 12% of autopsies with known malignancy.[39] Lung carcinoma, lymphomas, breast carcinomas, leukemia, gastric carcinomas, melanoma, hepatocellular carcinoma, and colon carcinoma are the most common malignancies that metastasize to the heart. Cardiac involvement may occur via four different routes of spread, including lymphatic, hematogenous, transvenous, and direct extension. Lymphatic spread is the most common route of metastasis and is observed in epithelial malignancies such as lung and breast cancers. Melanomas, sarcomas, and leukemia tend to deposit neoplastic cells via a hematogenous route to the myocardium. Metastasis to other organs, particularly lungs, is often present at the time of cardiac metastasis. Lung carcinoma, breast carcinoma, mesothelioma, and other thoracic malignancies may directly invade the heart and pericardium by contiguous growth. Transvenous spread to the right heart via systemic venous drainage is observed in renal, hepatic, adrenal, and uterine cancers. Lung cancers may also metastasize to the left atrium via pulmonary veins.

Cardiac metastases are often clinically silent and detected only on autopsy or can be encountered incidentally during cancer surveillance.[40] The clinical presentation of cardiac metastases depends on their location and route of spread. Arrhythmia is considered the most common symptom of myocardial metastasis due to the interruption of conduction pathways. Another typical clinical scenario is tamponade from neoplastic pericardial effusion, causing symptoms such as chest pain, dyspnea, tachycardia, and hypotension. Furthermore, congestive heart failure symptoms may be observed in patients with extensive myocardial involvement or obstruction of cardiac lymphatic drainage. Venous spread with contiguous involvement of the IVC and right atrium may lead to obstructive pathophysiology, including peripheral edema, cor pulmonale, and pulmonary hypertension.[41]

Imaging features of cardiac metastasis depend on the type of primary neoplasm and the route of extension. Similar to other cardiac masses, CMR is the first modality used, being isointense on T1-w images and hyperintense

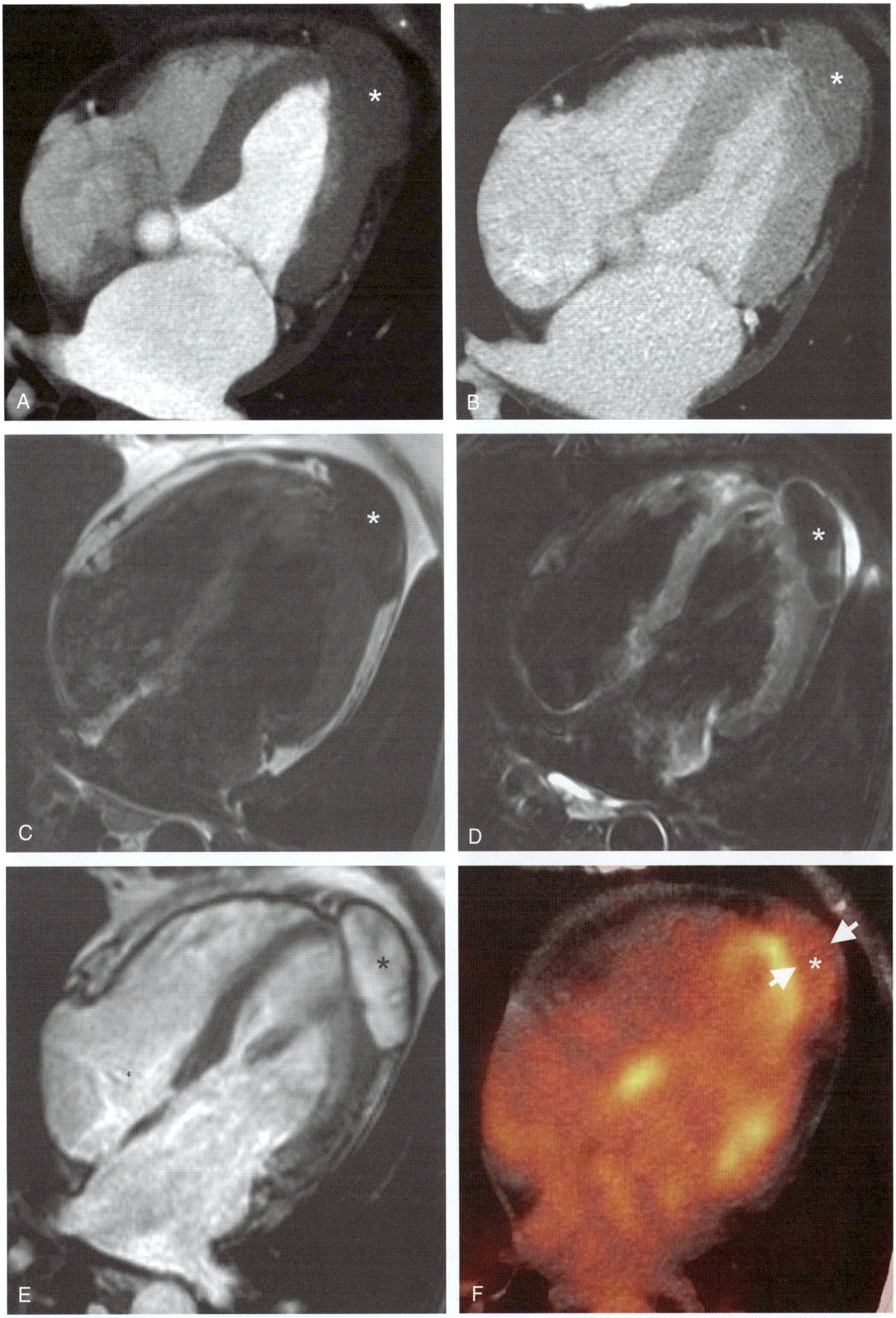

FIG. 21.8 A 52-year-old female presented with paroxysmal atrial fibrillation and underwent CCT to assess pulmonary veins. Four-chamber view arterial phase CCT image (A) shows a hypodense, large mass in the apical lateral wall (*asterisk*), with mild homogeneous enhancement on the delayed image (*asterisk*) (B). In CMR, the mass is hypointense both T1- (C) and T2-weighted (D) images (*asterisk*). LGE image (E) demonstrates homogeneously hyperintense mass due to avid gadolinium retention with the tumor, which is a classic imaging feature for fibroma. FDG-PET/CT image (F) demonstrates moderate FDG uptake* in the mass (*arrows*). *CCT*, Cardiac CT; *CMR*, cardiac magnetic resonance imaging; *FDG*, F-fluorodeoxyglucose; *PET/CT*, positron emission tomography/computed tomography; *LGE*, late gadolinium enhancement.

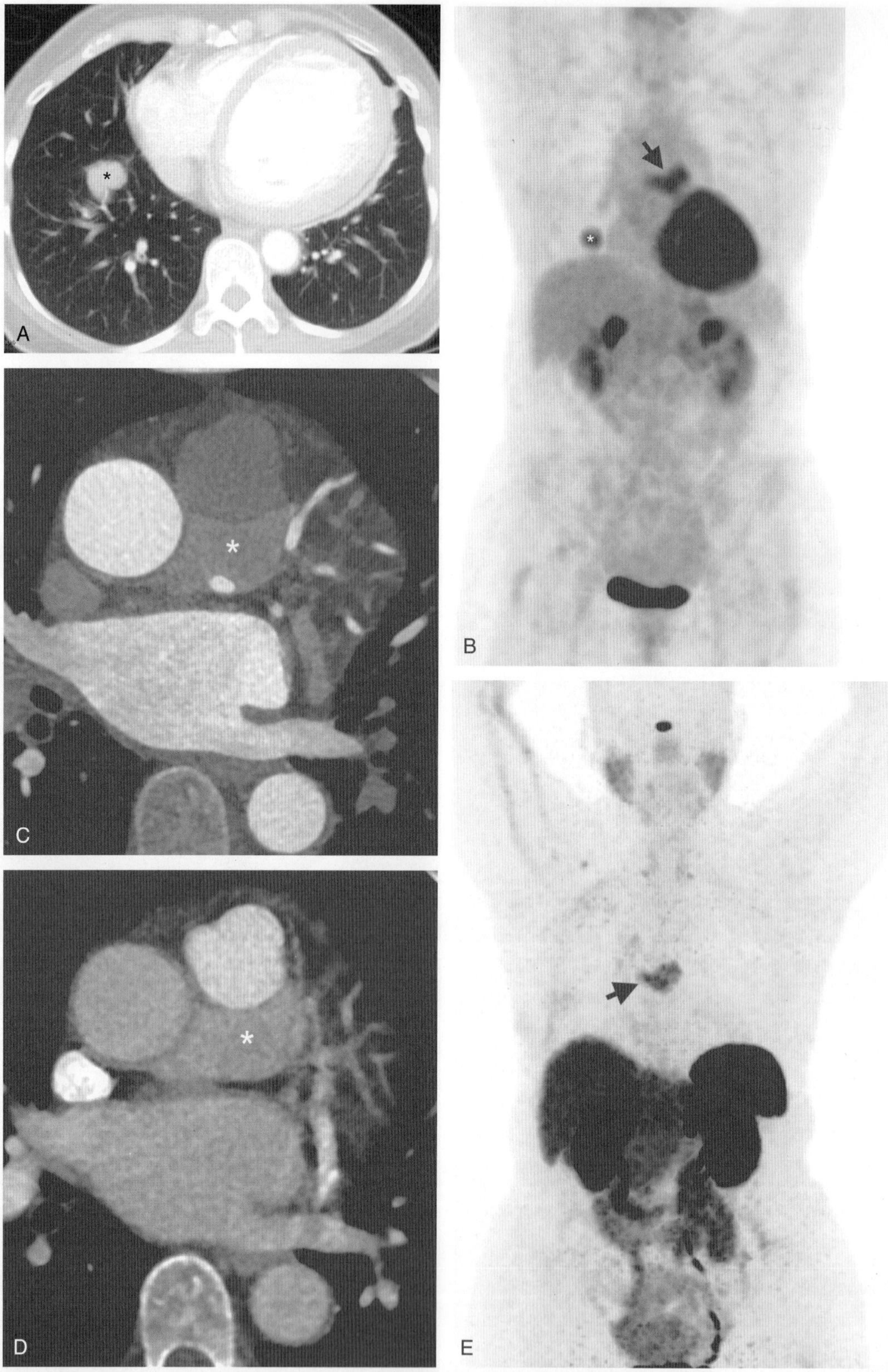

FIG. 21.9 A 60-year-old female with presented with left flank and abdominal pain. Chest CT (A) revealed a nodule in the right lung base (*asterisk*). The patient underwent FDG-PET/CT (B) that shows intense FDG uptake in the right lung base nodule and intense FDG uptake (*arrow*) in the heart/aortic root. CCT shows homogeneously enhancing mass in arterial (C) and delayed (D) images (*asterisk*). Given the location (aortopulmonary groove) and homogeneous enhancement, cardiac paraganglioma was suspected, and the patient underwent Ga-68-DOTATATE PET/CT (E), which revealed intense DOTATATE uptake associated with the mass (*arrow*). The patient underwent surgical resection of the right lower lobe mass and lymph node biopsy, and pathology confirmed the lung mass as stage I (T1cN0) invasive adenocarcinoma. *CCT*, Cardiac CT; *FDG*, F-fluorodeoxyglucose; *PET/CT*, positron emission tomography/computed tomography.

on T2-w images with heterogeneous enhancement due to the necrotic component.[42] It is difficult to differentiate primary malignant masses from metastases based on imaging features. In these clinical scenarios, FDG-PET/CT can help assess the primary source of the neoplasm. One important exception is melanoma metastasis, which shows hyperintensity on fat-suppressed T1-w images due to the shortening effect on melanin.[4] Furthermore, CCT is an alternative modality with multiphase image acquisition when CMR cannot be obtained[7] (Fig. 21.10). Besides its ability to provide a detailed evaluation of the heart, CCT can help evaluate the entire chest, including the lungs, mediastinum, soft tissues, and bones for the primary tumor, extracardiac metastatic disease, or both. CCT can demonstrate myocardial nodules or masses, multichamber involvement, valvular involvement, and pericardial involvement/effusion. Certain tumors may show calcification (osteosarcoma or chondrosarcoma) or fat (liposarcoma), which can be readily identified on CCT.

Lymphoma

Cardiac metastases from extracardiac lymphoma are more common than those from primary cardiac lymphoma. The incidence of cardiac involvement in patients with lymphoma has been reported to be between 8% and 20% in autopsy studies.[43] Approximately a quarter of patients with extracardiac lymphoma have cardiac involvement. In contrast, primary cardiac lymphomas are rare, accounting for ~2% of all primary cardiac tumors. Most primary cardiac lymphomas are aggressive B-cell type with slight male predominance and are usually present in the sixth decade of life. Patients may present with rapidly progressive cardiac failure, arrhythmias, cardiac tamponade, SVC syndrome, or sudden death. Primary cardiac lymphoma predominantly occurs in patients with immunocompromised conditions, particularly those with HIV infection. Furthermore, it can occur as part of posttransplant lymphoproliferative disorder.

Most primary cardiac and metastatic lymphomas involve the right atrium. However, any other cardiac chamber or pericardium can be involved. These lesions appeared on imaging as ill-defined infiltrative lesions or multiple polypoid masses involving the myocardium or pericardium, often with pericardial effusion. They are seen to cross the tissue borders. Unlike other malignant tumors, they lack central necrosis or hemorrhage. Therefore they are hypoattenuating or isoattenuating to the normal myocardium and demonstrate heterogeneous enhancement on CCT. Signal characteristics on CMR are usually homogeneous, isointense on T1-w images, and hyperintense on T2-w images, with diffuse progressive enhancement on postcontrast images.[42] The most important imaging finding on CCT or CMR is that lymphomas encase the adjacent coronary arteries without the obliteration of the lumen (Fig. 21.11).[44] FDG-PET/CT is an important imaging modality for staging. It usually demonstrates intense homogeneous FDG uptake throughout the mass.[15]

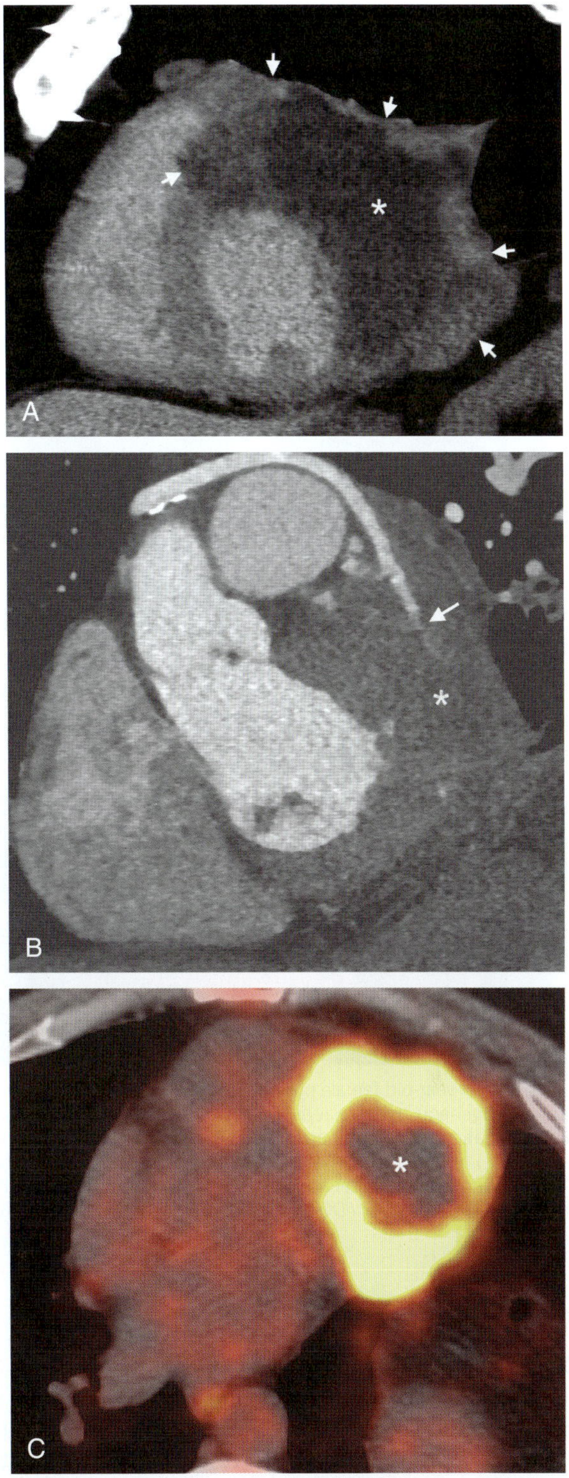

FIG. 21.10 A 62-year-old male with a history of coronary artery disease, prior coronary artery bypass grafts, and metastatic laryngeal squamous cell carcinoma presented with chest pain and shortness of breath. Short-axis delayed CCT image (A) shows metastatic infiltrative mass involving the anterior and lateral left ventricle extending to the right ventricle and pericardium. The mass is centrally hypodense (*asterisk*), likely due to necrosis with peripheral heterogeneous enhancement (*arrows*). As demonstrated in the multiplanar reformatted (MPR) coronary CCT image (B), the mass (*asterisk*) infiltrates the venous graft of the obtuse marginal branch, which is occluded (*arrow*). FDG-PET/CT image (C) shows a large, infiltrative cardiac mass with central necrosis (*asterisk*). *CCT*, Cardiac CT; *FDG*, F-fluorodeoxyglucose; *PET/CT*, positron emission tomography/computed tomography.

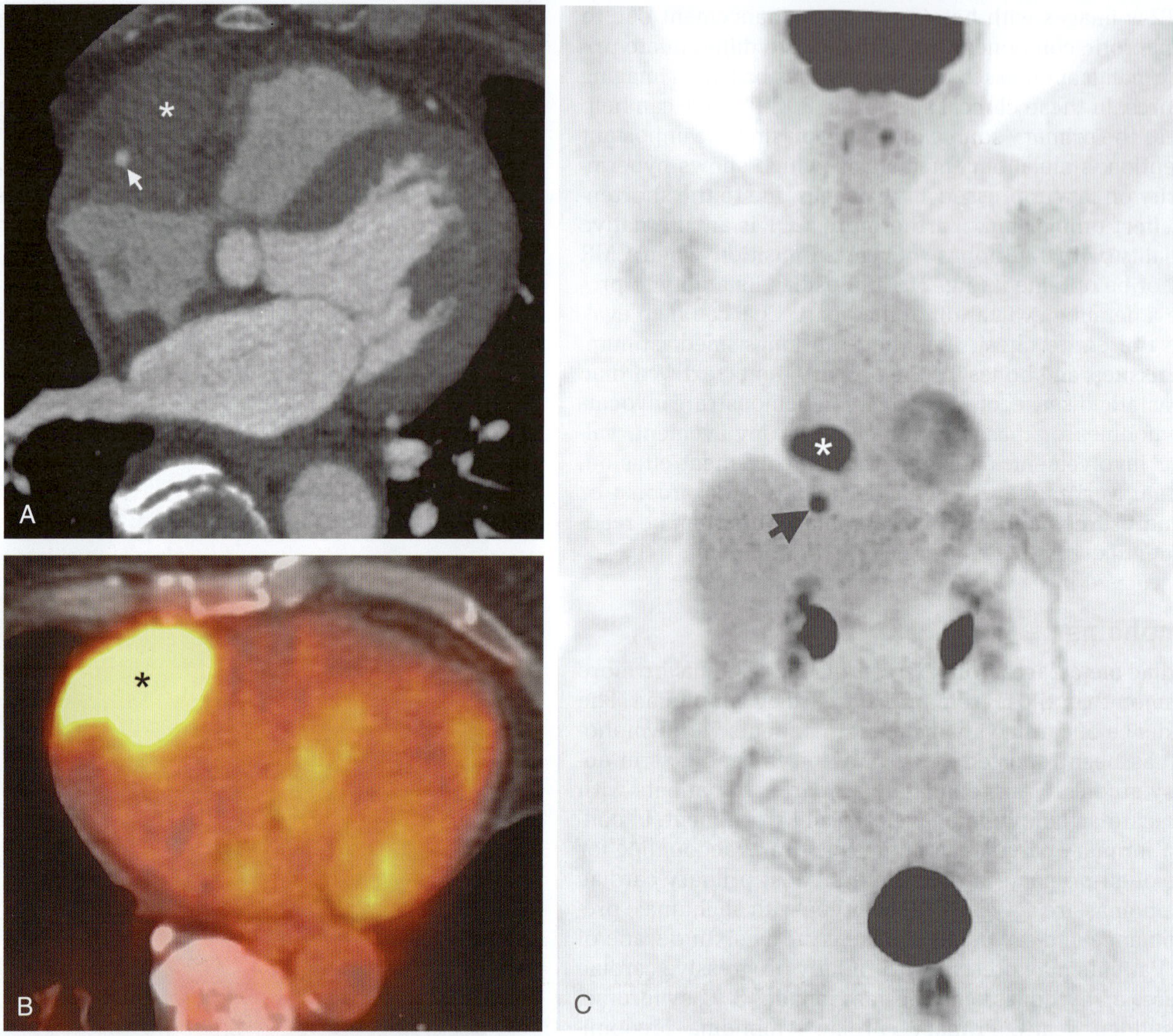

FIG. 21.11 A 75-year-old female presented with lower extremity edema. Echocardiography revealed a large mass in the right atrium. Axial CCT image (A) shows a homogeneous mass (*asterisk*) in the atrioventricular groove on the right, which is not obliterating the coronary artery (*arrow*). Given the imaging features, the patient underwent an FDG-PET/CT study that shows (B) intense FDG uptake associated with the mass; coronal maximum intensity projection (MIP) image (C) of the body demonstrates that in addition to the primary mass (*asterisk*), there is an additional small mass along the inferior border of the right heart. There were no other additional enlarged or FDG avid lymph nodes. The pathology of the mass was high-grade B cell lymphoma, primary cardiac lymphoma. *CCT*, Cardiac CT; *FDG*, F-fluorodeoxyglucose; *PET/CT*, positron emission tomography/computed tomography.

Sarcoma

ANGIOSARCOMA

Angiosarcoma is the most common primary cardiac malignancy in adults. It is a highly aggressive tumor, accounting for 37% of all sarcoma cases. A slight male predilection has been reported, with a male-to-female ratio of 2.5:1. The mean age of presentation is 40 years, ranging from 3 months to 80 years.[45] Patients usually present with right heart failure, hemorrhagic pericardial effusion, metastatic disease, or, in rare cases, rupture of pseudoaneurysm caused by angiosarcoma. In 66% to 89% of the patients, angiosarcomas have metastatic disease at presentation more often than other sarcomas.[45]

In contrast to most other subtypes of cardiac sarcomas, angiosarcomas are typically located in the right atrium near the atrioventricular groove.[46] They show sheet-like diffuse thickening along the cardiac mass borders when there is an extension and invasion of the pericardium. They may invade the right coronary artery and involve the IVC and tricuspid valve. They can form pseudoaneurysms in the right atrial or ventricular wall when the necrotic components grow larger. Angiosarcomas usually have heterogeneous density mass, depend on necrotic components, and are typically heterogeneously enhanced with associated pericardial thickening, nodularity, and effusion on CCT. On CMR, T1-w images demonstrate an isointense signal, and T2-w images demonstrate hyperintense signal intensities. Avid enhancement can be seen on the perfusion or postcontrast LGE images with necrotic/nonenhancing components. Similar to other malignant masses, FDG-PET/CT demonstrates intense FDG uptake in the solid component of the mass and associated pulmonary metastasis. CCT images can show pulmonary metastases with surrounding ground glass halo because of their hemorrhagic nature.

OTHER SARCOMAS

Other cardiac sarcomas, including undifferentiated sarcoma, rhabdomyosarcoma, osteosarcoma, leiomyosarcoma, fibrosarcoma, liposarcoma, and synovial sarcoma, are rare.

Undifferentiated sarcoma or undifferentiated pleomorphic sarcoma has no specific histological pattern and is the second most common primary cardiac malignancy, accounting for approximately one-third of all cardiac sarcomas.[47] Undifferentiated sarcomas have a similar imaging appearance to angiosarcoma. However, they have a predilection for the left atrium with reported biatrial and valvular involvement.[15] Undifferentiated pleomorphic sarcoma is usually the diagnosis of exclusion.

Rhabdomyosarcoma is the most common primary cardiac malignancy in children with a male predilection. Rhabdomyosarcomas have no chamber predilection, tend to involve cardiac valves more than other sarcomas, and are multifocal in 60% of the patients.[48] They tend to demonstrate infiltrative intramural multifocal or solitary masses on CCT, which are often hypodense to the normal myocardium.[49] Furthermore, on CMR, they have isointense signal intensity on T1-w images, hyperintense signal intensity on T2-w images, and heterogeneous enhancement on post-contrast images, including LGE.[33]

Osteosarcomas have a median age of presentation in the fourth decade with a female predilection. These tumors almost exclusively (>95%) arise from the left atrium and commonly involve the mitral valve.[50] These tumors may mimic cardiac myxoma on imaging. However, features that differentiate osteosarcomas include a broad-based attachment to the atrial wall, lack of association with fossa ovalis, and invasion of adjacent structures.[51] They can mimic undifferentiated sarcomas or cardiac metastasis based on CMR signal characteristics.[52] Furthermore, they may demonstrate a large amount of calcification on CCT, which is important imaging to differentiate from other entities. However, it is not a consistent feature, and calcification may be absent or minimal in the early stages.[53]

Liposarcoma usually occurs in the adult population. Metastatic liposarcoma is more common than primary cardiac liposarcoma. It tends to arise from the right side of the heart, particularly from the right atrium.[49] These lesions have been reported to manifest with signs and symptoms similar to those of other right-sided tumors, including right ventricular outflow obstruction, pulmonary embolism, valvular dysfunction, and arrhythmia.[54] CCT may not always demonstrate macroscopic fat, and cardiac liposarcoma is usually seen as heterogeneously enhanced soft tissue masses[54] (Fig. 21.12). Lesions may demonstrate hemorrhage and necrosis. Broad-based attachment and aggressive features, including the involvement of cardiac valves, may assist in the differentiation from benign masses such as myxoma.

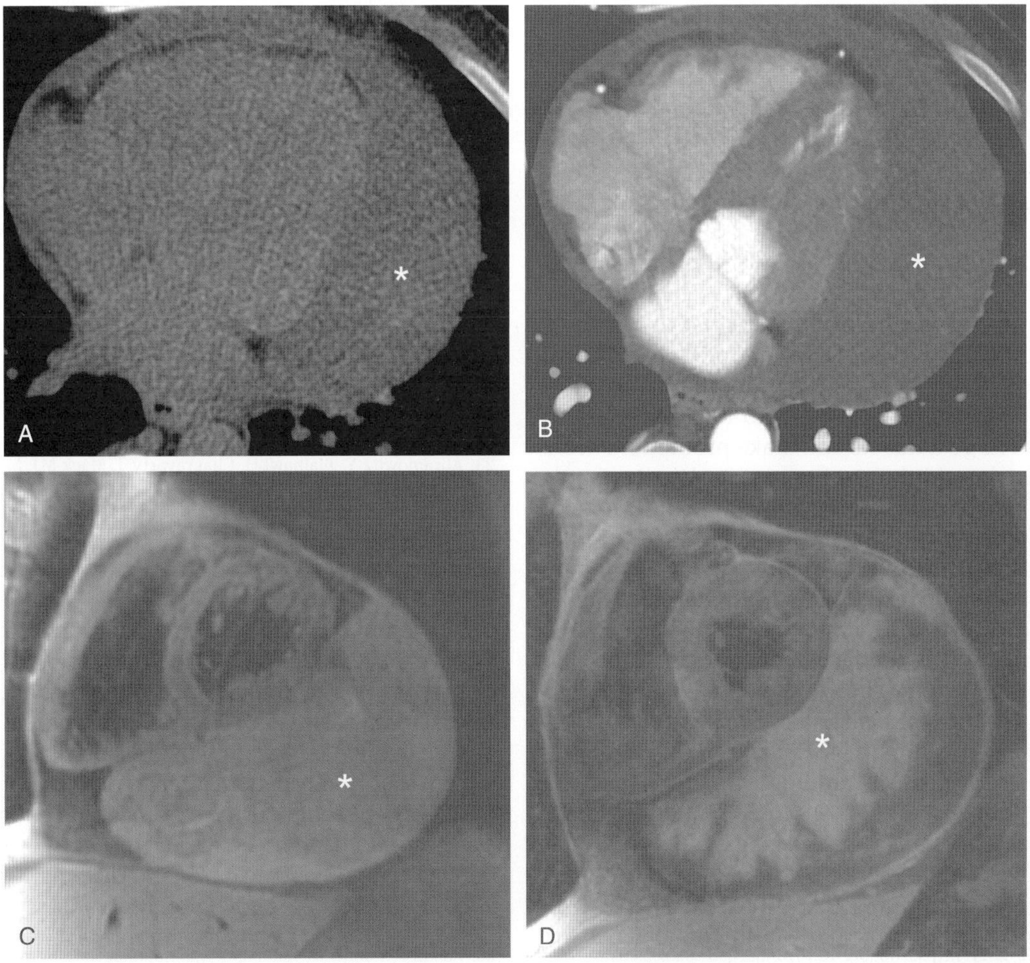

FIG. 21.12 A 46-year-old male with a history of right thigh myxoid liposarcoma with pericardial/cardiac mass. Axial noncontrast (A) and arterial phase (B) cardiac CT images show large homogeneous mass (*asterisk*) with no macroscopic fat. T2-weighted image (C) demonstrates homogeneous, hyperintense pericardial mass, which has heterogeneous enhancement in the central part of the mass (*asterisk*) on the postcontrast T1-weighted image (D).

FUTURE DIRECTIONS

Currently, CCT is underutilized for the assessment of cardiac masses. Existing strengths of CCT, such as high spatial resolution and multiplanar image reconstruction, when combined with recent technological development, including tissue characterization, iodine concentration, and perfusion assessment, further advance the capabilities of CCT. CCT also remains the best imaging test to evaluate cases where coronary involvement may be suspected.

Photon-counting CT (PCCT) can produce high spatial resolution images with increased contrast-to-noise ratio and reduced artifacts.[55,56] Besides these advantages, PCCT can help in several ways in imaging cardiac tumors. With the help of PCCT, perfusion imaging and iodine maps can be obtained without needing a baseline noncontrast scan, mitigating the potential of misregistration artifacts. Such techniques could help differentiate cardiac neoplasm from thrombus. Simultaneous multicontrast agent imaging and capturing multiple contrast phases on a single scan may further help tissue characterization. With PCCT, molecular CT imaging may become a reality,[55] allowing targeted imaging of different tumors.

High-resolution volumetric CT data enables three-dimensional (3D) printing, which may be helpful for presurgical planning. In complex cases, 3D printing provides accurate replication of the tumor and adjacent cardiac structures, which helps surgeons determine accurate resection planes, identify potential complications, and determine the suitable surgical strategy for resection.[57]

Advances in computing power and the availability of big data have enabled the emergence of artificial intelligence (AI) techniques for image analysis, including radiomics and deep learning (DL). Radiomics extracts a large amount of quantitative information from digital images, which is not distinguishable to the human eye, using advanced image analysis techniques.[58] Differentiating cardiac neoplasm from thrombus with the help of radiomics on CCT is an emerging technique.[59] DL is a type of machine learning that uses computer modeling, known as artificial neural networks, to identify complex relationships in large datasets and make predictions from new input data. In addition to improving the diagnostic performance, these techniques can be used to develop AI-enabled predictive or prognostic imaging biomarkers.[60] Using this approach with cardiac tumors may help predict outcomes and response to various treatments, assess disease progression and therapy-related cardiotoxicity, and support clinical decision-making.

REFERENCES

1. Butany J, Nair V, Naseemuddin A, Nair GM, Catton C, Yau T. Cardiac tumours: diagnosis and management. *Lancet Oncol.* 2005;6(4):219–228. https://doi.org/10.1016/S1470-2045(05)70093-0.
2. Rahouma M, Arisha MJ, Elmously A, et al. Cardiac tumors prevalence and mortality: a systematic review and meta-analysis. *Int J Surg.* 2020;76:178–189. https://doi.org/10.1016/j.ijsu.2020.02.039.
3. Pazos-Lopez P, Pozo E, Siqueira ME, et al. Value of CMR for the differential diagnosis of cardiac masses. *JACC Cardiovasc Imaging.* 2014;7(9):896–905. https://doi.org/10.1016/j.jcmg.2014.05.009.
4. Tyebally S, Chen D, Bhattacharyya S, et al. Cardiac tumors. *JACC: CardioOncol.* 2020;2(2):293–2311. https://doi.org/10.1016/j.jaccao.2020.05.009.
5. Wang JG, Han J, Jiang T, Li YJ. Cardiac paragangliomas. *J Card Surg.* 2015;30(1):55–60. https://doi.org/10.1111/jocs.12455.
6. Kassop D, Donovan MS, Cheezum MK, et al. Cardiac masses on cardiac CT: a review. *Curr Cardiovasc Imaging Rep.* 2014;7:9281. https://doi.org/10.1007/s12410-014-9281-1.
7. D'Angelo EC, Paolisso P, Vitale G, et al. Diagnostic accuracy of cardiac computed tomography and (18)F-fluorodeoxyglucose with positron emission tomography in cardiac masses. *JACC Cardiovasc Imaging.* 2020;13(11):2400–2411. https://doi.org/10.1016/j.jcmg.2020.03.021.
8. Young PM, Foley TA, Araoz PA, Williamson EE. Computed tomography imaging of cardiac masses. *Radiol Clin North Am.* 2019;57(1):75–84. https://doi.org/10.1016/j.rcl.2018.08.002.
9. Ye W, Ren G, Zhong X, et al. ECG-gated CT in aortic perivalvular abscess: comparison with transesophageal echocardiography and intraoperative findings. *Radiology.* 2020:200685. https://doi.org/10.1148/radiol.2020200685.
10. Motwani M, Kidambi A, Herzog BA, Uddin A, Greenwood JP, Plein S. MR imaging of cardiac tumors and masses: a review of methods and clinical applications. *Radiology.* 2013;268(1):26–43. https://doi.org/10.1148/radiol.13121239.
11. Weinsaft JW, Kim HW, Shah DJ, et al. Detection of left ventricular thrombus by delayed-enhancement cardiovascular magnetic resonance prevalence and markers in patients with systolic dysfunction. *J Am Coll Cardiol.* 2008;52(2):148–157. https://doi.org/10.1016/j.jacc.2008.03.041.
12. Rahbar K, Seifarth H, Schafers M, et al. Differentiation of malignant and benign cardiac tumors using 18F-FDG PET/CT. *J Nucl Med.* 2012;53(6):856–863. https://doi.org/10.2967/jnumed.111.095364.
13. Nensa F, Tezgah E, Poeppel TD, et al. Integrated 18F-FDG PET/MR imaging in the assessment of cardiac masses: a pilot study. *J Nucl Med.* 2015;56(2):255–260. https://doi.org/10.2967/jnumed.114.147744.
14. Qin C, Shao F, Hu F, et al. ^{18}F-FDG PET/CT in diagnostic and prognostic evaluation of patients with cardiac masses: a retrospective study. *Eur J Nucl Med Mol Imaging.* 2020;47(5):1083–1093. https://doi.org/10.1007/s00259-019-04632-w.
15. Aghayev A, Cheezum MK, Steigner ML, et al. Multimodality imaging to distinguish between benign and malignant cardiac masses. *J Nucl Cardiol.* 2022;29(4):1504–1517. https://doi.org/10.1007/s12350-021-02790-9.
16. Chang CA, Pattison DA, Tothill RW, et al. (68)Ga-DOTATATE and (18)F-FDG PET/CT in Paraganglioma and Pheochromocytoma: utility, patterns and heterogeneity. *Cancer Imaging.* 2016;16(1):22. https://doi.org/10.1186/s40644-016-0084-2.
17. Chan AT, Plodkowski AJ, Pun SC, et al. Prognostic utility of differential tissue characterization of cardiac neoplasm and thrombus via late gadolinium enhancement cardiovascular magnetic resonance among patients with advanced systemic cancer. *J Cardiovasc Magn Reson.* 2017;19(1):76. https://doi.org/10.1186/s12968-017-0390-2.
18. Werdan K, Dietz S, Loffler B, et al. Mechanisms of infective endocarditis: pathogen-host interaction and risk states. *Nat Rev Cardiol.* 2014;11(1):35–50. https://doi.org/10.1038/nrcardio.2013.174.
19. Erba PA, Pizzi MN, Roque A, et al. Multimodality imaging in infective endocarditis: an imaging team within the endocarditis team. *Circulation.* 2019;140(21):1753–1765. https://doi.org/10.1161/CIRCULATIONAHA.119.040228.
20. Swart LE, Gomes A, Scholtens AM, et al. Improving the diagnostic performance of (18)F-fluorodeoxyglucose positron-emission tomography/computed tomography in prosthetic heart valve endocarditis. *Circulation.* 2018;138(14):1412–1427. https://doi.org/10.1161/CIRCULATIONAHA.118.035032.
21. Scholtens AM, Swart LE, Verberne HJ, Tanis W, Lam MG, Budde RP. Confounders in FDG-PET/CT Imaging of Suspected Prosthetic Valve Endocarditis. *JACC Cardiovasc Imaging.* 2016;9(12):1462–1465. https://doi.org/10.1016/j.jcmg.2016.01.024.
22. Adel A, Jones E, Johns J, Farouque O, Calafiore P. Bacterial mural endocarditis. A case series. *Heart Lung Circ.* 2014;23(8):e172–e179. https://doi.org/10.1016/j.hlc.2014.03.026.
23. Abramowitz Y, Jilaihawi H, Chakravarty T, Mack MJ, Makkar RR. Mitral annulus calcification. *J Am Coll Cardiol.* 2015;66(17):1934–1941. https://doi.org/10.1016/j.jacc.2015.08.872.
24. Gupta S, Ge Y, Ghouri MA, Blankstein R, Steigner ML, Aghayev A. Caseous calcification of the mitral annulus with atrial and ventricular fistulization. *Circ Cardiovasc Imaging.* 2018;11(7):e007588. https://doi.org/10.1161/CIRCIMAGING.118.007588.
25. Fan CM, Fischman AJ, Kwek BH, Abbara S, Aquino SL. Lipomatous hypertrophy of the interatrial septum: increased uptake on FDG PET. *AJR Am J Roentgenol.* 2005;184(1):339–342. https://doi.org/10.2214/ajr.184.1.01840339.
26. Heyer CM, Kagel T, Lemburg SP, Bauer TT, Nicolas V. Lipomatous hypertrophy of the interatrial septum: a prospective study of incidence, imaging findings, and clinical symptoms. *Chest.* 2003;124(6):2068–2073.
27. Rajiah P, MacNamara J, Chaturvedi A, Ashwath R, Fulton NL, Goerne H. Bands in the heart: multimodality imaging review. *Radiographics.* 2019;39(5):1238–1263. https://doi.org/10.1148/rg.2019180176.
28. Akcay M, Bilen ES, Bilge M, Durmaz T, Kurt M. Prominent crista terminalis: as an anatomic structure leading to atrial arrhythmias and mimicking right atrial mass. *J the Am Soc Echocardiogr.* 2007;20(2):197.e9-10. https://doi.org/10.1016/j.echo.2006.08.037.
29. Grebenc ML, Rosado-de-Christenson ML, Green CE, Burke AP, Galvin JR. Cardiac myxoma: imaging features in 83 patients. *Radiographics.* 2002;22(3):673–689. https://doi.org/10.1148/radiographics.22.3.g02ma02673.
30. Rajiah P, Kanne JP, Kalahasti V, Schoenhagen P. Computed tomography of cardiac and pericardiac masses. *J Cardiovasc Comput Tomogr.* 2011;5(1):16–29. https://doi.org/10.1016/j.jcct.2010.08.009.

31. Burke AP, Rosado-de-Christenson M, Templeton PA, Virmani R. Cardiac fibroma: clinicopathologic correlates and surgical treatment. *J Thorac Cardiovasc Surg*. 1994;108(5):862–870.
32. O'Donnell DH, Abbara S, Chaithiraphan V, et al. Cardiac tumors: optimal cardiac MR sequences and spectrum of imaging appearances. *AJR Am J Roentgenol*. 2009;193(2):377–387. https://doi.org/10.2214/AJR.08.1895.
33. Esposito A, De Cobelli F, Ironi G, et al. CMR in the assessment of cardiac masses: primary malignant tumors. *JACC Cardiovasc Imaging*. 2014;7(10):1057–1061. https://doi.org/10.1016/j.jcmg.2014.08.002.
34. Masuda A, Manabe O, Oyama-Manabe N, et al. Cardiac fibroma with high (18)F-FDG uptake mimicking malignant tumor. *J Nucl Cardiol*. 2017;24(1):323–324. https://doi.org/10.1007/s12350-015-0362-6.
35. Li W, Teng P, Xu H, Ma L, Ni Y. Cardiac hemangioma: a comprehensive analysis of 200 cases. *Ann Thorac Surg*. 2015;99(6):2246–2252. https://doi.org/10.1016/j.athoracsur.2015.02.064.
36. Hrabak-Paar M, Hubner M, Stern-Padovan R, Lusic M. Hemangioma of the interatrial septum: CT and MRI features. *Cardiovasc Intervent Radiol*. 2011;34(Suppl 2):S90–S93. https://doi.org/10.1007/s00270-010-0062-1.
37. DeLellis RA, Lloyd RV, Heitz PU, Eng CPathology and Genetics of Tumours of Endocrine Organs8. IARC; 2004.
38. Taieb D, Hicks RJ, Hindie E, et al. European association of nuclear medicine practice guideline/society of nuclear medicine and molecular imaging procedure standard 2019 for radionuclide imaging of phaeochromocytoma and paraganglioma. *Eur J Nucl Med Mol Imaging*. 2019;46(10):2112–2137. https://doi.org/10.1007/s00259-019-04398-1.
39. Abraham KP, Reddy V, Gattuso P. Neoplasms metastatic to the heart: review of 3314 consecutive autopsies. *Am J Cardiovasc Pathol*. 1990;3(3):195–198.
40. Burazor I, Aviel-Ronen S, Imazio M, et al. Primary malignancies of the heart and pericardium. *Clin Cardiol*. 2014;37(9):582–588. https://doi.org/10.1002/clc.22295.
41. Chiles C, Woodard PK, Gutierrez FR, Link KM. Metastatic involvement of the heart and pericardium: CT and MR imaging. *Radiographics*. 2001;21(2):439–449. https://doi.org/10.1148/radiographics.21.2.g01mr15439.
42. Mousavi N, Cheezum MK, Aghayev A, et al. Assessment of cardiac masses by cardiac magnetic resonance imaging: histological correlation and clinical outcomes. *J Am Heart Assoc*. 2019;8(1):e007829. https://doi.org/10.1161/JAHA.117.007829.
43. O'Mahony D, Peikarz RL, Bandettini WP, Arai AE, Wilson WH, Bates SE. Cardiac involvement with lymphoma: a review of the literature. *Clin Lymphoma Myeloma*. 2008;8(4):249–252. https://doi.org/10.3816/CLM.2008.n.034.
44. Shah RN, Simmons TW, Carr JJ, Entrikin DW. Primary cardiac lymphoma diagnosed by multiphase-gated cardiac CT and CT-guided percutaneous trans-sternal biopsy. *J Cardiovasc Comput Tomogr*. 2012;6(2):137–139. https://doi.org/10.1016/j.jcct.2011.12.007.
45. Cina SJ, Smialek JE, Burke AP, Virmani R, Hutchins GM. Primary cardiac tumors causing sudden death: a review of the literature. *Am J Forensic Med Pathol*. 1996;17(4):271–281.
46. Herrmann MA, Shankerman RA, Edwards WD, Shub C, Schaff HV. Primary cardiac angiosarcoma: a clinicopathologic study of six cases. *J Thorac Cardiovasc Surg*. 1992;103(4):655–664.
47. Burke A, Jeudy Jr J, Virmani R. Cardiac tumours: an update: cardiac tumours. *Heart*. 2008;94(1):117–123. https://doi.org/10.1136/hrt.2005.078576.
48. Araoz PA, Eklund HE, Welch TJ, Breen JF. CT and MR imaging of primary cardiac malignancies. *Radiographics*. 1999;19(6):1421–1434. https://doi.org/10.1148/radiographics.19.6.g99no031421.
49. Shanmugam G. Primary cardiac sarcoma. *Eur J Cardiothorac Surg*. 2006;29(6):925–932. https://doi.org/10.1016/j.ejcts.2006.03.034.
50. Sparrow PJ, Kurian JB, Jones TR, Sivananthan MU. MR imaging of cardiac tumors. *Radiographics*. 2005;25(5):1255–1276. https://doi.org/10.1148/rg.255045721.
51. Syed IS, Feng D, Harris SR, et al. MR imaging of cardiac masses. *Magn Reson Imaging Clin N Am*. 2008;16(2):137–164. vii. https://doi.org/10.1016/j.mric.2008.02.009.
52. Trimble CR, Burke A, Kligerman S. Primary cardiac osteosarcoma: AIRP best cases in radiologic-pathologic correlation. *Radiographics*. 2015;35(5):1352–1357. https://doi.org/10.1148/rg.2015140265.
53. Burke AP, Virmani R. Osteosarcomas of the heart. *Am J Surg Pathol*. 1991;15(3):289–295.
54. Uemura S, Watanabe M, Iwama H, Saito Y. Extensive primary cardiac liposarcoma with multiple functional complications. *Heart*. 2004;90(8):e48. https://doi.org/10.1136/hrt.2004.036707.
55. Sandfort V, Persson M, Pourmorteza A, Noel PB, Fleischmann D, Willemink MJ. Spectral photon-counting CT in cardiovascular imaging. *J Cardiovasc Comput Tomogr*. 2021;15(3):218–225. https://doi.org/10.1016/j.jcct.2020.12.005.
56. Willemink MJ, Persson M, Pourmorteza A, Pelc NJ, Fleischmann D. Photon-counting CT: technical principles and clinical prospects. *Radiology*. 2018;289(2):293–312. https://doi.org/10.1148/radiol.2018172656.
57. Al Jabbari O, Abu Saleh WK, Patel AP, Igo SR, Reardon MJ. Use of three-dimensional models to assist in the resection of malignant cardiac tumors. *J Card Surg*. 2016;31(9):581–583. https://doi.org/10.1111/jocs.12812.
58. Xu P, Xue Y, Schoepf UJ, et al. Radiomics: the next frontier of cardiac computed tomography. *Circ Cardiovasc Imaging*. 2021;14(3):e011747. https://doi.org/10.1161/CIRCIMAGING.120.011747.
59. Lee JW, Park CH, Im DJ, et al. CT-based radiomics signature for differentiation between cardiac tumors and a thrombi: a retrospective, multicenter study. *Sci Rep*. 2022;12(1):8173. https://doi.org/10.1038/s41598-022-12229-x.
60. Bera K, Braman N, Gupta A, Velcheti V, Madabhushi A. Predicting cancer outcomes with radiomics and artificial intelligence in radiology. *Nat Rev Clin Oncol*. 2022;19(2):132–146. https://doi.org/10.1038/s41571-021-00560-7.

22 Endocarditis in Native and Prosthetic Valves

PAUL C. CREMER, NANDAN S. ANAVEKAR, MICHAEL A. BOLEN, AND ERIC E. WILLIAMSON

KEY POINTS

- Invasive endocarditis occurs when infection spreads beyond valve leaflets to involve adjacent structures and progresses from cellulitis to abscess and abscess cavity to pseudoaneurysm.
- Although cardiovascular CT angiography can identify vegetations, the strength of the modality is in the assessment of invasive complications, especially in the setting of prosthetic valve endocarditis.
- Noncontrast CT can be helpful in delineating hyperattenuating surgical material and calcification, whereas contrast-enhanced cardiac CT angiography with multiphase (cine) imaging is the primary means to assess for pathology, and delayed imaging can demonstrate peripheral enhancement of abscesses.
- Cardiovascular CT angiography in combination with a whole-body CT scan provides additive assessment of coronary arteries and extra cardiac embolic phenomena.

INTRODUCTION

Despite advances in cardiovascular medicine, morbidity and mortality related to infective endocarditis remains high. This morbidity and mortality is in part related to increased complexity of disease presentation—patients are older with more comorbidities and are more likely to have indwelling foreign material related to prior surgeries or interventions. In this setting, multimodality imaging is often necessary for diagnosis and appropriate management. Although echocardiography remains the mainstay for evaluation, the value of cardiovascular CT has been increasingly recognized over the past 15 years. Accordingly, the current chapter highlights anatomic considerations regarding the role of cardiovascular CT in infective endocarditis, provides guidance for CT protocols, discusses CT to evaluate vegetations and invasive complications, and emphasizes the value of CT for the assessment of coronary arteries and extra cardiac embolic phenomena.

DEFINITIONS AND ANATOMIC CONSIDERATIONS

Infective endocarditis is characterized by circulating microorganisms that adhere to damaged endocardium, endothelium, or foreign material. These organisms multiply and attract fibrin deposits and result in the hallmark feature of endocarditis, a vegetation. Characterized by independent, oscillating motion, vegetations are most commonly attached to the low-pressure side of abnormal valvular endocardium. Vegetations are the primary source of embolization, and this risk is related to size, mobility, and location.[1,2]

In addition, microorganisms produce specific enzymes which degrade tissue. This destruction can result in valve perforation with associated regurgitation. Bulky vegetations, in particular involving prosthetic leaflets that may be resistant to degradation, can also obstruct flow and result in stenosis. When this damage extends beyond the valve leaflets to involve the annulus or adjacent extravascular structures, patients are considered to have "invasive disease." Importantly, invasive disease follows a typical progression from cellulitis, to abscess and abscess cavity, and finally pseudoaneurysm formation.[3] The delineation of the extent of invasive disease and associated complications is essential to inform a definitive treatment plan.[4] For this assessment, cardiovascular CT is well suited given excellent spatial resolution, complete field-of-view of relevant structures, and readily available multiplanar reconstruction.[5]

In the management of infective endocarditis, classifications based on the duration of disease and the mode of acquisition are clinically relevant, though for the cardiovascular imager, anatomic classifications are more pertinent. These classifications include left-sided versus right-sided disease, native versus prosthetic valve, or cardiac device–related infections.[6] Within these anatomic classifications, the presence and degree of invasive disease are also important. Taken together, this categorization helps inform expected disease course and appropriate treatment. For example, compared with right-sided endocarditis, left-sided valvular destruction is more likely to result in hemodynamic embarrassment and decompensated heart failure requiring urgent or emergency surgery. The risk of devastating consequences from embolization is also higher with left-sided endocarditis and is increased with mitral valve compared with aortic valve endocarditis.[7] Moreover, for patients undergoing surgery, invasive disease on the right side of the heart is rare.[8] With left-sided endocarditis, invasive disease is more common, though direct extension into myocardium is unusual.[9]

Compared with native valve endocarditis, invasive disease is also more common with prosthetic valves. In fact, for patients undergoing surgery for prosthetic aortic valve endocarditis, a majority may have invasive disease.[8] With prosthetic valve endocarditis, infection often spreads along the sewing ring with development of an abscess, and this invasion can occur in the absence of large vegetations or leaflet destruction. Importantly, with the development of an aortic root abscess or pseudoaneurysm, cure with medical management is unlikely.[10] Similarly, infections on cardiac devices may develop biofilms that render them recalcitrant to antimicrobial therapy.[11]

Given the complexity of patients with endocarditis, these anatomic classifications aid in focusing evaluation and management. Oftentimes, multimodality imaging is informative, and given the hemodynamic information provided, echocardiography is essential in all patients. Transesophageal echocardiography (TEE) provides excellent spatial and temporal resolution in the near field, and when combined with Doppler color flow mapping, TEE generally provides superior evaluation of vegetations, fistulae, and leaflet perforations.[12] For certain patients, abnormal metabolism or inflammation adjacent to valves or foreign material, as seen with F18-fluorodeoxyglucose positron emission tomography, may help secure a diagnosis of infective endocarditis.[13] However, for patients with prosthetic valve involvement or suspected invasive disease, cardiovascular CT can also provide an excellent diagnostic performance.[14]

CT PROTOCOL

The advent of cardiac CT to aid in the diagnosis and management of infective endocarditis is relatively recent.[15] Continued technological improvements, especially related to ECG gating and temporal as well as spatial resolution, and increased availability of cardiac CT scanning with expert interpretation, have led to a greater application in suspected or known endocarditis. Importantly, in contrast to coronary CT angiography (CCTA), premedication with negative chronotropic agents or vasodilators is typically not performed in this setting given concern for potential hemodynamic instability if there is severe underlying valve disease. Based on the clinical context, when endocarditis is suspected, three CT phases can be considered, including (1) precontrast, (2) angiographic, and (3) delayed phase imaging (Fig. 22.1).

Precontrast images are helpful for identification of calcifications and surgical material.[16] In addition, aortic and mitral valves as well as the mitral annulus can often calcify, and this calcification may be better appreciated on noncontrast imaging. The ability of noncontrast CT to distinguish calcium and intrinsically dense surgical material from intravenous contrast can be helpful to assess the extent of disease. Precontrast CT images should be obtained with relatively high resolution (≤1 mm section thickness) and ECG synchronization. However, noncontrast 4D or cine images of cardiac motion are not typically needed. Accordingly, noncontrast imaging typically utilizes ECG-triggered, high-pitch, or prospective sequential imaging to cover the entire heart or chest, depending on the presence of surgical material and planned field-of-view for delayed images (see below).

Angiographic-phase images are the mainstay of CT diagnosis and allow delineation of the majority of anatomic findings associated with endocarditis, including vegetations, pseudoaneurysms, fistulae, and abscesses. Contrast timing can be tailored to the anatomic area suspected to be involved, if known.[5] In cases where the location of suspected endocarditis is unknown, a contrast injection protocol that allows for partial opacification of the right-sided cardiac structures (multiphase contrast injection with a blended flush of 50/50 iodinated contrast and saline) can be considered. CT angiography should be performed at high spatial resolution (<1 mm section thickness) using retrospective ECG-gating techniques that will allow for cine reconstruction of multiple cardiac phases.[17] These cine images, when obtained with submillimeter slice thickness, provide an isotropic dataset than can be reformatted according to clinical inquiry, and orientations analogous to standard echocardiographic short-axis and long-axis views can aid in interpretation and direct comparison. In younger patients, or when radiation dose from repeated examinations is of particular concern, ECG-triggered,

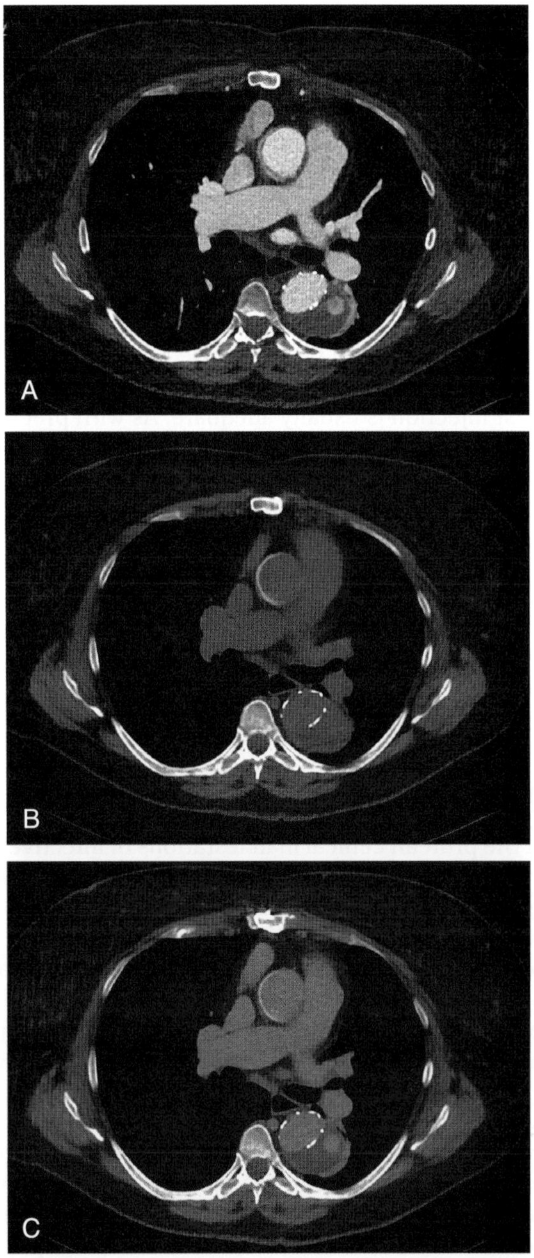

FIG. 22.1 Endocarditis CT protocol. Three phases may be helpful in the evaluation of endocarditis, including precontrast images, especially if prior surgical grafts or stents are present (A), angiographic phase images with retrospective ECG gating for cine reconstruction (B), and delayed images (C).

prospective sequential images with a wide temporal window that includes both systolic and diastolic phases can be used. Other methods to reduce radiation dose include low tube voltage scanning, iterative reconstruction, and ECG-controlled tube current modulation, though the latter may limit assessment of valve motion or vegetations during the phases of reduced current.

Delayed images can aid in distinguishing enhancing from nonenhancing tissue. This technique can be particularly helpful for periaortic abscesses and other extracardiac findings.[16] In general, contrast timing for delayed imaging does not need to be as precise as with angiographic phase images, and a fixed delay ~60 to 80 seconds after contrast injection is usually adequate. As with precontrast images, delayed images should be obtained with relatively high resolution (≤1 mm section thickness) and ECG synchronization, but cine reconstructions of cardiac motion are not necessary. Typically, delayed imaging is performed with ECG-triggered, high-pitch, or prospective sequential imaging to cover the heart, and often this series is extended to cover the entire chest. This expanded field of view can aid in surgical planning and is also helpful if septic emboli or other pulmonary complications are suspected.

EVALUATION OF VEGETATIONS

Given the protean clinical manifestations of infective endocarditis, diagnosis remains challenging. In 1994, a diagnostic algorithm, known as the Duke criteria, was established to qualify a diagnosis of IE as either definite, possible, or rejected. Subsequently, multiple clinical series have validated the high sensitivity, specificity, and negative predictive value of the Duke criteria when applied in the appropriate clinical context. As the role of transesophageal echocardiography in clinical practice evolved and the recognition of the importance of *Staphylococcus aureus* and the potential for endocarditis associated with *Coxiella burnetii* infection, the modified Duke criteria was proposed and is now central in clinical practice.[18] A major emphasis in these diagnostic pathways is the critical role of imaging, primarily echocardiography, to identify endocardial involvement with vegetations, perivalvular extension of infection, or evidence of disruption of the myocardial architecture.

Echocardiography has been regarded the gold standard for the diagnosis of infective endocarditis with a sensitivity of 80% for transthoracic echocardiography and 95% for transesophageal echocardiography.[18] Both transthoracic and transesophageal echocardiography are considered part of the typical algorithm in suspected endocarditis and have demonstrated efficacy in the identification of valvular vegetations (native and prosthetic), abscesses and extension of infection, valvular dysfunction as a result of the infectious process, and in the prediction of embolic risk.[19]

More recently, cardiac CT has emerged as an important consideration in the diagnostic evaluation of a patient with known or suspected native or prosthetic valve endocarditis. Although a strength of CT is detecting invasive disease, the spectrum of valvular involvement from leaflet thickening to perforation is feasible (Figs. 22.2–22.5).[20] In comparison to echocardiography, limitations of CT include suboptimal temporal resolution and limited insight into the hemodynamic consequences of valvular dysfunction. In addition, data comparing the diagnostic accuracy of the modalities for identifying vegetations have been predominantly limited to tertiary care centers with associated referral bias[14] (Fig. 22.6).

EVALUATION OF ABSCESS AND PSEUDOANEURYSM

As noted, invasive disease related to endocarditis typically progresses from cellulitis to abscess and abscess cavity and finally pseudoaneurysm. An abscess is a perivalvular purulent collection that may contain necrotic material and coalesces to form an abscess cavity. By definition, an abscess does not communicate with the cardiovascular lumen. When an abscess cavity ruptures into the cardiovascular lumen, a pseudoaneurysm is formed.

Clearly, these stages of invasive disease are on a continuum, and on CTA, cellulitis begins as heterogeneous soft

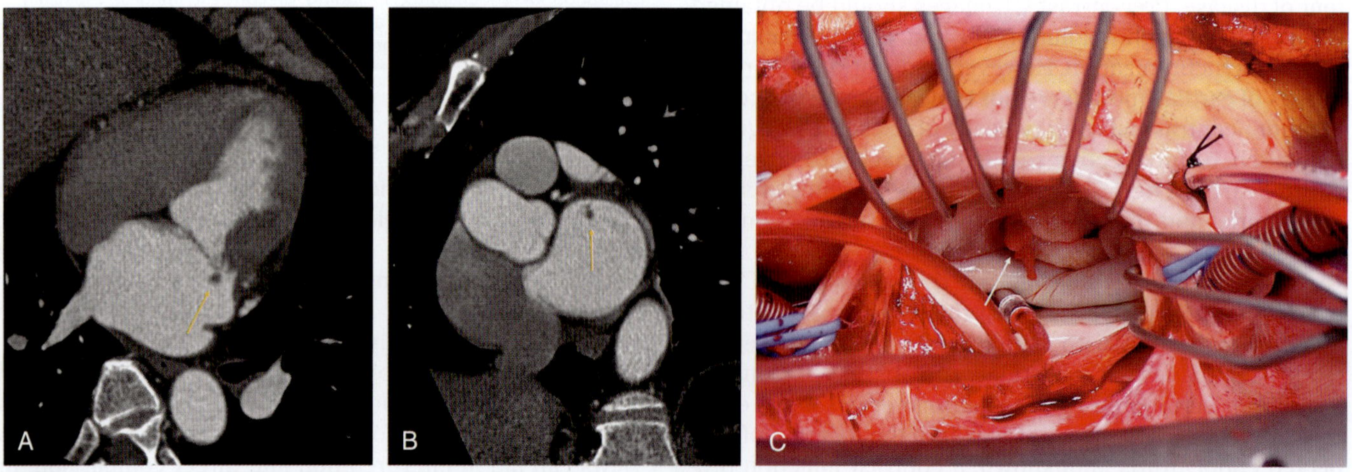

FIG. 22.2 Endocarditis of a native mitral valve. ECG-gated CT angiography with horizontal long-axis (A) and short-axis (B) left ventricular reconstructions demonstrating a small hypodensity at the lateral aspect of the posterior mitral valve leaflet (P1) in a patient with severe mitral regurgitation, pathologically confirmed as a vegetation (C).

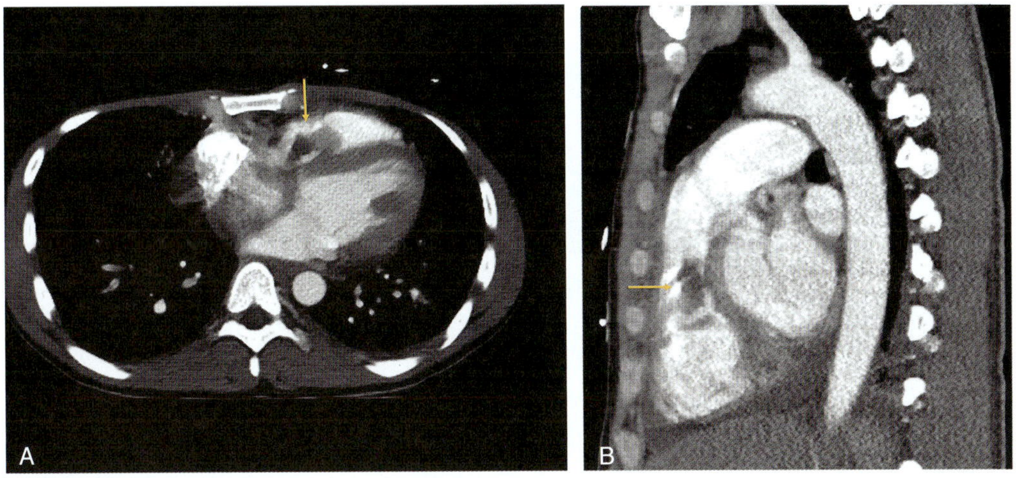

FIG. 22.3 Endocarditis of a native tricuspid valve. CT angiography with axial (A) and sagittal (B) images showing a large hypodensity associated with the tricuspid valve, compatible with a vegetation (*arrow*), in an intravenous drug user with *Staphylococcus aureus bacteremia*.

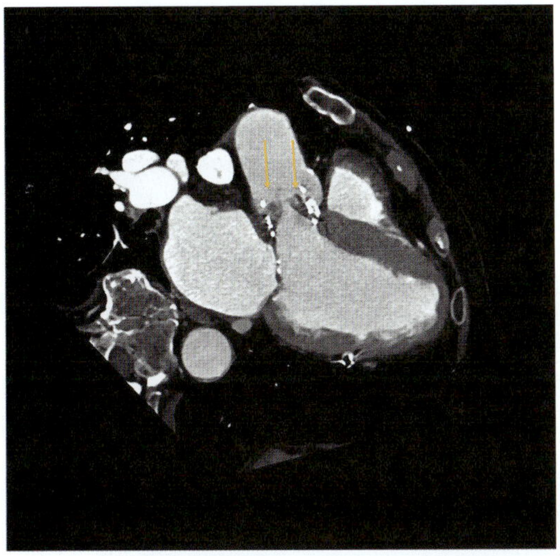

FIG. 22.4 Endocarditis of a transcatheter aortic valve. ECG-gated CT angiography with oblique reconstruction through the left ventricular outflow tract with hypodensities associated with the bioprosthetic leaflets (*arrows*) in a patient with definite infective endocarditis based on clinical diagnostic criteria.

tissue thickening. As the infection organizes to form an abscess, low-attenuation central necrosis may be present (Fig. 22.7). An abscess cavity can then form a peripheral enhancing rim, which may be particularly evident on delayed imaging (Fig. 22.8). With a pseudoaneurysm, CTA demonstrates a contrast-filled cavity, and a connection to the cardiovascular lumen is demonstrated (Figs. 22.9 and 22.10). In addition, the size and course of the pseudoaneurysm is well delineated on CTA (Figs. 22.10–22.12).

For aortic root abscess and pseudoaneurysm, CTA has an excellent diagnostic accuracy with reported sensitivity and specificity greater than 90% and may be even better for aortic prosthetic valve endocarditis.[14] However, the quality of data is generally limited to single-center retrospective cohort studies. Nonetheless, when compared with echocardiography, technical reasons for improved performance of CTA are readily apparent. First, prosthetic valves or significant calcifications, such as along the mitral annulus, may result in acoustic shadowing or reverberation artifacts with ultrasound that limit diagnostic yield. Second,

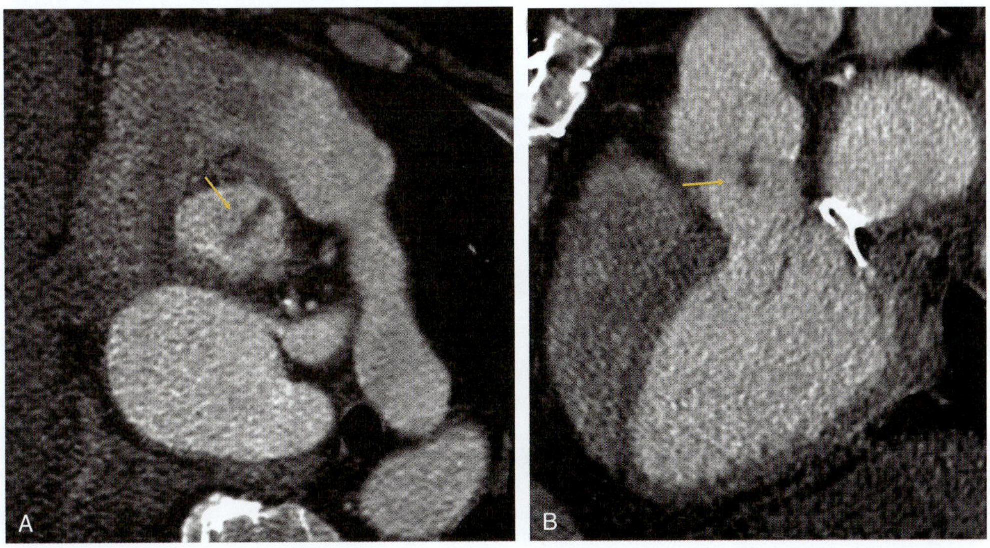

FIG. 22.5 Endocarditis of an aortic homograft. ECG-gated CT angiography with short-axis (A) and oblique reconstructions (B) of the left ventricular outflow tract (LVOT) demonstrates a hypodensity associated with an aortic homograft and prolapsing into the LVOT (*arrow*) in a patient who has also had prior mitral valve repair.

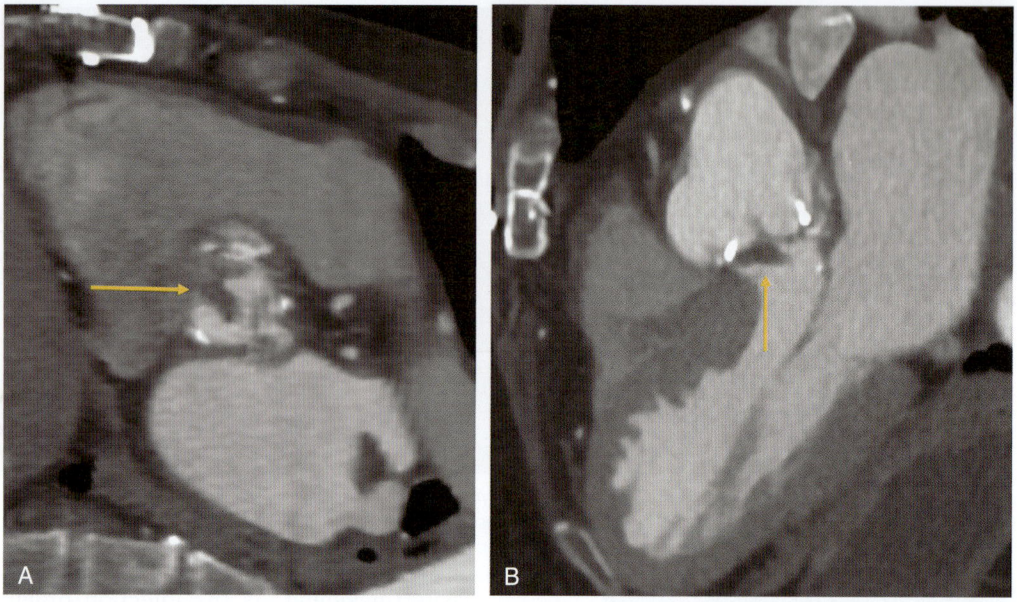

FIG. 22.6 Endocarditis of a stented surgical bioprosthesis. ECG-gated CT angiography with aortic valve short-axis (A) and oblique left-ventricular outflow tract (B) reconstructions with hypodensities involving the leaflets in the anatomic right and noncoronary cusp locations with a hypodensity prolapsing into the left ventricular outflow tract (*arrow*), compatible with vegetations.

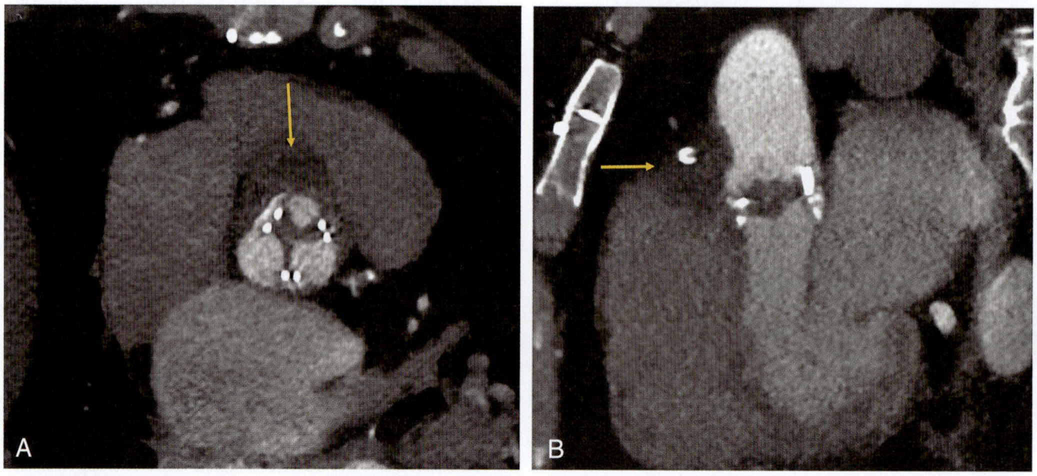

FIG. 22.7 Prosthetic valve endocarditis with an aortic root abscess. ECG-gated CT angiography with aortic valve short axis (A) and oblique left-ventricular outflow tract (B) reconstructions demonstrating abnormal bioprosthetic leaflet thickening and an abnormal heterogeneous and hypoattenuating collection involving the anterior aortic root adjacent to the right coronary artery.

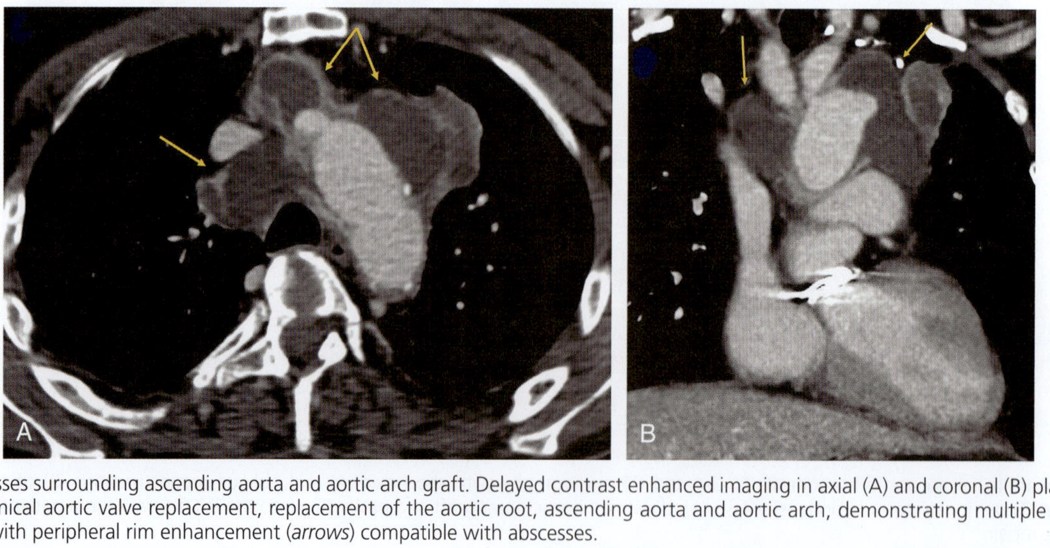

FIG. 22.8 Abscesses surrounding ascending aorta and aortic arch graft. Delayed contrast enhanced imaging in axial (A) and coronal (B) planes in a patient with prior mechanical aortic valve replacement, replacement of the aortic root, ascending aorta and aortic arch, demonstrating multiple hypoattenuated fluid collections with peripheral rim enhancement (*arrows*) compatible with abscesses.

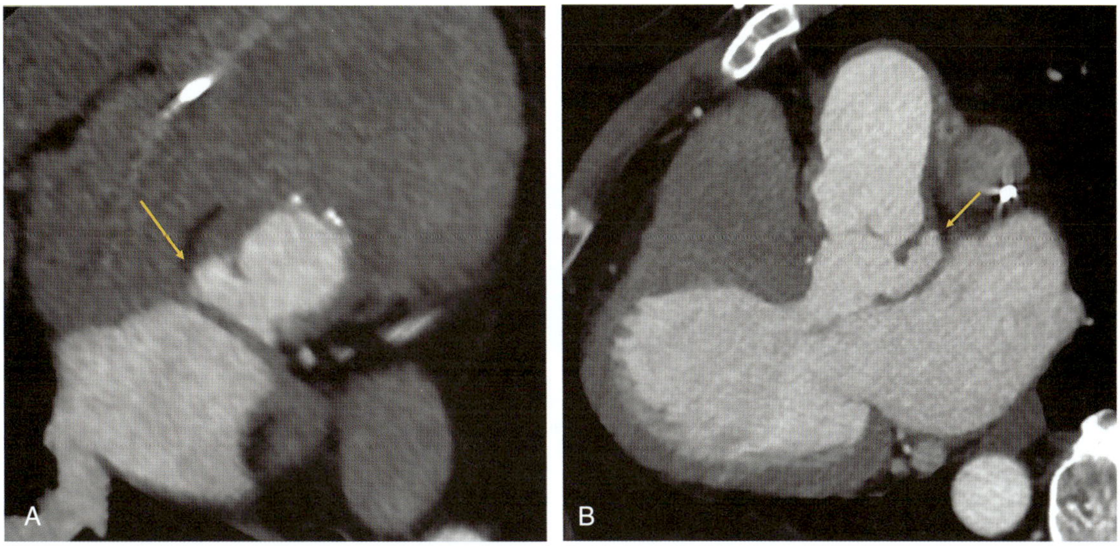

FIG. 22.9 Left ventricular outflow tract pseudoaneurysm in a patient with prior aortic homograft replacement. ECG-gated CT angiography (CTA) with aortic valve short-axis (A) and oblique left-ventricular outflow tract (B) reconstructions that show a small contrast-filled outpouching of the posterior left ventricular outflow tract (*arrow*) in a patient with prior aortic valve and ascending aortic replacement with a homograft. The connection to the left ventricle and course of the pseudoaneurysm is well defined with CTA.

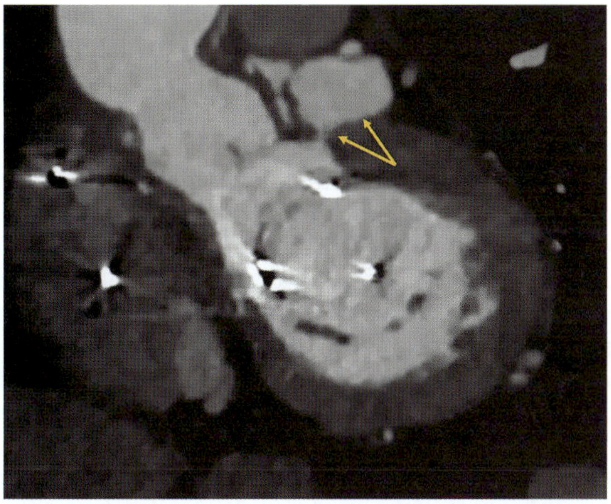

FIG. 22.10 Pseudoaneurysm in a patient with prior bioprosthetic mitral valve replacement. ECG-gated CTA angiography with an oblique basal left ventricular short-axis reconstruction demonstrating a large contrast-filled outpouching inferior to the left anterior descending coronary artery with a communicating channel to the left ventricle, compatible with a pseudoaneurysm (*arrows*).

the administration of intravenous contrast can help clearly distinguish an abscess from a pseudoaneurysm on CTA, though a pseudoaneurysm on echocardiography is often visualized as a pulsatile, anechoic space. Finally, the field of view with echocardiography is patient dependent and sonographer dependent with inherent limitations when there is intervening bone or air. CTA provides a much more uniform range across patients with generally fewer drawbacks when imaging through disparate tissue densities.

EVALUATION OF FISTULA, PERFORATION, AND OTHER COMPLICATIONS

As infection tracks along the fibrous skeleton of the heart, predictable complications can occur. For example, heart block typically results when infection spreads into the right atrium and triangle of Koch, destroying the atrioventricular node and upper end of the Bundle of His. In addition, infection can spread along the aortic-mitral continuity

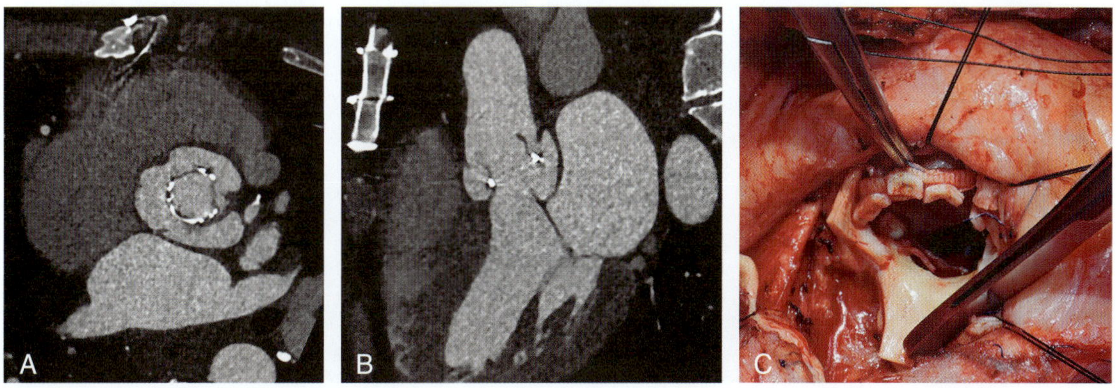

FIG. 22.11 Near circumferential pseudoaneurysm in a patient with a prior stented bioprosthetic aortic valve replacement. ECG-gated CT angiography with aortic valve short-axis (A) and oblique left ventricular outflow tract reconstructions (B) shows near circumferential contrast-filled outpouchings surrounding the bioprosthetic aortic valve, compatible with pseudoaneurysm. At surgery, the valve is almost completely dehisced and removed by cutting only a few sutures (C).

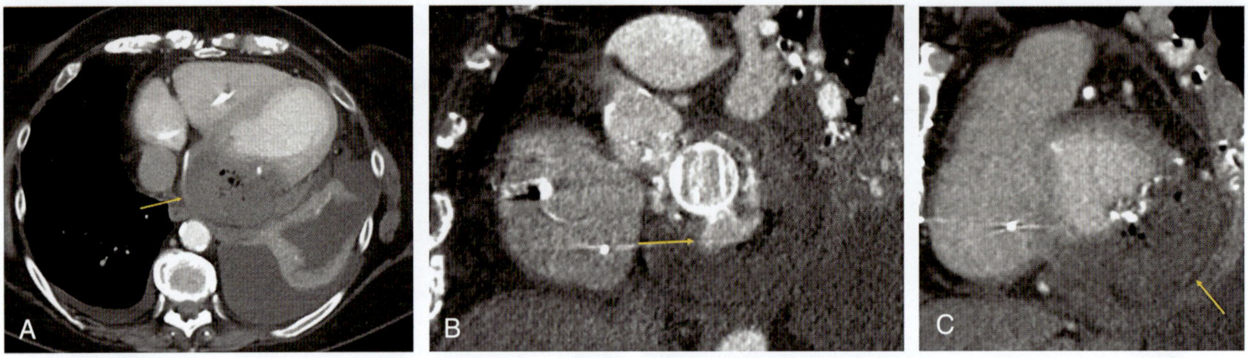

FIG. 22.12 Pseudoaneurysm and abscess cavity in a patient with prior mitral valve replacement with a bileaflet mechanical prosthesis. ECG-gated CT angiography with axial image (A), left ventricular short-axis reconstruction at the level of the mitral valve (B), and basal left ventricle (C). Short-axis mitral valve reconstruction (B) demonstrates a contrast-filled outpouching inferolaterally, consistent with a pseudoaneurysm. Adjacent to the pseudoaneurysm, there is a large collection eroding into the basal lateral and inferior myocardium and tracking inferiorly along the atrioventricular groove with numerous foci of air, consistent with an abscess cavity (*arrow*).

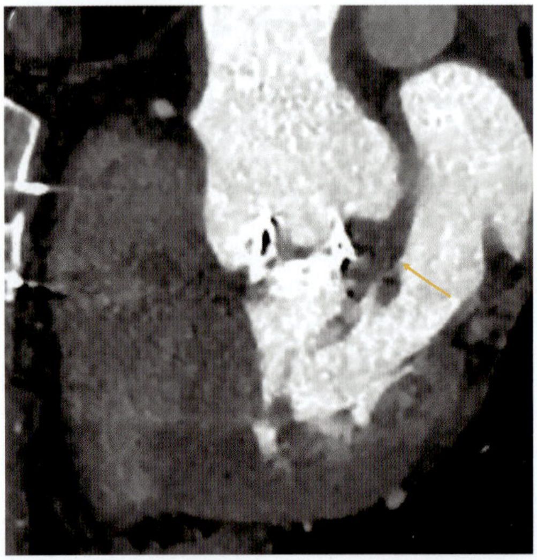

FIG. 22.13 Abscess of aortic-mitral continuity. ECG-gated CT angiography with oblique left ventricular outflow tract reconstruction in a patient with prior stented bioprosthetic aortic valve replacement demonstrates a lobulated hypodensity along the aortic-mitral intervalvular fibrosa (*arrow*) compatible with an abscess.

(Fig. 22.13). This invasive complication is important to define because definitive correction requires reconstruction of the intervalvular fibrosa, which increases operative complexity.[21]

Infection along the fibrous skeleton can also result in a fistula, defined as an abnormal communication between neighboring cavities. On CTA, a fistula is identified by a contrast-filled tract between two chambers. In endocarditis, when a fistula forms, it often occurs between the left ventricular outflow tract and right atrium, adjacent to the septal leaflet of the tricuspid valve. This lesion is referred to as an acquired Gerbode defect (Fig. 22.14).

Defects within valve leaflets are referred to as perforations. If a fistula or leaflet perforation is small, the defect may not be visualized with CTA. In addition to having excellent temporal resolution, echocardiography may be superior in this setting because the associated abnormal flow of a small defect with use of color Doppler is increased in conspicuity. However, for small defects involving the aorta, which could be related to surgical material or grafts, CTA may be better than echocardiography. In particular,

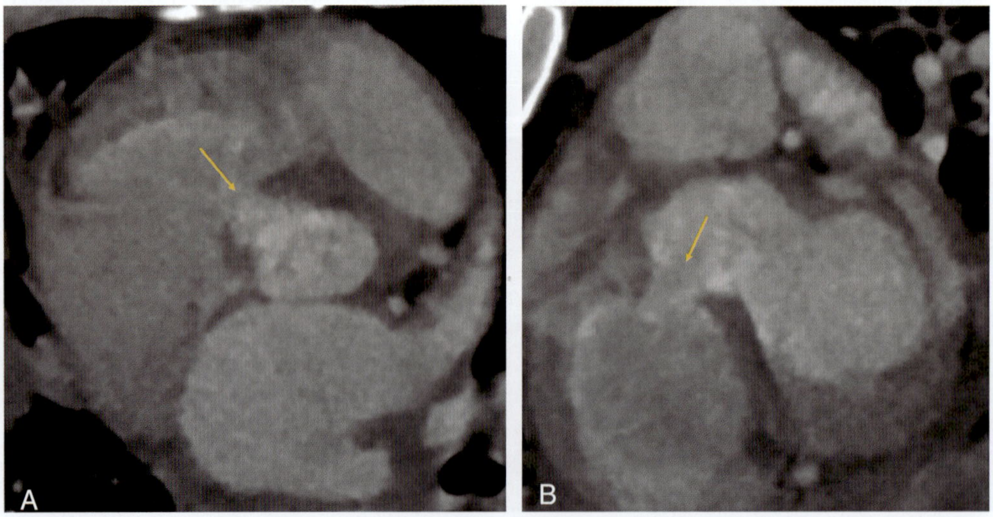

FIG. 22.14 Fistula between the left ventricular outflow tract and right atrium. ECG-gated CT angiography with aortic valve short-axis (A) and basal left ventricular short-axis (B) reconstructions in a patient with infective endocarditis. A large contrast-filled channel is noted between the left ventricular outflow tract and right atrium adjacent to the tricuspid valve. This fistula is referred to as an acquired Gerbode defect.

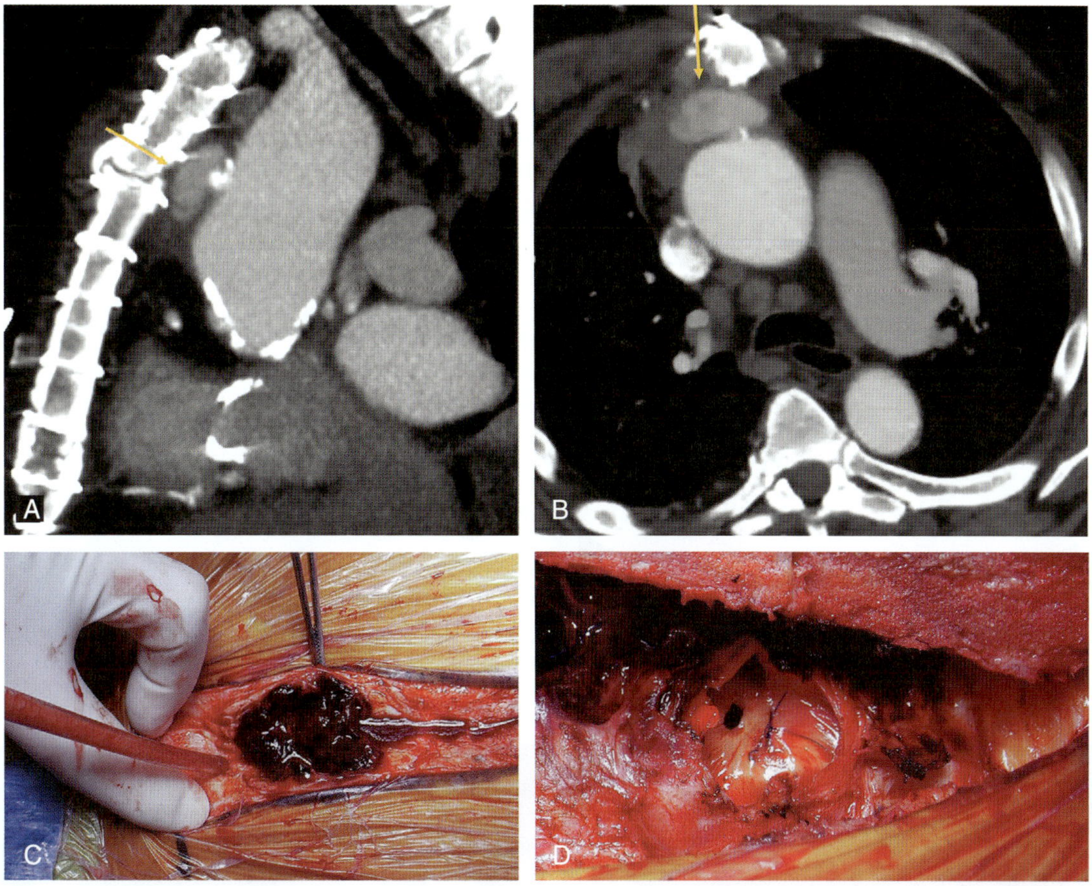

FIG. 22.15 Perforation with contained rupture at the site of prior aortic cannulation. ECG-gated CT angiography in sagittal (A) and axial (B) reconstructions in a patient with multiple prior cardiac surgeries and Staphylococcus aureus bacteremia demonstrates a perforation and contained rupture at the site of prior aortic cannulation (*arrow*), confirmed at surgery (C, D). This defect in the distal ascending aorta was not visualized with echocardiography.

motion artifacts are less problematic outside of the heart, and CTA allows more complete visualization of the aorta compared with echocardiography (Fig. 22.15).

Patients with endovascular cardiac device leads are also at increased risk of infection.[11] In comparison to echocardiography, vegetations on cardiac device leads may be more difficult to visualize with CTA due to small size, cardiac motion, or streak artifacts related to metallic leads. However, vegetations are occasionally visualized on cardiac device leads (Fig. 22.16). Moreover, CTA with delayed imaging may be helpful in planning percutaneous extraction of infected cardiac devices in order to visualize the course of endovascular leads, assess venous patency, and understand the relationship of cardiac and vascular structures to the sternum in patients with prior cardiac surgery.[22]

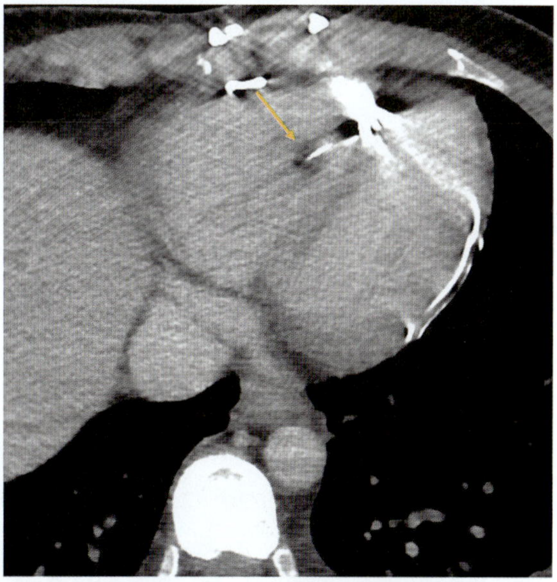

FIG. 22.16 Vegetation on right ventricular cardiac device lead. ECG-gated CT angiography in a patient with prior cardiac surgery and known bioprosthetic mitral valve endocarditis demonstrates a hypodensity on the right ventricular lead (*arrow*), compatible with a vegetation.

EXTRA CARDIAC FINDINGS

Given the capability to image the entire body, CT is a fundamental step in the assessment of extracardiac complications of infective endocarditis, which are driven primarily by embolic phenomena. These extracardiac findings can be divided into those from a left-sided versus a right-sided etiology. Extra cardiac manifestations of right-sided endocarditis are primarily related to pulmonary septic emboli (Fig. 22.17).

For left-sided emboli, there are several extracardiac complications that can be more acutely life threatening. These include central nervous system mycotic aneurysms, an infectious vasculitis. Mycotic aneurysms can rupture and result in intracranial hemorrhage (Fig. 22.18). Moreover, ischemic strokes from septic emboli can also undergo hemorrhagic transformation and lead to intracranial hemorrhage.[23] Septic emboli can also result in vascular emergencies with occlusion of visceral or peripheral arteries (Fig. 22.19). Although usually not as acutely devastating, the demonstration of visceral organ infarcts may lead to a suspicion of infective endocarditis, if the diagnosis is not already known (Fig. 22.20).

Finally, the retrospectively ECG-gated CTA of the heart that is obtained as part of an endocarditis protocol CT can be used to evaluate the coronary arteries for anatomic

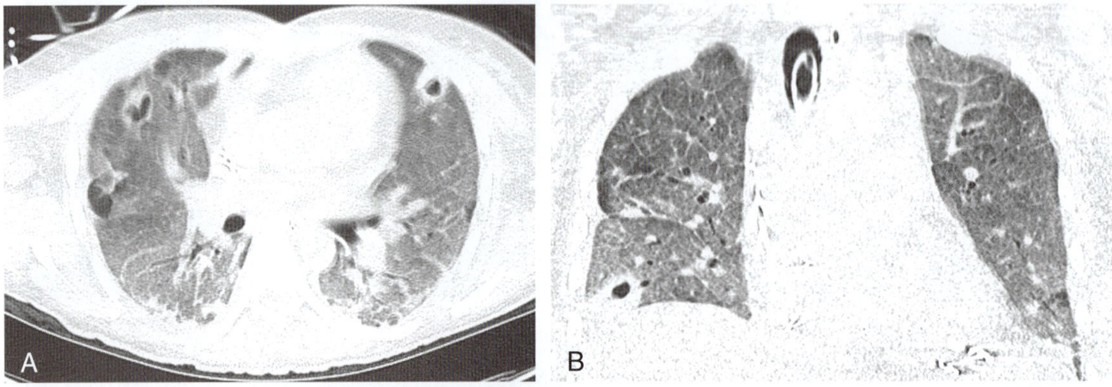

FIG. 22.17 Septic pulmonary emboli. Chest CT in an intubated patient with tricuspid valve endocarditis demonstrates numerous bilateral solid and cavitary nodules, compatible with septic pulmonary emboli, in a background of diffuse ground-glass opacification with associated interlobular septal thickening and interstitial thickening, in keeping with pulmonary edema.

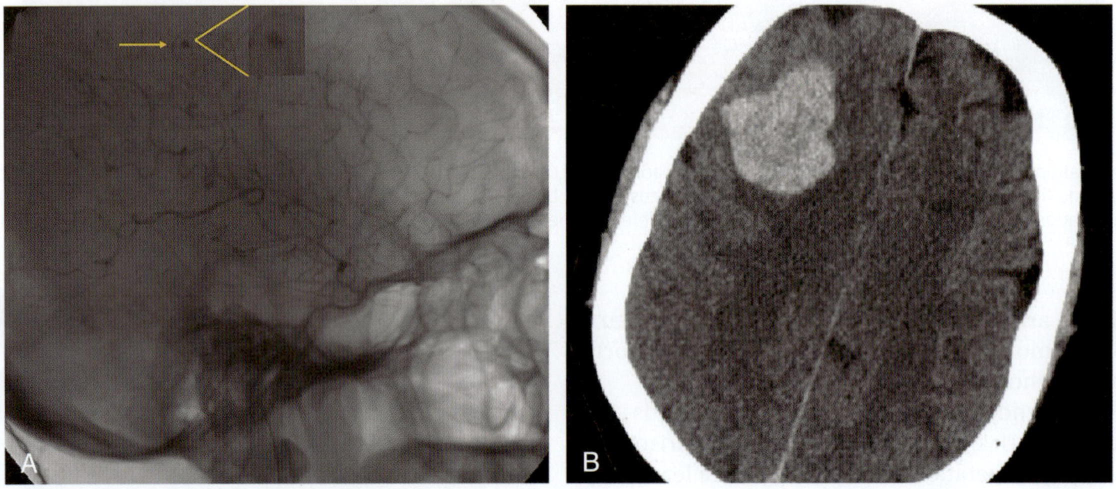

FIG. 22.18 Central nervous system complications of infective endocarditis. Cerebral angiogram (A) in a patient with infective endocarditis demonstrates a mycotic aneurysm (*arrow*). This infectious vasculitis can lead to rupture and intracranial hemorrhage (B).

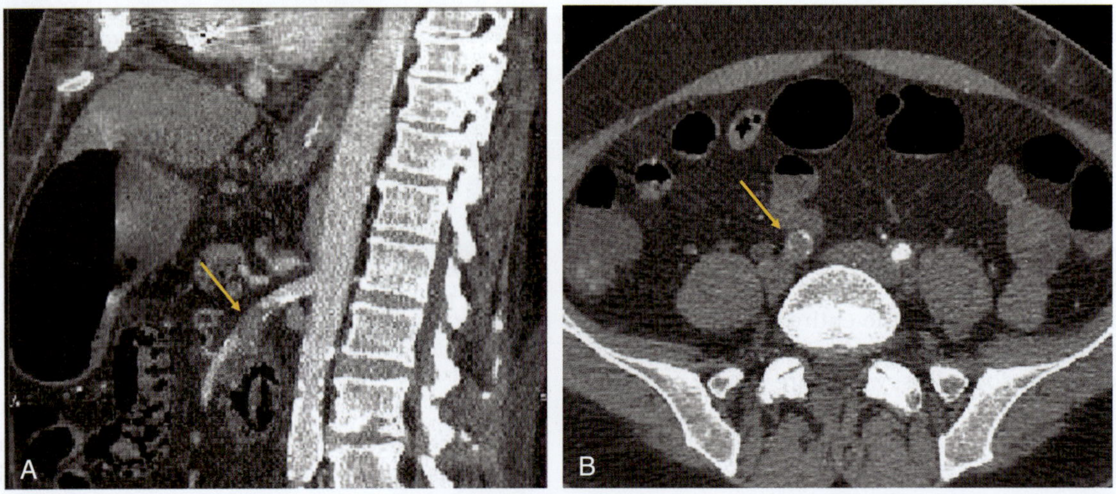

FIG. 22.19 Septic emboli resulting in arterial occlusion. Left-sided vegetations can embolize and result in vascular emergencies as shown in these patients with endocarditis and superior mesenteric artery occlusion (*arrow*) (A) and right common iliac artery occlusion (*arrow*) (B).

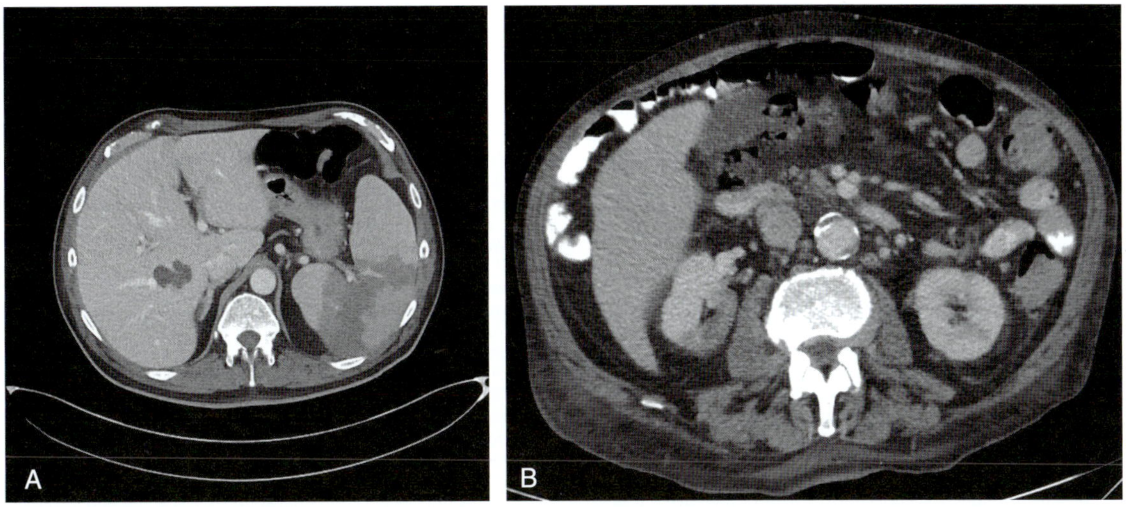

FIG. 22.20 Visceral organ infarcts due to septic emboli. CT angiographies in patients with infective endocarditis demonstrating hypodensity in the spleen consistent with splenic infarct (A) and hypodensity in the right kidney reflective of a renal infarct (B).

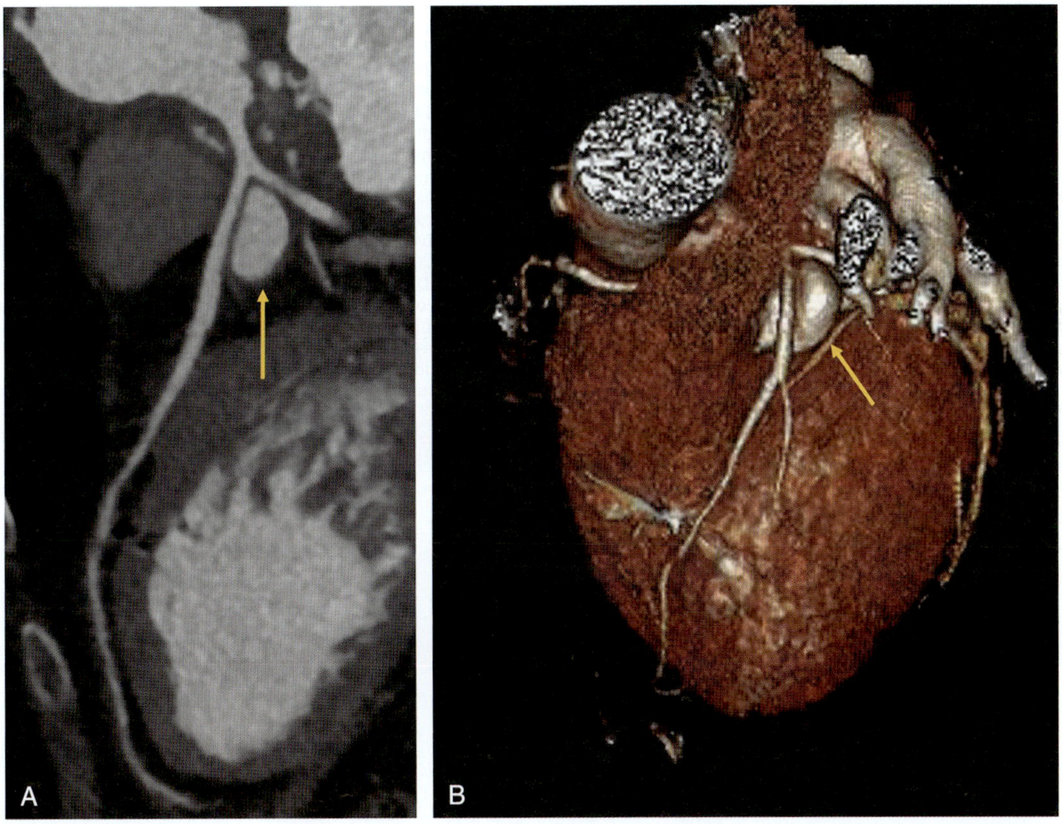

FIG. 22.21 Coronary assessment in infective endocarditis. ECG-gated CT angiography in a patient with endocarditis and a pseudoaneurysm posterior to the left anterior descending artery (*arrow*). Multiplanar reconstruction of the coronary arteries showed normal origins and courses with no significant stenotic or atherosclerotic disease (A). The relationship of the pseudoaneurysm (*arrow*) to the left coronary artery is also appreciated on the 3D virtual reconstruction (B).

course and atherosclerotic disease. Depending on the extent of underlying coronary atherosclerosis, these images may be sufficient for coronary artery assessment, even if the lack of premedication precludes optimal assessment of the distal vessels (Fig. 22.21).[20] In conclusion, by combining ECG-gated CTA with whole-body surveillance CT, a complete assessment can be obtained, including (1) understanding complex cardiac structure and involvement with infection, (2) extra cardiac foci and complications, and (3) preoperative coronary assessment.

CONCLUSION

Infectious endocarditis is a challenging and not uncommonly encountered clinical entity with potentially dire consequences. Imaging has long played a central role in the diagnosis and management of this disease process, though this has traditionally been dominated by echocardiography. Cardiac CT, with the benefit of improved temporal and spatial resolution in recent years, as well as a wide field of view and isotropic dataset, has played an increasingly important role in this process, though typically still complementary to echocardiography. In particular, cardiac CT, especially in patients with prosthetic valves, and in combination with extra cardiac CT scanning, identifies additional complications and foci of infection. Knowledge of typical imaging manifestations, relevant categorization schemes, and appropriate protocols allow the cardiovascular imager to optimize the use of cardiac CT as part of the evaluation and management of suspected or known endocarditis.

REFERENCES

1. Mohananey D, Mohadjer A, Pettersson, et al. Association of vegetation size with embolic risk in patients with infective endocarditis: a systematic review and meta-analysis. *JAMA Intern Med.* 2018;178(4):502–510.
2. Cahill TJ, Baddour LM, Habib G, et al. Challenges in infective endocarditis. *J Am Coll Cardiol.* 2017;69(3):325–344.
3. AATS Surgical Treatment of Infective Endocarditis Consensus Guidelines Writing Committee Chairs. 2016 The American Association for Thoracic Surgery (AATS) consensus guidelines: surgical treatment of infective endocarditis: executive summary. *J Thorac Cardiovasc Surg.* 2017;153(6):1241–1258 l.
4. Pettersson GB, Hussain ST. Current AATS guidelines on surgical treatment of infective endocarditis. *Ann Cardiothorac Surg.* 2019;8(6):630–644.
5. Saeedan MB, Wang TKM, Cremer P, et al. Role of cardiac CT in infective endocarditis: current evidence, opportunities, and challenges. *Radiol Cardiothorac Imaging.* 2021;3(1):e200378.
6. Habib G, Lancellotti P, Antunes MJ, et al. 2015 ESC Guidelines for the management of infective endocarditis: the task force for the management of infective endocarditis of the European Society of Cardiology (ESC). Endorsed by: European Association for Cardio-Thoracic Surgery (EACTS), the European Association of Nuclear Medicine (EANM). *Eur Heart J.* 2015;36(44):3075–3128.
7. Yanagawa B, Pettersson GB, Habib G, et al. Surgical management of infective endocarditis complicated by embolic stroke: practical recommendations for clinicians. *Circulation.* 2016;134(17):1280–1292.
8. Hussain ST, Shrestha NK, Witten J, et al. Rarity of invasiveness in right-sided infective endocarditis. *J Thorac Cardiovasc Surg.* 2018;155(1):54–61.
9. Witten JC, Tan CD, Rodriguez ER, et al. Invasive aortic valve endocarditis: clinical and tissue findings from a prospective investivation. *Ann Thorac Surg.* 2022;113(2):535–545.
10. Pettersson GB, Hussain ST, Shrestha NK, et al. Infective endocarditis: at atlas of disease progression for describing, staging, coding, and understanding the pathology. *J Thorac Cardiovasc Surg.* 2014;147(4):1142–1149.
11. Blomstrom-Lundqvist C, Traykov V, Erba PA, et al. European Heart Rhythm Association (EHRA) international consensus document on how to prevent, diagnose, and treat cardiac implantable electronic device infections-endorsed by the Heart Rhythm Society (HRS), the Asia Pacific Heart Rhythm Society (APHRS), the Latin American Heart Rhythm Society (LAHRS), International Society for Cardiovascular Infectious Diseases (ISCVID), and the European Society of Clinical Microbiology and Infectious Diseases (ESCMID) in collaboration with the European Association for Cardio-Thoracic Surgery (EACTS). *Eur Heart J.* 2020;41(21):2012–2032.
12. Fagman E, Flinck A, Snygg-Martin U, Olaison L, Bech-Hanssen O, Svensson G. Surgical decision-making in aortic prosthetic valve endocarditis: the influence of electrocardiogram-gated computed tomography. *Eur J Cardiothorac Surg.* 2016;50(6):1165–1171.
13. Wang TKM, Sanches-Nadales A, Igbinomwanhia E, Cremer P, Griffin B, Xu B. Diagnosis of infective endocarditis by subtype using 18F-fluorodeoxyglucose positron emission tomography/computed tomography: a contemporary meta-analysis. *Circ Cardiovasc Imaging.* 2020;13(6):e010600.
14. Vardhmaan J, Wang TKM, Bansal A, et al. Diagnostic performance of cardiac computed tomography versus transesophageal echocardiography in infective endocarditis: a contemporary comparative meta-analysis. *J Cardiovasc Comput Tomogr.* 2021;15(4):313–321.
15. Feuchtner GM, Stolzmann P, Dichtl W, et al. Multislice computed tomography in infective endocarditis: comparison with transesophageal echocardiography and intraoperative findings. *J Am Coll Cardiol.* 2009;53:436–444.
16. Faure ME, Swart LE, Dijkshoorn ML, et al. Advanced CT acquisition protocol with a third-generation dual-source CT scanner and iterative reconstruction technique for comprehensive prosthetic heart valve assessment. *Eur Radiol.* 2018;28:2159–2168.
17. Entrikin DW, Gupta P, Kon ND, Carr JJ. Imaging of infective endocarditis with cardiac CT angiography. *J Cardiovasc Comput Tomogr.* 2012;6:399–405.
18. Li JS, Sexton DJ, Mick N, et al. Proposed modifications to the duke criteria for the diagnosis of infective endocarditis. *Clinical Infectious Diseases.* 2000;30:633–638.
19. Erba PA, Pizzi MN, Roque A, et al. Multimodality imaging in infective endocarditis: an imaging team within the endocarditis team. *Circulation.* 2019;140:1753–1765.
20. Sims JR, Anavekar NS, Chandrasekaran K, et al. Utility of cardiac computed tomography scanning in the diagnosis and pre-operative evaluation of patients with infective endocarditis. *Int J Cardiovasc Imaging.* 2018;34:1155–1163.
21. Navia JL, Elgharably H, Hakim AG, et al. Long-term outcomes of surgery for invasive valvular endocarditis involving the aortomitral fibrosa. *Ann Thorac Surg.* 2019;108(5):1314–1323.
22. Patel D, Sripariwuth A, Abozeed M, et al. Lead location as assessed on cardiac computed tomography and difficulty of percutaneous transvenous extraction. *JACC Clin Electrophysiol.* 2019;5(12):1432–1438.
23. Garcia-Cabrera E, Fernandez-Hidalgo N, Almirante B, et al. Neurological complications of infective endocarditis: risk factors, outcome, and impact of cardiac surgery: a multicenter observational study. *Circulation.* 2013;127:2272–2284.

Index

Note: Page numbers followed by "*f*" indicate figures, "*t*" indicate tables, and "*b*" indicate boxes.